Series Editors:
Steven F. Warren, Ph.D.
Marc E. Fey, Ph.D.

and Language
Intervention
Series

Interventions for

Speech
Sound
Disorders

in Children

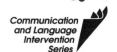

Communication
and Language
Intervention
Series

Interventions for
Speech
Sound
Disorders
in Children

edited by

A. Lynn Williams, Ph.D.
East Tennessee State University
Johnson City, Tennessee

Sharynne McLeod, Ph.D.
Charles Sturt University
Bathurst, New South Wales
Australia

and

Rebecca J. McCauley, Ph.D
The Ohio State University
Columbus, Ohio

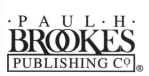

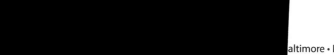

altimore • London • Sydney

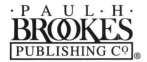

Paul H. Brookes Publishing Co.
Post Office Box 10624
Baltimore, Maryland 21285-0624
USA

www.brookespublishing.com

Typeset by Integrated Publishing Solutions, Grand Rapids, Michigan.
Manufactured in the United States of America by
Sheridan Books, Inc., Chelsea, Michigan.

Video finishing and DVD authoring by Daniel Santiago and Harold "Buddy" Arnold,
East Tennessee State University, Johnson City, Tennessee.

The individuals described in this book are composites or real people whose situations are masked and are based on the authors' experiences. In all instances, names and identifying details have been changed to protect confidentiality.

The accompanying DVD contains a video segment for most of the interventions discussed in *Speech Sound Disorders in Children* (see the DVD icons in the table of contents). The video clips were supplied by the chapter authors, and permission was obtained for all individuals shown in footage contained in the DVD.

Library of Congress Cataloging-in-Publication Data

Interventions for speech sound disorders in children / edited by A. Lynn Williams, Sharynne McLeod, and Rebecca J. McCauley.
    p. ;   cm. – (Communication and language intervention series ; v. 16)
Includes bibliographical references and index.
ISBN-13: 978-1-59857-018-2 (pbk. with dvd)
ISBN-10: 1-59857-018-8
1. Speech therapy for children.   2. Speech disorders in children.   I. Williams, A. Lynn.
II. McLeod, Sharynne.   III. McCauley, Rebecca Joan, 1952–   IV. Series: Communication and language intervention series ; 16.
[DNLM: 1. Articulation Disorders–therapy.   2. Child.   3. Speech Therapy–methods. W1 CO4272C
v.16 2010 / WL 340.2 I612 2010]
RJ496.S7I58   2010
618.92'85506–dc22   2009036352

British Library Cataloguing in Publication data are available from the British Library.

2019 2018 2017 20[ ]

10   9   8   7

Contents

Series Preface

The purpose of the *Communication and Language Intervention Series* is to provide meaningful foundations for the application of sound intervention designs to enhance the development of communication skills across the life span. We are endeavoring to achieve this purpose by providing readers with presentations of state-of-the-art theory, research, and practice.

In selecting topics, editors, and authors, we are not attempting to limit the contents of this series to viewpoints with which we agree or that we find most promising. We are assisted in our efforts to develop the series by an editorial advisory board consisting of prominent scholars representative of the range of issues and perspectives to be incorporated in the series.

Well-conceived theory and research on development and intervention are vitally important for researchers, educators, and clinicians committed to the development of optimal approaches to communication and language intervention. The content of each volume reflects our view of the symbiotic relationship between intervention and research: Demonstrations of what may work in intervention should lead to analysis of promising discoveries and insights from developmental work that may in turn fuel further refinement by intervention researchers. We trust that the careful reader will find much that is of great value in this volume.

An inherent goal of this series is to enhance the long-term development of the field by systematically furthering the dissemination of theoretically and empirically based scholarship and research. We promise the reader an opportunity to participate in the development of this field through debates and discussions that occur throughout the pages of the *Communication and Language Intervention Series*.

About the Editors

A. Lynn Williams, Ph.D. /lɪn wɪljəmz/ Professor, Department of Communicative Disorders, Associate Director, Center of Excellence in Early Childhood Learning and Development, East Tennessee State University, Box 70434, Johnson City, TN 37614

Dr. Williams joined the Communicative Disorders faculty of East Tennessee State University in 1995 following academic positions at Oklahoma State University and California State University at Fullerton. Most of her research over the past decade has involved clinical investigations of models of phonological treatment for children with severe to profound speech disorders. She developed an alternative model of phonological intervention, called *multiple oppositions*, which she has examined in National Institutes of Health (NIH)–funded treatment efficacy studies and recently has compared with other models of contrastive phonological intervention. Dr. Williams is the author of SCIP: Sound Contrasts in Phonology, a phonological intervention software program that was funded through the National Institute of Deafness and Communicative Disorders.

Sharynne McLeod, Ph.D. /ˈʃæɹən məˈklaʊd/ Professor in Speech and Language Acquisition, School of Teacher Education, Charles Sturt University, Panorama Avenue, Bathurst, New South Wales 2795, Australia

Dr. McLeod is a professor in speech and language acquisition in the School of Teacher Education at Charles Sturt University (CSU), Australia. She is a Fellow of the American Speech-Language-Hearing Association and Speech Pathology Australia as well as Vice President of the International Clinical Linguistics and Phonetics Association. Dr. McLeod is currently editor of *International Journal of Speech-Language Pathology*. Dr. McLeod's translational research has primarily focused on children's speech and foregrounds the right of everyone (particularly children) to participate fully in society. Recently she has been awarded an Australian Learning and Teaching Council Citation for Outstanding Contribution to Student Learning "For sustained dedication, innovation and enthusiasm in university teaching that has had local, national and international impact."

Rebecca J. McCauley, Ph.D. /ɹəˈbɛkə ʤe məˈkɔli/ Board Recognized Specialist in Child Language, Professor, Department of Speech and Hearing Science, The Ohio State University, Department of Speech & Hearing Science, 1070 Carmack Road, 105 Pressey Hall, Columbus, OH 43210

Dr. McCauley joined the faculty of The Ohio State University in 2008 after 23 years at the University of Vermont. She is an American Speech-Language-Hearing Association Fellow and a Board-Recognized Specialist in Child Language. She has served as an associate editor for the *American Journal of Speech-Language-Pathology* and has produced four books on child communication disorders in addition to this one. She is currently working on editing a book of this type in the area of autism spectrum disorders with Dean Patricia Prelock of the University of Vermont. Her research focuses on severe speech disorders in children, especially childhood apraxia of speech, and on strategies for understanding and improving clinical practice related to children's communication disorders.

Contributors

Penelope Bacsfalvi, Ph.D.   /pʰəˈnɛləpi ˌbatʃfɑːlvi/   Certified Speech Language Pathologist, Department of Linguistics, University of British Columbia, 2613 West Mall, Vancouver, BC V6T 1Z4, Canada

Dr. Bacsfalvi is a researcher and clinician and the Speech Sciences Undergraduate Advisor at the University of British Columbia. Her research program concerns articulatory feedback. Her current clinical work focuses on hearing loss in children, cochlear implants, visual feedback technologies, and a team approach to auditory and verbal interventions. Email: penbacs @interchange.ubc.ca

Elise Baker, Ph.D.   /əlis beɪkə/   Discipline of Speech Pathology, The University of Sydney, 75 East Street, Lidcombe, NSW 2141, Australia

Dr. Baker is a speech-language pathologist (SLP), lecturer, and clinical researcher with The University of Sydney. She is interested in how theoretical principles of phonology guide intervention research, and how SLPs put research into practice. She is particularly interested in the effect of SLP feedback and instruction on children's speech. Email: e.baker@usyd .edu.au

B. May Bernhardt, Ph.D.   /ˈbi ˈmeɪ bɹ̩nˌhaɹt/   Professor, School of Audiology and Speech Sciences, University of British Columbia, 2177 Wesbrook Mall, Vancouver, BC V6T 1Z3, Canada

Dr. (Barbara) May Bernhardt is a professor in the School of Audiology and Speech Sciences at the University of British Columbia focusing on language acquisition and intervention in children. A major component of her research program has been the application of nonlinear phonological theories to assessment and intervention. Email: bernharb@interchange.ubc.ca

Karen D. Bopp, Ph.D.   /ˈkʰæːɹn̩ ˈdiː ˈbɑːp/   Research Associate, Educational Psychology and Special Education, University of British Columbia, 2125 Main Mall, Vancouver, BC V6T 1Z4, Canada

Karen D. Bopp is a postdoctoral fellow and SLP who has worked extensively with children with developmental disabilities. She teaches courses in language development and special education at the University of British Columbia. Dr. Bopp's major research interests include speech and language development patterns in young children with autism. Email: bopp@interchange .ubc.ca

Caroline Bowen, Ph.D. /kæɹəˈlaɪn ˈboʊʷən/ Speech Pathology Practice, and Honorary Associate in Linguistics, Macquarie University, 9 Hillcrest Road, Wentworth Falls, NSW 2782, Australia

An Honorary Associate in Linguistics at Macquarie University, and a dedicated internationalist, Dr. Bowen has devoted much of her long speech-language pathology career to understanding and bridging the theory—therapy and research—practice gaps in our profession and spreading the word, worldwide, about what we do. Find her on the Internet at www.speech-language-therapy.com. Email: cbowen@ihug.com.au

Françoise Brosseau-Lapré, M.Sc.CA. /fRɑ̃sˈwɑz ˈbRɔso ˈlæpRe/ Doctoral Student, School of Communication Sciences and Disorders, McGill University, 1266 Pine Avenue West, Montréal, QC H3G 1A8, Canada

Françoise Brosseau-Lapré obtained her master's degree in speech-language pathology from McGill University in 2002. She has practiced as a pediatric SLP since then and began her doctoral studies at McGill in 2007 under the supervision of Dr. Susan Rvachew. Ms. Brosseau-Lapré is investigating the efficacy of interventions for SSD. Email: francoise.brosseau-lapre@mail.mcgill.ca

Stephen M. Camarata, Ph.D. /stivən kæməɹatə/ Professor, Vanderbilt University School of Medicine, 1215 21st Avenue South, Room 8310, Nashville, TN 37232

Dr. Camarata is Professor of Hearing and Speech Sciences at Vanderbilt University School of Medicine and an investigator at the John F. Kennedy Center for Research on Development and Disorders. His research focuses on diagnosis and treatment of speech and language disorders in children with disabilities, including autism, Down syndrome, phonological disorder, and expressive and receptive language disorder. Email: stephen.m.camarata@vanderbilt.edu

Heather M. Clark, Ph.D. /hɛðəɹ klɑɹk/ Appalachian State University, ASU Box 32085, Boone, NC 28608

Dr. Clark teaches courses in adult and pediatric oral motor speech and swallowing disorders. Her research explores sensorimotor function and its relationship to speech/swallowing integrity. Her article, "Neuromuscular Treatments for Speech and Swallowing: A Tutorial" was awarded the *American Journal of Speech-Language Pathology* Editor's Award. Email: clarkhm@appstate.edu

Sharon Crosbie, Ph.D. /ʃæɹən kɪɒzbi/ Research Fellow, University of Queensland Centre for Clinical Research, Royal Brisbane and Women's Hospital, University of Queensland, Brisbane, QLD 4029, Australia

Sharon Crosbie is an SLP and Australian Research Council Postdoctoral Fellow. Her research has explored subtypes of specific language impairment, and assessment and intervention for children with phonological disorders. Her current research focus is the communication outcomes of children born preterm at the Perinatal Research Centre at The University of Queensland. Email: s.crosbie@uq.edu.au

Bonnie Daudlin, M.A. /bɑː.niˈdɑːd.lɳ/ Registered Speech-Language Pathologist, BC Centre for Ability, 2805 Kingsway, Vancouver, BC V5R 5H9, Canada

Ms. Daudlin is a registered SLP. She has worked with preschoolers with communicative impairments since 1991. She participated as a clinician-researcher with four children from 1993 to 1998 as part of two nonlinear phonological intervention projects coordinated by Professor (Barbara) May Bernhardt. Email: bdaudlin@centreforability.bc.ca

Barbara Dodd, Ph.D. /babərə dɒd/ Professor, Perinatal Research Centre, Queensland University Centre for Clinical Research, Royal Brisbane and Women's Hospital, Butterfield Street, Brisbane, QLD 4029, Australia

Barbara Dodd, Australian Research Council Research Professor at The University of Queensland, is an SLP, teacher, and researcher who has worked in universities in Australia and the United Kingdom. She has written extensively on differential diagnosis of subtypes of speech disorders, including evidence from clinical efficacy studies. Email: b.dodd@uq.edu.au

Susan M. Edwards, M.Sc. /ˈsuː.zn̩ ˈɛd.wɪdz/ Private Practice, 3829 Cumberland Road, Victoria, BC V8P 3J1, Canada

Ms. Edwards is an SLP in private practice. Her master's degree thesis (1995) was a project in nonlinear phonological intervention. She was a research coordinator on a nonlinear phonological intervention project in 1997 and has worked on several other research projects with Professor (Barbara) May Bernhardt relating to language development. Email: susanedwards @cripps.net

Jennifer Eigen, M.S. /jenifeɹ aigin/ Speech-Language Pathologist, Private Practice, 26 Court Street, Suite 902, Brooklyn, NY 11242

Ms. Eigen is a private practitioner who specializes in pediatrics. Areas of particular interest include the treatment of motor-speech disorders as well as language-learning disorders. She is also a PROMPT instructor and is involved in PROMPT treatment research studies. Email: jennifer_eigen@yahoo.com

Fiona E. Gibbon, Ph.D. /fiəʊnə ɡɪbən/ Professor, Department of Speech and Hearing Sciences, Brookfield Health Sciences Complex, University College Cork, College Road, Cork, Ireland

Dr. Gibbon is a speech and language therapist and Head of Department of Speech and Hearing Sciences, University College Cork in Ireland. Her research focuses on using instrumentation to improve the diagnosis and treatment of children with speech disorders. She has published more than 70 book chapters and papers in professional-scientific journals and has been awarded numerous research council and charity funded grants. The research presented in Chapter 21 was awarded the Queen's Anniversary Prize for excellence in 2002. Dr. Gibbon is a Fellow of the Royal College of Speech and Language Therapists. Email: fgibbon@qmu .ac.uk

Allison M. Haskill, Ph.D.   /ˈælɪsɑn ˈhæskl̩/   Assistant Professor, Augustana College, 639 38th Street, Rock Island, IL 61201

Dr. Haskill is an assistant professor in the Department of Communication Sciences and Disorders at Augustana College, where she teaches courses and completes research in the areas of child language development and disorders. Email: csdhaskill@augustana.edu

Deborah A. Hayden, M.A.   /ˈdɛbɔɹɑ æn ˈheidɪn/   Executive Director, The PROMPT Institute, 4001 Office Court Drive, Suite 305, Santa Fe, NM 87507

Ms. Hayden is Founder and Executive Director of the PROMPT Institute. Her primary research interests are developmental and acquired speech production disorders. Primary author of the *Verbal Motor Production Assessment for Children* (Pearson PsychCorp, 1999) and the soon to be released *Early Motor Control Scales* (Paul H. Brookes Publishing Co., in press), Ms. Hayden lectures extensively and presents internationally. Email: deb@promptinstitute.com

Anne Hesketh, Ph.D.   /æn ˈhɛskəθ/   Senior Lecturer in Speech Language Therapy, The University of Manchester, Oxford Road, Manchester, England M13 9PL

Dr. Hesketh qualified as a speech and language therapist in the United Kingdom in 1981 and worked in hospitals and clinics before joining the University of Manchester. Her teaching, research, and clinical work are now all focused on children with SSD and on the effective practice of speech-language pathology. Email: anne.hesketh@manchester.ac.uk

Megan M. Hodge, Ph.D.   /ˈmɛgn̩ ˈhɑdʒ/   Professor, Department of Speech Pathology and Audiology, University of Alberta, Room 2-70, Corbett Hall, Edmonton, AB T6G 2G4, Canada

Dr. Hodge is a professor and SLP. She brings an interdisciplinary approach to linking theory with practice for serving children with motor speech disorders and understanding how these children meet the challenge of mastering intelligible speech. Email: megan.hodge@ualberta.ca

Barbara Williams Hodson, Ph.D.   /ˈbɑɚˈbɚɹə ˈhɑdsən/   Professor, Wichita State University, 1845 Fairmount, Wichita, KS 67260

Dr. Hodson is a professor at Wichita State University and has been directly involved with phonology clients for more than 30 years. Her major professional goal has been to develop more effective assessment and remediation procedures for children with highly unintelligible speech. In 2004 she received the American Speech-Language-Hearing (ASHA) Foundation Kleffner Lifetime Clinical Career Award, and in 2009 she received the ASHA Honors of the Association. Email: barbara.hodson@wichita.edu

Paul R. Hoffman, Ph.D.   /pɔl ˈhɔfmən/   Professor and Chair, Department of Communication Sciences & Disorders, Louisiana State University, Baton Rouge, LA 70803

Dr. Hoffman is an American Speech-Language-Hearing Association (ASHA) Fellow and two-time winner of the Editor's Award for work in *Language, Speech, and Hearing Services in Schools*. He researches children's SSD in the context of broader language disorders. Email: phoffmanlsu@gmail.com

Alison Holm, Ph.D.   /ˈæləsən hɒlm/   Research Fellow, University of Queensland Centre for Clinical Research, Royal Brisbane and Women's Hospital, Brisbane, QLD 4029, Australia

Dr. Holm is a speech-language pathology researcher funded by the National Health and Medical Research Council at the Perinatal Research Centre at The University of Queensland. Her research interests include the communication outcomes of children born preterm, phonological development and disorders of bilingual and monolingual children, and phonological awareness and literacy development. Email: a.holm@uq.edu.au

Ann P. Kaiser, Ph.D.   /æn keɪzɻ/   Susan W. Gray Professor of Education and Human Development, Vanderbilt University, MR 314 Magnolia Circle, Nashville, TN 37203

Dr. Kaiser is the Susan W. Gray Professor of Education and Human Development and has been conducting research for 30 years on treatment efficacy of enhanced milieu teaching. She has adapted this approach for use with children with developmental delays, autism, and language delays and now for children with both speech and language impairments. Email: Ann.p.kaiser@vanderbilt.edu

Beth McIntosh, Ph.D.   /bɛθ mækɪntɒʃ/   University of Queensland Centre for Clinical Research, Royal Brisbane and Women's Hospital, Herston, QLD 4029, Australia

Dr. McIntosh is a research SLP and primary school teacher. Her research interests include literacy learning in children from socially disadvantaged backgrounds and the phonological development of 2-year-olds. Email: b.mcintosh@uq.edu.au

Adele W. Miccio, Ph.D.   /ədɛl miʔtʃoʊ/   Associate Professor, Pennsylvania State University, 308 Ford Building, University Park, PA 16802

Adele Miccio died in March 2009. Having completed her Ph.D. degree in Speech and Hearing Sciences at Indiana University in Bloomington, she was a distinguished Professor at The Pennsylvania State University since 1995. Her research, funded by the National Institutes of Health and the U.S. Department of Education, focused on interventions for children with SSD and phonological development of bilingual children and children with chronic middle-ear infections. In 2002, she was a visiting scholar and guest lecturer at Harvard University, and in 2006 she was named the Director of the Penn State Center for Language Science. A beloved and cherished colleague, Adele is greatly missed by all of us who had the privilege of knowing her.

Janet A. Norris, Ph.D.   /ˈʤænət ˈnɔɚ-əs/   Professor, Department of Communication Sciences & Disorders, Louisiana State University, Baton Rouge, LA 70803

Dr. Norris is an ASHA Fellow and two-time winner of ASHA's Clinical Achievement Award. In 2009 she was awarded the ASHA Certificate of Recognition for Special Contributions in Higher Education. She uses principles of whole language to develop specific assessment and intervention strategies for children with speech and language disorders. Email: jnorrislsu @gmail.com

Lisa Olsen, M.A.   /lisə olsɪn/   Speech-Language Pathologist, Private Practice, Buffalo, New York; PROMPT Institute, Santa Fe, NM; 406 Huntington Avenue, Buffalo, NY 14214

Ms. Olsen is a PROMPT instructor and maintains a pediatric private practice in Buffalo. She is particularly interested in treatment of children with motor speech deficits and sensory integrative dysfunction and of children with disorders on the autism spectrum. E-mail: lisaolsen@verizon.net

Michelle Pascoe, Ph.D.   /ˈmɪʃæl ˈpæskɛʊ/   Division of Communication Sciences and Disorders, University of Cape Town, F45 Old Main Building, Groote Schuur Hospital, Observatory, Cape Town, 7925 South Africa

Dr. Pascoe is a senior lecturer in Speech and Language Pathology in the Division of Communication Sciences and Disorders, University of Cape Town. She received her Ph.D. degree in 2004 from the University of Sheffield. Her research focuses on intervention for children with speech, language, and literacy difficulties. Email: michelle.pascoe@uct.ac.za

Raúl F. Prezas, Ph.D.   /raul presəs/   Assistant Professor, Texas Christian University, TCU Box 297450, Fort Worth, TX 76129

Dr. Prezas is an assistant professor at Texas Christian University, specializing in Spanish phonology and bilingual children. He has investigated the intelligibility of bilingual preschool children in Spanish and English and compared measures of performance in both languages. Email: r.prezas@tcu.edu

Sue Roulstone, Ph.D.   /su ɹolstən/   Professor of Speech & Language Therapy, University of The West of England, Bristol; Speech & Language Thereapy Research Unit, Frenchay Hospital, Frenchay, Bristol, England B516 1LE

Sue Roulstone is a professor of speech and language therapy at the University of The West of England, Bristol, and is Director of the Speech and Language Therapy Research Unit. Her research interests are in evaluation of speech and language therapy interventions, children and family perspectives on speech and language impairment, the epidemiology of speech and language impairment, and professional judgment and decision making. Email: sue@speech-therapy .org.uk

Susan Rvachew, Ph.D. /ˈsuzən ɹəˈvæʃu/ Associate Professor, School of Communication Sciences & Disorders, McGill University, 1266 Pine Avenue West, Montréal, QC H3G 1A8, Canada

Dr. Rvachew is an associate professor in the Faculty of Medicine at McGill University. Her research focuses on the relationship between speech perception and speech production in first and second language learning and on the development of effective interventions for the treatment of SSD. Email: susan.rvachew@mcgill.ca

Nancy J. Scherer, Ph.D. /næntsi ʃɪɹɪ / Dean, Clinical and Rehabilitation Health Sciences, East Tennessee State University, 100 CR Drive, Box 70282, Johnson City, TN 37614

Dr. Scherer is a professor and Dean of Clinical and Rehabilitative Health Sciences. Her research has focused on longitudinal studies of speech and language development in children with cleft palate and craniofacial conditions and on studies of early intervention treatment efficacy. Email: scherern@etsu.edu

Joy Stackhouse, Ph.D. /ˈʤɔɪ ˈstækhaʊs/ Professor, Department of Human Communication Sciences, University of Sheffield, 31 Claremont Crescent, Sheffield, England S10 2TA

Dr. Stackhouse is Head of the Department of Human Communication Sciences at the University of Sheffield and a registered speech and language therapist, chartered psychologist, and teacher of children with specific literacy difficulties. Her research focuses on children with speech and literacy difficulties, social disadvantage, intervention, and training others. Email: j.stackhouse@sheffield.ac.uk

Joseph P. Stemberger, Ph.D. /ˈʤoʊsəf ˌpʰi ˈstɛmbəɹɡəɹ/ Professor, University of British Columbia, Department of Linguistics, Totem Field Studios, 2613 West Mall, Vancouver, BC V6T 1Z4, Canada

Dr. Stemberger is a professor in the Department of Linguistics at the University of British Columbia who studies adult language processing and first language acquisition. His research program focuses on phonology and morphology (and their interaction) in language production, with current projects on English, Zapotec, and Slovene.

Hilary Stephens, B.Sc. /hɪləɹi stivənz/ Principal Speech and Language Therapist, Nuffield Hearing and Speech Centre, RNTNE Hospital, 330 Gray's Inn Road, London, England WC1X 8DA

Ms. Stephens has worked at the Nuffield Speech and Language Unit for more than 20 years. She has developed highly specialized clinical skills working with young children with the most severe speech disorders, on an intensive basis. With Pam Williams, she coauthored the *Nuffield Centre Dyspraxia Programme, Third Edition* (The Miracle Factory, 2004). She has a particular interest in the relationship between spoken and written language. Email: Hilary.stephens@royalfree.nhs.uk

Ann A. Tyler, Ph.D.   /æn taɪleɹ/   Professor and Chair, Western Michigan University, 1903 West Michigan Avenue, Kalamazoo, MI 49008

Dr. Tyler is an ASHA Fellow and Professor and Chair at Western Michigan University, where she teaches courses in childhood SSD. Her clinical and research interests focus on efficient interventions for children with speech-language impairments. Email: ann.tyler@wmich.edu

Anne Walker, B.Sp.Path.   /æn wɑkɚ/   Speech-Language Pathologist, S.P.E.E.C.H. Pty Ltd. (Private Practice), University of Queensland (Masters Student), 16 Esplanade, Upper Coomera, QLD 4209, Australia

Ms. Walker is a pediatric SLP working in private practice. Areas of special interest include speech-motor disorders, developmental delay/disability, as well as language-based learning difficulties. She is a PROMPT instructor and is currently enrolled in a master's/Ph.D. degree program at the University of Queensland investigating the nature of speech-motor learning in PROMPT. Email: annewalker0@telstra.com

Susan E. Wastie, M.A.   /ˈsuː.zn̩ ˈweɪ.sti/   Speech-Language Pathologist, Provincial Resource Program for Auditory Outreach-Deaf/Hard of Hearing, 210-5021 Kingsway, Burnaby, BC V5H 4A5, Canada

Ms. Wastie, a speech therapist, emigrated to Canada in 1977 from the United Kingdom. She has worked primarily with children. She participated in the first community nonlinear phonological intervention project. Recently retired as a supervisor with the health department, she now provides services to children with cochlear implants or autism. Email: swastie@sd47.bc.ca

Nicole Watts Pappas, Ph.D.   /nəˈkoʊl wɒts pæpəs/   Speech-Language Pathologist, Charles Sturt University/Queensland Health, Panorama Avenue, Bathurst, NSW 2795 Australia

Dr. Watts Pappas is an adjunct lecturer at Charles Sturt University as well as a speech pathologist with Queensland Health in Australia. She has focused her research on the topic of working with families in intervention for SSD. She is co-editor of a book titled *Working with Families in Speech-Language Pathology* (Plural Publishing, 2009) and has written and spoken extensively on the subject of working with families. In addition to her research, Dr. Watts Pappas has 12 years of clinical experience working with families in intervention for young children. To ensure the clinical applicability of her research, she continues to work in a community health clinic. Email: nwattspappas@hotmail.com

Pam Williams, M.Sc. /pæm wɪljəmz/ Consultant Speech and Language Therapist, Nuffield Hearing and Speech Centre, RNTNE Hospital, 330 Gray's Inn Road, London, England WC1X 8DA

Ms. Williams qualified as a speech and language therapist 30 years ago. She was involved in the creation of the original Nuffield Centre Dyspraxia Programme (1985) and has managed the Nuffield therapy team since 1993. Although primarily a clinician, her research interests include childhood apraxia of speech, intervention studies, and diadochokinetic skills. Email: Pamela.williams@royalfree.nhs.uk

Sara E. Wood, Ph.D. /sɛəɹə wʊd/ Queen Margaret University, Queen Margaret University Drive, Musselburgh, Edinburgh, East Lothian, Scotland EH21 6UU

Dr. Wood is Senior Lecturer in Speech and Hearing Sciences at Queen Margaret University, Edinburgh. She is a speech and language therapist who qualified from The University of Reading in 1991 and is a member of both the Royal College of Speech and Language Therapists and The Health Professions Council. Dr. Wood was awarded her Ph.D. degree in 1997 for a study titled "An Electropalatographic Study of Speech Sound Errors in Adults with Acquired Aphasia." Her research has focused on instrumental analysis and treatment of intractable speech sound difficulties. She has spent many years working with electropalatography with a range of client groups, including those with stammering, Down syndrome, cerebral palsy, hearing impairment, and functional articulation difficulties. Dr. Wood regularly reviews for a wide variety of journals (United Kingdom and international). Email: swood@qmu.ac.uk

Yvonne Wren, Ph.D. /ɪvon ɹen/ Speech and Language Therapy Research Unit, North Bristol NHS Trust, Frenchay Hospital, Frenchay, Bristol, England BS16 1LE

Dr. Wren is a senior research fellow at the Speech and Language Therapy Research Unit, Bristol. Her research interests are in the field of children's speech development, impairment, and intervention. She is a coauthor of the Phoneme Factory software series and has investigated how software can assist in collaboration between teachers and SLPs. Email: yvonne@speech-therapy.org.uk

Foreword

The treatment of children's developmental speech sound disorders (SSD) has been a principal concern from the very beginning of our still-youthful profession of speech-language pathology. From the earliest efforts to teach perception and production of individual speech sounds, to more current efforts to foster systemwide changes in children's phonologies, a great deal of evidence varying widely in level and quality has shown that, in general, "treatment works." Perhaps the strongest single indicator of this broad claim of efficacy comes from the landmark meta-analysis of randomized controlled trials by Law, Garrett, and Nye (2004). But even this general evidence-based claim made by these investigators had to be qualified in many ways. For example, by design, only studies of children with primary SSD were included; children with notable sensory or motor disorders, including hearing impairment, dysarthria, apraxia of speech, and cleft palate were not considered. More important, the small number of available trials made it impossible to determine whether certain types of intervention may be more suitable than others for children who differ on potential moderators, such as speech symptoms, presence and severity of broader nonspeech language impairment, psychological and emotional status, and family circumstances, including language and cultural background.

The lack of a comprehensive, high-quality evidentiary record cannot stop clinicians from plying their trade, however. As to be expected, then, there has been a substantial proliferation of intervention philosophies, procedures, and general approaches or models, accompanied by claims of effectiveness based on everything from clinical anecdotes to careful experimental trials. Textbooks that cover developmental SSD must cut a broad swath across the discipline, including information on typical development, evaluation, assessment, and intervention. Consequently, their coverage of specific treatments is always limited, even in recent volumes that have devoted more space to the concerns of interventionists than is historically typical. This is unfortunate, especially for clinicians and students, because the rich details underlying intervention decision making can rarely be found in peer-reviewed reports of treatment studies; those who venture to this literature are often disappointed to find that the details of the interventions tested are poorly described, even in otherwise well-designed, well-implemented, and well-presented studies. More detailed accounts of these interventions are often available in book chapters and clinical journals, but these are scattered about, making them hard for clinicians and students to obtain. Furthermore, they are written for different purposes and in different voices, making comparisons between interventions difficult and the rationales for selecting one over the other unclear.

Fortunately for clinicians, students, and even parents of children with SSD, many of these issues have been addressed by A. Lynn Williams, Sharynne McLeod, and Rebecca J. McCauley in their book, *Interventions for Speech Sound Disorders in Children*. This outstanding volume, which is dedicated solely to the treatment of children's SSD, differs from all of its competitors in both breadth and depth of the coverage of its topic. On its first full page, the editors present explicitly its two primary purposes: 1) to thoroughly describe, analyze, and generally expose readers to a broad spectrum of intervention approaches designed for all types of SSD and what is known about their efficacy, and 2) to provide clinicians with enough information to enable them to select an appropriate and, perhaps, the *most* appropriate intervention for a specific child with whom they are working. These are lofty objectives, indeed. Taken together, however, they separate this book, even in principle, from all others to date.

Readers will be pleased to find that these goals are met, often in exquisite fashion, both within the book's individual chapters and across chapters, throughout the book. This success stems largely from four crucial design innovations. First, the book covers a large, if not exhaustive, set of intervention approaches designed for children with primary SSD and SSD related to organic factors such as childhood apraxia of speech, dysarthria, and cleft palate. Each chapter is written by noted authorities in the profession around the world who are developers or have been users of their approach. Second, each chapter follows a standard template for describing and exemplifying its topic intervention. This not only makes the content of each chapter more uniform and, thus, easier for readers to process; it encourages readers to compare and contrast interventions on a large set of common variables that recur across chapters, and it maximizes the efficiency of their efforts to do so. Third, as part of the template, each chapter author provides a narrative review of the published and unpublished evidence relevant to the approach. These reviews vary in the comprehensiveness of their coverage of available evidence and in the extent to which the evidence is critically analyzed. They should not be mistaken for systematic reviews or meta-analyses. Nevertheless, the level of attention each author places on the evidence base is unprecedented for books in our field. Finally, the book is accompanied by a DVD that presents demonstrations of key components of nearly all of the target interventions and quite literally brings them to life. It is hard to imagine a more valuable supplement to the chapters of the volume than a live demonstration of the interventions, enacted in most cases by the chapter authors themselves.

It has been a pleasure to see this volume grow over many months from the seeds of an idea to its present form, a book with 25 separate parts that cohere nicely into a meaningful and clinically valuable whole. It stands not just as a contribution to the literature on speech sound intervention but as a testament to the growing maturity of our field of speech-language pathology.

Marc E. Fey, Ph.D.
University of Kansas Medical Center

REFERENCE

Law, J., Garrett, Z., & Nye, C. (2004). The efficacy of treatment for children with developmental speech and language delay/disorder: A meta-analysis. *Journal of Speech, Language, and Hearing Research, 47*(4), 924–943.

Acknowledgments

Interventions for Speech Sound Disorders in Children has evolved due to the generosity and expertise of the chapter authors, who have carefully crafted their knowledge of and insights on each intervention into the organizational structure of this book. We have enjoyed the international collaborations and collegiality among the team and are grateful for their contributions to the book and to interventions for speech sound disorders (SSD) in children around the world.

The first person who believed this book should and could be assembled was our colleague and friend, Marc E. Fey. He has been a terrific sounding board at various stages in the development of this book, and we are hugely grateful for his helpful and timely comments that often pushed us to think outside the traditional articulation-phonology paradigm. We also want to thank Ronald B. Gillam for his encouragement to pursue this book and for making the initial contact to Paul H. Brookes Publishing Company on our behalf.

We wish to express our gratitude and appreciation to the many wonderful people at Brookes Publishing who worked closely with us every step of the way. A very special thank you to Astrid Zuckerman, who provided steady guidance and encouragement through all stages of development. Her work helped us to do our best work. We couldn't have had a better editor! We also appreciate the good work of Julie Chávez, who kept everything well organized and moving smoothly. Finally, Jan Krejci was an outstanding production editor; the careful and thorough editing brought out the best in all the chapters.

In Tennessee, Lynn received resolute support from her colleagues in the Center of Excellence in Early Childhood Learning and Development at East Tennessee State University (ETSU). A very heartfelt thank you is also due to Daniel Santiago and Harold "Buddy" Arnold in the ETSU Broadcast Studio for their creative and tireless work in producing the exceptional DVD that accompanies this book. Their work helps make the interventions described in the book come to life. Several personal notes of thanks are due to people who have influenced and supported Lynn's life and work in so many ways. Mary Elbert provided her with a solid and strong foundation that has been the basis of her research and teaching for the past 20 years. Mary's influence is clearly evident in this book. And to her family—Jim, Alison, and Nora; their supportive presence in Lynn's life has been her bedrock.

In Australia, Sharynne and Lynn acknowledge the assistance of the Charles Sturt University Global Alliance Development Scheme and the Research Institute for Professional Practice, Learning and Education (RIPPLE) for their generous support of our collaboration that launched this book. We are grateful for the progressive philosophy that underlies these two support systems to assist and encourage international collaborations in the construction of knowledge. Sharynne also acknowledges the constant support of her family—David, Brendon, and Jessica.

In Ohio, Rebecca wants to give her special thanks to Ralph Shelton, who introduced her to the fascinating topic of SSD intervention and helped her recognize how very important it is. In addition she would like to acknowledge the contribution that Vasile Mulligan has made to her understanding of SSD and so many other things, such as courage and persistence. Finally, she wishes to thank the friends and colleagues in Vermont and Ohio who have supported her as she worked on this book.

In the end, we thank the children and their families who continually inspire us to learn more and continue our efforts to make a difference to improve communication for all children.

We dedicate this book to our friend and colleague

Dr. Adele W. Miccio
1951–2009

In memory and appreciation for her many contributions
to interventions for speech sound disorders in children

Introduction to *Interventions for Speech Sound Disorders in Children*

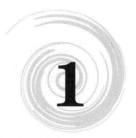

A. Lynn Williams, Sharynne McLeod, and Rebecca J. McCauley

ABSTRACT

Speech sound disorders (SSD) are a widespread problem in preschool and school-age children. For most, the cause of SSD is unknown; however, for others, SSD can encompass a variety of etiologies (e.g., cleft lip and/or palate, cerebral palsy, Down syndrome). In addition, SSD often involves concomitant disabilities (e.g., language and literacy impairments). This diversity presents a considerable challenge for understanding SSD and how best to design intervention that also meets the standards of evidence-based practice (EBP). It also prods us as professionals to move beyond the articulation-phonology dichotomy and debate that has been a central tenet of SSD in children. As part of the *Communication and Language Intervention Series* and as a companion book to *Treatment of Language Disorders in Children* (McCauley & Fey, 2006), this book makes use of a prescribed template; a device that we believe facilitates critical comparisons across interventions in terms of client populations and key elements, as well as levels of evidence. Given this organization, the book may be useful for diverse groups of readers who would probably be reading it for different reasons, with different goals in mind. In particular, we anticipate four primary categories of readers who may be especially interested in this book: 1) students of speech-language pathology, 2) clinical practitioners who work with children with SSD, 3) professors who teach in the area of SSD in children, and 4) parents of children with SSD. To prepare all readers to use the book to its fullest advantage, we begin this chapter with a general description of the book's purpose and a delineation of the template that guided the preparation of individual intervention chapters. Then, we address each of the four primary categories of readers separately, offering suggestions for how each can get the most out of their interactions with this book. Finally, we present a structural framework for intervention that facilitates readers' understanding of the components of each intervention, and provides a mechanism for comparing intervention components across the various approaches.

THE PURPOSE OF THIS BOOK

In a clinical forum on EBP, Kamhi (2006) stated that it is "often troubling to clinicians and researchers who want there to be a 'gold standard' treatment approach that works for all children with SSD" (p. 272). He continued that the problem is that "there seem to be too many ways to improve children's speech, and these approaches are often theoretically incompatible with one another" (p. 272). As Kamhi reported, a number of different reviews indicated that the range of intervention approaches has been shown to be effective in modifying children's sound systems. So the question is, How do clinicians determine which intervention approach is the best one to use with their client? That is where this book comes in.

A primary purpose of this book is to describe and critically analyze a spectrum of intervention approaches used for SSD in children (see Table 1.1). A second, equally important, or even *more* important, purpose is to help readers learn skills that will enable them to examine and critically evaluate these and other approaches *for themselves*. Thus, in response to the previous question, our goal with this book is to provide speech-language pathologists (SLPs) with sufficient information about each intervention approach so that they can align the clinical characteristics of their client's SSD to the intervention approach that best addresses those needs. Furthermore, we do not believe that a single intervention approach will be the sole intervention for any child with SSD. As readers will learn through reading about the various approaches in this book, several interventions are designed as transitional methods to help children progress from emerging sound systems to elaborating their sound systems.

Both of these purposes provide compelling rationales for a book because SSD in children is frequently occurring and often has broad and long-lasting effects. In fact, SSD is considered the most prevalent communication disability diagnosed among preschool and school-age children, affecting approximately 10%–15% of preschoolers and 6% of school-age children in Grades 1–12 (American Speech-Language-Hearing Association [ASHA],

Table 1.1.   Breadth of speech sound disorders included in this book

Primary populations	Children with:
	Articulation delay/disorder
	Phonological delay/disorder
	Inconsistent speech disorder
	Speech impairment
	Phonological/morphological disorder
	Childhood apraxia of speech
	Motor speech disorders, including childhood apraxia of speech and developmental dysarthria
Secondary populations	Children with:
	Craniofacial anomalies
	Hearing loss
	Sensorimotor impairments
	Cerebral palsy
	Tongue thrust
	Intellectual impairment, including children with Down syndrome
	Congenital conditions associated with developmental dysarthria, such as conditions affecting the cranial nerves, and early onset muscular dystrophy

2000; Jessup, Ward, Cahill, & Keating, 2008; Law, Boyle, Harris, Harkness, & Nye, 2000; McLeod & Harrison, 2009). There is a high correlation between some forms of SSD and difficulties with written language including reading, writing, spelling, and mathematics (Bird, Bishop, & Freeman, 1995; Catts, 1993; Clark-Klein & Hodson, 1995; Harrison, McLeod, Berthelsen, & Walker, 2009; Leitão & Fletcher, 2004; Sices, Taylor, Freebairn, Hansen, & Lewis, 2007). Furthermore, 50%–70% of children with SSD exhibit general academic difficulty through high school (Felsenfeld, Broen, & McGue, 1994; Overby, Carrell, & Bernthal, 2007; Shriberg & Kwiatkowski, 1988) and socialization difficulties are not uncommon among these children (Rice, Hadley, & Alexander, 1993). In short, although SSD presents focal challenges of relatively short duration for some children, for others, they are associated with difficulties that are neither confined to speech nor to early childhood (McCormack, McLeod, McAllister, & Harrison, 2009).

To introduce readers to an extensive range of interventions for SSD, we invited 23 groups of authors from around the world to write chapters about interventions they have developed and/or tested. Consequently, the book contains chapters by the world's foremost SLP researcher-clinicians from the United States, Canada, Scotland, Ireland, England, and Australia. The interventions were selected based on their empirical evidence, or potential efficacy, as well as their widespread use across ages, severity levels, and populations. Included are approaches encompassing interventions that focus on sound production accuracy, systemwide restructuring of the child's phonology, motor speech, and perceptual training, as well as computer-based interventions and family-focused interventions.

THE BOOK'S OVERALL ORGANIZATION

The book is divided into three major sections: Direct Speech Production Interventions, Interventions in Broader Contexts, and Interventions for Achieving Speech Movements. In Section I, Direct Speech Production Interventions, we have included seven approaches that address speech sound production goals within a focused and explicit context. Section II, Interventions in Broader Contexts, includes a large number of approaches—12 in fact. Although diverse in their goals and implementation, these approaches similarly occur in broader contexts, in which "broader contexts" refers either to additional domains that are also at risk in children with SSD (e.g., perception, lexical/sentential stress, morphology, syntax) or to a broader service delivery context (e.g., parent-administered interventions). Section III, Interventions for Achieving Speech Movements, contains four approaches, all of which share a focus on helping children achieve the movements required for appropriate speech sound productions. This focus has particular relevance for children with motor speech disorders, but the section as a whole includes information that is also valuable to intervention for other types of SSD.

Although these three sections may not fit every reader's preconception about how to classify interventions for SSD (e.g., McCauley, 2004), this organization grew out of discussions with contributing authors about how they viewed their own intervention and other interventions they considered similar in scope and/or intent. We offer this organization, then, not as a definitive classification (or even as an attempt that completely satisfied all of the participants in this project, including ourselves), but rather as a heuristic approach used to group interventions for comparison and study within this book. The many, many variables that can influence the nature of interventions for SSD placed the identification of an ideal classification beyond our grasp. Nonetheless, we believe that readers will find this classification useful for many of their purposes.

Each of the three sections comprises an overview and several additional chapters dedicated to specific interventions. The overviews provide a critical integration of the approaches included in that section in order to guide the reader to a more thorough understanding. Summary tables provide easy reference and comparison.

Each intervention chapter incorporates two features of special interest:

1. Standard headings that enable comparisons among interventions, including practical requirements and key features—These headings should also facilitate implementation of interventions once they are chosen as appropriate for a given child.

2. Evaluation of each approach within an EBP framework that examines the levels of evidence for each approach—This information helps readers gauge the strength of an intervention's empirical base, thus allowing them to determine an intervention's likely benefit for appropriate children.

In addition, video demonstrations of almost all intervention approaches are available on an accompanying DVD. This kind of visual documentation can help readers consider an intervention, its implementation, and its suitability to their specific needs from a vivid perspective not offered by even the best-written textual account.

THE ORGANIZATION OF INDIVIDUAL INTERVENTION CHAPTERS

In order to encourage greater uniformity across approaches, authors of individual intervention chapters were invited to use the same template, with its prescribed specific headings and expected content. The standardization of headings across chapters promotes easy access to and evaluation of important information about each approach, thus facilitating decisions concerning treatment efficacy, clinician expertise, and clients' preferences—the triad of considerations within EBP (Dollaghan, 2007; Sackett, Rosenberg, Gray, Hayes, & Richardson, 1996). The current template was modified from one used in the companion book, *Treatment of Language Disorders in Children* (McCauley & Fey, 2006). Consequently, use of this template across these two volumes also facilitates the examination of synergies between interventions for SSD and language disorders. Table 1.2 describes the current template in terms of the headings and content.

Target Populations

Following an abstract and brief introduction, each chapter describes the primary populations for which the intervention is designed, as well as any secondary populations—especially those for which there is empirical support or theoretical support for its use. Client populations are described in terms of age or developmental range and prerequisite skills required for use of the approach or program.

Assessment Methods for Determining Intervention Relevance

In this section of their chapter, authors describe any assessment methods used to establish the appropriateness of the intervention for the individual child. When assessment methods associated with determining the appropriateness of the approach to the child

Table 1.2. The template: Components of each chapter

Section heading	Content
Target Populations	Description of population(s) for which empirical and/or theoretical support of the intervention is available (e.g., in terms of age, major disability, prerequisite skills)
Assessment Methods for Determining Intervention Relevance	Assessments used to determine that the intervention is appropriate
Theoretical Basis	The dominant rationale for the intervention
	Assumptions made about the deficits, compensatory strategies, or strengths that are targeted
	Nature of outcomes targeted (e.g., positive effect on social roles, decreased functional limitation)
	Area of functioning being targeted (e.g., intelligibility, movement for speech)
Empirical Basis	Summary and interpretation of studies supporting the intervention's use
	Study descriptions including information about participants and the study design
	Level of evidence table providing a quick reference to the strength of the designs included in this section
Practical Requirements	Time demands
	Personnel demands, including training, for both professionals and family members
	Type of sessions (e.g., group, individual)
	Frequency and duration of sessions (dosage)
Key Components	Types of goals targeted (e.g., production of a specific sound, improved phonological awareness)
	Strategy for addressing multiple goals (sequential, cyclic, simultaneous)
	Procedures (therapeutic actions of the primary clinician, who may be a professional or family member depending on the approach)
	Activities in which procedures are embedded (e.g., storybook reading, play, conversation, structured repetition)
	Materials used in the intervention
	Roles of secondary personnel (e.g., teachers, family members, the clinician for family-based interventions)
Assessment and Progress Monitoring to Support Decision Making	Recommendations for data collection and for how decisions are made regarding the alteration of goals, methods, stimuli, termination of therapy, and so forth
Considerations for Children from Culturally and Linguistically Diverse Backgrounds	Applicability of approach to children of different linguistic and cultural backgrounds
	Recommended ways in which the intervention can be adapted to better meet child and caregiver needs
Case Study	Description of one or more children for whom the intervention was helpful (used to illustrate children's responses to the intervention and ongoing decision making)
Study Questions	Three to five questions to help readers integrate their understanding of the intervention
Future Directions	Recommendations for areas of further study regarding the intervention; these may include additional populations for which it may be useful
Suggested Readings	Three to five readings providing additional information about the intervention's theoretical or empirical basis or its procedures

are particularly detailed, authors use citations to supplement a brief overview of the methods.

Theoretical Basis

In this section, authors discuss the dominant theoretical explanation or rationale for the intervention approach or program, including the underlying assumptions regarding the nature of 1) the impairment being addressed or 2) compensatory strategies being developed via the intervention. Authors provide information about whether the intervention approach focuses solely on speech output and/or on other domains (e.g., perception, literacy, morphosyntax). Each chapter's placement in one of the three sections also provides the reader with clues about the focus of the intervention approach.

Typically, the authors also provide information about the level of consequences being addressed—for example, whether the intervention is targeting a functional limitation directly or the social skill, activity, or social role restrictions that result from it. Interest in this distinction arises from work by the World Health Organization (WHO; 2007) in the form of the *International Classification of Functioning, Disability and Health for Children and Youth* (ICF-CY). The ICF-CY is a framework that provides an international interdisciplinary language of health and health-related issues for children that allows for the holistic consideration of the biopsychosocial issues facing children.

Over the past 30 years, WHO has been working to create a common language for comparison of data across countries, health care disciplines, services, and time; to provide a systematic coding scheme for health information systems; and to provide a scientific basis for consequences of health conditions. In 2001, WHO launched the *International Classification of Functioning, Disability and Health* (ICF). The ICF presents a holistic approach for all people, of all ages, across all nations, from a perspective of health and wellness. It has been endorsed by many professional associations throughout the world including ASHA in the *Scope of Practice in Speech-Language Pathology* (ASHA, 2007) and the *Scope of Practice in Audiology* (ASHA, 2004), the Royal College of Speech and Language Therapists (RCSLT), the Canadian Association of Speech-Language Pathologists and Audiologists (CASLPA), and Speech Pathology Australia (SPA).

The ICF and ICF-CY comprise the following interrelated components: Body Functions, Body Structures, Activities and Participation, Environmental Factors, and Personal Factors. Each of these factors relates to children with SSD who are the focus of this book. An example of the application of the ICF-CY to a 7-year-old boy with unintelligible speech is found in McLeod (2006). Table 1.3 describes the components of the ICF.

Empirical Basis

This section of each chapter presents the empirical basis for the intervention through summaries and interpretation of studies that provide evidence to support the use of the intervention. Authors have been encouraged to distinguish among the following three types of study: 1) *exploratory studies* of a potential intervention (sometimes consisting of observational or feasibility studies; Fey, 2002, 2004), 2) *efficacy studies* of the intervention (i.e., studies illustrating its usefulness under conditions allowing for greater experimental control), and 3) *studies of effectiveness* (i.e., studies illustrating its usefulness under the conditions of everyday practice, following the definitions described by Robey

Table 1.3. Components of the *International Classification of Functioning Disability and Health* (ICF)

Component	Definition	Difficulty
Body Functions	Physiological functions of body systems (including psychological functions) Eight chapters describe Body Functions including: Chapter 1: Mental functions (e.g., memory functions, intellectual functions) Chapter 3: Voice and speech functions (e.g., articulation functions)	Impairment: Problems in body function such as significant deviation or loss
Body Structures	Anatomical parts of the body such as organs, limbs, and their components Eight chapters describe Body Structures including: Chapter 2: The eye, ear, and related structures (e.g., structure of inner ear) Chapter 3: Structures involved in voice and speech (e.g. structure of mouth)	Impairment: Problems in body structure such as significant deviation or loss
Activities and Participation	Activity: The execution of a task or action by an individual Participation: Involvement in a life situation Nine chapters describe Activities and Participation including: Chapter 3: Communication (e.g., speaking, conversation) Chapter 7: Interpersonal interactions and relationships (e.g., relating with strangers)	Activity limitation: Difficulties an individual may have in executing activities Participation restriction: Difficulties an individual may experience in involvement in life situations
Environmental Factors	The physical, social, and attitudinal environment in which people live and conduct their lives Five chapters describe Environmental Factors including: Chapter 3: Support and relationships (e.g., support from siblings) Chapter 4: Attitudes (e.g., attitude of friends)	Environmental factors are either barriers to or facilitators of the person's functioning
Personal Factors	These are not specified within the ICF; however, factors may include age, sex, and indigenous status	

Source: World Health Organization (2001).

& Schultz, 1998; cf., Olswang, 1998). In authors' descriptions of the evidence for their intervention approach, the nature of outcome data are reported; for example, standardized testing versus naturalistic probes.

This section of each chapter is considered of the utmost importance because of its relevance to EBP. Although EBP was initially developed within medicine, it has become shorthand for the assumption that clinical services are improved when practitioners become "data seekers, data integrators, and critical evaluators of the application of new knowledge to clinical cases" (Bernstein Ratner, 2006, p. 257–258). Furthermore, EBP encompasses specific steps by which professionals not only seek and evaluate research evidence in support of their practice but also actively integrate such evidence with their own expertise (including clinical data gathering) and client preferences (e.g., Dollaghan, 2007).

Within this section, authors analyze the research conducted for their approach and describe this research in terms of levels of evidence—a summary of evidence quality, in order to facilitate readers' effective and appropriate implementation of the interventions

Table 1.4. Levels of evidence for studies of treatment

Level	Description
Ia	Meta-analysis of > 1 randomized controlled trial
Ib	Randomized controlled study
IIa	Controlled study without randomization
IIb	Quasi-experimental study
III	Nonexperimental studies, i.e., correlational and case studies
IV	Expert committee report, consensus conference, clinical experience of respected authorities

Adapted from the Scottish Intercollegiate Guideline Network (http://www.sign.ac.uk).

in clinical practice. A table is included in each intervention chapter that indicates the level of evidence for the journal articles and other sources cited by the authors to support the intervention approach. The levels-of-evidence system used here comes from a system selected by ASHA (which appears on its website http://www.asha.org/docs/html/TR2004-00001.html#sec2.2; see Table 1.4 for a brief introduction). This system was adapted from the Scottish Intercollegiate Guideline Network.

Although widely used, this system and many other commonly used systems for evidence evaluation have been criticized for inadequate evaluation of the rigor and importance of single-subject experimental designs in applied behavioral sciences (Beeson & Robey, 2006). Especially for those interventions that are in early stages of development (as are a number of those in this book), single-subject experimental designs can be considered both appropriately conserving of time and resources, yet also sufficiently rigorous to offer important causal insights (Robey & Schultz, 1998; Robey, Schultz, Crawford, & Sinner, 1999). Therefore, although studies that make use of single-subject experimental designs are likely to appear toward the bottom of the levels-of-evidence table for a given intervention (indicating lower quality evidence), readers are cautioned to consider the maturity of the intervention and the claims being made by the authors. When claims of efficacy are modest and appropriate to an intervention with a persuasive theoretical base but relatively few empirical supports, such studies deserve special consideration.

Practical Requirements

In this section, authors describe the nature, frequency, and length of sessions, as well as whether the sessions are individual, group, school-based, or home-based. In addition, authors describe the personnel demands by identifying the primary clinician and other participants, as well as the training required of those involved, and the dosage of the intervention (e.g., frequency and length of sessions). Where appropriate, the authors have included the nature of involvement of participants beyond the clinician and child (e.g., parents, peers, siblings, teachers). In the case of parent-administered interventions, the clinician's role is specified.

Key Components

This section describes the nature of goals (e.g., broad goals of intervention and basis of target selection) and goal attack strategies (e.g., sequential, simultaneous, cyclical). In addition, there is a description of the activities undertaken during the intervention approach, procedures implemented by the clinician, and what materials and equipment are required.

Assessment and Progress Monitoring to Support Decision Making

In each chapter, authors provide recommended assessment techniques and data collection used for decision making within each intervention approach. This includes discussion regarding techniques for determining whether progress is being made, when changes should be made to the intervention plan, and when treatment should be terminated. For some interventions, this section may be relatively brief, usually because it is assumed that these methods are independent of the specific approach and may differ by setting or clinician.

Considerations for Children from Culturally and Linguistically Diverse Backgrounds

This section highlights the applicability of each intervention approach to children who are from linguistically and culturally diverse backgrounds. Authors provide ways in which their intervention approach might be modified to be more appropriate for children across the world. The length of this section can be relatively brief when authors believe that their approach poses few challenges associated with cultural and linguistic differences. When appropriate, the authors also document countries where their approach has been adopted and languages in which their approach has been translated. This searching was facilitated with reference to *The International Guide to Speech Acquisition* (McLeod, 2007), a resource documenting speech acquisition, assessment, and intervention practices across 24 languages and 12 English dialects.

CASE STUDY

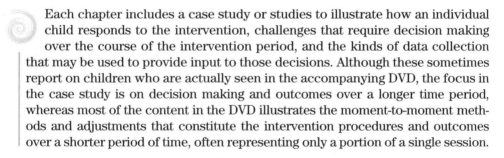

Each chapter includes a case study or studies to illustrate how an individual child responds to the intervention, challenges that require decision making over the course of the intervention period, and the kinds of data collection that may be used to provide input to those decisions. Although these sometimes report on children who are actually seen in the accompanying DVD, the focus in the case study is on decision making and outcomes over a longer time period, whereas most of the content in the DVD illustrates the moment-to-moment methods and adjustments that constitute the intervention procedures and outcomes over a shorter period of time, often representing only a portion of a single session.

Study Questions

In this section, authors propose three to five questions that may be used by readers to foster their own active engagement with the chapter content. When this text is being read as part of a course, professors may choose to use these questions to spur class discussion or to structure in-class writing assignments.

Future Directions

This section provides authors with the opportunity to draw on their current research and clinical experiences with their approach and point the way toward further, productive development of that approach. Therefore, readers can use this section to confirm their impressions about current gaps in the research evidence and the theoretical underpinnings of a given approach. Furthermore, readers can consider how they themselves might address those gaps—through data collection designed to provide local evidence that the intervention is useful to a specific client or group of clients, if they decide to adopt the intervention despite its limitations, or through their own research efforts, if they are interested in and able to conduct more formal research.

Suggested Readings

Because book chapters are necessarily limited in space and some of the interventions are quite complex, we include this section in each chapter so that authors can direct readers to additional readings. Whereas many of these readings will provide further information about intervention procedures, stimuli, and materials, others represent the primary scholarly sources in which important studies were first reported. Readers who become particularly intrigued by a given approach should consider these sources as their next logical step in learning about the intervention.

HOW TO USE THIS BOOK: COMMENTS TO SPECIFIC AUDIENCES

This book may be useful for diverse groups of readers who would probably be reading it for different reasons, with different goals in mind. As noted earlier in this chapter, we anticipate four primary categories of readers who may be especially interested in this book:

- Students of speech-language pathology
- Clinical practitioners who work with children with SSD
- Professors who teach in the area of SSD in children
- Parents of children with SSD

Because each audience will probably approach the book from different needs and perspectives, this section suggests strategies, as well as specific chapters and sections within chapters, that may address each group's special needs and interests.

Students

We realize that you are probably reading this book as part of a course requirement, but we hope that the following suggestions will increase your access to and understanding of the information that you need in order to successfully grasp the material, integrate it, and ultimately apply it clinically. We also hope the book will continue to be a useful resource for you after you move from the role of student to that of practicing clinician. Consequently, it may be valuable for you to read beyond this section in order to view our suggestions to other groups of readers, such as practicing clinicians and parents. And, yes, it may even be helpful to read our comments to professors of classes on SSD, because it never hurts to gain insight into influences on an instructor's perspective on course readings.

Getting Started

A primary question that students often have is, What is the best intervention approach to implement with a particular client who has an SSD? In this book we have compiled chapters on 23 different interventions that have been used in treating SSD with different origins—for example, phonological impairments, articulation impairments, and motor speech disorders in children. It can be a daunting task for a student to sort through all of these interventions. That's where we can help.

Several clinical decision-making points help determine which intervention is best. Obviously, in your student role, you will receive additional input about treatment selection from your clinical instructor or supervisor. In fact, you may even be told exactly what approach to adopt and be required to read a chapter or two for background. Even in that case, however, we encourage you to remain as active as possible at each step we outline below so that you will judge the probable fit between your client and the intervention—only then are you likely to maximize your gains as a clinician.

First, you need to examine your client's needs, which are identified through your assessment and analysis of the child's speech; the case history; and other sources of information about that child's experiences with speech, communication, and possibly academic settings. This information will include severity and overall intelligibility, age, consistency of error, and stimulability (the ease with which the child can produce the sound with input from the clinician). It will also include information about differential diagnosis of motor speech disorders from other types of SSD. The breadth of the child's problems (e.g., whether they also include several areas of language) further determines which interventions you may want to consider.

Second, you need to decide which of the approaches have the strongest evidence given your client's needs, your level of clinical abilities, and the support available to you to implement it. That's where this book helps readers critically evaluate intervention options in terms of evidence supporting their effectiveness. Each author has summarized the strongest evidence for their intervention and then, in the section overviews , we have examined the levels of evidence and strength of recommendation for each intervention. Your clinical abilities may be at a novice level at this point in implementing any of these interventions. We hope the structured template, along with guidance from your clinical educator or supervisor, will give you the support you need to get started.

Third, consider how you will examine the actual value of an intervention once it has been selected for use with a given client. What probe data, standardized testing, and other methods will you adopt in order to document the child's response? Although chapter authors have been encouraged to describe methods they would generally recommend for this purpose, it is important to consider whether there are measures that will mean more to the child or to his or her family as indicators of progress. These may depend on the specific reasons that intervention was sought (e.g., ability to perform in a school play without fear of unintelligibility, greater clarity in producing the names of school friends) and therefore may lie outside of those described here.

Recommended Chapters and Sections

As academic faculty, we've learned that students often focus on different things when reading a chapter. Consequently, learning from a text is often more effective when it is done across multiple readings and while accompanied by suggestions (from us and your professors) about how to first overview information before diving in for more careful study. The suggestions provided in the following list will guide you in reading the chapters so that you will know the focus of particular chapters and can therefore structure your reading to meet your specific questions or learning needs.

1. Read this introduction chapter first to get an idea how the intervention chapters are organized, as well as information on ways to think about the nature of different inter-

ventions and how their relative merits can be evaluated—especially the quality of the evidence available to suggest that they are effective (a cornerstone of EBP.)

2. Before reading individual chapters dedicated to specific interventions, read the overview of the section to which they belong. The section overviews are intended to provide you with the "big picture" to which you can attach all of the details that differentiate interventions from each other, thus, taking them from generalities to the specifics that can actually be acted on in intervention sessions. Even if your professor only requires you to know about one or two intervention chapters in a section, reading the section overview can help you gain perspective and later retain details with minimal confusion.

3. Read individual chapters by previewing sections that can help prepare you for the whole. For many students, this may simply require a very thoughtful reading of the Introduction; for others, it may entail an examination of key words from the glossary and the list of references as well. Examination of the chapter template outlined in Table 1.2 can help you anticipate what sections to include in your prereading.

Clinical Practitioners

As a professional, you almost certainly have considerable experience with children with SSD because of their ubiquity and the frequent breadth of their clinical needs. However, you may recognize a gap between your practice and the exciting array of interventions that have been refined or developed since you were trained. It is easy to let oneself develop clinical practices by accretion—gradually adding a few new "tricks" here and there as they are passed along by colleagues or picked up at conferences or from reading. However, a fresh look at more cohesive approaches can provide resources for renewing one's methods and even one's outlook on this frequently served population. In addition, you realize that many of the approaches described here will have been studied for effectiveness to a degree that your practice and, indeed, many older interventions have not.

Even if you have endeavoured to keep abreast of important developments in interventions for children with SSD and worked to make EBP a bedrock of your work, it is likely that you have confined your regrettably limited time for reading and conference attendance to sources that are relatively convenient. In this book, therefore, we have attempted to provide a concise but broad introduction to the international scope of developments in this area of speech-language pathology. Whereas many of the authors whose work we include are probably well known to you, others whose work is of equal merit are likely to be new to you because they work abroad and have published in journals that are less familiar to you.

Getting Started

In this chapter, we have synthesized the information across all 23 approaches in a grid format (see Table 1.5), which we believe should be among the first things you read. Because this table synthesizes and summarizes many of the most salient features of each intervention approach (e.g., Developmental Level, Targeted Stage of Production, and Targeted Outcomes), we believe that it will help you identify approaches that you will want to explore further in your reading. Then in each section overview, we included an additional summary table that recaps features of the interventions that are included in that section based on the primary section headings of the chapter template (e.g., Primary Client Populations, Key Components, Broad Goals, etc.). This strategy will give you the "big picture" of all 23 approaches so that you can then move to more focused reading of a specific category of intervention approaches, and finally read in detail those specific approaches of particular interest.

Recommended Chapters and Sections

If you choose to read several chapters, and especially if you are considering several interventions that fall within the same section in this book, the section overviews should provide a rapid orientation to some of the dimensions along which comparisons are likely to be productive.

Individual sections within intervention chapters that may be most valuable to you are likely to be those related to the Theoretical Basis and Empirical Basis for the intervention because these will probably help you identify an intervention's possible advantages over those you currently use. However, the chapter sections on Key Components, Practical Requirements, and the Case Study—along with examination of the video clips associated with the intervention—will provide you with information that helps you determine the extent to which the intervention fits your own clinical style and the constraints of your work setting. Finally, both the Case Study and section on Considerations for Children from Culturally and Linguistically Diverse Backgrounds may help you anticipate how well the intervention will fit the needs and situations of children you encounter in your practice.

Professors

In preparing this book, we attempted to balance a focus on theoretical and research considerations associated with EBP with attention to practical matters that readers need to grasp in order to move from ideas to clinical actions based on them. Nonetheless, depending on your orientation to the subject of SSD in children and, perhaps, the experience level of your students, you may lean more heavily toward one end of the theory/research-practicalities continuum than the other. In this section, we endeavour to make suggestions that you will find helpful no matter where you fall on the continuum.

Getting Started

In order to determine how you will use this book in your teaching, we recommend that you begin by scanning the tables we have included in the section overviews, including this one. By doing this, you will obtain a quick sense of the types of problems addressed by the interventions included and the amount of attention paid to those interventions you consider important, as well as major principles to consider as they evaluate intervention quality and feasibility.

Recommended Chapters and Sections

Obviously, we hope that you will assign most, if not all, of the chapters in this book. However, if you've decided to incorporate this book as a supplementary text, you may choose to limit your use to those intervention chapters describing interventions with the great-

Table 1.5. Intervention approaches for children with speech sound disorders

Approach	Author(s)	Emerging	Developing	Elaborating	Key components	Technology and/or materials	Interventions for specific diagnoses	Planning	Programming	Execution	Speech Production	Speech Perception	Phonological Awareness	Other Oral Language	Literacy
Minimal Pair Intervention	Baker		✓	✓	Contrastive word pairs (error ~ target) Intervention phases typically include familiarization, identification, and production at imitative and spontaneous levels	Some computer programs are available, but not required Commercial illustrations/Internet resources	SSD			✓	✓				
Multiple Oppositions Intervention	Williams		✓		Large integrated contrastive treatment sets across a phoneme collapse Treatment paradigm that includes focused practice at imitation and spontaneous levels, naturalistic activities, and contrasts within communicative contexts	SCIP software program Clip art or compiled illustrations	SSD			✓	✓				

Approach	Authors								Description	Materials	Population
Complexity Approaches to Intervention	Baker & Williams	✓				✓	✓		Maximally distinctive word pairs that include one or two phonologically complex phonemes absent from phonetic inventory; Nonsense words are recommended and assigned lexical meaning; Intervention conducted in two phases: imitation and spontaneous	Nonsense pictures from Internet or SCIP software program	SSD
Core Vocabulary Intervention	Dodd, Holmes, Crosbie, & McIntosh	✓	✓	✓		✓	✓		Consistent production of < 50 functionally powerful words; Sound-by-sound and syllable-by-syllable dense response drill with pictures	Picture stimuli	SSD
The Cycles Phonological Remediation Approach	Prezas & Hodson	✓	✓		✓	✓	✓	✓[a]	Ordering of phonological patterns within cycles, auditory bombardment, facilitating contexts, active involvement, and self-monitoring; Home program	Amplification device; 5 × 8-inch index cards; Motivational/experiential play items	SSD; Inconsistent speech; Childhood apraxia of speech

(continued)

15

Table 1.5. *(continued)*

Approach	Author(s)	Emerging	Developing	Elaborating	Key components	Technology and/or materials	Interventions for specific diagnoses	Planning	Programming	Execution	Speech Production	Speech Perception	Phonological Awareness	Other Oral Language	Literacy
Nuffield Centre Dyspraxia Programme	P. Williams & Stephens		✓		Focuses on building speech processing skills from the bottom up through the establishment of motor programs for single sounds in isolation and increasing phonotactic complexity. Includes auditory discrimination and specific nonspeech oral motor skills within repetitive practice	NDP3 manual and pictorial intervention materials and worksheets	SSD Childhood apraxia of speech	✓	✓	✓	✓		✓		
Stimulability Approach Intervention	Miccio & Williams	✓			Stimulable and nonstimulable sounds are targeted. Sounds are paired with alliterative characters and body motions	Alliterative sound character card illustrations (http://www .brookes publishing.com /williams/miccio .htm)	SSD Very young children with limited sound inventory			✓	✓		✓		

Intervention	Author	Description	Resources	Population
Psycholinguistic Intervention	Stackhouse & Pascoe	Speech input (e.g., auditory discrimination), lexical representations (e.g., semantic, phonological, motor), speech output (e.g., programming and production of speech)	All resources can be used in a psycholinguistic way; new or specific materials not required	SSD, Speech and literacy difficulties
Metaphonological Intervention	Hesketh	Emphasis on phonological awareness including rhyming, syllable clapping, alliteration, blending, and segmenting activities followed by production of contrasting sounds and minimally paired words	Can include some computer-based resources (e.g., PFSS or SAILS), but not required; written letters linked to picture; standard clinical materials	SSD
Computer-Based Interventions	Roulstone, Wren, & Williams	Key components vary depending on program. Provide ease and accessibility, efficiency, data management, and report generation	Computer software programs (variety)	SSD
Speech Perception Intervention	Rvachew & Brosseau-Lapré	Phonemic perception training	SAILS computer program	SSD

(continued)

Table 1.5. *(continued)*

Approach	Author(s)	Emerging	Developing	Elaborating	Key components	Technology and/or materials	Interventions for specific diagnoses	Planning	Programming	Execution	Speech Production	Speech Perception	Phonological Awareness	Other Oral Language	Literacy
		Developmental level						**Targeted stage of production**			**Targeted outcomes**				
Nonlinear Phonological Intervention	Bernhardt, Bopp, Daudlin, Edwards, & Wastie		✓	✓	Constraint-based nonlinear approach targeting prosodic structures and segments by considering individual phonological units and interactions between phonological units	Audio and video recording; creative materials, including costumes and props can be included to dramatize certain speech elements	SSD Range of etiologies	✓		✓	✓	✓	✓		
Dynamic Systems and Whole Language Intervention	Hoffman & Norris		✓	✓	Addresses discourse structure, semantic, syntactic, morphological, and letter-sound knowledge	Illustrated books; Phonic Face books and cards; MorphoPhonic Face cards	SSD Concomitant speech and language impairment	✓		✓	✓			✓	✓
Morphosyntax Intervention	Tyler & Haskill		✓	✓	Cycles targeting speech sounds and grammatical morphemes	Months of morphemes that include scripts with lists for activities and materials	SSD Phonological and morphological difficulties			✓	✓			✓	

Approach	Author(s)	Description/Goals	Materials	Population
Naturalistic Intervention for Speech Intelligibility and Speech Accuracy	Camarata	Recasts of child productions during naturalistic activities	No special materials or equipment required; materials that are used must support child initiations	SSD; Secondary populations of Down syndrome, autism, stuttering
Parents and Children Together (PACT) Intervention	Bowen	Parents/family education; Metalinguistic training; Phonetic production training; Multiple exemplar training (minimal contrasts therapy and auditory bombardment); Homework	Audio recorder for recorded home segments; computer for educative slide-shows and *Quick Screener*; vowel and consonant pictures on cards; toys and craft supplies	SSD
Enhanced Milieu Teaching with Phonological Emphasis: Application for Children with Cleft Lip and Palate	Scherer & Kaiser	Vocabulary and speech sound production; Phonological recasting	Materials and toys of interest to child; occasional limited use of low resistance blowing toys (e.g., bubbles)	SSD
PROMPT	Hayden, Eigen, Walker, & Olsen	Addresses motor phonemes (via auditory-tactual input) and lexicon within broader linguistic context	No specific materials required; toys, books, academic resources; also some PROMPT intervention materials, including computer software, stimulus cards, and web site resources (SmarTalk)	SSD; Childhood apraxia of speech

(continued)

Table 1.5. *(continued)*

Approach	Author(s)	Developmental level			Key components	Technology and/or materials	Interventions for specific diagnoses	Targeted stage of production				Targeted outcomes			
		Emerging	Developing	Elaborating				Planning	Programming	Execution	Speech Production	Speech Perception	Phonological Awareness	Other Oral Language	Literacy
Family-Friendly Intervention	Watts Pappas	✓	✓	✓	Involvement of parents in intervention via parent-as-therapist, family-centered, and/or family-friendly practices	No specific materials required	SSD. Varies depending on specific intervention approach	✓[c]	✓[c]	✓[c]	✓[c]	✓[c]	✓[c]	✓[c]	✓[c]
Visual Feedback Therapy with Electropalatography	Gibbon & Wood			✓	Real time and static displays of tongue activity displayed through EPG. Practice organized to take motor learning into account	EPG hardware and software; custom-made palatal plate	SSD, including children with cleft palate or Down syndrome			✓	✓				
Vowel Intervention	Bernhardt, Stemberger, & Bacsfalvi			✓	Ultrasound to provide visual feedback on articulation combined with intervention strategies. Goal setting based on nonlinear phonology	Ultrasound equipment; audiovisual recording equipment	SSD. Including children and adults with hearing impairment or other causes of vowel disorders			✓	✓				

Intervention	Author							Population
Developmental Dysarthria Intervention	Hodge	✓	✓	Bite block use followed by phonemic practice Two additional interventions described including intensive voice intervention and phonetic placement via electromyography	Bite block and associated materials for its safe use	✓	✓	Developmental dysarthria resulting from cerebral palsy, congenital conditions affecting the cranial nerves, and early onset muscular dystrophy
Nonspeech Oral Motor Intervention	Clark	✓	✓	Variable exercises depending on specific oral motor (OM) program, including bite-block and continuous positive airway pressure (CPAP)	Numerous materials are available but generally are unsupported by empirical evidence	✓	✓	Sensorimotor impairments, including children with Down syndrome, cerebral palsy, or tongue thrust

[a]Indirectly addressed through approach
[b]Varies depending on software program
[c]Varies depending on the specific intervention approach

est amount of supporting research (e.g., Chapter 2 on minimal pairs). Alternatively, you may suggest that students contrast chapters that differ in the amount of evidence they provide as a means of having them work through some of the thornier issues raised by EBP, such as when an intervention appears to be theoretically promising or is preferred by a child's parent but as yet has little in the way of empirical support. For either approach, you may find it helpful to include both section overviews and individual chapters in your assigned reading. You may also decide to have students focus on those interventions (from Sections I and III primarily) that focus on traditional, speech-related goals, holding off assigning chapters about interventions that target outcomes from other domains (e.g., perception, morphosyntax, phonological awareness) until later in a course, or even until a different course in which broader communication needs are considered.

Regardless of whether you are using this book as a main or supplementary textbook, there are certain sections of each intervention chapter that you will find particularly helpful. You may, for example, suggest that students use the Introduction, the Glossary (see p. 615), and the Study Questions to help them cement their understanding of the intervention approach. Furthermore, these sections can help you identify topics for class discussion or test question preparation. Suggested Readings represent sources of enrichment that you can use to expand and solidify your own understanding of a technique or that you can assign in addition to text readings as a means of having students delve more deeply into the methods, theoretical basis, or research associated with one or more intervention. Finally, the DVD accompanying this text provides you with clips that you may ask students to use to develop their observation or critical thinking skills—either in class or as part of assignments to be completed outside of class.

Parents

Although you may be the smallest of our anticipated groups of readers, we nonetheless hope that this book can help you work with an SLP in thinking about how your child's needs can best be met and how you can contribute to that process as an intervention is selected and implemented. Because you are experts concerning your child and because you often have the greatest and emotionally most important access to the child, as a parent you are considered a key decision maker and agent for change in your child's SSD interventions. Parents can either contribute directly by being involved in the intervention procedures or indirectly by consulting with the SLP and supporting the child's gains at home. However, interventions differ in the extent to which parental expertise is sought on a moment-to-moment basis during intervention sessions and, of course, parents also differ in the extent and nature of involvement they seek. Therefore, although we encourage you to read as much as possible of this book and other materials concerning intervention, we do expect you to make your own choices about the depth and breadth of your reading.

Getting Started

This chapter gives you a map for the layout of all the intervention chapters, which will guide your reading as well as provide a basis for comparing the various components of each of the intervention approaches. Although the summary table in this chapter provides more technical information than may be useful for parents (see Table 1.5), the overview of all 23 approaches will present the scope and range of available interventions for treating SSD in children. Then in each section overview, the additional summary tables recap the unique features of the interventions that are included.

Recommended Chapters and Sections

If you choose to read several chapters, and especially if you are considering several interventions that fall within the same section in this book, the section overviews should provide a rapid orientation to some of the dimensions along which comparisons are likely to be productive.

Once you've selected an intervention or interventions to read about, we suggest you begin by reading the Introduction and Case Study sections of the appropriate chapter, then look at the video clip associated with it on the accompanying DVD. Those steps could help you decide whether to read further or, instead, approach the SLP with questions or concerns based on what you have read and seen thus far. For those approaches that have family members actively engaged in the intervention, all of the practically oriented sections (i.e., Practical Requirements, Key Components) will assume particular importance.

After an intervention or combination of interventions has been adopted for your child, you may want to read further still—to increase your understanding of the intervention's methods or rationale. As SLPs ourselves, the editors of this book have always welcomed parents who want to understand the process by which we are seeking to help their child—and we've regularly benefited from suggestions that they have made based on their reading. That said, we have also benefited greatly from parents' suggestions that are based on no technical reading at all, but simply on their observations of their child, of our intervention sessions, or on their individual insights into the nature of learning to speak. In short, our final suggestion to you as a parent is to read as much of this book as seems helpful but to trust that your value in the intervention process is not dependent upon it!

A STRUCTURAL FRAMEWORK FOR INTERVENTION

Intervention approaches are implemented within a framework that encompasses a number of components that comprise an "intervention package," so to speak. To better understand the individual components of the package, it is helpful to separate the parts to determine how they fit within a structural framework of intervention. One framework that has been described and commonly referenced is a model developed by Fey and his colleagues (Fey, 1986, 1990, 1992, 2008; Fey, Catts, & Larrivee, 1995; Fey & Cleave, 1990). This framework provides a broad-based structure for conceptualizing intervention and therefore is not tied to a specific theoretical perspective or intervention approach. We present it here in Figure 1.1 as a structural framework for readers to understand the various components of the intervention package, as well as to provide a scheme for comparisons across the 23 intervention approaches presented in this book.

As shown in Figure 1.1, this model includes the following components: 1) *goals* (hierarchy of specificity that advances from broad to specific goals in terms of basic, intermediate, specific, and subgoals), 2) *intervention context* (clinic, classroom, or home), 3) *intervention agent* (clinician, teacher, or parent), 4) *dosage of intervention* (frequency and intensity of sessions), 5) *procedures* (the various intervention components that com-

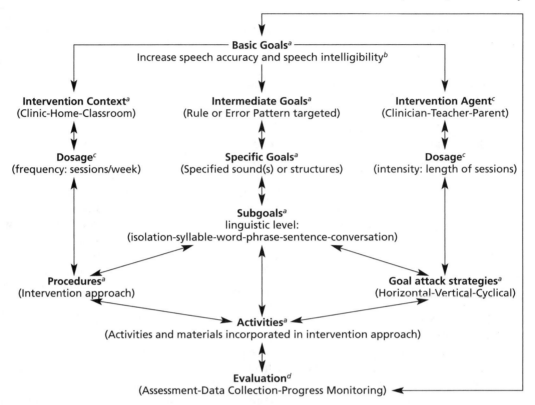

Figure 1.1.   Structure of intervention focused on speech sound disorders (based on Fey, 1986, 2008). [a]Key Components (Goals-Goal Attack Strategy-Procedures-Activities-Materials). [b]Including interrelated goals of language and/or literacy. [c]Practical Requirements (Personnel-Dosage). [d]Assessment and Progress Monitoring (Evaluation-Data Collection)

prise a specific intervention approach), 6) *goal attack strategies* (plan for addressing multiple goals), 7) *activities* (the specific activities and materials used to address a goal within a session), and 8) *evaluation* (data collection procedures and methods for progress monitoring and decision making relevant to alteration of goals, methods, stimuli, activities, and so forth). This figure links each intervention component represented in the diagram to the chapter section that addresses those components. This will facilitate readers' connection of the intervention components to the chapter template sections for each intervention approach, as well as allow comparisons to be easily made between and among the approaches.

CONCLUDING COMMENTS

We believe this book has the potential to positively impact speech-language pathology through the advancement of effective practices for the intervention of SSD with individual children in the present day, as well as with children who will be served by future generations of clinical practitioners. By making EBP and interventions for which evidence is being sought accessible to practicing clinicians, we hope to facilitate increased intervention effectiveness, as well as increased efficiency, by significantly decreasing the amount of time these children require services.

REFERENCES

American Speech-Language-Hearing Association. (2000). *Communication facts*. Rockville, MD: Author.

American Speech-Language-Hearing Association. (2004). *Scope of practice in audiology* [Scope of Practice]. Available from http://www.asha.org/policy

American Speech-Language-Hearing Association. (2007). *Scope of practice in speech-language pathology* [Scope of Practice]. Available from http://www.asha.org/policy

Beeson, P.M., & Robey, R.R. (2006). Evaluating single-subject treatment research: Lessons learned from the aphasia literature. *Neuropsychological Review, 16*(4), 161–169.

Bernstein Ratner, N. (2006). Evidence-based practice: An examination of its ramifications for the practice of speech-language pathology. *Language, Speech, and Hearing Services in Schools, 37*, 257–267.

Bird, J., Bishop, D.V.M., & Freeman, N.H. (1995). Phonological awareness and literacy development in children with expressive phonological impairments. *Journal of Speech and Hearing Research, 38*, 446–462.

Catts, H. (1993). The relationship between speech-language disabilities and reading disabilities. *Journal of Speech and Hearing Research, 36*, 948–958.

Clark-Klein, S., & Hodson, B. (1995). A phonological based analysis of misspellings by third graders with disordered-phonology histories. *Journal of Speech and Hearing Research, 38*, 839–849.

Dollaghan, C.A. (2007). *The handbook for evidence-based practice in communication disorders*. Baltimore: Paul H. Brookes Publishing Co.

Felsenfeld, S., Broen, P.A., & McGue, M. (1994). A 28 year follow-up of adults with a history of moderate phonological disorder: Educational and occupational results. *Journal of Speech and Hearing Research, 37*(6), 1341–1353.

Fey, M.E. (1986). *Language intervention with children*. Boston: Allyn & Bacon.

Fey, M.E. (1990). Understanding and narrowing the gap between treatment research and clinical practice with language impaired children. *ASHA Reports, 20*, 31–40.

Fey, M.E. (1992). Articulation and phonology: An addendum. *Language, Speech, and Hearing Services in Schools, 23*, 277–282.

Fey, M.E. (2002, March). *Intervention research in child language disorders: Some problems and solutions*. Paper presented at the 32nd Annual Mid-South Conference on Communicative Disorders, Memphis, TN.

Fey, M.E. (2004, May). *EBP in child language intervention: Some background and some food for thought*. Presentation to the Working group on EBP in Child Language Disorders, Austin, TX.

Fey, M.E. (2008, November). *Practice in child phonological disorders: Tackling some common clinical problems*. Seminar presentation at the American Speech-Language-Hearing Association Convention, Chicago.

Fey, M.E., Catts, H., & Larrivee, L.S. (1995). Preparing preschoolers for the academic and social challenges of school. In S.F. Warren & J. Reichle (Series Eds.) & M.E. Fey, J. Windsor, & S.F. Warren (Vol. Eds.), *Communication and language intervention series: Vol. 5. Language intervention: Preschool through the elementary years* (pp. 3–37). Baltimore: Paul H. Brookes Publishing Co.

Fey, M.E., & Cleave, P.L. (1990). Efficacy of intervention in speech-language pathology: Early language disorders. *Seminars in Speech and Language, 11*, 165–182.

Harrison, L.J., McLeod, S., Berthelsen, D., & Walker, S. (2009). Literacy, numeracy and learning in school-aged children identified as having speech and language impairment in early childhood. *International Journal of Speech-Language Pathology, 11*(5), 392–403.

Jessup, B., Ward, E., Cahill, L., & Keating, D. (2008). Prevalence of speech and/or language impairment in preparatory students in northern Tasmania. *International Journal of Speech-Language Pathology, 10*(5), 364–377.

Kamhi, A.G. (2006). Treatment decisions for children with speech-sound disorders. *Language, Speech, and Hearing Services in Schools, 37*, 271–279.

Law, J., Boyle, J., Harris, F., Harkness, A., & Nye, C. (2000). Prevalence and natural history of primary speech and language delay: Findings from a systematic review of the literature. *International Journal of Language and Communication Disorders, 35*(2), 165–188.

Leitão, S., & Fletcher, J. (2004). Literacy outcomes for students with speech impairment: Long-term follow-up. *International Journal of Language and Communication Disorders, 39*, 245–256.

McCauley, R.J. (2004). Description and classification of child speech disorders. In R.D. Kent (Ed.), *MIT encyclopedia of communication disorders* (pp. 218–220). Cambridge, MA: The MIT Press.

McCauley, R.J., & Fey, M.E. (Vol. Eds.). (2006). In S.F. Warren & M.E. Fey (Series Eds.), *Communication and language intervention series: Treatment of language disorders in children*. Baltimore: Paul H. Brookes Publishing Co.

McCormack, J., McLeod, S., McAllister, L., & Harrison, L.J. (2009). A systematic review of the association between childhood speech impairment and participation across the lifespan. *International Journal of Speech-Language Pathology, 11*(2), 155–170.

McLeod, S. (2006). A holistic view of a child with unintelligible speech: Insights from the ICF and ICF-CY. *Advances in Speech-Language Pathology, 8*(3), 293–315.

McLeod, S. (Ed). (2007). *The international guide to speech acquisition.* Clifton Park, NY: Thomson Delmar Learning.

McLeod, S., & Harrison, L.J. (2009). Epidemiology of speech and language impairment in a nationally representative sample of 4- to 5-year-old children. *Journal of Speech, Language, and Hearing Research, 52,* 1213–1229.

Olswang, L.B. (1998). Treatment efficacy research. In C.M. Frattali (Ed.), *Measuring outcomes in speech-language pathology* (pp. 134–150). New York: Thieme.

Overby, M., Carrell, T., & Bernthal, J. (2007). Teachers' perceptions of students with speech sound disorders: A quantitative and qualitative analysis. *Language, Speech, and Hearing Services in Schools, 38*(4), 327–341.

Rice, M.L., Hadley, P.A., & Alexander, A.L. (1993). Social biases toward children with speech and language impairments: A correlative causal model of language limitations. *Applied Psycholinguistics, 14*(4), 445–471.

Robey, R.R., & Schultz, M.C. (1998). A model for conducting clinical outcome research: An adaptation of the standard protocol for use in aphasiology. *Aphasiology, 12,* 787–810.

Robey, R.R., Schultz, M.C., Crawford, A.B., & Sinner, C.A. (1999). Single-subject clinical-outcome research: Designs, data, effect sizes, and analyses. *Aphasiology, 13,* 445–473.

Sackett, D.L., Rosenberg, W.M.C., Gray, J.A.M., Hayes, R.B., & Richardson, W.S. (1996). Evidence-based medicine: What it is and what it isn't. *British Medical Journal, 312,* 71–72.

Shriberg, L.D., & Kwiatkowski, J. (1988). A follow-up study of children with phonological disorders of unknown origin. *Journal of Speech and Hearing Disorders, 47,* 256–270.

Sices, L., Taylor, G., Freebairn, L., Hansen, A., & Lewis, B. (2007). Relationship between speech-sound disorders and early literacy skills in preschool-age children: Impact of comorbid language impairment. *Journal of Developmental and Behavioral Pediatrics, 28*(6), 438–447.

World Health Organization. (2001). *International classification of functioning, disability and health.* Geneva: Author.

World Health Organization. (2007). *International classification of functioning, disability and health: Children and youth version.* Geneva: Author.

I

Direct Speech
Production Interventions

Direct Speech Production Interventions

A. Lynn Williams, Sharynne McLeod, and Rebecca J. McCauley

As the chapters in this book indicate, a number of evidence-based interventions are available for children with speech sound disorders (SSD). The interventions target different stages of speech production and have different targeted outcomes. Often, no single approach is used as the sole intervention for children with SSD. Rather, different approaches provide a better match to a client's needs and speech characteristics at specific points in his or her acquisition of the phonology of a language. This can be seen across the interventions included in this section, in which some are designed to facilitate a skill or knowledge that then transitions the child's development to a different level and, consequently, makes them candidates for a different intervention approach.

Section I includes chapters on the following intervention approaches that directly and explicitly address goals of speech sound production:

- Minimal pair intervention (Chapter 2)

- Multiple oppositions intervention (Chapter 3)

- Complexity approaches to intervention (Chapter 4)

- Core vocabulary intervention (Chapter 5)

- Cycles phonological remediation approach (Chapter 6)

- Nuffield Centre Dyspraxia Programme (Chapter 7)

Although these intervention approaches share similarities, particularly with regard to directly targeting speech production, this overview will also point out the unique differences among them with regard to the following 10 factors: client age, primary client populations, key intervention agents, key components, broad goals, basis of target selection, level of focus, session type, technology and/or materials required, and key codes from the International Classification of Functioning, Disability and Health: Children and Youth Version (ICF-CY; World Health Organization [WHO], 2007). These factors are important within an evidence-based practice framework to select an appropriate intervention that aligns with client factors (age, type of speech sound disorder), as well as family and clinician factors (key intervention agents, key components, broad goals, level of focus, session type, and technology/materials required). Table I.1 provides a comparative summary of these 10 factors across the seven intervention approaches. Before discussing each of these factors, however, it is important to summarize each approach with regard to the available levels of evidence (LOE).

LEVELS OF EVIDENCE

The authors used the Scottish Intercollegiate Guideline Network (SIGN; http://www.sign .ac.uk) as a common framework for characterizing the scientific evidence available for each intervention approach. A summary of the authors' findings in Table I.2 indicates that there are no examples of the highest LOE (Ia: meta-analysis of more than one randomized controlled trial) and only two examples of the lowest level (IV: expert committee report, consensus conference, clinical experience of respected authorities) across the seven intervention approaches. The majority of research falls between these two extremes within Level III (nonexperimental, including correlational and case studies; 32 research studies) and Level IIb (quasi-experimental, which includes mostly single-subject experimental research studies; 27 research studies).

This distribution of the research that has been conducted with intervention approaches that directly target speech production is both characteristic of the state of intervention research within our discipline, as well as reflective of the stages of research undertaken within a particular intervention approach. One hallmark of science is the accumulation of evidence, which is the development of an evidentiary and knowledge base that utilizes a variety of methodological tools and research designs to address questions of study (Justice & Fey, 2004). Although different research designs allow researchers to answer different kinds of research questions, the single-subject experimental designs are a common and important research tool in communicative disorders. These research designs provide in-depth examination of behavior over time, which are particularly suited to developing and testing specific interventions (Mullen, 2007). Given this, it is not surprising that the majority of research evidence has been in the categories of nonexperimental case studies and quasi-experimental single-subject study designs.

Similarly, the LOE incorporates a continuum of stages of research that represents a logical progression of research within the examination of a particular intervention approach. In the earliest stage of research, *exploratory studies*, such as Level III nonexperimental correlational and case studies, are conducted to determine whether or not an intervention shows promise of being efficacious (Mullen, 2007). The second stage of research involves *efficacy studies*, which test promising interventions in rigorous and controlled conditions to examine the resulting outcomes of the intervention under ideal conditions. This would correspond to Levels IIa and IIb, controlled studies without randomization and quasi-experimental studies. Finally, *effectiveness studies* examine the positive outcomes from the highly controlled studies under more "real world" clinical settings (Level Ib). Again, it is not surprising that the majority of the research within these seven intervention approaches has fallen within exploratory and efficacy studies.

Taken together, the LOE for the seven intervention approaches that directly address speech sound production within a focused and explicit manner suggests that each of the interventions represents a promising intervention with probable efficacy.

COMPARATIVE FACTORS

Client Age

The intervention approaches in Section I are primarily aimed at preschool children who are 3;0 to 6;0 years of age. However, some approaches include younger children at age 2;0

Table I.1.   Characteristics of interventions featured in Section I

Intervention approach (chapter)	Client age	Primary client populations	Key intervention agents	Key components	Broad goals
Minimal pair intervention (2)	Typically 3;0–6;0	Children with mild to moderately delayed and/or disordered speech; consistent errors; normal hearing, oromotor, and language skills	Typically SLPs	Contrastive word pairs involving child's error and target sound typically in five contrastive word pairs; intervention phases frequently include familiarization, identification, and production (at imitative then spontaneous levels)	Reduce homonymy: differentiated production of minimally contrastive words; primarily consonants, but can also address vowel errors
Multiple oppositions intervention (3)	Typically 3;6–6;0	Children with moderate to severely delayed and/or disordered speech; unintelligible speech from a nonorganic basis	SLPs	Large integrated contrastive treatment sets across a phoneme collapse. Treatment paradigm that includes focused practice at imitative and spontaneous levels, naturalistic activities, contrast within communicative contexts	Reduce homonymy by eliminating phoneme collapse and promote systemwide phonological restructuring

Basis of target selection	Level of focus	Session type	Technology and/or materials required	Key ICF-CY codes[a]
Developmental: frequency of occurrence of phonological processes; non-stimulable excluded sounds from phonetic inventory	Speech output skills; primarily at word level	Individual and/or small-group sessions; generally 45 minutes twice weekly	Some computer programs are available, but not required; commercial illustrations; Internet resources	b320: Articulation Functions
Distance metric that includes two parameters: 1) maximal classification and 2) maximal distinction; based on identification of phoneme collapses	Speech output skills; primarily at word level	Individual and/or small-group sessions; generally 30–45 minutes twice weekly	SCIP software program; clip art	b320: Articulation Functions

(continued)

Table I.1.   *(continued)*

Intervention approach (chapter)	Client age	Primary client populations	Key intervention agents	Key components	Broad goals
Complexity approaches to intervention (4)	Range in age from 2;8–7;11, with mostly 4;0	Functional SSD with ≥6 sounds across 3 manners excluded from phonetic inventory	SLPs	Maximally distinctive word pairs involving one or two phonologically complex phonemes that are absent from the child's inventory; 8 NSW pairs for contrastive approaches, 16 NSW pairs for complex clusters assigned lexical meaning and addressed in two intervention phases (imitation–spontaneous)	Promote broad systemwide generalization through hierarchically complex units cascading to simpler linguistic units
Core vocabulary intervention (5)	Children across a wide age range, though typically preschool to school age	Children with inconsistent speech errors	SLPs, caregivers , and teachers	Consistent production of ≥50 functionally powerful words supported by sound-by-sound and syllable-by-syllable dense response drill with pictures	Establish consistency of production and enhance consonant and vowel accuracy
Cycles phonological remediation approach (6)	2;6–14;0, though primarily prior to kindergarten	Children with delayed and/or disordered speech, particularly highly unintelligible speech, including CAS	SLPs, paraprofessionals, and caregivers	Ordering of phonological patterns within cycles, auditory bombardment, facilitating contexts, active involvement, self monitoring, generalization, home program	Expedite intelligibility gains in order for child to succeed in school

Basis of target selection	Level of focus	Session type	Technology and/or materials required	Key ICF-CY codes[a]
Consonants and clusters that are linguistically complex, later developing, consistently in error, and represent least knowledge within nonsense words	Speech output skills that focus on the phoneme primarily at nonsense-word level	Individual sessions 30–60 minutes three times weekly	Nonsense pictures from the Internet, SCIP software program	b320: Articulation Functions
Functionally powerful words	Speech output skills via stable phonological representations at the word level	Individual 30-minute sessions twice weekly for approximately 8 weeks	Picture stimuli	b320: Articulation Functions
Developmental: ≥40% occurrence of phonological patterns; primary and secondary target patterns that are consistent deviations and stimulable targets based on HAPP-3 assessment	Speech output skills primarily involving phonological patterns; also auditory awareness, speech perception, language, and literacy skills	Individual 60-minute sessions once a week (cycle)	Amplification device; 5x8 inch index cards; motivational, experiential play items	b320: Articulation Functions; b2304: Speech Discrimination

(continued)

Table I.1.   *(continued)*

Intervention approach (chapter)	Client age	Primary client populations	Key intervention agents	Key components	Broad goals
Nuffield Centre Dyspraxia Programme (7)	3;0–7;0	Severe SSD, primarily CAS	SLPs with daily practice with parents at home	Build speech processing skills from the bottom up through the establishment of motor programs for single sounds in isolation and increasing phonotactic complexity; includes auditory discrimination, specific nonspeech oral motor skills within repetitive practice	Primary focus is to establish accurate motor programs, programming, and planning skills
Stimulability intervention (8)	2;0–4;0	Very young children with very limited phonetic inventories and poor stimulability skills	SLPs, parents, teachers	Target stimulable and nonstimulable sounds by pairing consonants with alliterative characters and body motions	Increase the number of stimulable sounds in the child's phonetic inventory

Key: CAS, childhood apraxia of speech; HAPP-3, Hodson Assessment of Phonological Patterns-3; ICF-CY, *International Classification of Functioning, Disability and Health: Children and Youth Version;* NDP3, *Nuffield Centre Dyspraxia Programme-3;* NSW, nonsense words; SLP, speech-language pathologist; SLPAs, speech-language pathology assistants; SSD, speech sound disorders.

[a]Within the ICF-CY, Articulation Functions includes phonological functions.

Basis of target selection	Level of focus	Session type	Technology and/or materials required	Key ICF-CY codes[a]
Goals selected on basis of Nuffield Centre Dyspraxia Programme-3 assessment	Speech output skills and phonological awareness skills	Individual 30- to 60-minute sessions once weekly (or twice weekly or daily for more severe disorders); generally lasting 12 months to 4 years depending on severity	NDP3 manual and pictorial intervention materials and worksheets	b320: Articulation Functions; b2304: Speech Discrimination; b176: Mental Function of Sequencing Complex Movements
Stimulability probe to identify stimulable and nonstimulable sounds	Speech output skills at the phoneme level in isolation and syllable	Primarily individual 45- to 50-minute sessions twice weekly for 12 sessions	Alliterative sound character illustrations (http://www.brookespublishing.com/williams/miccio.htm)	b320: Articulation Functions

Table I.2. Number of published research studies pertaining to each level of evidence for direct speech production interventions identified by chapter authors in Section I

Intervention approach (chapter)	Ia: Meta analysis of > 1 randomized controlled trial	Ib: Randomized controlled study	IIa: Controlled study without randomization	IIb: Quasi-experimental study	III: Non-experimental study	IV: Expert report, consensus conference, clinical experience of respected authorities
Minimal pair intervention (2)	0	0	0	28	11	0
Multiple oppositions intervention (3)	0	0	1	2	4	0
Complexity approaches to intervention (4)	0	2	1	17	2	0
Core vocabulary intervention (5)	0	1	0	1	4	0
Cycles phonological remediation approach (6)	0	1	1	0	6	2
Nuffield Centre Dyspraxia Programme (7)	0	0	0	0	2	0
Stimulability intervention (8)	0	1	0	7	3	0
TOTAL	0	5	3	55	32	2

(particularly stimulability intervention , but also the cycles approach, core vocabulary intervention, and complexity approaches), as well as older children up to 7 years of age (the complexity approaches, cycles approach, core vocabulary intervention, and Nuffield Centre Dyspraxia Programme). With the ages primarily involving preschool children, these intervention approaches focus principally on the developmental levels of emerging and developing sound systems.

Primary Client Populations

The primary population of children that is the basis for the direct speech production interventions include predominantly functional SSD of unknown origin, specifically children with multiple speech errors and unintelligible speech. The core vocabulary intervention specifies a diagnostic category of SSD that includes children who have inconsistent speech errors. Another subpopulation of SSD that was specified was childhood apraxia of speech, which comprised the primary population of the Nuffield Centre Dyspraxia Programme and was included within the population of children for whom the cycles approach would be appropriate.

Key Intervention Agents

For each of the interventions in Section I, a speech-language pathologist was the key intervention agent. Supplemental intervention assistants included parents or caregivers (cycles approach, stimulability intervention, core vocabulary intervention, and Nuffield Centre Dyspraxia Programme), paraprofessionals (cycles approach), and teachers (stimulability intervention, core vocabulary intervention).

Key Components

The direct speech production interventions within Section I specifically target speech sound production in a focused and explicit manner. The approaches address speech production chiefly at the word level using meaningful words. Exceptions to this include the complexity approaches, which recommend using nonsense words that are assigned meaning, and the Nuffield Centre Dyspraxia Programme, which begins at the level of the sound in isolation and progresses to words, phrases/sentences, and connected speech.

Given the emphasis on direct sound production, the approaches presented in Section I describe an intervention structure that supports the establishment of a new sound production or phonemic contrast. Specifically, most of the intervention approaches structure intervention around two phases of production: imitation and spontaneous levels of production. In addition, dense response rates of 60–100 responses per session were recommended, with even denser rates of up to 170 responses suggested for the core vocabulary intervention. Although all approaches focus on speech production skills, some approaches addressed auditory awareness (cycles approach) or auditory discrimination (Nuffield Centre Dyspraxia Programme).

Broad Goals

The main goal of all approaches in Section I is to increase speech intelligibility. Some interventions specified reduction or elimination of homonymy as the goal to increase overall speech intelligibility (minimal pair intervention, multiple oppositions intervention, complexity approaches). Other approaches incorporated goals that were particular to that approach. For example, the goal of the stimulability intervention is to increase the number of stimulable sounds; the goal of the core vocabulary intervention is to increase consistent productions; and the goal of the Nuffield Centre Dyspraxia Programme is to establish accurate motor programs, programming, and planning skills. Still other approaches, such as the cycles approach, stated increased intelligibility as a means to the ultimate goal of the child being successful in school due to the strong link between SSD and literacy.

Basis of Target Selection

A range of target selection approaches was incorporated across the seven interventions in Section I. Some approaches included a developmental approach to target selection (e.g., cycles approach), others included a linguistic approach using phonological complexity factors (e.g., complexity approaches) or a distance metric that selects targets having the greatest phonetic distance from the child's error and from the other targeted sounds (multiple oppositions). The stimulability intervention incorporates all consonants, both stimulable and nonstimulable, in order to encourage vocal practice and ensure early success. Rather than a specific sound target, the core vocabulary intervention targets functionally powerful words that contain inconsistently produced sounds.

Level of Focus

Similar to the key components of the approaches in Section I, the level of focus of these approaches involve principally speech output skills, with production being the targeted outcome. Some of the approaches expanded the level of focus to the representation and planning stage of speech production (e.g., core vocabulary intervention focused on speech output via stable phonological representations, and the Nuffield Centre Dyspraxia Programme focused on establishing speech processing skills from the bottom up). Likewise, the approaches chiefly addressed production of phonemes within words, but some approaches expanded the production focus of intervention to include auditory awareness (cycles approach), auditory discrimination (Nuffield Dyspraxia Centre Programme), and, indirectly, language (cycles approach, core vocabulary intervention, Nuffield Centre Dyspraxia Programme) and literacy (stimulability intervention, cycles approach).

Session Type

The direct speech production intervention approaches represented in Section I incorporated intensive individual 30- to 60-minute sessions that largely met twice weekly. This is consistent with the explicit and focused intervention of these approaches on direct speech sound production.

Technology and/or Materials Required

Each of the approaches incorporated illustrations into intervention activities. Many of the approaches specified use of commercial illustrations or pictures from the Internet or software programs, such as Sound Contrasts in Phonology (SCIP; Williams, 2006). Some approaches used specific illustrations, such as the alliterative sound character cards for the stimulability approach (see http://www.brookespublishing.com/williams/miccio.htm) or the Nuffield Centre Dyspraxia Programme-3 (NDP3) set of pictorial intervention materials and worksheets. The complexity approaches recommend nonsense illustrations that can be obtained from the Internet or the SCIP software program. With regard to technology, the SCIP software program is designed to be used with the contrastive approaches of minimal pairs, multiple oppositions, and the complexity approaches of maximal oppositions and treatment of the empty set. The cycles approach requires an amplification device for auditory bombardment.

Key Codes from the *International Classification of Functioning, Disability and Health: Children and Youth Version*

The ICF-CY codes specify the Body Structure, Body Function, and Activities and Participation that are addressed by individual intervention approaches. Given the focus on direct speech sound production of the intervention approaches within Section I, it is not surprising that all of the approaches address Body Functions, and specifically Articulation Functions (b320: "Functions of the production of speech sounds"; WHO, 2007, p. 71). Other aspects of Body Functions were addressed by the Nuffield Centre Dyspraxia Programme and included Speech Discrimination (b2304: "Sensory functions relating to determining spoken language and distinguishing it from other sounds"; WHO, 2007, p. 65) and Mental Function of Sequencing Complex Movements (b176: "Specific mental functions of sequencing and coordinating complex, purposeful movements"; WHO, 2007, p. 60).

REFERENCES

Justice, L.M., & Fey, M.E. (2004). Evidence-based practice in schools: Integrating craft and theory with science and data. *The ASHA Leader*, 4–5, 30–32.

Mullen, R. (2007). The state of the evidence: ASHA develops levels of evidence for communication sciences and disorders. *The ASHA Leader*, *12*(3), 24–25.

Williams, A. L. (2006). SCIP: Sound Contrasts in Phonology. [Computer software Version 1.0]. Greenville, SC: Thinking Publications.

World Health Organization. (2007). *International classification of functioning, disability and health: Children and youth version.* Geneva: Author.

Minimal Pair Intervention

Elise Baker

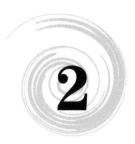

ABSTRACT

The minimal pair approach is one of the oldest, most well-known, and widely used approaches for phonological intervention. Words produced as homonyms by children are paired. Presentation of the word pairs via communication-based activities helps children learn to produce the contrast between the word pairs in order to be understood. Empirical support for the approach (including one effectiveness study, 26 efficacy studies, and 15 exploratory case studies) suggests that the approach is effective. Children most suited to the approach have a mild or mild-to-moderate phonological impairment characterized by one or two age-inappropriate phonological processes or one or two speech sounds consistently in error. The approach has been implemented in a variety of ways by different researchers internationally.

INTRODUCTION

Intervention for speech sound disorders (SSD) in children has a fascinating history. Prior to the 1970s, a child who said [pʊt] for *foot* and [ti] for *see* was usually taught how to articulate the problematic sounds in the words. Although this approach seemed reasonable, it did not make sense for a child who could articulate speech sounds but failed to use them contrastively in words, such as saying [θɪŋk] for *sink* but [fɪŋk] for *think*. In a major paradigm shift, Ingram's (1976) seminal work, *Phonological Disability in Children*, changed the focus of SSD to the phonological system. This shift motivated researchers to develop new approaches based on phonological (rather than articulatory) principles such as reorganizing children's phonological systems; facilitating phonological generalization; deemphasizing articulation training; and highlighting the contrastive function of phonemes, syllables, and word shapes in speech (e.g., Fey, 1985; Grunwell, 1983; Stoel-Gammon & Dunn, 1985; Weiner, 1981, 1984). The minimal pair approach, otherwise known as *the method of meaningful minimal contrast* (Weiner, 1981), *conventional minimal pair treatment* (Barlow & Gierut, 2002), or *minimal opposition contrast treatment* (Gierut, 1990), was one of the first approaches designed to adhere to phonological principles of intervention. Indeed, McCauley described the minimal pair approach as "quintessentially phonologic in nature" (1993, p. 156).

What is a minimal pair? According to Barlow and Gierut, a minimal pair is "a set of words that differ by a single phoneme, whereby that difference is enough to signal a change in meaning" (2002, p. 58). Using this definition, the words *tip* and *sip* are minimal pairs (containing few or minimally opposing features between /s/ and /t/) as are *tip* and *rip* (containing many or maximal opposing features between /t/ and /ɹ/). Words that differ by the presence or absence of one phoneme, as in *tip* and *trip*, are near minimal pairs. Conventional minimal pair intervention, as reported by Weiner (1981), pairs meaningful words produced as homonyms by a child. The word pairs typically contain few or minimally opposing features (e.g., *tip* and *sip*) or are near minimal pairs (e.g., *tip* and *trip*). Minimal pair words containing maximally opposing features (e.g., *tip* and *rip*) form the basis of the maximal opposition intervention approach (see Chapter 4), as developed by Gierut (1989, 1990). The present chapter focuses on the original or conventional minimal pair intervention approach. For the remainder of this chapter, the terms *minimal pair* and *minimal pair approach* assume this conventional usage.

Historical Background

The use of minimal pairs in intervention was first reported by Cooper in 1968 and later by Ferrier and Davis in 1973. These two studies primarily used paired contrasts in words not so much to reorganize children's phonological systems, but in Cooper's case to improve "defective articulation" (1968, p. 18), and in Ferrier and Davis's case to increase a child's vocabulary size in the hope that it would decrease final consonant omissions. Ferrier's (1963) ideas were revolutionary at the time, suggesting that functional defective articulation might reflect an underlying language problem. One of the earliest intervention studies to use minimal pairs within a phonological framework was reported by Weiner in 1981. Weiner used minimal pairs to highlight loss of phonemic contrast in two boys ages 4;4 and 4;10. Weiner reported that the procedure facilitated phonological generalization and as such reduced the frequency of the phonological processes exhibited by the children. Blache, Parsons, and Humphreys (1981) reported a similar study with seven children, ages 5;4 to 6;7, using a distinctive feature framework. Like Weiner (1981), Blache et al. considered that minimal pairs helped to highlight for the children a need to produce a contrast between word pairs.

Since the publication of the early works by Weiner (1981) and Blache et al. (1981), numerous investigations and commentaries on the minimal pair approach have been published (e.g., Barlow & Gierut, 2002; Crosbie, Holm, & Dodd, 2005; Elbert, Dinnsen, Swartzlander, & Chin, 1990; Tyler, Edwards, & Saxman, 1987, 1990). The minimal pair approach has served as the basis from which other intervention approaches have developed (e.g., maximal oppositions [Gierut, 1990; see Chapter 4]; treatment of the empty set [Gierut, 1991; see Chapter 4]; multiple oppositions [Williams, 2000; see Chapter 3]). Minimal pairs have also been used as a component within other approaches containing multiple components (e.g., PACT therapy [Bowen & Cupples, 2006; see Chapter 17]; Metaphon [Howell & Dean, 1994]; metaphonological intervention [Hesketh, Adams, Nightingale, & Hall, 2000; see Chapter 10]; imagery [Klein, 1996]; cycles [Hodson, 2007; see Chapter 6]). The minimal pair approach, unlike many other approaches to phonological intervention, has evolved and diversified for more than 25 years. No particular researcher is associated with the approach, and as Saben and Costello-Ingham pointed out, "there seems to be no consensus on the ideal form minimal pairs treatment should take" (1991, p. 1032). The information presented in this chapter subsequently reflects this diversity within the minimal pair literature.

TARGET POPULATIONS

Primary Populations

The minimal pair approach was originally developed for children with "unintelligible speech" (Weiner, 1984, p. 87). In Weiner's 1981 study, the participants, ages 4;4 and 4;10, were reported to have unintelligible speech characterized by at least six different phonological processes. Blache et al. (1981) used minimal pairs with seven children with a moderate-to-severe phonological disability. Since the publication of Weiner's (1981) work and that of Blache et al. (1981), more than 200 children have served as participants across 42 peer-reviewed published investigations of the minimal pair approach (see Table 2.1). The number of participants per investigation has ranged from 1 to 34, with a mean of 6 and mode of 1. Across this literature, the children have ranged in age from 2;1 to 10;5, with 4;0 to 5;0 being the most common range. The children participating in this research have typically been monolingual (English speaking) with a moderate, moderate-to-severe, or severe phonological impairment; normal hearing; age-appropriate receptive language; and no evidence of oral-motor difficulties or neurological, socioemotional, or general developmental problems (e.g., Baker & McLeod, 2004; Elbert et al., 1990; Elbert, Powell, & Swartzlander, 1991; Forrest, Dinnsen, & Elbert, 1997; Miccio, Elbert, & Forrest, 1999; Powell, Elbert, & Dinnsen, 1991; Tyler, 1995; Tyler, Figurski, & Langsdale, 1993). Although children with these characteristics may have been appropriate for the minimal pair approach, the findings from more recent phonological intervention research suggest that minimal pairs may not be the most appropriate approach for the children for whom it was originally designed. A number of key studies make special mention as to the type of children and type of phonological impairment primarily suited to the minimal pair approach (see Table 2.1).

Tyler et al. (1987) compared minimal pairs with cycles (Hodson & Paden, 1991), and reported that although "both treatment procedures were found to be not only effective but efficient," the cycles approach was reported to be better suited to "children who exhibit a large number of inappropriate phonological processes that occur frequently and significantly reduce intelligibility," whereas "children who have one particularly pervasive process or only a few age-inappropriate phonological processes seem to be better candidates for the perception-production minimal pairs procedure because it involves concentration on one process at a time" (1987, p. 405).

Saben and Costello-Ingham (1991) raised a different issue for consideration in determining whether a child is suited to the minimal pair approach. In a study of two children, they suggested that "minimal pairs treatment might be appropriate for phonemes for which a child has some degree of productive knowledge and may not be appropriate for error phonemes for which productive knowledge is absent" (p. 1035). Gierut, Elbert, and Dinnsen's (1987) findings countered Saben and Costello-Ingham's suggestion. As part of a minimal pair investigation into the impact of selecting targets associated with more or less productive phonological knowledge, Gierut et al. recommended that intervention "should be structured such that sounds of which a child has least knowledge be treated first" (p. 475).

Rvachew's (1994) research suggested that children's perceptual (rather than just productive) phonological knowledge may influence the efficiency of intervention. Although it would seem that children with a phonological impairment may be suited to the minimal pair approach irrespective of the degree of their productive phonological knowledge of

Table 2.1.   Levels of evidence for studies of treatment efficacy for minimal pairs

Level	Description	References
Ia	Meta-analysis of > 1 randomized controlled trial	—
Ib	Randomized controlled study	Dodd et al. (2008); Ruscello et al. (1993)
IIa	Controlled study without randomization	—
IIb	Quasi-experimental study	Abraham (1993); Baker & McLeod (2004); Blache et al. (1981); Crosbie et al. (2005); Dinnsen et al. (1992); Dodd & Barker (1990); Elbert et al. (1990); Elbert et al. (1991); Forrest et al. (1997); Gierut (1990, 1991); Gierut et al. (1987); Gierut & Neumann (1992); Miccio et al. (1999); Miccio & Ingrisano (2000); Powell (1993); Powell & Elbert (1984); Powell et al. (1991); Powell et al. (1998); Tyler et al. (1987); Tyler et al. (1990); Tyler et al. (1993); Tyler & Sandoval (1994); Weiner (1981); Williams (2005)
III	Nonexperimental studies, i.e., correlational and case studies	Dodd & Iacono (1989); Fey & Stalker (1986); Grunwell & Dive (1988); Grunwell & Russell (1990); Grunwell et al. (1988); Hoffman et al. (1990); Holm & Dodd (2001); Holm et al. (1997); Leahy & Dodd (1987); Masterson & Daniels (1991); Powell (1991); Ray (2002); Robb et al. (1999); Saben & Costello-Ingham (1991); Tyler (1995)
IV	Expert committee report, consensus conference, clinical experience of respected authorities	—

Adapted from the Scottish Intercollegiate Guidelines Network (http://www.sign.ac.uk).

an intervention target, the role of perceptual phonological knowledge in determining suitability for the minimal pair approach remains to be better understood. See Chapter 12 for further discussion on the role of perception training in phonological intervention.

With regard to consistency of error, Forrest et al. (1997) reported that a minimal pair approach was better suited to children who had a consistent substitution pattern, ideally within a word position and/or across a word position. In a study of the relative benefits of the minimal pair approach versus a core vocabulary approach for a group of 18 children with either consistent or inconsistent speech disorder, Crosbie et al. reported that "core vocabulary therapy resulted in greater change in children with inconsistent speech disorder and phonological contrast therapy resulted in greater change in children with consistent speech disorder" (2005, p. 485).

In summary, in light of the research by Tyler et al. (1987), minimal pair may not be the ideal approach for children with a moderate-to-severe or severe phonological impairment who need to make multiple changes to their phonological system. Rather, it would seem that these children may be better suited to other approaches such as multiple oppositions (see Chapter 3), complexity approaches to intervention (see Chapter 4), cycles (see Chapter 6), PACT therapy (see Chapter 17), nonlinear phonological intervention (see Chapter 13), psycholinguistic intervention (see Chapter 9), perceptual intervention (see Chapter 12), or metaphonological intervention (see Chapter 10). According to Williams, the "minimal pair therapy approach may be better suited for children who exhibit a mild-to-moderate level of phonological impairment" (2000, p. 291); that is, children with one or two sounds in error (that may or may not be associated with least productive phonological knowledge) or one or two age-inappropriate phonological processes. In light of the research by Forrest et al. (1997) and Crosbie et al. (2005), the errors that characterize such children's phonological impairment need to be consistent, and they need to create a collapsed contrast between the child's production and the target. Finally, given the clinical characteristics of most children involved in minimal pair research, the primary population would seem to be children between 3;0 and 6;0 without concomitant hearing, oro-motor, or language difficulties.

Secondary Populations

According to Elbert, Rockman, and Saltzman, whereas the primary population most obviously suited to the minimal pair approach is "young children who are not acquiring the phonological system" (1980, p. 9), "other populations with problems involving the sound system can also profit from contrast training" (p. 9). The efficacy of the minimal pair approach has been examined with a variety of other populations. In a study by Abraham (1993), the minimal pair approach was compared with a traditional phonetic approach in four children with a moderate-to-severe sensorineural hearing impairment who were trained orally. Abraham reported that the "meaningful minimal contrast procedure proved to be a viable phonological speech training procedure" (p. 26); however, by contrast, "no consistent pattern of improvement in training or in generalization" (p. 26) was observed for the traditional phonetic approach. A minimal pair approach was also incorporated within an effective intervention program for a child with a concomitant intermittent conductive hearing loss (Grunwell, Yavaş, Russell, & Le Maistre, 1988). In a study of a girl (age 5;3) with a severe phonological impairment and concomitant gross and fine motor delay and language impairment, Miccio and Ingrisano found that "a linguistic treatment approach was applied successfully to the treatment of a phonological disorder in a child with concomitant problems in other domains" (2000, p. 225). Grunwell and Dive (1988) reported two case studies in which phonological intervention characterized by the perception and production of minimal pairs in conjunction with traditional articulation therapy was used to successfully treat what they referred to as "cleft palate speech." One case reported by Grunwell and Dive included a child with a repaired submucous cleft, whereas the other included a child diagnosed with velopharyngeal insufficiency, a concomitant fluctuating conductive hearing loss, and mild sensorineural hearing loss.

Published investigations into the minimal pair approach have also included children with concomitant expressive language difficulties (e.g., Hoffman, Norris, & Monjure, 1990; Saben & Costello-Ingham, 1991; Tyler & Sandoval, 1994) and bilingual phonological difficulties (e.g., Holm, Ozanne, & Dodd, 1997). Further information about the efficacy of intervention for these two different populations is provided later in this chapter in the section on the empirical basis for the approach and in the section on considerations for children from culturally and linguistically diverse backgrounds.

ASSESSMENT METHODS FOR DETERMINING INTERVENTION RELEVANCE

A variety of assessment tools and analysis methods can be used to determine whether an individual child is suited to the minimal pair approach. Across published intervention research, various combinations of standardized and nonstandardized single-word and connected speech sampling tools have been used, in combination with phonological process analysis (e.g., Crosbie et al., 2005; Dodd & Iacono, 1989; Leahy & Dodd, 1987; Ray, 2002;

Ruscello, Cartwright, Haines, & Shuster, 1993; Saben & Costello-Ingham, 1991; Tyler et al., 1987; Tyler & Sandoval, 1994; Weiner, 1981), distinctive feature analysis (e.g., Blache et al., 1981), systemic phonological analysis (e.g., Williams, 2005), and comprehensive generative analysis evaluating productive phonological knowledge (e.g., Elbert et al., 1990, 1991; Gierut, 1990, 1991; Gierut et al., 1987; Powell et al., 1991).

Once a child's speech production skills have been sampled, the severity of a child's impairment and the nature of the speech errors determine whether a child is suited to the minimal pair approach. Severity of impairment may be derived from either the percentile rank or standard score obtained from a standardized test or, alternatively, from calculating the percentage of consonants correct (PCC). According to Shriberg and Kwiatkowski (1982), a mild phonological impairment is consistent with a PCC of 85%–100%, whereas a mild-to-moderate phonological impairment is consistent with a PCC of 65%–84.9%.

In conjunction with a mild or mild-to-moderate severity rating, the child's speech production errors need to be phonological rather than articulatory. There needs to be a loss of contrast between minimal pair words (e.g., *sea* and *tea* both produced as [ti]) or near minimal pair words (e.g., *ski* and *key* both produced as [ki]). For example, if a child says *sea* as [θi] and *tea* as [ti], maintaining a contrast between the word pairs, then a minimal pair approach would not be appropriate. However, if a child consistently says *sea* as [ti] and *tea* as [ti], resulting in a loss or collapse of contrast, then a minimal pair approach would be appropriate. Barlow and Gierut (2002) added that a child who substitutes sounds that are not part of the ambient phonological system (e.g., [x] for /ʃ/ in English) would not be appropriate for the minimal pair approach.

Although Saben and Costello-Ingham (1991) suggested that only those children who have some degree of productive phonological knowledge of or association with an intervention target are suited to the minimal pair approach, other research does not clearly support productive phonological knowledge as a prerequisite (e.g., Gierut et al., 1987; Powell, Elbert, Miccio, Strike-Roussos, & Brasseur, 1998). Rather, it would seem that as long as a child has a loss of contrast, whether it be segmental (e.g., /k, t/ [t]) or syllable/word shape (CCV and CV CV), minimal pairs would be appropriate. The actual steps or procedures needed within the approach account for whether a child needs help learning how to articulate the contrast.

THEORETICAL BASIS

Dominant Theoretical Rationale for the Intervention Approach

The minimal pair approach, as described by Weiner (1981, 1984) was based on two theoretical tenets: Stampe's (1979) theory of natural phonology and Greenfield and Smith's (1976) pragmatic principle of informativeness. Weiner (1981) used Stampe's theory of natural phonology to guide *what* to target and monitor over a course of intervention and used Greenfield and Smith's pragmatic principle of informativeness to guide *how* the targets might be worked on and changed during intervention sessions.

Theory of Natural Phonology

Stampe proposed that children are born with an innate set of phonological processes or rules in which an opposition (e.g., stops and fricatives) in the adult phonology is realized as "that member of the opposition which least tries the restrictions of the human speech capacity" (Stampe, 1969, p. 443). In other words, Stampe considered that children are born with patterns of easier ways of saying words, such as stopping of fricatives and deletion of final consonants. Over time, children presumably learn to suppress these processes to make way for adult-like speech. Weiner (1981) proposed that intervention based on the basic tenets of natural phonology would target the suppression of the phonological processes present in a child's speech, rather than the articulation of individual speech sounds across word positions, so that entire classes of sounds might change, thus expediting intelligibility gains.

At the time of Weiner's (1981) work, phonological processes were considered to be a construct with psychological reality. Despite phonological process terminology becoming a widespread framework for describing error patterns in children's speech for more than 20 years, it could be argued that the idea of the suppression of a phonological process is somewhat untenable. Phonological processes, although helpful terms for describing speech patterns, have not been identified nor widely accepted as real constructs (Stoel-Gammon & Dunn, 1985). Alternative theoretical frameworks, such as distinctive features (Blache et al., 1981) or constraint-based nonlinear phonology (Bernhardt & Stemberger, 2000), might suggest that minimal pair intervention exposes children to the segment, feature, or word shape they need to learn via lexical contrasts highlighting a child's production with a targeted phonological skill. In a linguistic commentary on one of the first minimal pair clinical resources, *Contrasts: The Use of Minimal Pairs in Articulation Training* by Elbert et al. (1980), Dinnsen aptly suggested that

> While phonological theory has been subjected to divergent theoretical perspectives over the years . . . and . . . while there are currently a number of competing theories of phonology . . . one construct survives as central to any theory of phonology and as fundamental to any and all particular sound systems—and that is the construct phonemic contrast. (1980, p. vi)

Thirty years later, such a comment continues to make sense among theoretical discussion and debate. A minimal pair approach seems to expose children to what they need to learn about the ambient phonological system via contrasting word pairs.

Pragmatic Principle of Informativeness

The second theoretical tenet underlying the minimal pair approach was the pragmatic principle of informativeness (Greenfield & Smith, 1976). According to Weiner, "pragmatic factors present in the speaker–listener interaction can have a positive effect on communication including improved production of speech" (1984, p. 87). The pragmatic principle of informativeness suggests that speakers accommodate to their listeners' needs by helping to resolve uncertainties and miscommunication. Gallagher (1977) reported that typically developing children from an average age of 1;9 show the ability to revise an utterance phonologically (e.g., "hit kit ball" "he kick ball") in response to requests for clarification. According to Weiner and Ostrowski (1979), children attempt to revise their pronunciation following a request for clarification in an effort to repair communication breakdown. Within a therapy context, in which an intervention target might be gliding of /ɹ/ to [w], the presentation of minimal pair words *right* and *white* would create speaker–listener uncertainty when the words are produced by the child. The ensuing communication breakdown creates an opportunity for the child to experience a need to produce a contrast between two phonological oppositions and in turn resolve the miscommunication. Essentially, the presentation of minimal pairs produced as homonyms by a child confronts the child with a need to produce a difference between the words in order to be understood. The desire to be understood facilitates the change in the child's speech during the intervention session, which in turn facilitates the suppression of the phonological process within the child's phonological system. Theoretically, Weiner's (1984) perspective provided "an intuitively appealing functional account of phonological change" (Gierut, 1991, p. 120).

In contrast to Weiner's (1984) theoretical rationales, Gierut (1991) suggested that homonymy is not essential for motivating phonological change. Gierut reported that non-homonymous word pairs facilitated more widespread change in three children's phonological systems compared with homonymous word pairs. Gierut (2005) argued that what is targeted may be more important in facilitating widespread change than bringing children's attention to the homonymy in their speech (i.e., how an intervention target is treated). Gierut (1991) suggested that the *structure* of the constituent phonemes that make up nonhomonymous paired contrasts provides children with more information about the phonological system they are learning than the *functional* impact of homonymous word pairs. The findings of a more recent comparative study by Dodd et al. (2008) failed to unequivocally support Gierut's position. Dodd et al. compared the performance of 19 children randomly assigned to one of two intervention conditions: homonymous and nonhomonymous word pairs (referred to as *minimal* and *nonminimal pairs*). Dodd et al. reported "no difference between the progress made by children receiving minimally or nonminimally paired intervention stimuli" (p. 341).

In contrast to Gierut's and colleagues' work, Williams's (2000) evidence for the multiple opposition approach, which contrasts a child's production of one sound for many adult-target sounds or clusters (e.g., [t] versus [k, s, tɹ, tʃ]), suggested that both the *structural* and *functional* role of homonymy in phonological learning may be relevant for children with a phonological impairment (see Chapter 3). Thus, although minimal pair may no longer be the approach of choice for a child with a moderate-to-severe or severe impairment, minimal pairs would still seem to have a place as a suitable intervention approach for a child with a mild or mild-to-moderate phonological impairment. Exactly how minimal pair works, in terms of the role of an intervention target in effecting change within a child's phonological system, and the role of communication breakdown in facilitating change during intervention sessions, the relative importance of these two notions remains to be clearly understood.

Levels of Consequences Being Addressed

The minimal pair approach, like most approaches for targeting unintelligible speech, was designed to help children become better communicators. According to Weiner, minimal pair is "a conceptual approach based on increasing communication ability" (1981, p. 102). Blache et al. offered "the need for 'making words different' in a communicative paradigm" (1981, p. 294) as the main functional goal of minimal pair intervention. The International Classification of Functioning, Disability and Health for Children and Youth (ICF-CY; World Health Organization [WHO], 2007) provides a framework for thinking about SSD in children in a broader context. According to McLeod and McCormack, application of the "ICF-CY to children with speech impairment requires consideration of every component: Body Functions, Body Structures, Activities and Participation, Environmental Factors, and Personal Factors" (2007, p. 255).

McLeod and Threats (2008) suggested that the minimal pair approach focuses primarily on the ICF-CY component of Body Functions and the ICF-CY domain of Articulation Functions (b320). In light of the functional goals offered by Weiner (1981) and Blache et al. (1981), it could be added that the minimal pair approach indirectly addresses a child's activity and participation, specifically with reference to the domain of Communication (d3). Furthermore, although the full range of possible consequences of having a phonological impairment may not have been directly addressed in minimal pair intervention research, changes in consequences have been monitored and considered a result of intervention. For instance, in a case study of a boy named Neil, Grunwell and Russell noted that their intervention program (which included minimal pairs) led to improvements across a range of domains within the ICF-CY: "Neil became a better communicator not only with his therapist but also with his teachers, his peers in the school, and his mother. It was our impression that he also became more confident and outgoing" (1990, p. 34).

Is it enough then that the minimal pair approach focuses exclusively on Body Function, with the potential to have indirect benefits on children's activities and participation? McLeod and McCormack (2007) suggest not. The ICF-CY provides a helpful framework for thinking about how the minimal pair approach might be used in a more deliberate and concerted way to help the whole child—not just the child with a mild or mild-to-moderate phonological impairment, but the child with a mild or mild-to-moderate phonological impairment who enjoys playing and talking with his sister at home but resists playing and talking with peers at preschool. A tool such as the Speech Participation and Activity of Children (SPAA-C; McLeod, 2004) may be a useful starting point for guiding a holistic minimal pair intervention plan. The SPAA-C contains a series of questions "about the daily lives of children and impact of having speech impairment" (McLeod & McCormack, 2007, p. 259). The SPAA-C could be used to guide intervention that not only directly targets body function but also directly targets individual children's activity and participation in light of environmental and personal factors. In doing so, Weiner's (1981) original goal for minimal pair intervention to increase children's "communication ability" would take on a new level of meaning.

Target Areas of Intervention

The minimal pair approach primarily targets speech production in children with a phonological impairment. Speech production skills include the production of consonants (e.g., [ki]:[ti]), vowels (e.g., [bed]:[bæd]), words (e.g., [mi]:[mit]), and syllable shapes (e.g., [noʊ]:[snoʊ]) within real words. Although auditory discrimination or speech perception has also been a target of some minimal pair investigations (e.g., Blache et al., 1981; Dodd et al., 2008; Grunwell & Dive, 1988; Ruscello et al., 1993; Tyler et al., 1987; Tyler & Sandoval, 1994), it has not been a feature of all published studies of the approach. To date, the necessity of targeting speech perception as part of the minimal pair approach has not been resolved. It should be noted, however, that Rvachew's (1994) research and intervention framework (see Chapter 12) supports the inclusion of speech perception training in conjunction with production training for children with phonological impairment.

In a study of the literacy outcomes of children with SSD, Nathan, Stackhouse, Goulandris, and Snowling suggested that "the literacy development of children with preschool speech impairments will be normal if their speech difficulties have resolved when they begin to receive literacy instruction and phoneme awareness is adequate" (2004, p. 389). According to Gillon, 3- and 4-year-old children with a phonological impairment would benefit from "the clinical practice of integrating phoneme awareness and letter knowledge activities into therapy sessions" (2005, p. 322) in an effort to support successful early reading and spelling outcomes. Although phonemic awareness and letter knowledge activities are not an integral feature within minimal pair intervention, Gillon's findings suggested that it might be beneficial to target these areas alongside regular minimal pair intervention.

EMPIRICAL BASIS

Forty two intervention studies published across 18 internationally refereed journals were identified for a review of the empirical basis of the minimal pair approach for treating phonological impairment in children (see Table 2.1). At the outset of the identification process, a selection criteria was specified whereby studies were only included if they either labeled the approach *minimal pairs; minimal opposition contrast;* or *meaningful minimal contrast therapy, treatment,* or *intervention;* or used minimal pairs as a principle component within a published intervention study on an unnamed phonological approach. This meant that studies that incorporated minimal pairs within a named approach, such as Metaphon (Howell & Dean, 1994), PACT therapy (Bowen & Cupples, 2006), or cycles (Hodson, 2007) were not included in the review.

Evaluation of the level of evidence for each study based on a framework adapted from the Scottish Intercollegiate Guidelines Network (see http://www.sign.ac.uk) revealed two randomized controlled studies, 25 quasi-experimental studies, and 15 case studies. Of the quasi-experimental studies, the majority (84%) were single-case experimental designs (SCED), with a smaller portion (16%) being quasi-experimental group investigations. Of the SCED research, 57% used a multiple baseline design across participants or behaviors, 24% reported using an alternating treatments design with or without a concomitant multiple baseline design across participants, 9.5% reported using a multiple probe design, and the remaining 9.5% reported using a simple AB design.

An adequate summary and interpretation of the findings from the research on the minimal pair approach requires identification and evaluation of the methodological procedures used within and across the studies. Why? It is of little value to know that the approach works if you do not know how to implement it. When researchers used a minimal pair approach, what did their approach involve? Across the 42 studies, the majority used a combination of the following seven distinct procedural components:

1. *Speech production activities:* Activities began with either imitation or spontaneous production of minimal pair words.

2. *Semantic confusion:* Participants were confronted with the homonym in their speech and were given feedback in the form of a request for clarification containing the target word and the minimal pair cognate.

3. *Articulation instruction:* Participants were offered articulatory instruction on how to say the target word or sound. (*Note:* The use of articulation instruction was either explicit or implied based on the description of the intervention procedure.)

4. *Phonetic accuracy:* Speech production responses were defined as correct if they contained a phonemic contrast and were phonetically accurate.

5. *Auditory discrimination:* Children were shown pictures of minimal pair words and given instruction to identify the picture spoken by the clinician.

6. *Phrase and sentence level:* Children were requested to use minimal pair words in phrases or sentences once a predetermined performance criterion had been met at word level.

7. *Parent involvement:* Parents administered the intervention following a period of training, assisted with the administration of the intervention, or completed follow-up activities at home.

Across the 42 studies in Table 2.1

- 65% began with imitation of the target stimulus (typically single words), while 23% began with spontaneous production

- 53% capitalized on the semantic confusion that arises when contrasting words are spoken as homonyms, while 7% did not

- 7% provided articulation instruction, while 2% did not

- 40% required a phonologically and phonetically accurate response, while 16% required a phonologically accurate response only

- 3% included auditory discrimination/perception training, while 53% did not

- 33% included phrase and/or sentence-level activities, while 47% targeted word level only

- 37% involved parents either directly within a session or via the provision of homework, while 7% clearly stated that parents were not involved in an effort to minimize the impact of external variables on the manipulation of experimental variables

One of the striking findings from evaluating and comparing the components of intervention was the lack of methodological detail. For instance, it was difficult to discern whether articulation instruction was used across 51% of studies and whether parents were or were not involved in some way across 56% of studies. Figure 2.1 provides a visual summary of the variation in use of these common components of intervention across the studies.

The variation in components used across minimal pair intervention research supports Saben and Costello-Ingham's (1991) observation that there seems to be no standard procedure for conducting minimal pairs intervention. If speech-language pathologists (SLPs) are to draw meaningful conclusions about the empirical basis for the minimal pair approach, then the particular combination of components used by individual investigations needs to be considered.

Minimal Pair Research Outcomes

Across the 42 studies, the majority reported that intervention was effective. In Weiner's (1981) study, two children were shown pictures of pairs of words that they produced as homonyms (e.g., [boʊ] for both *boat* and *bow*). During a game-like activity, each child was to tell the researcher which picture to pick up. In Weiner's description of the intervention procedure, the children were offered instructions on how to complete the task after two

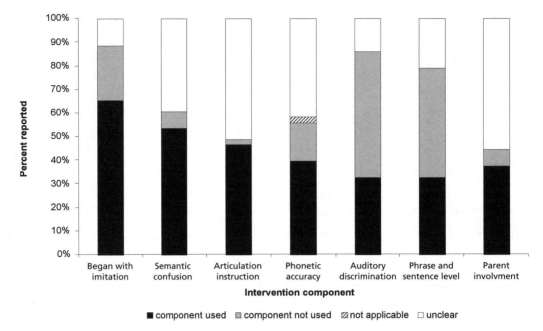

Figure 2.1. Proportion of intervention components used, not used, or indeterminately used across published minimal pair research.

consecutive errors. Verbal and tangible reinforcement was provided, as was auditory stimulation. Auditory stimulation took the form of an auditory model of the pairs of words during feedback. Using a multiple baseline design across behaviors, Weiner reported that the approach was "highly efficient" (p. 102) at reducing the frequency of the three targeted phonological processes per participant given, with one participant showing generalized improvement within 2 weeks of intervention (six sessions three times per week), and another within approximately 5 weeks of intervention (14 sessions three times per week). Blache et al. (1981) reported that all seven participants in their study showed signs of generalized acquisition of the targeted distinctive feature given three to five minimal pair intervention sessions. Dodd and Iacono (1989) reported that PCC scores for six of the seven children involved in their study improved post intervention and that there was a significant decrease in the number of unusual processes. Duration of intervention varied across participants from 3 to 16 months, with one participant still receiving intervention at the conclusion of the study. Grunwell and Russell (1990) reported that a child progressed over 12 months of phonological development in a quarter of the time given an intervention program involving minimal pairs. Powell (1991) reported that a participant showed generalized acquisition of $+/-$ voiced fricatives and voiced stops in final position, with no change on control behavior of /ɹ/, given 15 sessions each consisting of 100 minimal pair word trials.

Minimal pair research has also addressed a number of specific questions regarding the effect of different components of intervention within the approach and the relationship between participant characteristics and response to intervention. Powell and colleagues explored the role of stimulability in facilitating phonological change using a minimal pair approach. Using a multiple baseline design across six participants, Powell et al. (1991) selected two targets per participant and monitored the remaining sounds excluded from the participants' phonetic inventories for phonological generalization. Although all participants showed an improvement in their production of the targeted sounds, patterns of generalization seemed to vary in accordance with each participant's preintervention stimulability. Specifically, "subjects' productions of stimulable sounds tended to improve regardless of treatment target, but generalization of nonstimulable sounds was rarely observed" (p. 1326). In an in-depth reanalysis of the data, Powell (1993) reported that 21 of the 28 sounds monitored had been added to the participants' phonetic inventories by the end of the study. Of the 12 sounds targeted for intervention, 9 were added to participants' phonetic inventories. Of the 16 untreated sounds, 12 were added to the participants' phonetic inventories. With regards to stimulability, of the 14 sounds that were stimulable prior to intervention, 13 were added to the participants' inventories post intervention, while only 8 of the 14 nonstimulable sounds were acquired. Of the seven sounds that were still absent from the participants' inventories at the end of the study, six of the seven were nonstimulable. Powell et al. (1991) recommended that minimal pair intervention prioritize nonstimulable over stimulable phonemes to maximize phonological learning.

Elbert et al. (1990) examined the issue of whether minimal pair intervention at word level only would be sufficient to facilitate generalization to conversational speech. Minimal pair words (ranging from 3 to 10 pairs) were used to contrast the child's error with the target sound, initially through imitation activities, then through the spontaneous production of single words. At no time were phrases, sentences, or conversational speech skills targeted. Elbert et al. identified a statistically significant difference in PCC during conversational speech at a follow-up visit 3 months post intervention and concluded that "many phonologically disordered children are able to extend their correct production to conversation without direct treatment on spontaneous speech" (p. 694).

In a study exploring the number of words required to facilitate phonological generalization, Elbert et al. (1991) began intervention with three exemplars (treatment words). Additional words were provided if generalization criterion had not been met at predetermined intervals, up to a total of 10 words. Elbert et al. reported that "three exemplars were sufficient for generalization to occur in 17 (59%) of the 29 test cases" (p. 84). An additional 21% required 5 exemplars, a further 14% required 10 exemplars, and 7% needed more than 10 exemplars. Elbert et al. concluded that "most subjects generalized to untrained words in the same position after receiving treatment on a relatively small number of exemplars" (1991, p. 86).

In an interesting study examining the necessity of a specific component of intervention, Powell, Elbert, Miccio, Strike-Roussos, and Brasseur (1998) compared the effect of minimal pair intervention with and without production practice. The intervention that did not involve any production practice was identified as the conceptual approach, whereas the intervention that included production practice was identified as the motoric approach. Powell et al. described their motoric approach as traditional in that it targeted phonemes in a hierarchy beginning with isolation, syllables, words, carrier phrases, and then sentences. The feedback provided to the participants during the motoric approach was consistent with conceptual aspects of minimal pair intervention (e.g., "Oh, oh, I heard you say [ti], not [si]"; p. 133). Eighteen children were assigned to one of the two treatment groups. Powell et al. reported that although improvements were noted for both approaches, the motoric approach (incorporating instructional feedback containing minimal pairs) was more effective overall. Powell et al. concluded that "it is advantageous to include some form of motor practice as part of the treatment process, especially when the targeted sound is absent from an individual's phonetic inventory" (p. 142).

Forrest et al. (1997) considered the issue of the variability of children's speech and response to minimal pair intervention. Of 14 children in the study, those with a consistent substitute across word positions showed generalized acquisition of the target across positions. The children who had a consistent substitute within a position only (i.e., used another substitute across other positions), only learned the targeted word position. The children who had inconsistent substitutes within and across positions did not learn the targeted sound in any word position. Forrest et al. suggested that the minimal pair approach for these children with inconsistent substitution patterns was not effective.

Tyler et al. (1990) reported that of four participants who received minimal pair intervention, the one who had place and voicing contrasts (acoustically) prior to intervention showed 78% accuracy in generalization probes 2 weeks (four sessions) after starting intervention. Two participants required 8 weeks (16 sessions) to achieve a similar outcome. The fourth participant (control) in the study showed no progress over 8 weeks of study. The results from Tyler et al. suggest that pretreatment productive knowledge of a treatment target may influence rate of progress.

In contrast with the overall positive findings in the literature, Saben and Costello-Ingham (1991) reported that minimal pair intervention for two children with a severe phonological impairment (and in one of the cases concomitant expressive language impairment) was not effective. Saben and Costello-Ingham's minimal pair approach did not bring the homonymy to the attention of the children via semantic confusion. They concluded that although both children learned to produce the treatment words given motoric placement cues and models to imitate, "neither subject generalized modified speech-sound production to treated phonemes in untreated words or to untreated phonemes affected by the target phonological process" (p. 1023). Saben and Costello-Ingham speculated that their omission of semantic confusion may have contributed to the participants' slow progress.

Across the 42 studies, the efficiency of the minimal pair approach compared with other approaches has also been explored. In a study of two brothers from identical triplets, Hoffman et al. (1990) compared a minimal pair approach with a whole-language approach. The participant assigned to the minimal pair approach was instructed to name minimal pair words pointed to by a clinician. This meant that semantic confusion arising from the homonymy in the child's speech did not occur. Hoffman et al. found that although "similar improvements were seen in the phonological performance of both children . . . the child in the whole language treatment showed greater improvements in expressive language performance" (p. 102). Hoffman et al. recommended that a whole language approach be used for children with concomitant phonology and expressive language difficulties. Work by other researchers with children who have a concomitant profile has failed to provide unequivocal support for the findings of Hoffman et al. In a study involving six children with moderate-to-severe phonological and language impairment, Tyler and Sandoval (1994) examined the effect of a minimal pair approach, language intervention characterized by an indirect narrative approach with focused stimulation, and a combined intervention involving features from both approaches. Tyler and Sandoval reported that the combined approach followed by the minimal pair approach was associated with better outcomes than the language intervention approach. They added that "children with severely disordered phonologies make more gains if they receive direct phonological treatment than if they do not" (p. 229). In a randomized controlled trial by

Fey et al. (1994) in which a grammar facilitation approach was used with children with concomitant phonology and expressive language difficulties, the participants' phonology did not show a statistically significant improvement post intervention. The findings from Tyler and Sandoval, and Fey et al., coupled with the fact that the Hoffman et al. minimal pair approach did not use semantic confusion as a component of minimal pair intervention, tempers the original recommendation by Hoffman et al.

Using an alternating treatments design, Gierut (1990) compared minimal pairs with maximal oppositions in three children with a phonological impairment characterized by the exclusion of at least six sounds from both phonetic and phonemic inventories. Gierut reported that

> In general, maximal oppositions enhanced production of excluded but treated sounds to a greater degree than minimal oppositions. Maximal oppositions also supported changes in untreated sounds, with elaboration and expansions of a child's inventory at least within an existing level of phonetic complexity. (p. 547)

In an extension of this work, Gierut (1991) compared minimal pairs (homonymous condition) with the empty or unknown set (nonhomonymous condition pairing two unknown sounds) in another three children with a phonological impairment. Gierut reported that "treatment of the unknown set appeared to motivate more extensive change in treated sounds excluded from a child's pretreatment inventory than did conventional minimal pair treatment" (1991, p. 127). In all three minimal pair conditions, the intervention target was an interdental fricative. It was possible that the use of this target for all three participants confounded the results. The nonhomonymous condition may have resulted in greater learning because this condition targeted two new phonemes (Subject 6 /tʃ/:/dʒ/, Subject 8 /s/:/dʒ/, Subject 9 /s/:/ʃ/) rather than one new later developing presumably more difficult phoneme (/θ/ or /ð/). In an extension of this work, Gierut and Neumann (1992) reported a case study in which a child (age 4;8) was taught /θ/ paired with /ʃ/ in a nonhomonymous condition. Using an alternating treatments design, the child was also exposed to conventional minimal pairs in a homonymous condition targeting /s/:/t/. Gierut and Neumann reported that the greatest probe accuracy was observed in the nonhomonymous condition, associated with /θ/. These results suggest that perhaps a nonhomonymous intervention (e.g., maximal oppositions, treatment of the empty set) may be more efficient than traditional minimal pairs.

In light of Gierut's (1990, 1991) research, should minimal pairs be seen as an interesting yet antiquated approach for children with phonological impairment? Proponents of effective intervention approaches that explicitly capitalize on the effects of communication failure and heighten children's communication awareness through the use of minimal pairs (e.g., Metaphon [Howell & Dean, 1994]; metaphonological intervention [Hesketh et al., 2000]) might suggest not. Although the target of intervention or what is treated is important (Gierut, 2005, 2007), this does not necessarily negate consideration of how a target is treated. Before concluding that maximal oppositions is definitively more efficient than minimal pairs, it would be important to understand the role of semantic confusion within this body of research. Across minimal pair investigations by Gierut and colleagues (Gierut, 1990, 1991; Gierut, Elbert & Dinnsen, 1987; Gierut & Neumann, 1992), intervention began with imitation of real or nonsense words (that had been assigned meaning). It was unclear whether a request for clarification was provided to the participants once the participants were up to the stage of spontaneous production of treatment words. Had the participants been given the opportunity to experience the communicative consequence of homonymy and been given instructional feedback to facilitate their own discovery of the need to use a phonological contrast from the outset of the study, would the results have been different?

At present, although the findings from the comparative research lean toward the use of nonhomonymous word pairs over minimal pairs for children with a moderate or moderate-to-severe phonological impairment characterized by a limited phonetic inventory, additional comparative research with larger numbers of participants replicated by other researchers examining the inclusion of semantic confusion would seem to be needed before definitive conclusions could be made. Given discussions regarding the impact of complex target selection on phonological generalization, it would also be germane to compare intervention using nonhomophonous word pairs targeting complex targets with conventional minimal pairs targeting equally complex targets on widespread phonological change.

Dodd et al. (2008) began this task by comparing homonymous with nonhomonymous contrasts in a between-groups study of 19 children. In the homonymous condition, consonant clusters (considered to be more complex than singleton consonants) were paired with children's productions (e.g., /st/:/t/), whereas in the nonhomonymous condition, singletons or clusters were paired with singleton consonants in the children's preintervention grammars. Dodd et al. reported that progress (as measured by increase in PCC, decrease in number of error patterns, and increase in the number of singleton consonants and clusters in each participant's phonetic inventory) was similar between groups. Although the Dodd et al. results add empirical support for the minimal pair approach, it is difficult to draw meaningful conclusions in contrast with Gierut's research, due to the theoretical and practical differences underlying their respective approaches to target selection. Dodd et al. prioritized stimulable nondevelopmental (unusual) patterns followed by stimulable developmental error patterns. Gierut (1989, 1990, 1991) considered the participants' levels of productive phonological knowledge, and prioritized singleton consonants excluded from participants' phonetic and phonemic inventories, pairing them in varying combinations according to the number and nature of the feature differences. If the debate surrounding the relative efficacy of minimal pairs versus maximal (nonhomonymous) oppositions is to be resolved, then researchers need to use a consistent approach for describing and measuring change in children's phonological systems.

The minimal pair approach has also been compared with the multiple opposition approach. In an experimental case study involving one participant, Williams reported that "greater system-wide change occurred following the multiple oppositions approach than the minimal pair approach" (2005, p. 239). The participant in this investigation had a moderate phonological impairment. These preliminary findings suggest that further comparative research is needed to confirm the efficiency of the multiple opposition approach over the minimal pair approach for children with moderate or more severe phonological impairment.

In the Tyler et al. comparison of cycles and minimal pairs with four children with a moderate-to-severe phonological impairment, each intervention "facilitated dramatic changes . . . within 2 ½ months" (1987, p. 405). As noted in the Primary Populations section earlier in this chapter, Tyler et al. suggested that minimal pairs may be better suited to children with one or two age-inappropriate phonological processes, whereas cycles may be better suited to children with a more severe phonological impairment. Like Tyler's work, Crosbie et al. (2005) conducted a comparative study on children with different types of SSD. In the Crosbie et al. investigation, the focus was on consistent versus inconsistent speech patterns rather than severity of impairment. Using a multiple baseline design with alternative treatments, 18 children were randomly assigned to an 8- to 9-week block of intervention, either minimal pairs or core vocabulary. Following a 4-week break, the participants received intervention on the alternate approach for another 8- to 9-week block. Crosbie et al. reported that "core vocabulary therapy resulted in greater change in children with inconsistent speech disorder and phonological contrast therapy resulted in greater change in children with consistent speech disorder" (p. 485). Thus, although empirical evidence supports the use of minimal pairs with children who have consistent patterns of phonological difficulty, it does not support the use of the approach with children who have inconsistent phonological difficulties. (See Chapter 5 for further information on the core vocabulary approach.)

Summary of Levels of Evidence

The minimal pair approach has an empirical basis spanning more than 25 years (see Table 2.1). It is one of the few phonological intervention approaches to have been investigated by different researchers internationally. Of the 42 investigations identified, the majority were efficacy studies, (including 25 quasi-experimental investigations [either single-case experimental research designs or pre/post group investigations] and one small scale randomized controlled trial) implemented under controlled conditions, usually within university clinic settings. An additional 15 investigations were exploratory case studies. Only one study (Dodd et al., 2008) could be considered a study of clinical effectiveness, as the intervention was administered by eight practicing SLPs working in community clinics. A team of university-based researchers managed the study (e.g., randomly allocated participants to one of two treatment groups, selected participants' intervention targets, provided therapy materials, monitored progress). Together the majority of the research suggests that the minimal pair approach is effective for children with consistent phonological speech errors. In making this statement, it is important to understand that the approach covers a range of permutations and combinations of intervention components. The components that seem to be important in contributing to positive and efficient outcomes include production practice at word level using three to five minimal pair words containing nonstimulable targets. Although some studies accepted phonologically accurate responses regardless of phonetic accuracy, the impact of accepting such responses on the efficiency of intervention is not well understood. Saben and Costello-Ingham (1991) suggested that acceptance of phonetic variations may have impeded their participants' progress. Effective intervention dialogue may need to include articulation instruction in conjunction with a request for clarification following semantic confusion, however this remains to be experimentally validated. The effect of other components of intervention such as auditory discrimination and parental input also remains to be clearly understood. Further efficacy studies exploring the effect of such intervention components would seem to be needed.

What also remains to be better established is the effectiveness of the approach under everyday clinical conditions. As Fey and Finestack (2009) point out, effectiveness studies are a logical extension of efficacy research. It would seem that minimal pair research needs to move on to this next logical extension and better establish the effectiveness of the approach, beginning with children with mild or mild-to-moderate phonological impairment without any concomitant difficulties. For this to happen, SLPs working in everyday clinical environments, such as in schools, community health centers, and private practice, need to work together with researchers in university-based clinics, such as in Dodd et al. (2008), to construct well-designed randomized controlled trials that compare one particular combination of minimal pair components with another combination of minimal pair components. The minimal pair approach could also be compared with another phonological approach, considered suitable for children with mild or mild-to-moderate phonological impairment, such as metaphonological intervention (see Chapter 10), perceptual intervention (see Chapter 12) or PACT therapy (see Chapter 17).

PRACTICAL REQUIREMENTS

Nature of Sessions

Minimal pair intervention may be implemented within a variety of session frameworks. Across the 42 minimal pair studies listed in Table 2.1, the most frequently chosen model of service delivery was individual intervention in a university-based clinic with a clinician. A smaller portion of the studies reported positive outcomes for childcare, school, home, and hospital settings. Using case-study data, Grunwell and Dive (1988) also reported positive outcomes with an intensive group format. Across the 42 studies, session durations ranged from 20 minutes to $4\frac{1}{2}$ hours, with the majority being between 30 and 60 minutes. Session frequency ranged from each weekday to fortnightly, with a median of twice weekly sessions. No particular service delivery option has emerged as better than another. This is an area of research that could be further explored in effectiveness studies of the minimal pair approach.

Personnel

Minimal pair intervention has typically been administered by a clinician. Two investigations have evaluated the effect of intervention administered by agents of intervention other than clinicians. In the Ruscello et al. (1993) study on the issue of service delivery, 12 children were randomly assigned to one of two treatment groups: minimal pair intervention administered by a clinician or minimal pair intervention administered by a combination of a clinician and the child's parent using the IBM SpeechViewer system (IBM, 1988). Following 16 sessions (8 weeks of 1-hour sessions twice weekly), Ruscello et al. reported that both groups showed a statistically significant improvement on a measure of phonological generalization for the targeted phonological processes. Importantly, there was no significant difference between the groups, suggesting that parent-administered minimal pair intervention using the IBM SpeechViewer system was equally effective as clinician-delivered intervention.

Dodd and Barker (1990) examined the efficacy of a minimal pair approach using parents and teachers as the agents of intervention. The group parent training involved weekly 2-hour training sessions for 11 weeks, while the preschool teacher training involved a 2-day workshop followed by 3 $\frac{1}{2}$-hour workshops at 3 weekly intervals. A number of measures of the participants' ability were obtained, including PCC. Dodd and Barker reported a significant difference in PCC scores between pre- and postintervention. At the conclusion of the study, only 3 of the 11 participants did not require any further intervention. These three participants received parent training. The preschool teachers reported difficulty finding time to do the intervention with the children. Thus, although minimal pair intervention may be administered by agents other than clinicians, the efficacy of such intervention seems equivocal. What also remains to be established is the empirical basis for parental involvement, either within a session or between sessions in the form of administering homework. See Chapter 17 and Chapter 20 for further discussion on the role of personnel, particularly families, in the management of phonological impairment in children.

Dosage

Dosage of intervention is a difficult construct to meaningfully quantify. Of the 42 investigations, the dosage in hours could be determined for 26 (62%) of the studies in Table 2.1. Of these studies, the dosage in hours ranged from $4^1/2$ to 45 hours, with a mean of approximately 18 hours. These hours of intervention were delivered over weeks, ranging from 2 to 27 weeks, with a mean of 9 $^1/2$ weeks. A closer inspection of this literature shows the difficulty of extracting meaning to identify an evidence-based recommended dosage. First, published minimal pair research has typically been conducted for a predetermined period of time (e.g., 20 sessions, 8 weeks) or until participants met a predetermined performance criteria, rather than from the point of referral to the point of dismissal. This restriction in duration is typical of the wider body of published phonological intervention research (Baker & McLeod, 2008). Second, published minimal pair research has reported different schedules of service using varying outcome measures. For example, of a selection of investigations reporting a total duration of 8 weeks, Crosbie et al. (2005) provided 8 hours of minimal pair intervention (30 minutes twice weekly), reporting improvements in PCC; Tyler et al. (1990) provided 12 hours (45 minutes twice weekly), reporting improvements in voice onset time differences for stop contrasts; and Ruscello et al. (1993) provided 16 hours (60 minutes twice weekly), reporting improvements in percent correct production on a probe task. The issue is further complicated by individual variation. For example, Baker and McLeod (2004) reported that what took one child 7 weeks to achieve, took another child 5 months. To date, the average amount of intervention required to treat a mild or mild-to-moderate phonological impairment in a child from the time of referral to the time of dismissal is unknown.

Meaningful dosage for minimal pairs also needs to be contextualized within overall intervention programs in which children with more severe impairments may receive more than one approach over time, and in which children may receive additional input from parents or caregivers at home. For example, Williams (2000) reported that of 10 children with a moderate, severe, or profound phonological impairment, 6 children received minimal pair intervention following multiple oppositions. It would seem that dosage for minimal pairs may vary depending on a child's initial presentation of severity and the context in which minimal pairs may or may not be one part of a child's overall intervention program. Research is needed to provide SLPs with clear evidence-based guidelines on this important clinical issue.

KEY COMPONENTS

Nature of Goals

Across the 42 investigations of the minimal pair approach, the goals of intervention varied and included:

- Common structural and systemic developmental phonological processes, such as cluster reduction or velar fronting (e.g., Baker & McLeod, 2004; Crosbie et al., 2005;

Dodd et al., 2008; Saben & Costello-Ingham, 1991; Tyler et al., 1987; Tyler & Sandoval, 1994; Weiner, 1981)

- Nondevelopmental or unusual phonological processes (e.g., Dodd et al., 2008; Leahy & Dodd, 1987; Saben & Costello-Ingham, 1991)

- Distinctive features, such as continued versus interrupted, grave versus acute, and strident versus mellow (Blache et al., 1981)

- Sounds consistently in error or excluded from phonetic/phonemic inventories (e.g., Dinnsen, Chin, & Elbert, 1992; Elbert et al., 1990, 1991; Gierut, 1990, 1991; Gierut et al., 1987; Miccio et al., 1999)

Gibbon and Beck (2002) also suggested that vowel disorders (typically [ɛ] [æ] confusion) can be contrasted using minimal pairs.

The ways in which goals have been identified and prioritized have also varied. Some investigations have prioritized phonological processes according to developmental factors, effect on intelligibility, and stimulability (e.g., Dodd et al., 2008; Dodd & Iacono, 1989; Tyler, 1995). By contrast, other studies have prioritized nonstimulable intervention targets (e.g., Powell, 1993; Powell et al., 1991). The empirical evidence for the minimal pair approach seems to support the prioritization of nonstimulable speech sounds excluded from children's phonetic inventories in an effort to facilitate more widespread change. These sounds may be used within syllable or word shapes that have been prioritized for intervention.

Goal Attack Strategies

Intervention goals have most frequently been implemented within a sequential goal attack strategy (one phoneme or pattern at a time) (e.g., Dodd & Iacono, 1989; Miccio et al., 1999; Miccio & Ingrisano, 2000; Powell et al., 1998; Tyler, 1995; Tyler et al., 1990). A simultaneous goal attack strategy (remediation of two or more phonemes or patterns at a time) has also been used (e.g., Abraham, 1993; Fey & Stalker, 1986; Gierut, 1991; Gierut & Neumann, 1992; Grunwell & Dive, 1988; Weiner, 1981), with the cyclical goal attack strategy (targeting a range of processes or error patterns sequentially from one session to the next for a block of time) being used infrequently (e.g., Tyler & Sandoval, 1994). Some studies have also reported modifying their strategy partway through an investigation in an effort to facilitate progress (e.g., Baker & McLeod, 2004; Powell, 1993). To date, although there is evidence to support the use of either a vertical, simultaneous, or cyclical goal attack strategy, there is no clear indication that one strategy is better than another across published investigations of the minimal pair approach.

Description of Activities

Most approaches to phonological intervention are composed of a unique combination of components or procedures developed by a single researcher or research team (e.g., multiple oppositions, cycles, PACT therapy). This makes the task of providing an operational description relatively straightforward. One of the problems for the minimal pair approach is that there are various unique combinations of intervention components across the published literature reflecting a minimal pair approach. The problem for the SLP is identifying and implementing a version of minimal pairs supported by empirical evidence. This task becomes difficult when there is insufficient methodological detail within a published study to replicate the approach. Consequently, what follows is a description of two distinct versions of minimal pairs derived from a review of the intervention components and procedures across the 42 studies: 1) a meaningful minimal pair approach, based on research by Abraham (1993), Blache et al. (1981), and Weiner (1981), and 2) a perception-production minimal pair approach, based on research by Crosbie et al. (2005), Elbert et al. (1990, 1991), and Tyler et al. (1987, 1990). The main way in which the versions differ is *how* the minimal pairs are introduced to the child. Within the meaning-based minimal pair approach the child is challenged to produce a contrast between word pairs in the first intervention session. If a child needs help producing a contrast, the SLP provides that help within the context of teaching the child how he or she can provide a repair in response to a request for clarification. Within the perception-production approach, the child receives perception training followed by imitation speech production practice before starting spontaneous speech production practice, so that when he or she is given a request for clarification, the child may be more likely to produce a successful repair. Prior to starting either approach, the SLP selects five pictures of meaningful minimal pair words representing the selected intervention target whether it be a phonological process, consonant, consonant feature, syllable, or word shape. Using gliding of /ɹ/ as an example, suitable words would be *ring:wing; right:white; rip:whip; rock:wok; read:weed*. The SLP could then create two copies of each picture for each word, totaling 20 pictures. A description of the two versions of minimal pairs follows.

Meaningful Minimal Pair Intervention

The meaningful minimal pair approach consists of three steps. Steps one and two are completed within the first session while step three is begun during the first session and continues in subsequent sessions until predetermined phonological generalization performance criteria are met.

Step 1: Familiarization. The SLP and child sit together at a small table facing each other at eye level. The SLP shows the child the picture for each word, saying, for example, "This is a *ring*, we wear it on our finger. This is a *wing* on a bird."

Step 2: Listen, and pick-up. Once the child has been familiarized with the pictures, the SLP spreads out one picture for each word on the table and asks the child to listen and pick up one picture at a time (e.g., "Pick up the picture of the *ring*"). This process continues until the child picks up all 10 pictures. The SLP provides praise for a correct response (e.g., "Great listening, that's the *ring*") and instructional feedback following an incorrect response (e.g., "The *wing*? The word I said sounds a bit like *wing*, but it's different. Listen again, pick up the picture of the *ring*").

Step 3: Production of minimal pair words. During the third and final step, the child is given a turn to be the teacher. The child is instructed to tell the SLP which picture to pick up. It is during this step that the child is likely to experience semantic confusion and is challenged to produce a contrast between the word pairs in order to be understood. The SLP provides praise for a correct response (e.g., "The *ring*, I know what you mean!") and instructional feedback following semantic confusion (e.g., "I'm not sure what you mean. Do you mean *wing* or *ring*? Tell me again"). If on a second attempt the child does not make a contrast between the word pairs, the SLP provides instructional feedback regarding the articulation of the target word. The moment the child accurately produces or approximates the target word, the SLP provides meaning-based praise (e.g., "Oh, I can understand you now! You meant the *ring* didn't you, not the *wing*, the *ring* with the growling /ɪ/ sound").

Step 3 of the meaningful minimal pair approach continues at word level until a performance-based phonological generalization criterion has been met. Following the first session, subsequent sessions would typically consist of 20 trials of each of the five target words (with or without the pictures of the minimal pair cognates, as the instructional feedback already contains the minimal pair cognate), totaling 100 trials. Production practice activities could include three to five games, each lasting approximately 10 minutes, in which multiple opportunities are provided to say the target words within a meaningful context. The activities are structured such that the child requests the target word (e.g., barrier games, magnetic fishing for words, playing shops).

Perception-Production Minimal Pair Intervention

The perception-production minimal pair approach consists of five steps:

Step 1: Familiarization and perception training. The SLP and child sit at a small table at eye level. The SLP shows the child the minimal pair pictures (e.g., "This is *ring*, and this is *wing*"). The 20 treatment words (two copies of each of the five target items and two copies of each of the five cognate pairs) are spread out on a table, and the child is asked to pick up the word the SLP says. A child moves on to Step 2 once he or she identifies the picture corresponding to each treatment word with 90% accuracy. Crosbie et al. (2005) included a sorting activity at this step, in that the child is expected to listen to and sort the word pairs into their respective categories (e.g., compiling /ɪ/ pictures versus /w/ pictures). The SLP provides praise for correct responses (e.g., "Great listening, yes, that's the *ring*") and instructional feedback for incorrectly identified or sorted pictures (e.g., "Uh oh, that's the *wing* that starts with the /w/ sound. Listen again, and find the ring that starts with the /ɪ/ sound").

Step 2: Production—word imitation. Of the five minimal pairs (five target words and five cognate pairs), the child is to imitate each of the five target words given auditory models and articulation instruction as necessary from the SLP. The SLP provides praise regarding the articulatory accuracy of the word for correct responses (e.g., "Great /ɪ/ sound when you said *ring*") and instructional feedback for incorrect responses (e.g., "Try again. Watch me and listen, *ring*, remember to use the growly /r/ sound when you say *ring*"). This step continues until the child can imitate the target words with 90% accuracy in at least 50 trials. This step is reminiscent of traditional articulation therapy at word level.

Step 3: Production—independent naming. Using the five target words, the child is instructed to name each picture without a model. The SLP provides praise and instructional feedback, similar to Step 2, as necessary. This step continues until the child achieves 50% accuracy independently producing the target words in at least 50 trials.

Step 4: Production—minimal pairs. This step is identical to Step 3 of the meaningful minimal pair approach, in which the child is given the opportunity to request either a target word or a minimal pair cognate of a target word. Meaning-based feedback is provided in conjunction with instructional cues as necessary. According to Tyler et al. (1987), the inclusion of imitation and independent naming of the target words prior to the child naming the minimal pairs in this final step facilitates success. Presumably, if a child has the phonetic ability to produce the word, then the frustration sometimes experienced by children when confronted with the homonym in their speech might be minimized using the perception-production approach.

Materials and Equipment Required

Many resources are available for conducting minimal pair intervention. As discussed previously, the SLP requires picture stimuli, in addition to any games or toys for conducting the production practice activities. A selection of commercially available minimal pair resources include Daly (1999), Flahive and Lanza (1998), Frederick (2005), Hall (2006), Krupa (1995), LinguiSystems (2007), Pavlovic, (2007), Rippon (2001), Webber (2005), and Williams (2006). Minimal pair picture stimuli are also freely available on the Internet (e.g., http://speech-language-therapy.com/txresources.html). The SLP needs to be mindful of the language of origin on the minimal pair stimuli, as dialect differences can influence whether word pairs are minimally contrastive.

ASSESSMENT AND PROGRESS MONITORING TO SUPPORT DECISION MAKING

Although there is literature supporting the efficacy of the minimal pair approach, the clinical application of the approach to an individual child is not a guarantee that the approach will work. Using Dollaghan's (2007) helpful evidence-based practice framework, E^3BP, the empirical evidence examined so far in this chapter provides one of three types of evidence to be conscientiously, explicitly, and judiciously integrated in the conduct of evidence-based practice. The other two types of evidence include the "best available evidence *internal* to clinical practice, and . . . best available evidence concerning the preferences of a fully informed patient" (Dollaghan, 2007, p. 2). This section explores how SLPs can apply external evidence to develop internal evidence to guide everyday clinical decision making for individual children receiving minimal pair intervention.

Internal evidence is a measure of an individual's response to intervention in a clinical as opposed to a research context. Measures of an individual's response to minimal pair intervention can be derived from quantitative and qualitative treatment, generalization, and control data (Baker & McLeod, 2004). These data can then be used to answer four clinically important questions proposed by Olswang and Bain (1994) and articulated by Baker and McLeod (2004):

1. Is the child responding to the intervention program?

2. Is clinically significant and important change occurring?

3. Is intervention responsible for the change?

4. How long should a therapy target be treated? (p. 263)

Treatment data help determine whether a child is responding to minimal pair intervention. Stimulus and response generalization data, and in particular phonological response generalization data (often referred to as *probe data* in the research literature), can be used to determine whether clinically significant and important change is occurring in a child's phonological system. Ideally, for minimal pairs to have worked, a child needs to exhibit generalized acquisition of a targeted speech skill and any implicationally related speech skills, during conversational speech. Understanding of a child's preintervention productive phonological knowledge of or association with selected intervention targets (such as knowledge of the constituents of consonant clusters when targeting clusters), may guide anticipated changes to a child's phonological system and as such the type of probe used to monitor progress (Powell & Elbert, 1984). Phonological generalization data are also important for determining how long an intervention target needs to be worked on. Finally, control data provide the information necessary for determining whether the minimal pair approach is responsible for the change in the child's speech. Together, data-driven answers to the four clinically important questions provide SLPs with the internal evidence to justify ongoing intervention, changes to intervention, or the cessation of intervention. Table 2.2 provides a sample data management plan for a minimal pair approach targeting gliding of /ɹ/, guided by the work of Baker and McLeod (2004) and Olswang and Bain (1994).

According to Baker and McLeod (2004), although treatment data might suggest that intervention is working, the most important measure of the efficacy of intervention for the minimal pair approach is whether phonological generalization is evident during conversational speech. In the event that a child shows limited phonological generalization, intervention would need to be modified. Two cases (Cody and James) discussed by Baker and McLeod illustrate when and how a minimal pair approach might be modified. In Cody's case, minimal pairs was effective with Cody reaching the generalization criterion of 70% correct production of the intervention target during conversational speech, following 12 intervention sessions (equivalent to 7 weeks). This dismissal criterion was similar to previous minimal pair research (Tyler, 1995; Tyler et al., 1993). Visual inspection of Cody's generalization data showed distinct signs of generalization within 4 weeks of receiving twice-weekly intervention. Although the treatment data for James suggested that he was responding to intervention, clinically significant and important changes were not evident in his conversational speech across the same period of time.

If minimal or slow progress is apparent within approximately 1 month to 6 weeks of starting minimal pair intervention, steps need to be taken to facilitate the child's progress, such as working at phrase or sentence level, increasing the number of treatment words and trials completed per session, increasing session frequency, and changing from a vertical attack strategy to a horizontal attack strategy (if there are other intervention targets to be treated). Alternatively, a different approach to analysis, goal selection, and intervention could be trialed, as discussed by Baker and Bernhardt (2004). See Baker and McLeod (2004) for case study examples on the development and implementation of data collection plans for children with a phonological impairment receiving minimal pair intervention.

CONSIDERATIONS FOR CHILDREN FROM CULTURALLY AND LINGUISTICALLY DIVERSE BACKGROUNDS

Internationally, the minimal pair approach has been reported to be used with children who speak General American English (Smit, 2007), Canadian English (Bernhardt & Deby, 2007), British English (Howard, 2007), Australian English (McLeod, 2007), Finnish (Kun-

Table 2.2. Minimal pairs data management plan for gliding of /ɹ/

Question asked	What to measure?	Category and type of data	When?	Where?	Who?
(Q1) Is the child responding to the minimal pairs intervention program?	Production of word-initial /ɹ/ on treatment words	*Quantitative treatment data:* Percentage correct of /ɹ/ on treatment words *Qualitative treatment data:* Rating of child's production of /ɹ/ on treatment words (range from 1 to 5, with 5 being clear [ɹ] and 1 being [w])	Every session	In the clinic setting	SLP
(Q2) Is clinically significant and important change occurring? and (Q3) How long should a therapy target be treated?	Production of /ɹ/ in a variety of linguistic and social contexts	*Quantitative phonological response generalization probe data:* Percentage correct of /ɹ/ in initial and medial position in single-word probe and conversational speech *Qualitative stimulus and phonological response generalization probe data:* Rating of child's production of /ɹ/ by other listeners in other environments	Every 4th session	In the clinic, at home, and in (pre)school settings	SLP, caregiver, and teacher
	Production of implicationally related targets	*Quantitative phonological response generalization probe data:* PCC and phonetic inventory based on conversational speech sample to measure broad changes in child's phonological system. (*Note:* Specific targets anticipated to change by implication depend on analysis of child's speech sample prior to starting intervention.)			
(Q4) Is intervention responsible for the change?	Unrelated speech or language ability to be targeted for intervention	*Quantitative control data:* Percentage correct production of unrelated speech target (e.g., θ, ð) or language target (e.g., production of morpheme in error) requiring intervention during single-word and/or conversational speech probe	Every 4th session	In the clinic	SLP

Based on Baker & McLeod (2004) and Olswang & Bain (1994).
Key: PCC, percent consonants correct; SLP, speech-language pathologist.

nari & Savinainen-Makkonen, 2007), German (Fox, 2007), Greek (Mennen & Okalidou, 2007), Israeli Hebrew (Ben-David & Berman, 2007), Japanese (Ota & Ueda, 2007), Korean (Kim & Pae, 2007), Maltese (Grech, 2007), and Turkish (Topbaş, 2007). Evidence also supports the use of the minimal pair approach with speakers who use a language in addition to English. Ray (2002) used the minimal pair approach to successfully treat a phonological impairment in a child who was learning three languages: English, Hindi, and Gujarati. Ray reported that "the successful treatment of MC's phonological disorder required 40 sessions, coupled with regular work at home" (p. 312). Improvements were noted in the target language (English) and the child's other two languages not targeted during intervention. Holm and colleagues (Holm & Dodd, 2001; Holm et al., 1997) also reported on a series of case studies in which a minimal pair approach was used to treat a phonological impairment in children learning two languages. Holm et al. reported on a boy age 5;2 with articulatory and phonological errors in both English and Cantonese. Traditional articulation therapy was used to target distorted [s], whereas a minimal pair approach was used to target cluster reduction and gliding of /ɹ/ and /l/. Holm et al. reported that although intervention was successful in English (the targeted language), there were no obvious improvements in Cantonese. They suggested that the child had two separate phonological systems, each requiring direct intervention. Although a minimal pair approach was reported to be successful in both reports, the conflicting findings with regard to generalization across languages highlights a need to better understand bilingual phonological difficulties in children and how they might best be treated within a minimal pair approach.

CASE STUDY

Leonardo (age 5;2) was an Australian-English speaking boy referred by his parents for a speech assessment because of concerns about his immature pronunciation of words containing /ʃ/ and /ɹ/. Leonardo's parents had particularly noticed his production of /s/ for /ʃ/ in the word *finished* and the phrases *show me* and *I'll show you.* An initial SLP assessment revealed that Leonardo's receptive and expressive language, phonological awareness, and oral musculature structure and function were within normal limits; his hearing was normal with no history of otitis media with effusion; and he had received no prior intervention for speech or language impairment. Leonardo's medical and developmental histories were unremarkable. Based on a 200 single-word sample, Leonardo's PCC was 83%, equivalent to a mild-to-moderate phonological impairment. There were three distinct phonological processes evident in his speech: palatal fronting of /ʃ, ʒ, tʃ, dʒ/ to [s, z, ts, dz], gliding of /ɹ/ to [w], and fricative simplification of /θ, ð/ to [f, v]. Leonardo produced /ɹ/ on one occasion in the 200 single-word sample. Identical patterns were evident during conversational speech, with the exception of /ð/. Occasionally, albeit deliberately, Leonardo said [ðæt] for *that* (rather than his more typical form of [æt] or [væt]). Leonardo was stimulable for all speech sounds that were absent from his phonetic inventory (/ʃ, ʒ, tʃ/). Baseline data were collected, comprising a sample of 45 words containing singleton palatal fricatives and affricates across initial, medial, and final position in addition to the initial consonant cluster /ʃɹ/. This task subsequently served as the response phonological generalization probe. A meaningful minimal pair approach was selected to target palatal fronting using the consonant target of /ʃ/. Pictures of five minimal pair treatment words (*sew:show; sock:shock; sour:shower; save:shave;* and *sell:shell*) were selected. In consultation with Leonardo's family, Leonardo was seen twice weekly for individual sessions with the clinician. A session consisted of 100 single-word trials across two or three games and lasted approximately 45 minutes. Leonardo's parents were instructed to select one 10-minute period of time during each day to listen to Leonardo's speech, provide praise when they heard him use the target sound /ʃ/ during conversational speech, and provide a request for clarification containing his production and the adult-like production (e.g., "Do you mean *sew* or *show?*") when they heard him use /s/ for /ʃ/.

During the first intervention session, Leonardo was able to change his production of /s/ to /ʃ/ in response to semantic confusion and a request for clarification. Quantitative generalization probe data (45-item single-word probe and 5-minute conversational speech sample) were collected every fourth session by the author. Qualitative ratings of Leonardo's production of /ʃ/ during conversational speech were collected by his father once every 2 weeks. Leonardo reached the discontinuation criterion (70% correct production of all sounds affected by palatal fronting during the single-word probe) by the third probe (12th session), which was equivalent to 6 weeks after starting intervention. Follow-up of Leonardo's production of /ʃ, ʒ, tʃ, dʒ/ during conversational speech 2 months later revealed that palatal fronting was no longer evident. Leonardo's family had continued to provide praise and feedback in the form of a request for clarification during daily 10-minute conversational periods over this time. Leonardo's family, including grandparents, commented that his speech was easier to understand and sounded more mature. Frequently heard utterances, such as *I'm finished, I'll show you,* and *watch me* had become adult-like. Gliding of /ɹ/ served as the control behavior. Over the period of intervention and follow up, there was minimal change in Leonardo's use of gliding of /ɹ/, suggesting that the minimal pair intervention had been effective.

STUDY QUESTIONS

1. A meaningful minimal pair approach was used with the child in the case study, Leonardo. In what ways would a perception-production minimal pair approach differ?

2. In light of the research on service delivery by Ruscello et al. (1993), how could Leonardo's intervention been made more efficient?

3. The speech sound /ʃ/ was used to work on the phonological process of palatal fronting. Using a complexity approach to target selection (Gierut, 2007), what other intervention target(s) might have been suitable for Leonardo, and what impact might these targets have had on the efficiency of his intervention?

4. What other phonological intervention approaches are suitable for children such as Leonardo?

FUTURE DIRECTIONS

Minimal pairs is one of the most widely used and widely investigated approaches for treating phonological impairment in children. A relatively large empirical basis supports the efficacy of the approach. In controlled environments such as university clinics with researchers, children with moderate-to-severe and severe phonological impairments have been reported to show generalized improvement in their phonological systems. The approach has also been successfully used with children with a concomitant hearing loss, developmental difficulties, and cleft palate speech. The efficiency of minimal pairs relative to other phonological intervention approaches, however, has been questioned (Williams, 2003). It would seem that minimal pairs might be primarily suited to children with a mild or mild-to-moderate phonological impairment. Four challenges remain ahead for the minimal pair approach. First, experimentally controlled efficacy studies of the approach need to be conducted for children with a mild or mild-to-moderate phonological impairment compared with other approaches reported to be suitable for similar children. Second, the clinical effectiveness of the approach in less controlled yet more externally valid clinical environments needs to be established. Such investigations could also evaluate the efficiency of the approach using alternate service delivery models, such as parent training. The results from Ruscello et al. (1993) indicate that this is a promising line of inquiry. In light of Gillon's (2005) research, studies of the clinical effectiveness of minimal pairs could also evaluate the impact of including phoneme awareness and letter-sound knowledge training as an adjunct to minimal pair intervention. Third, the effect and necessity of the different components that comprise minimal pair intervention requires ongoing investigation. Although a number of studies have begun this task (e.g., Powell et al., 1998; Saben & Costello-Ingham, 1991), more carefully controlled experimental investigations manipulating the interactive and additive effectives of the different components of intervention are needed. A randomized controlled comparison of the two approaches to minimal pair intervention offered in this chapter might be a helpful place to start. Finally, in light of the ICF-CY (WHO, 2007) framework, it would seem timely to more formally consider the consequences of a phonological impairment as experienced by children. Although the literature has indirectly considered the benefits of minimal pair intervention on children's communication skills, future investigations could measure the impact of intervention on children's activities and participation and explore how the approach could be modified and refined to better consider the whole child. In one of the first investigations of the minimal pair approach, Blache et al. stated "the simultaneous teaching of the structure and function of the phoneme may open new paths of research" (1981, p. 295). It would seem that the research path, although paved with many research findings, is still open for inquiry.

SUGGESTED READINGS

Baker, E., & McLeod, S. (2004). Evidence-based management of phonological impairment in children. *Child Language Teaching and Therapy, 20*(3), 261–285.

Barlow, J.A., & Gierut, J.A. (2002). Minimal pair approaches to phonological remediation. *Seminars in Speech and Language, 23*(1), 57–67.

Bernthal, J.E., Bankson, N.W., & Flipsen, P. (Eds.). (2009). *Articulation and phonological disorders: Speech sound disorders in children* (6th ed.). Boston: Allyn & Bacon.

Blache, S.E., Parsons, C.L., & Humphreys, J.M. (1981). A minimal-word-pair model for teaching the linguistic significant difference of distinctive feature properties. *Journal of Speech and Hearing Disorders, 46,* 29–296.

Crosbie, S., Holm, A., & Dodd, B. (2005). Intervention for children with severe speech disorder: A comparison of two approaches. *International Journal of Language and Communication Disorders*, *40*, 467–491.

Dodd, B., Crosbie, S., McIntosh, B., Holm, A., Harvey, C., Liddy, M., et al. (2008). The impact of selecting different contrasts in phonological therapy. *International Journal of Speech-Language Pathology*, *10*(5), 334–345.

Saben, C.B., & Costello-Ingham, J. (1991). The effects of minimal pairs treatment on the speech-sound production of two children with phonologic disorders. *Journal of Speech and Hearing Research*, *34*, 1023–1040.

Weiner, F.F. (1981). Treatment of phonological disability using the method of meaningful minimal contrast: Two case studies. *Journal of Speech and Hearing Disorders*, *46*, 97–103.

REFERENCES

Abraham, S. (1993). Differential treatment of phonological disability in children with impaired hearing who were trained orally. *American Journal of Speech-Language Pathology*, *2*, 23–30.

Baker, E., & Bernhardt, B.H. (2004). From hindsight to foresight: Working around barriers to success in phonological intervention. *Child Language Teaching and Therapy*, *20*(3), 287–318.

Baker, E., & McLeod, S. (2004). Evidence-based management of phonological impairment in children. *Child Language Teaching and Therapy*, *20*(3), 261–285.

Baker, E., & McLeod, S. (2008, November). *EBP and speech sound disorders: What do we know?* Paper presented at the American Speech-Language-Hearing Association Convention, Chicago.

Barlow, J.A., & Gierut, J.A. (2002). Minimal pair approaches to phonological remediation. *Seminars in Speech and Language*, *23*(1), 57–67.

Ben-David, A., & Berman, R.A. (2007). Israeli Hebrew speech acquisition. In S. McLeod (Ed.), *The international guide to speech acquisition* (pp. 437–456). Clifton Park, NY: Thomson Delmar Learning.

Bernhardt, B.M.H., & Deby, J. (2007). Canadian English speech acquisition. In S. McLeod (Ed.), *The international guide to speech acquisition* (pp. 177–187). Clifton Park, NY: Thomson Delmar Learning.

Bernhardt, B.M.H., & Stemberger, J.P. (2000). *Workbook in nonlinear phonology for clinical application.* Austin, TX: PRO-ED.

Bernthal, J.E., Bankson, N.W., & Flipsen, P. (Eds.). (2009). *Articulation and phonological disorders: Speech sound disorders in children* (6th ed.). Boston: Allyn & Bacon.

Blache, S.E., Parsons, C.L., & Humphreys, J.M. (1981). A minimal-word-pair model for teaching the linguistic significant difference of distinctive feature properties. *Journal of Speech and Hearing Disorders*, *46*, 29–296.

Bowen, C., & Cupples, L. (2006). PACT: Parents and children together in phonological therapy. *Advances in Speech-Language Pathology*, *8*(3), 245–260.

Cooper, R. (1968). The method of meaningful minimal contrasts in functional articulation problems. *Journal of the Speech and Hearing Association of Virginia*, *10*, 17–22.

Crosbie, S., Holm, A., & Dodd, B. (2005). Intervention for children with severe speech disorder: A comparison of two approaches. *International Journal of Language and Communication Disorders*, *40*, 467–491.

Daly, G.H. (1999). *Scissors, glue, and phonological processes, too!* East Moline, IL: LinguiSystems.

Dinnsen, D.A. (1980). Linguistic commentary. In M. Elbert, D. Rockman, & D. Saltzman (Eds.), *Contrasts: The use of minimal pairs in articulation training* (pp. v–vi). Austin, TX: PRO-ED.

Dinnsen, D.A., Chin, S.B., & Elbert, M. (1992). On the lawfullness of change in phonetic inventories. *Lingua*, *86*, 207–222.

Dodd, B., & Barker, R. (1990). The efficacy of utilizing parents and teachers as agents of therapy for children with phonological disorders. *Australian Journal of Human Communication Disorders*, *18*, 29–44.

Dodd, B., Crosbie, S., McIntosh, B., Holm, A., Harvey, C., Liddy, M., et al. (2008). The impact of selecting different contrasts in phonological therapy. *International Journal of Speech-Language Pathology*, *10*(5), 334–345.

Dodd, B., & Iacono, T. (1989). Phonological disorders in children: Changes in phonological process use during treatment. *British Journal of Disorders of Communication*, *24*, 333–351.

Dollaghan, C.A. (2007). *The handbook for evidence-based practice in communication disorders.* Baltimore: Paul H. Brookes Publishing Co.

Elbert, M., Dinnsen, D.A., Swartzlander, P., & Chin, S.B. (1990). Generalization to conversational speech. *Journal of Speech and Hearing Research*, *55*, 694–699.

Elbert, M., Powell, T.W., & Swartzlander, P. (1991). Toward a technology of generalization: How many exemplars are sufficient? *Journal of Speech and Hearing Research*, *34*, 81–87.

Elbert, M., Rockman, B., & Saltzman, D. (1980). *Contrasts: The use of minimal pairs in articulation training.* Austin, TX: Exceptional Resources.

Ferrier, E.E. (1963). *An investigation of the psycholinguistic abilities of children with functional defects of articulation.* Urbana, IL: University of Illinois.

Ferrier, E., & Davis, M. (1973). A lexical approach to the remediation of final sound omissions. *Journal of Speech and Hearing Disorders, 38,* 126–131.

Fey, M.E. (1985). Articulation and phonology: Inextricable constructs in speech pathology. *Human Communication Canada, 9*(1), 7–16.

Fey, M.E., Cleave, P.L., Ravida, A.I., Long, S.H., Dejmal, A.E., & Easton, D.L. (1994). Effects of grammar facilitation on the phonological performance of children with speech and language impairments. *Journal of Speech and Hearing Research, 37,* 594–607.

Fey, M.E., & Finestack, L.H. (2009). Research and development in child language intervention: A 5-phase model. In R.G. Schwartz (Ed.), *Handbook of child language disorders* (pp. 513–529). New York: Psychology Press.

Fey, M., & Stalker, C.H. (1986). A hypothesis-testing approach to treatment of a child with an idiosyncratic (morpho)phonological system. *Journal of Speech and Hearing Disorders, 51,* 309–324.

Flahive, L.K., & Lanza, J.R. (1998). *Just for kids: Phonological processing.* East Moline, IL: LinguiSystems.

Forrest, K., Dinnsen, D.A., & Elbert, M. (1997). Impact of substitution patterns on phonological learning by misarticulating children. *Clinical Linguistics and Phonetics, 11,* 63–76.

Forrest, K., Elbert, M., & Dinnsen, D.A. (2000). The effect of substitution patterns on phonological treatment outcomes. *Clinical Linguistics and Phonetics, 14*(7), 519–531.

Fox, A.V. (2007). German speech acquisition. In S. McLeod (Ed.), *The international guide to speech acquisition* (pp. 386–397). Clifton Park, NY: Thomson Delmar Learning.

Frederick, M. (2005). *Webber Spanish phonology cards.* Greenville, SC: Super Duper Publications.

Gallagher, T.M. (1977). Revision behavior in the speech of normal children developing language. *Journal of Speech and Hearing Research, 20,* 303–318.

Gibbon, F.E., & Beck, J.M. (2002). Therapy for abnormal vowels in children with phonological impairment. In M.J. Ball & F.E. Gibbon (Eds.), *Vowel disorders* (pp. 217–248). Woburn, MA: Butterworth-Heinemann.

Gierut, J.A. (1989). Maximal opposition approach to phonological treatment. *Journal of Speech and Hearing Disorders, 54,* 9–19.

Gierut, J.A. (1990). Differential learning of phonological oppositions. *Journal of Speech and Hearing Research, 33,* 540–549.

Gierut, J.A. (1991). Homonymy in phonological change. *Clinical Linguistics and Phonetics, 5,* 119–137.

Gierut, J.A. (2005). Phonological intervention: The how or the what? In S.F. Warren & M.E. Fey (Series Eds.), &

A.G. Kamhi & K.E. Pollock (Vol. Eds.), *Communication and language intervention series: Phonological disorders in children—Clinical decision making in assessment and intervention* (pp. 201–210). Baltimore: Paul H. Brookes Publishing Co.

Gierut, J.A. (2007). Phonological complexity and language learnability. *American Journal of Speech-Language Pathology, 16*(1), 6–17.

Gierut, J.A, Elbert, M., & Dinnsen, D. (1987). A functional analysis of phonological knowledge and generalization learning in misarticulating children. *Journal of Speech and Hearing Research, 30,* 462–479.

Gierut, J.A., & Neumann, H.J. (1992). Teaching and learning: A non-confound. *Clinical Linguistics and Phonetics, 6*(3), 191–200.

Gillon, G. (2005). Facilitating phoneme awareness development in 3- and 4-year-old children with speech impairment. *Language, Speech, and Hearing Services in Schools, 36*(4), 308–324.

Grech, H. (2007). Maltese speech acquisition. In S. McLeod (Ed.), *The international guide to speech acquisition* (pp. 483–494). Clifton Park, NY: Thomson Delmar Learning.

Greenfield, P., & Smith, J. (1976). *Communication and the beginnings of language: The development of semantic structure in one-word speech and beyond.* New York: Academic Press.

Grunwell, P. (1983, August). *Phonological therapy: Premises, principles and procedures.* Paper presented at the XIX Congress of International Association of Logopedics and Phoniatrics, University of Edinburgh.

Grunwell, P., & Dive, D. (1988). Treating 'cleft palate techniques': Combining phonological techniques with traditional articulation therapy. *Child Language Teaching and Therapy, 4,* 193–210.

Grunwell, P., & Russell, J. (1990). A phonological disorder in an English speaking child: A case study. *Clinical Linguistics and Phonetics, 4,* 29–38.

Grunwell, P., Yavaş, M., Russell, J., & Le Maistre, H. (1988). Developing a phonological system: A case study. *Child Language Teaching and Therapy, 4*(2), 142–153.

Hall, A. (2006). *Have you ever . . . ? Eight interactive books for phonological processes.* Greenville, SC: Super Duper Publications.

Hesketh, A., Adams, C., Nightingale, C., & Hall, R. (2000). Phonological awareness therapy and articulatory training approaches for children with phonological disorders: A comparative outcome study. *International Journal of Language and Communication Disorders, 35*(3), 337–354.

Hodson, B.W. (2007). *Evaluation and enhancing children's phonological systems: Research and theory to practice.* Greenville, SC: Thinking Publications.

Hodson, B.W., & Paden, E.P. (1991). *Targeting intelligible speech: A phonological approach to remediation* (2nd ed.). Austin, TX: PRO-ED.

Hoffman, P.R., Norris, J.A., & Monjure, J. (1990). Comparison of process targeting and whole language treatments for phonologically delayed preschool children. *Language, Speech, and Hearing Services in Schools, 21*, 102–109.

Holm, A., & Dodd, B. (2001). Comparison of cross-language generalization following speech therapy. *Folia Phoniatrica et Logopaedica, 53*, 166–172.

Holm, A., Ozanne, A., & Dodd, B. (1997). Efficacy of intervention for a bilingual child making articulation and phonological errors. *International Journal of Bilingualism, 1*(1), 55–69.

Howard, S. (2007). English speech acquisition. In S. McLeod (Ed.), *The international guide to speech acquisition* (pp. 188–203). Clifton Park, NY: Thomson Delmar Learning.

Howell, J., & Dean, E. (1994). *Treating phonological disorders in children: Metaphon theory to practice* (2nd ed.). London: Whurr.

IBM. (1988). *IBM Personal System/2 SpeechViewer: A guide to clinical and educational applications.* Atlanta, GA: International Business Machines Corporation.

Ingram, D. (1976). *Phonological disability in children.* New York: Elsevier.

Kim, M., & Pae, S. (2007). Korean speech acquisition. In S. McLeod (Ed.), *The international guide to speech acquisition* (pp. 472–482). Clifton Park, NY: Thomson Delmar Learning.

Klein, E. (1996). *Clinical phonology: Assessment and treatment of articulation disorders in children and adults.* San Diego: Singular.

Krupa, L. (1995). *Minimal contrast stories.* Greenville, SC: Super Duper Publications.

Kunnari, S., & Savinainen-Makkonen, T. (2007). Finnish speech acquisition. In S. McLeod (Ed.), *The international guide to speech acquisition* (pp. 351–363). Clifton Park, NY: Thomson Delmar Learning.

Leahy, J., & Dodd, B. (1987). The development of disordered phonology: A case study. *Language and Cognitive Processes, 2*, 115–132.

LinguiSystems. (2007). *Preschool phonology cards.* East Moline, IL: LinguiSystems.

Masterson, J., & Daniels, D. (1991). Motoric versus contrastive approaches to phonology therapy: A case study. *Child Language Teaching and Therapy, 7*(2), 127–140.

McCauley, R.J. (1993). A comprehensive phonological approach to the assessment and treatment of sound systems disorders. *Seminars in Speech and Language, 14*(2), 153–165.

McLeod, S. (2004). Speech pathologists' application of the ICF to children with speech impairment. *Advances in Speech-Language Pathology, 6*, 75–81.

McLeod, S. (2007). Australian English speech acquisition. In S. McLeod (Ed.), *The international guide to speech acquisition* (pp. 241–256). Clifton Park, NY: Thomson Delmar Learning.

McLeod, S., & McCormack, J. (2007). Application of the ICF and ICF-Children and Youth in children with speech impairment. *Seminars in Speech and Language, 28*, 254–264.

McLeod, S., & Threats, T.T. (2008). The ICF-CY and children with communication disabilities. *International Journal of Speech-Language Pathology, 10*(1–2), 92–109.

Mennen, I., & Okalidou, A. (2007). Greek speech acquisition. In S. McLeod (Ed.), *The international guide to speech acquisition* (pp. 398–411). Clifton Park, NY: Thomson Delmar Learning.

Miccio, A.W., Elbert, M., & Forrest, K. (1999). The relationship between stimulability and phonological acquisition in children with normally developing and disordered phonologies. *American Journal of Speech-Language Pathology, 8*, 347–363.

Miccio, A.W., & Ingrisano, D.R. (2000). The acquisition of fricatives and affricates: Evidence from a disordered phonological system. *American Journal of Speech-Language Pathology, 9*(3), 214–229.

Nathan, L., Stackhouse, J., Goulandris, N., & Snowling, M.J. (2004). The development of early literacy skills among children with speech difficulties: A test of the "critical age hypothesis." *Journal of Speech, Language, and Hearing Research, 27*(2), 377–391.

Olswang, L., & Bain, B. (1994, September). Data collection: Monitoring children's treatment progress. *American Journal of Speech-Language Pathology, 3*, 55–66.

Ota, M., & Ueda, I. (2007). Japanese speech acquisition. In S. McLeod (Ed.), *The international guide to speech acquisition* (pp. 457–471). Clifton Park, NY: Thomson Delmar Learning.

Pavlovic, S. (2007). *Spanish preschool phonology cards.* East Moline, IL: LinguiSystems.

Powell, T.W. (1991, September). Planning for phonological generalization: An approach to treatment target selection. *American Journal of Speech-Language Pathology, 1*, 21–27.

Powell, T.W. (1993). Phonetic inventory constraints in young children: Factors affecting acquisition patterns during treatment. *Clinical Linguistics and Phonetics, 7*, 45–57.

Powell, T.W., & Elbert, M. (1984). Generalization following the remediation of early- and later-developing consonant clusters. *Journal of Speech and Hearing Disorders, 49*, 211–218.

Powell, T.W., Elbert, M., & Dinnsen, D.A. (1991). Stimulability as a factor in the phonological generalization of misarticulating preschool children. *Journal of Speech and Hearing Research, 34*, 1318–1328.

Powell, T.W., Elbert, M., Miccio, A.W., Strike-Roussos, C., & Brasseur, J. (1998). Facilitating [s] production in young children: An experimental evaluation of motoric and conceptual treatment approaches. *Clinical Linguistics and Phonetics, 12*(2), 127–146.

Ray, J. (2002). Treating phonological disorders in a multilingual child: A case study. *American Journal of Speech-Language Pathology, 11*(3), 305–315.

Rippon, H. (2001). *Pairs in pictures 1: Fronting/backing, gliding.* Yorks, England: Black Sheep Press.

Robb, M.P., Bleile, K.M., & Yee, S.S.L. (1999). A phonetic analysis of vowel errors during the course of treatment. *Clinical Linguistics and Phonetics, 13*(4), 309–321.

Ruscello, D.M., Cartwright, L.R., Haines, K.B., & Shuster, L.I. (1993). The use of different service delivery models for children with phonological disorders. *Journal of Communication Disorders, 26,* 193–203.

Rvachew, S. (1994). Speech perception training can facilitate sound production learning. *Journal of Speech and Hearing Research, 37,* 347–357.

Saben, C.B., & Costello-Ingham, J. (1991). The effects of minimal pairs treatment on the speech-sound production of two children with phonologic disorders. *Journal of Speech and Hearing Research, 34,* 1023–1040.

Shriberg, L.D., & Kwiatkowski, J. (1982). Phonological disorders I: A diagnostic classification system. *Journal of Speech and Hearing Disorders, 47,* 226–241.

Smit, A.B. (2007). General American English speech acquisition. In S. McLeod (Ed.), *The international guide to speech acquisition* (pp. 128–147). Clifton Park, NY: Thomson Delmar Learning.

Stampe, D.L. (1969). *The acquisition of phonetic representation.* Paper presented at the Fifth Regional Meeting of the Chicago Linguistic Society, Chicago.

Stampe, D.L. (1979). *A dissertation on natural phonology.* New York: Garland.

Stoel-Gammon, C., & Dunn, C. (1985). *Normal and disordered phonology in children.* Baltimore: University Park Press.

Topbaş, S. (2007). Turkish speech acquisition. In S. McLeod (Ed.), *The international guide to speech acquisition* (pp. 566–579). Clifton Park, NY: Thomson Delmar Learning.

Tyler, A.A. (1995). Durational analysis of stridency errors in children with phonological impairment. *Clinical Linguistics and Phonetics, 9*(3), 211–228.

Tyler, A.A., Edwards, M.L., & Saxman, J.H. (1987). Clinical application of two phonologically based treatment procedures. *Journal of Speech and Hearing Disorders, 52,* 393–409.

Tyler, A.A., Edwards, M.L., & Saxman, J.H. (1990). Acoustic validation of phonological knowledge and its relationship to treatment. *Journal of Speech and Hearing Disorders, 55,* 251–261.

Tyler, A.A., Figurski, G.R., & Langsdale, T. (1993). Relationships between acoustically determined knowledge of stop place and voicing contrasts and phonological treatment progress. *Journal of Speech and Hearing Research, 36,* 746–759.

Tyler, A.A., & Sandoval, K.T. (1994). Preschoolers with phonological and language disorders: Treating different linguistic domains. *Language, Speech, and Hearing Services in Schools, 25,* 215–234.

Webber, S.G. (2005). *Webber photo phonology minimal pair cards.* Greenville, SC: Super Duper Publications.

Weiner, F.F. (1981). Treatment of phonological disability using the method of meaningful minimal contrast: Two case studies. *Journal of Speech and Hearing Disorders, 46,* 97–103.

Weiner, F.F. (1984). A phonologic approach to assessment and treatment. In J. Costello (Ed.), *Speech disorders in children* (pp. 75–91). San Diego: College-Hill Press.

Weiner, F.F., & Ostrowski, A.A. (1979). Effects of listener uncertainty on articulatory inconsistency. *Journal of Speech and Hearing Disorders, 44,* 487–493.

Williams, A.L. (2000). Multiple oppositions: Case studies of variables in phonological intervention. *American Journal of Speech-Language Pathology, 9,* 289–299.

Williams, A.L. (2003). *Speech disorders resource guide for preschool children.* Clifton Park, NY: Thompson Delmar Learning.

Williams, A.L. (2005). Assessment, target selection, and intervention: Dynamic interactions within a systemic perspective. *Topics in Language Disorders, 25*(3), 231–242.

Williams, A.L. (2006). *SCIP—Sound Contrast in Phonology: Evidence-based treatment program.* Greenville, SC: Super Duper Publications.

World Health Organization. (2007). *International classification of functioning, disability and health for Children and youth version (ICF-CY).* Geneva: Author.

Multiple Oppositions Intervention

A. Lynn Williams

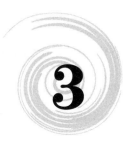

ABSTRACT

Multiple oppositions is a variation of the minimal pair contrastive approach that addresses moderate-to-severe speech disorders in children with speech intelligibility impairments. For children who exhibit sound substitution preferences or error patterns that result in phoneme collapses of several adult targets to a single error production, multiple oppositions provides a systemic approach to target selection and intervention across a rule set, which results in larger contrastive treatment sets. A series of exploratory and efficacy studies indicates that multiple oppositions is a promising intervention in efficiently facilitating systemwide change.

INTRODUCTION

Since the 1990s, greater emphasis has been focused on developing newer models of intervention for children who have speech sound disorders (SSD). This emphasis has largely been in response to the earlier identification of younger children with highly unintelligible speech. It has become increasingly important to find ways to effectively and efficiently remediate SSD given research that has shown the link between SSD and later reading difficulties. In fact, Bishop and Adams (1990) hypothesized that there is a critical age of 5;6 by which unintelligible speech must be resolved in order to significantly reduce academic problems that are often associated with speech disorders. One area of intervention that has been studied since the 1990s has been in the extension of the contrastive approach of minimal pairs (see Chapter 2). Specifically, alternative contrastive approaches have been developed that extend not only what is being contrasted but also how many new target sounds are contrasted simultaneously. Although there is evidence that supports the effectiveness of these approaches (Gierut, 1998; Kamhi, 2006), the question becomes, which is more efficient and therefore most effective? One answer to that question appears to lie in the selection of the targets themselves that are involved in the contrastive intervention (see Chapter 4). In this chapter, the contrastive approach of multiple oppositions is described as an approach that represents an extension of minimal pair therapy but also prescribes the selection of targets that are addressed in intervention through larger treatment sets of contrastive word pairs.

TARGET POPULATIONS

Primary Populations

The multiple oppositions approach has been used primarily with children who have multiple sound errors that originate from a nonorganic basis. According to Shriberg's (1994) classification, this population of children with SSD is characterized as childhood SSD of unknown origin, or simply *speech delay* (SD). The characteristic that distinguishes this subgroup of children from other subgroups of children with SSD is the absence of "clinical involvement of the speech-hearing mechanism or psychosocial processes" (Shriberg, 1994, p. 41). Shriberg and colleagues (2005) reported that SD is the most prevalent subtype of childhood SSD (60%) and proposed that the neurodevelopmental processes that are affected are cognitive-linguistic. Thus, this population of children is likely to have comorbid speech, language, and/or reading impairments.

For this population of children with SSD, the primary concern is speech intelligibility. These children are frequently characterized as having limited sound inventories, often with restricted distribution of available sounds across all word positions and in consonant clusters. Speech unintelligibility results from the presence of homonymy that occurs when the child produces one sound for several different target sounds. For example, a child's production of [tu] could represent a number of different words, such as *two, Sue, shoe, coo, chew,* and *stew.*

In intervention studies, Williams (2000a, 2006c) specifies that the children must be between 36 and 72 months of age and produce at least six sounds in error across three different manner classes of sound production. This represents at least a moderate level of severity of the SSD. In addition to age and severity, the children exhibit typical hearing and intelligence and have normal structure and function of the speech mechanism. Many of the children have concomitant expressive language delays in addition to their SD.

Secondary Populations

Although the majority of children exhibit expressive phonology and language impairments, Donehew and Williams (2005) reported the treatment outcomes of a child, age 7;8, who had a concomitant mixed receptive-expressive language impairment and SSD. Treatment outcomes revealed that although the intervention was effective, the extent of generalization and systemwide change was much lower when compared with children who did not have a receptive language impairment. Specifically, this child increased her productive phonological knowledge (PPK) by 19% compared with an average of 50.8% increase for children without a receptive language impairment. This case reflects similar outcomes to children from a larger intervention study who exhibited receptive language impairments in which the average increase in PPK was 18.1% (Williams & Kalbfleisch, 2001). These findings suggest that although multiple oppositions was an effective approach with these children, mixed receptive-expressive language impairment impacts treatment outcomes.

The contrastive approach, on which multiple oppositions is based, as a broad-based approach that addresses homonymy, has been used within a larger group of children with SSD. Consequently, there would be theoretical support for the application of multiple oppositions to other subtypes of SSD, including Speech Delay-Otitis Media with Effusion (SD-OME), some children characterized as Speech Delay-Apraxia of Speech (SD-AOS), as well as children whose SSD is of known origin, such as Down syndrome. Various studies support the use of contrastive approaches in treating childhood apraxia of speech

(CAS; Forrest, 2002; Forrest & Morrisette, 1999; Williams, Epperly, Rodgers, & Feltes, 1999). Modifications would likely be needed, such as shorter and more frequent sessions, when implementing multiple oppositions with children who represent these other subtypes of SSD.

ASSESSMENT METHODS FOR DETERMINING INTERVENTION RELEVANCE

Multiple oppositions is based on a systemic analysis of a child's speech that provides a child-based description of the error patterns rather than an adult-based description. The Systemic Phonological Analysis of Child Speech (SPACS; Williams, 2003) is a broad-based phonological analysis that includes an independent and relational analysis of the child's speech. Although the SPACS can be completed on smaller single-word samples, such as the Goldman-Fristoe Test of Articulation-2 (GFTA-2; Goldman & Fristoe, 2000), the published intervention studies incorporated the Systemic Phonological Protocol (SPP; Williams, 2003) that includes 245 words that sample all English sounds at least five times in each word position. Based on this single-word sample, an independent analysis provides a description of the child's phonetic inventory, distribution of sounds, and phonotactic constraints (Williams, 1993; 2003). A relational analysis maps the child's system onto the adult system in terms of phoneme collapses, which represent a rule set. The phoneme collapses provide a visual representation of the one-to-many correspondence between the child and adult sound systems that has been described as a characteristic of phonological impairment (Grunwell, 1997), and results in homonymy. These phoneme collapses are viewed as compensatory strategies developed to accommodate a limited sound system. In addition, they reflect the phonetic characteristics of the target sounds that are collapsed to the child's error substitute (Grunwell, 1997; Williams, 2006a). Grunwell referred to this systematicity in a child's sound system as "the order in the disorder" (p. 61). The phoneme collapses provide the basis for designing intervention using a multiple oppositions approach. Finally, the child's PPK is evaluated to determine the percentage of correct underlying representations (PCUR), which quantifies the proportion of the child's sound system that is "known" relative to the adult sound system (Gierut, Elbert, & Dinnsen, 1987; Williams, 1991). PCUR values can then be related to severity categories (Williams, 2000a), which Forrest and Morrisette (1999) reported to be highly correlated to another commonly used measure of severity, the percentage of consonants correct (PCC; Shriberg & Kwiatkowski, 1982), suggesting it provides a valid index of severity (Flipsen, Hammer, & Yost, 2005).

In addition to the SPP single-word sample, a 20-minute conversational speech sample is elicited to examine consistency and overall speech intelligibility. Stimulability testing is also completed using a stimulability probe to evaluate the child's ability to imitate all English consonants in isolation and in syllables (Miccio, 2002; Powell & Miccio, 1996).

THEORETICAL BASIS

Dominant Theoretical Rationale for the Intervention Approach

Grunwell (1997) claimed that sound systems have a phonological function to signal meaning differences. The contrastive elements of language, or the phonological oppositions of a language, are the essential components of languages that make them meaningful. When the contrastivity of phonemes is lost, as in the case of phoneme collapses, homonymy results. That is, two or more words are pronounced alike but have different meanings. The more extensive the phoneme collapse (i.e., the more sounds produced as a single sound by the child), the greater the impact on speech intelligibility. Multiple oppositions directly addresses homonymy through the use of larger treatment sets of contrastive word pairs using sounds that were selected from across the rule set or phoneme collapse.

The larger treatment sets of the multiple oppositions approach incorporate the child's rule, or phoneme collapse, more systemically than would be accomplished by singular contrastive approaches. A singular contrastive approach, such as minimal pairs, selects only one sound to be contrasted, and learned, at a time. Williams (2000b) presented two competing hypotheses that can be considered between singular oppositions, such as minimal pairs, and multiple oppositions. One hypothesis suggests that single oppositions are easier to learn because there is only a single contrast to be learned, so the focus in treatment is greater; there is less semantic load in terms of treatment exemplars; and there are fewer demands on attention and memory. These models of intervention are based on the premise that the target contrast is generalizable to other phonetically similar sounds that are affected by the child's error pattern. Alternatively, the opposing hypothesis suggests that single oppositions would be relatively more difficult to learn and integrate phonemically. Although the child would have only a single new contrast to learn, it is fragmented from a larger, more diverse rule pattern and thus is more difficult to integrate into a new rule set. This second hypothesis suggests that multiple oppositions would present the child with the range and diversity of the new contrasts, which would therefore facilitate discovery of the extent of the new rule to be learned and increase generalization.

The case study reported by Williams (2000b) of a girl (age 3;5) who produced the idiosyncratic error pattern of continuants /w, s, ʃ/ as [l] provides an illustration for these two opposing hypotheses. The implementation of minimal pair therapy, as a test of the first hypothesis, predicts that it would be easier for the child to learn the single new contrast and generalize it to other phonetically similar sounds that were affected by the idiosyncratic error pattern. As the data bear out, however, this was not the case. It was only after the target sounds were integrated into a larger treatment set of contrastive word pairs across the child's error pattern that immediate and significant change occurred. Thus, the alternative second hypothesis correctly predicted that it was easier for the child to integrate the new contrasts phonemically from the diverse rule pattern using multiple oppositions. As shown in this case, learnability of multiple sound contrasts made it easier for the child to systematically reorganize her sound system than when intervention was provided on a single contrast that was isolated from her rule set. Although learning several contrastive oppositions simultaneously requires greater focus and attention to learn the range and extent of the new phonological rule, multiple oppositions directed the child's attention to the entire rule, which appeared to facilitate her learning and integration of the contrasts more efficiently into her sound system.

Although homonymy is a central theoretical tenet underlying the multiple oppositions approach, there is a second critical component; namely the functional and structural aspects of the sounds selected to be contrasted with the child's error substitute. Recall that phoneme collapses were described earlier as reflecting "the order in the disorder" by representing the phonetic resemblance between the target sounds collapsed to the child's error substitute. As such, the phoneme collapses represent compensatory strategies that a child creates to accommodate a limited phonetic inventory. In the case study example provided in the previous paragraph, the child's phonetic inventory restricted the production of fricatives /s, ʃ/ and the glide /w/. It appears that the child attended to the phonetic characteristics that were similar among these target sounds (i.e., continuancy) and grouped them together with a sound within her inventory that had that same phonetic feature of continuancy /l/.

Looking at error patterns from this perspective allows us to see what function, or purpose, these patterns serve in a child's sound system. Intervention that is directed at the functional characteristics of the error patterns will select targets based on the child's organizational strategies in order to more efficiently restructure his or her phonological system. Consequently, targets are not selected based on the dichotomous characteristics of the individual sounds themselves as being early or later developing sounds, stimulable or nonstimulable sounds, or known versus unknown sounds. Rather, selection of the targets directs intervention across the rule set, or phoneme collapse, using a distance metric that emphasizes the phonetic distance among the targets and enlarges the relevant frame of learning that is required (Williams, 2005a; 2005b; 2006a). Specifically, targets are chosen to represent different manner, place, and voice characteristics in order to reflect the range of contrasts that the child must learn. Thus the structural properties of the targets are considered in relation to each other and to the child's error as they function within a phoneme collapse and not as the characteristics of the sounds by themselves. It is assumed that the greater phonetic distance among the targets will fill in the gaps of the child's inventory while also making the targets more salient from each other and from the child's error substitute.

Maximal distinction is a construct advocated by Gierut (1990a) and described as a linguistic principle for clinical intervention (Gierut, 1990b). Specifically, Gierut postulated that it was better to "teach sound pairs that involve maximal oppositions and major class distinctions" (1990b, p. 11) because greater widespread improvement is expected when the trained sounds differ by many features. This principle is based on research that Gierut conducted with the maximal oppositions intervention approach in which she contrasted sound pairs that differed minimally versus maximally and involved major versus nonmajor class distinctions. She reported that the greatest change occurred with maximal oppositions that involved major class distinctions. Although the construct of the sound pairs in maximal oppositions is quite different from multiple oppositions in that maximal oppositions *indirectly* address homonymy, the principle of maximal distinction is still relevant to multiple oppositions.

To conclude, the theoretical basis of the multiple oppositions approach involves two constructs: 1) the function of a phonology to signal differences in meaning through contrastive phonemes in order to avoid homonymy; and 2) selection of intervention targets from across a rule set that represent the function of the phoneme collapse and are maximally distinct from each other in terms of place, voice, and manner, as well as maximally distinct from the child's error substitute, which will serve to increase the saliency of the targets and expand the relevant frame of learning that is required. This theoretical orientation addresses the importance of not only *how* we design intervention, but also the importance of *what* we train as part of the intervention approach.

Levels of Consequences Being Addressed

The International Classification of Functioning, Disability, and Health (ICF; World Health Organization, 2001) provides a framework that integrates social and impairment models in broadening our decision making in considering the health and well-being of adults and children.

The goals within a multiple oppositions approach primarily address Articulation functions (b320) within the compoment of Body Funcions with the goal of improving "speech functions" (McLeod & Threats, 2008). The use of contrastive word pairs has the direct goal of decreasing homonymy, which increases speech intelligibility. In turn, improving intelligibility impacts the child's Activities and Participation by increasing their effectiveness within the domains of Communication (d3), as well as Learning and Applying Knowledge (d1). Although not directly addressed as an intervention goal, a secondary impact of more effective communication involves the personal factor of improving the child's self-confidence.

Target Areas of Intervention

The multiple oppositions approach directly focuses on speech output through the production of contrastive word pairs. Intervention can address substitution errors through production of vowels or singleton consonants, or syllable structure errors involving consonant clusters or deletion of consonants word-initially or word-finally. The following contrastive multiple opposition sets illustrate the types of substitution and syllable structure patterns that can be addressed for target consonants, vowels, and clusters:

1. Substitution errors

    a. Consonant production: *tea:key, see, she*

    b. Vowel production: *eat:it, at*

2. Syllable structure errors

    a. Cluster reduction: *tuck:stuck, truck, cluck*

    b. Word-initial deletion: *eat:Pete, feet, meat, wheat*

    c. Word-final deletion: *bee:beat, beef, bees, beach*

EMPIRICAL BASIS

A framework for evaluating the level of empirical support of effectiveness is to consider studies as part of a programmatic continuum of research (Dollaghan, 2007; Fey, 2002, 2006; McCauley & Fey, 2006). Based on this framework, a distinction is made among exploratory studies, efficacy studies, and effectiveness studies. Intervention approaches that have empirically demonstrated efficacy or effectiveness are classified as evidence-based approaches.

Exploratory Studies

A series of intervention studies investigating the multiple oppositions approach have been conducted. A number of these investigations were exploratory studies that involved case studies. The first case study, Williams (2000b), was described previously as the genesis of the multiple oppositions approach. The girl (3;5 years) demonstrated a moderate-to-severe functional speech disorder. As noted earlier, she exhibited an idiosyncratic substitution error pattern in which she produced [l] for /w, s, ʃ/ word-initially. Following 5 weeks of minimal pair intervention, or 10 sessions, the child exhibited some improvement on target /w/, which was already at 60% accuracy during baseline, with little to no improvement on /s, ʃ/. At that point, intervention was redesigned to address the three targets within larger, integrated contrastive treatment sets of multiple oppositions involving a four-way contrast across the rule set. Significant and immediate improvement occurred in the first session with multiple oppositions. The child met the treatment criterion by the second session for all target sounds, and intervention shifted from word to sentence level with generalization criterion obtained following the third treatment session with multiple oppositions. A second phonological analysis was completed at the end of the academic semester, or 15 intervention sessions (10 minimal pair sessions; 5 multiple oppositions sessions). Systemwide restructuring of her sound system occurred, which involved both treated and untreated sounds. The original phoneme collapses that involved idiosyncratic substitution errors for target fricatives in all three word positions (1:5 phoneme collapse to [l] word-initially; 1:8 phoneme collapse to [h] word-medially; 1:6 phoneme collapse to [x] word-finally) were eliminated ([h] and [x] collapses) or significantly reduced (1:2 collapse to [l]). The child restructured her sound system to incorporate the new fricatives that she added to her phonetic inventory. In addition, the postintervention phoneme collapses reflected a more developmental error pattern as compared with the idiosyncratic collapses before treatment. Although the child's phonological learning was likely facilitated by the initial intervention with minimal pairs for the first 10 sessions, the immediate and significant changes that occurred following the introduction of multiple oppositions suggests that there was validity in implementing a systemic approach that directed intervention across a rule set.

A second case study reported by Cathell and Ruscello (2004) involved a child (age 4;0) who exhibited a severe phonological impairment characterized by a small consonant and vowel inventory, with predominantly deletion errors. Multiple oppositions were introduced to eliminate the word-initial 1:34 phoneme collapse of consonants to null (i.e., initial consonant deletion). Generalization probes and posttreatment measures showed that the child expanded her consonant inventory following twenty-four 50-minute intervention sessions. This, in turn, resulted in the reduction of the 1:34 phoneme collapse of word-initial consonant deletion to a 1:7 phoneme collapse, with phonological restructuring that reflected additional phonetic differentiation from her incorporation of the new sounds into her phonetic repertoire.

Additional exploratory case studies were completed that examined the application of the multiple oppositions approach with children who exhibited co-morbid SSD with language impairment (Marcum & Williams, 2005) and mixed phonetic-phonemic speech disorder (Liles & Williams, 2006). Marcum and Williams reported the outcomes of multiple oppositions with a kindergarten child, LC, age 5;5, who exhibited a severe speech disorder concomitant with moderate expressive language impairment. Multiple oppositions were constructed to address the extensive 1:16 phoneme collapse of nonlabial obstruents and clusters to [d] word-initially. Systemwide change was noted on trained and untrained aspects of her sound system. Particularly, LC's PPK was assessed with a PCUR of 57% prior to intervention, which increased to 83% following the 21 sessions of multiple oppositions. Similarly, the original 1:16 phoneme collapse was eliminated.

In another case study, Liles and Williams (2006) reported the outcome of multiple oppositions with George, age 5;5, a kindergartner who exhibited a severe mixed phonetic-phonemic SSD. George scored below the 1st percentile on the GFTA-2 (Goldman & Fristoe, 2000). His errors consisted primarily of dentalization and stopping of fricatives and affricates in all positions, gliding of liquids, and cluster reduction. Stimulability testing indicated that George was not stimulable on any of his error sounds. A 5-point intelligibility rating scale developed by Bleile (1995) was administered to George's mother, his classroom teacher, and his speech-language pathologist (SLP) prior to intervention. His overall rating was 3.67, which included his mother's rating of 3 (somewhat intelligible) and his teacher and SLP's independent ratings of 4 (mostly unintelligible). Following intervention with multiple oppositions that targeted three primary error patterns in two separate goals, George's postintervention GFTA-2 results indicated that his speech improved from 44 errors initially to 25 errors, which corresponded to a change from the 1st to 6th percentile. This improvement was also reflected in the decrease of the phoneme collapses in which both phoneme collapses were eliminated and his phonological restructuring revealed the presence of smaller 1:2 phoneme collapses that involved stopping of interdental fricatives (i.e., d/ð and t/θ). Intelligibility rating scales completed by his mother, SLP, and kindergarten and first-grade teachers following intervention revealed an average rating of 2.5 (mostly intelligible).

Although these case studies do not provide empirical validation of the effectiveness of the multiple oppositions approach, they are important in demonstrating a replication of treatment effects. Collectively, the case studies describe the course of intervention across different children who represent different profiles with intervention directed at different error patterns and sound targets.

Efficacy Studies

In an experimental study, Williams and Kalbfleisch (2001) used a combined single-subject design of multiple baseline across subjects and across behaviors (Behavior 1 and 2) to investigate the efficacy of the multiple oppositions approach. Fourteen children (mean age 4;9) with moderate-to-severe phonological impairments served as participants in this study and were randomly assigned to the treatment or delayed treatment condition for the multiple baseline across subjects component of the experimental design. Based on the phonological analysis, two error patterns were selected for intervention for each child. Treatment consisted of five contrastive multiple oppositions for each error pattern, and intervention continued for a maximum of 21 sessions or until 90% generalization was achieved on the target sound in untrained items.

For each target, the end-of-treatment mean was compared with the baseline mean with the t-test. The results indicated that the majority of sounds showed significant improvement in 21 treatment sessions or less. Specifically, 77% (37/48) of the sounds treated within Behavior 1 and 97% (38/39) of the sounds in Behavior 2 achieved statistical significance. The pre-post comparison of means for PPK was tested with the paired t-test. Systemwide phonological change was observed as the PPK significantly increased from a mean of 38.7% (pretreatment) to a mean of 62.5% (posttreatment). An increase was observed for each study participant. These results represent an empirical replication of the results reported across the case studies and indicate that the multiple oppositions approach resulted in significant changes on trained as well as untrained aspects of the children's sound systems within a relatively short time period.

Williams (2006a) conducted a comparative study of the efficacy of the multiple oppositions approach relative to minimal pairs. These two approaches provide an examination of complexity of learning with regard to the *size* (larger treatment sets of multiple oppositions versus smaller treatment sets for minimal pairs) and *nature* of the treatment sets (integrated treatment sets of multiple oppositions versus divergent treatment sets of minimal pairs). Further, the teachability of different target sound selection approaches was examined with regard to distributed versus mass practice of targets selected from the children's error patterns. The purpose of the investigation was to examine these two parameters in tandem in the learning outcomes of children with moderate-to-severe SSD.

In a multiple baseline across behaviors design, six children (mean age 5;4) with moderate-to-severe SSD participated in this study. Two phonological goals were selected for each child with the order of the treatment approaches (multiple oppositions and minimal pairs) counterbalanced. Children were randomly assigned to a treatment order. The number of target sounds trained under each treatment approach was controlled in order to avoid differences related simply to the number of sounds trained within each approach. With the multiple oppositions approach, a maximum of four targets were selected from *one rule set*. All multiple oppositions targets necessarily involve distributed practice (targets are distributed across different classes, place, and linguistic unit, yet are integrated within the same rule set). With the minimal pair approach, an equivalent number of targets were selected either from *one error pattern* (massed) or from *different error patterns* (distributed). The distributed or massed practice approach was also randomly assigned but was limited by the presenting error patterns of each child. As a consequence, two children received massed practice whereas four children received distributed practice with the minimal pair approach.

The results were evaluated with regard to three measures of global change: 1) percentage of new or expanded knowledge following each treatment approach, which indicated the proportion of the sound system that moved from *unknown* to *known* level of knowledge relative to ambient sound system; 2) number of sounds that became stabilized after each treatment approach, which is the number of prior sounds produced inconsistently that were then consistently produced correctly; and 3) number of untreated sounds added to each child's phonetic inventory following each treatment approach, which reflected changes in inventory constraints that were not directly treated. Two main results were obtained. First, greater *systemwide change* occurred following multiple oppositions intervention, as indicated by the percentage of new/expanded knowledge (multiple oppositions average percentage of new/expanded knowledge was 17% compared with 4.6% for minimal pairs), as well as by the number of untreated sounds added to the inventory (average of two new untrained sounds for multiple oppositions compared with average of 0.7 new untrained sounds for minimal pairs). Second, greater *stabilization* of inconsistently produced sounds occurred following minimal pair intervention. Specifically, the average number of stabilized sounds after minimal pairs was 3.7 compared with 1.7 following multiple oppositions. That is, whereas multiple oppositions resulted in new knowledge, minimal pairs resulted in *stabilization* of existing knowledge. These findings suggest that the larger, integrated treatment sets of multiple oppositions that involve distributed treatment across classes of sounds within a rule set result in the greatest amount of systemwide change, whereas the divergent treatment sets of minimal pairs result in greater sound stabilization.

Finally, Pagliarin (2009) conducted an efficacy study in Brazil that examined phonological severity and treatment outcomes across three contrastive approaches. Nine Portuguese-speaking children (ages 4;2–6;6) who represented three different levels of severity (mild-to-moderate, moderate-to-severe, and severe), as determined by PCC-revised (PCC-R; Shriberg, Austin, Lewis, McSweeny, & Wilson, 1997), were assigned to one of three intervention groups: minimal pairs (Weiner, 1981), maximal oppositions with two target sounds (also referred to as the empty set; Gierut, 1989, 1991, 1992), or multiple oppositions (Williams, 2000b). One child in each treatment group represented each of the three severity levels, which resulted in crossing the intervention approach with severity. Each child received thirty 45-minute individual sessions in their assigned treatment approach. Pre- and posttreatment phonological analyses were completed to evaluate treatment outcomes across the three approaches with regard to phonetic factors (number of sounds acquired in the phonetic inventory) and phonemic factors (number of phonemes established in the phonological system and number of distinctive features established). The results indicated that although all three approaches were effective, there were differences in treatment outcomes with regard to the phonetic and phonemic measures. Specifically, the minimal pair and empty set approaches resulted in greater phonetic gains with an increase of sounds in phonetic inventory occurring for children with moderate-to-severe and severe impairments. Conversely, the multiple oppositions approach resulted in greater phonemic changes as indicated by the largest acquisition of phonemes in the phonological system and the establishment of more distinctive features for children with moderate-to-severe and severe phonological impairments.

Since the first published study in 2000, the empirical support for multiple oppositions encompasses seven studies, which include a total of 33 children (16 girls, 17 boys) ranging in age from 3;5 to 6;6. Twenty-nine of the thirty-three children participated in experimental efficacy studies whereas the other four children were part of exploratory case studies. All of the children exhibited functional SSD that ranged in severity from mild-to-moderate to profound. The studies included a range of error patterns and sound targets, and in the Pagliarin (2009) study, included Brazilian Portuguese-speaking children in addition to the American English-speaking children of the other studies.

Summary of Levels of Evidence

The level of evidence for studies of multiple oppositions is summarized in Table 3.1. The available evidence base indicates that multiple oppositions is a promising intervention with probable efficacy for creating systemwide change that increases speech intelligibility in children with multiple sound errors.

PRACTICAL REQUIREMENTS

Nature of Sessions

Multiple oppositions has been primarily employed within individual 30–45 minute sessions, although this approach can be implemented within a small-group format. (See SCIP video demonstration in the accompanying DVD [see the videos for Chapter 11] for an example of the multiple oppositions approach within a small group using computer-based intervention). Although the majority of the research studies were conducted in university clinics with a clinician, some of the case studies were carried out in a public school setting.

Personnel

Multiple oppositions intervention is provided by an SLP. In most of the research studies, the treating clinician was a first or second semester graduate student in communicative disorders who was under the direct supervision of a certified SLP clinic supervisor.

Table 3.1. Levels of evidence for studies of treatment efficacy for multiple oppositions

Level	Description	References
Ia	Meta-analysis of > 1 randomized controlled trial	—
Ib	Randomized controlled study	—
IIa	Controlled study without randomization	Pagliarin (2009)
IIb	Quasi-experimental study	Williams (2006c); Williams & Kalbfleisch (2001)
III	Nonexperimental studies, i.e., correlational and case studies	Cathell & Ruscello (2004); Liles & Williams (2006); Marcum & Williams (2005); Williams (2000a)
IV	Expert committee report, consensus conference, clinical experience of respected authorities	—

Adapted from the Scottish Intercollegiate Guidelines Network (http://www.sign.ac.uk).

Although not empirically studied, parents have been engaged as supplementary agents to facilitate change in more naturalistic play activities that are designed to be implemented within typical family routines. Williams (2003) described a parent involvement program in which parents provided models and recasts of the child's target sound(s) during typical daily routines (e.g., meal time, driving to school, going to the grocery store, setting the table, cleaning the dishes, bathtime, bedtime). The activities usually involved turn-taking activities that included a high proportional frequency of occurrence of the target sound(s) and typically lasted about 5–10 minutes. Parents were encouraged to elicit 10–20 responses in each activity. Weekly activities were given to the parents along with a questionnaire on which they reported the previous week's activities, such as frequency of activities, general accuracy and number of responses, what worked or did not work, and any questions or problems that arose.

Dosage

The frequency of the therapy sessions is typically twice weekly. The number of sessions in the intervention studies varied, but typically involved 21 to 42 sessions, as required by the research design. Williams (2000a) reported the longitudinal intervention histories of 10 children (ages 4;0–6;5) with moderate to profound phonological impairments from entry in the university clinic services until dismissal from therapy. All 10 of the children initiated therapy with multiple oppositions, with implementation of other intervention approaches during later phases of intervention (including minimal pairs [see Chapter 2] and naturalistic speech intelligibility training [see Chapter 16]) as the children progressed in therapy and their sound systems improved. The average length of intervention was 60 sessions over 3.4 semesters (approximately 14 months). As expected, children with greater severity generally required longer periods of intervention than children with less severity.

KEY COMPONENTS

Nature of Goals

Research over the past several years has indicated that the decision of what to address in intervention plays an important role in intervention outcomes (Dinnsen & Elbert, 1984; Gierut et al., 1987; Gierut, Morrisette, Hughes, & Rowland, 1996; Rvachew & Nowak,

2001). In the multiple oppositions approach, target selection is directly related to the intervention approach, and both follow directly from the phonological analysis of a child's sound system. Recall that the phonological analysis, SPACS, involves a systemic approach to describing children's sound systems. It is logical, therefore, that target selection and intervention are consistent and congruent with that perspective. In other words, if we analyze a child's sound system from a systemic perspective, theoretical and practical coherence is achieved if we also select intervention targets from a systemic perspective and design intervention to achieve systemic change.

Williams (2003, 2005b, 2006a) described the distance metric as a *systemic approach* to target selection. Essentially two parameters are involved with the distance metric of target selection: 1) maximal classification and 2) maximal distinction. Based on maximal classification, target sounds are chosen that differ with regard to manner of production, place of production, voicing, and linguistic unit. Maximal distinction involves selecting a target sound that is maximally different from the child's error substitute. These represent guidelines for selecting treatment targets and do not prescribe specific sound targets. Other considerations, such as frequency of occurrence of a target sound in English, may result in selection of a target within the guidelines of maximal distinction. However, the primary principle of the distance metric is to choose targets that represent the greatest phonetic distance in order to expand the relevant frame of learning required (maximal classification), as well as to increase the saliency of the contrasts (maximal distinction and maximal classification).

The principle goal of multiple oppositions is to eliminate homonymy by inducing multiple phonemic splits across a phoneme collapse, or rule set. Consequently, the multiple oppositions approach addresses several target sounds from a phoneme collapse, or rule set, within larger contrastive treatment stimuli. Using maximal classification and maximal distinction, up to four target sounds are chosen from one rule set. Depending on the severity of the child's phonological impairment, a phoneme collapse might be relatively small (e.g., 1:4 phoneme collapse) or quite extensive (e.g., 1:17 phoneme collapse). Using the distance metric, two, three, or four targets are selected from one phoneme collapse, which represents one phonological goal in intervention.

It is believed that phonological learning across a rule set increases the relevant frame of learning for the child that is not possible when target sounds are addressed individually within single goals (Williams, 2004). This reveals the part-whole learning dichotomy in which it is assumed that learning of the whole is greater than the sum of its parts (Williams, 2000b). Intervention is directed at phonological reorganization through the systemic selection of several target sounds from the phoneme collapse using a distance metric.

Goal Attack Strategies

In the longitudinal intervention study reported previously (Williams, 2000a), different goal attack strategies (Fey, 1986; McCauley & Fey, 2006) were used throughout the course of each child's intervention program. The horizontal strategy was used at some point with all 10 children, the vertical strategy with one child, and the cyclical strategy with four children. Across the entire intervention period for all children, the horizontal strategy was used for 76% of the treated goals, the cyclical strategy for 18% of the goals, and the vertical strategy for 6% of the targeted goals. Although there is evidence that supports the use of vertical, horizontal, or cyclical goal attack strategies, there are no studies that have examined the comparative benefit of one strategy over another. Williams (2000a), however, proposed a developmental structure in intervention that utilizes different goal attack strategies at different stages of intervention. Specifically, a higher degree of focus using a vertical strategy might be required to establish new productions in the early phases of learning a new sound contrast, although lessening the degree of focus (horizontal or cyclical strategies) might be required to facilitate generalization and help the child expand his or her learning to trained and untrained aspects of their sound system.

Description of Activities

Williams (2000a; 2003) described a treatment paradigm as a structure for implementing the multiple oppositions intervention approach. The paradigm, illustrated in Figure 3.1, provides a framework for establishing criterion levels in therapy to determine when to progress to more complex linguistic levels, as well as generalization criterion levels that provide guidelines for discontinuing intervention on a particular goal. The treatment paradigm is based on the following principles of intervention:

- Opportunities are provided for the child to discover the rule that is being trained.

- Unusually focused therapeutic input is incorporated to reduce the child's search for the new contrast and also reduce demands on attention and memory. This is achieved through a high proportional frequency of occurrence of the target contrast(s) in salient contexts using stress and intonation paired with physical prompts of the new contrast to be learned (e.g., contrasting long and short arm movements coinciding with the production of fricative and stop sounds).

- Opportunities for the child to produce the new contrast in both focused and play intervention activities are provided in order to expose the child to the range and application of the new rule. Meaningful, naturalistic play activities bridge the focused practice of the contrasts.

- Linguistic/communicative feedback is given with regard to the semantic meaning of the child's production.

These psycholinguistic principles address the dual nature of phonologic learning: 1) learning of the new linguistic rule (conceptual) *and* 2) learning of the new articulatory pattern (motoric). The duality of phonologic learning is addressed through the focused practice of the new contrasts with dense response rates in order for the new contrast to become automatic.

The four phases in the treatment paradigm include the following:

1. Familiarization and Production of the Contrasts

2. Production of the Contrasts (Focused Practice) + Interactive Play (Naturalistic Activities)

3. Production of Contrasts with Communicative Contexts

4. Conversational Recasts

The first two phases of the paradigm emphasize familiarization and focused practice, with intervention initiated at an imitative level. In Phase 1, the SLP creates a meaningful context for intervention by familiarizing the child to three important aspects of the inter-

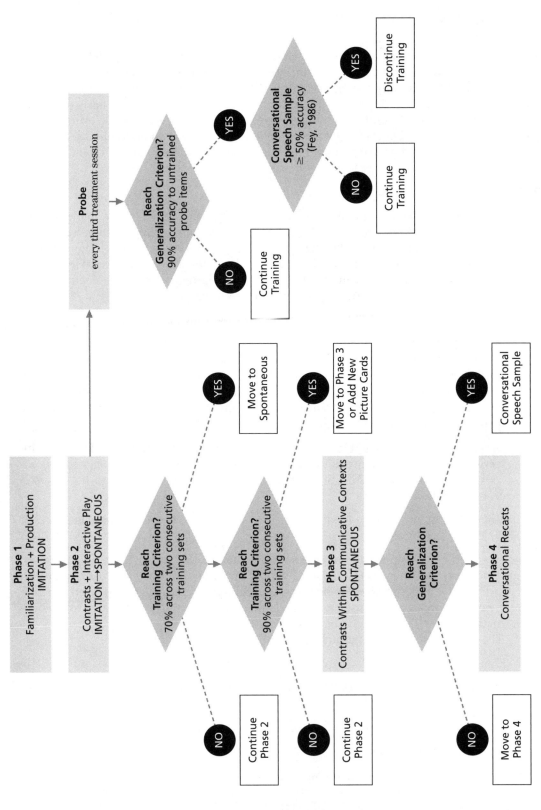

Figure 3.1. Treatment paradigm. (From Williams, A.L. [2000]. Multiple oppositions: Theoretical foundations for an alternative contrastive intervention approach. *American Journal of Speech-Language Pathology, 9,* 282–288; reprinted by permission.)

vention: 1) familiarization of the rule, 2) familiarization of the target sounds, and 3) familiarization of the pictured stimuli and vocabulary. Phase 2 emphasizes the phonetic aspects of sound learning through dense response rates of imitative productions. However, the phonetic practice is linked to the use of the new sound contrast in naturalistic play activities within each session. The later phases (Phase 3 and Phase 4) place more emphasis on the contrastive function of the target sounds within communicative and conversational contexts.

Training and generalization criteria are established within the paradigm to govern progression throughout intervention and determine ultimate discontinuation of intervention on a particular target. A *training criterion* is specified for changing from imitative to spontaneous production in Phase 2, which is 70% accuracy across two consecutive training sets. A training set consists of 20–30 responses depending on the number of contrasts that are being trained. Once the training criterion is achieved at this level, intervention switches to spontaneous production. The new training criterion at this level is 90% spontaneous production across two consecutive training sets. Williams and Kalbfleisch (2001) reported that the majority of target sounds reached the spontaneous level of production by the end of the maximum 21 intervention sessions in an intervention study with 14 children. Specifically, 58% of the targets trained in the first goal reached spontaneous production, and 90% of the targets in the second goal were at the spontaneous level.

Two types of *generalization criteria* are specified within the treatment paradigm: a *narrow generalization* measure based on untrained probe words and a *broad generalization* measure based on conversational speech. The probe, then, serves as a gateway to the conversational sample. If the child achieves 90% accuracy on the 10 untrained probe words, a conversational sample is obtained. This serves as the final criterion for discontinuation of intervention for a specific target. Based on Fey's (1986) recommendation, if the child produces the sound with at least 50% accuracy in spontaneous connected speech, treatment for that sound is terminated.

It is not only important to *measure* generalization, but we must also *program* generalization within intervention in order for it to be achieved by the child. Culatta and Horn (1982) claimed that generalization from clinically structured tasks to conversational speech is achieved by simultaneously programming two aspects of intervention: 1) gradually increasing the situational complexity of the task, and 2) gradually decreasing modeled support provided by the SLP. To facilitate generalization from the focused stimulation of the contrastive oppositions to conversational speech, Figure 3.2 illustrates a continuum that systematically adjusts these two aspects with regard to three components: feedback, focus, and functionality. Specifically, *feedback* in the early phases of intervention (Phase 1 and early Phase 2) is immediate with modeling and recasts (Level I), whereas in the later phases of intervention (later Phase 2, Phase 3, and Phase 4), the feedback is delayed using semantic confusion and wrong clinician models to encourage self-monitoring (Level III). The *focus* of early intervention activities (Phases 1 and 2) is highly salient with increased stress and intonation of the target sounds in salient positions (Level I) and then moves to conversationally appropriate and embedded contexts in low salience activities (Level III) during Phases 3 and 4. Finally, the *functionality* of the early activities involves high communicative structure that require formulaic responses within a closed response set (Level I) in Phases 1 and 2 and later changes to a diverse response set of open-ended responses that require minimal support in low commu-

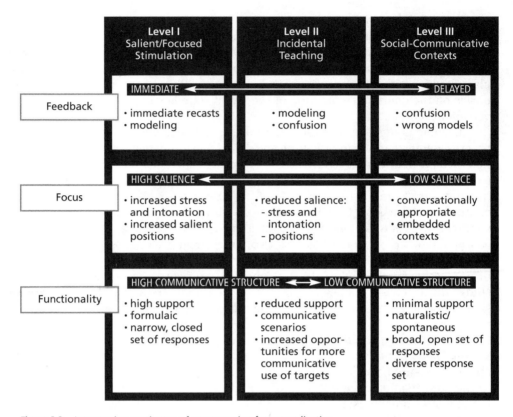

Figure 3.2. Intervention continuum of programming for generalization.

nicatively structured activities (Level III), which are more spontaneous and naturalistic (Phases 3 and 4).

In summary, a treatment paradigm provides a structure for implementing the multiple oppositions approach using clinically structured tasks of focused stimulation within a context that facilitates generalization to spontaneous conversational speech.

Materials and Equipment Required

The multiple oppositions approach incorporates pictured stimuli of real words, although occasionally nonsense words are used to extend available rhyme sets of contrastive target sounds. Based on the findings from Elbert, Powell, and Swartzlander (1991) regarding the number of exemplars children needed to achieve response generalization to a larger, untrained set of items, the number of treatment exemplars used in multiple oppositions intervention is five contrastive sets. Resources for developing the treatment materials include *40,000 Selected Words* (Blockcolsky, Frazer, & Frazer, 1987) to aid in identifying rhyming word pairs for the larger contrastive treatment sets, and card files of pictured stimuli, clip art, or Boardmaker (DynaVox Mayer-Johnson, Pittsburgh, PA) can be sourced for pictures of the words identified for the contrastive rhyme sets. An intervention software program, Sound Contrasts in Phonology (SCIP; Williams, 2006b), was published as a resource for all the contrastive phonological approaches, including multiple oppositions. It includes a database of more than 2,000 real-word illustrations and more than 100 nonsense-word illustrations that the SLP can use to create the larger contrastive rhyme sets for individual intervention goals of targeted sounds contrasted with the child's erred production. Intervention can be conducted at the computer (see Chapter 11), or the illustrations can be printed out for traditional table-top intervention.

ASSESSMENT AND PROGRESS MONITORING TO SUPPORT DECISION MAKING

As described earlier, the treatment paradigm is a data-driven framework that prescribes careful monitoring of the child's therapy performance and generalization learning. Appendix 3A includes a multiple oppositions data sheet that was completed for Adam (a pseudonym). The left side of the data sheet provides space to list the five sets of multiple opposition exemplars. For Adam, the contrastive sets are listed for his goal of [g] ~ /d, f, ʧ, st/ in word-initial position. These five sets are repeated twice for one treatment set of 20–40 responses depending on the number of targets addressed from a rule set (i.e., two, three, or four target sounds). The treatment sets are separated by bold lines with dated columns to indicate the session date. Accuracy of Adam's responses was indicated with a +/− scoring, although the clinician noted accurate though segmented productions with a special notation. At the bottom of each treatment set, space is provided to list the percent accuracy and response level (I: imitative or S: spontaneous) for each target. The data sheet helps structure the therapy sessions to track the number of responses that are obtained and to determine when the child has achieved the training criterion to move from imitation to spontaneous production (Phase 2) or to move to practice within communicative contexts (Phase 3). Because data are collected on each target, the sounds can progress independently through the treatment paradigm.

Generalization learning is monitored through the construction of 10 untrained probe words of each target sound in the trained position. Adam's probe would include 10 untrained words each for word-initial /d, f, ʧ, st/ for a total of 40 words. The probe is administered prior to intervention to establish a baseline of performance and then at the end of every third therapy session. As noted earlier, the probe provides a narrow measure of generalization, which serves as a gateway to obtaining a broad measure of generalization through a conversational speech sample. If the child achieves 90% accuracy on a target sound, then a conversational sample is obtained that provides frequent opportunities to elicit the target. If 50% accuracy in conversational speech is achieved, intervention on that target sound is discontinued.

CONSIDERATIONS FOR CHILDREN FROM CULTURALLY AND LINGUISTICALLY DIVERSE BACKGROUNDS

Although multiple oppositions has primarily been used in the United States with American English-speaking children, it also has been used in Brazil with Brazilian Portuguese-speaking children (Pagliarin, 2009). The contrastive constructs, however, would be applicable for any language.

CASE STUDY

A case study to illustrate the multiple oppositions approach is taken from data presented in Williams (2006c) that included six children with moderate-to-severe phonological impairment. Here, a clinical case involving Adam, a boy age 4;6, will be presented as demonstration of an intervention effect for multiple oppositions. The SPACS (Williams, 2003) was completed on the SPP (Williams, 2003), which revealed a limited phonetic inventory that resulted from the presence of phonotactic inventory, positional, and sequence constraints. Mapping Adam's sound system to the adult system revealed two primary phoneme collapses that represented mirror rules. Specifically, Adam exhibited a 1:17 phoneme collapse of obstruents and stop clusters to [g] word-initially, whereas sonorants and fricative clusters were collapsed to [w] in a 1:6 phoneme collapse word-initially. These two phoneme collapses reflect the symmetry in Adam's sound system between the major sound classes of obstruents and sonorants. Furthermore, these phoneme collapses highlight the phonetic resemblance between the adult sounds and his error substitute: Obstruents and stop clusters were produced as an obstruent stop ([g]), and sonorants and continuant clusters were produced as a continuant sonorant ([w]). Adam's PPK was assessed with a PCUR of 37%, which corresponds to a severity rating of profound. Adam exhibited age-appropriate language skills, as demonstrated by a standard score of 113 on the Peabody Picture Vocabulary Test–Revised (PPVT-III; Dunn & Dunn, 1981) and a mean length of utterance of 3.9, which is within 1 standard deviation for his chronological age.

Based on Adam's SPACS, the 1:17 obstruent and cluster collapse to [g] was addressed. Using the distance metric, the targets /d, f, ʧ, st/ were targeted in contrast to his error substitute, [g], using multiple oppositions. Four sets of multiple opposition exemplars were constructed and included *gear:deer, fear, cheer, steer; go:doe, foe, /ʧoʊ/, stow; goo:dew, foo, chew, stew; gill:dill, fill, chill, still;* and *gain:Dane, feign, chain, stain.* Adam was seen twice weekly for seven individual 50-minute sessions. A dense response rate was achieved with 80–100 responses per session.

Effectiveness of intervention was tested by comparing the baseline mean with treatment performance and calculating effect size using percentage of nonoverlapping data (PND). An intervention effect is observed when there is a clear increase following a stable baseline with little overlap occurring between the baseline and intervention phases. For Adam, he had a baseline mean of 0% accuracy and achieved 100% accuracy on all targeted sounds in seven sessions. The proportion of data points that exceeded the baseline value (i.e., PND) was 70% (52/74), which corresponds to an *effective treatment* (Scruggs & Mastropieri, 1998).

Systemwide change was also examined by calculating the percentage of new or expanded knowledge following intervention and the number of untreated sounds added to Adam's phonetic inventory at the end of intervention. From the assessment of PPK, Adam's PCUR of 37% prior to intervention increased dramatically to 86% following multiple oppositions intervention. This represents a 49% increase in new or expanded phonological knowledge. Interestingly, although narrow measures of generalization learning did not show change, the global measure of learning indicated that intervention affected both trained and untrained aspects of Adam's sound system with the addition of seven new phonemes to his phonetic inventory that were not trained.

Based on the intervention and pre- and posttreatment phonological analysis data, multiple oppositions was an effective approach in restructuring Adam's sound system. Systemwide change occurred within a short time period across both trained and untrained aspects of his sound system.

STUDY QUESTIONS

1. In what ways is the multiple oppositions approach different from the other contrastive intervention approaches?

2 For what children would the multiple oppositions approach be appropriate?

3. How does the distance metric expand the frame of learning for a child?

FUTURE DIRECTIONS

Future research is focused on extending current findings of multiple oppositions to different populations of children with SSD (e.g., children with Down syndrome, cleft palate, hearing impairment) to identify the learning characteristics and determine modifications that may be required. Another area of research is scaling up to larger sample effectiveness studies within school-based environments, in individual and group therapy formats. Finally, comparative research between different intervention models and service delivery formats (computer-based intervention versus traditional table-top intervention) is planned.

SUGGESTED READINGS

Williams, A.L. (2005a). A model and structure for phonological intervention. In S.F. Warren & M.E. Fey (Series Eds.), & A.G Kamhi & K.E. Pollock (Vol. Eds.), *Communication and language intervention series: Phonological disorders in children—Clinical decision making in assessment and intervention* (pp. 189–199). Baltimore: Paul H. Brookes Publishing Co.

Williams, A.L. (2005b). Assessment, target selection, and intervention: Dynamic interactions within a systemic perspective. *Topics in Language Disorders*, *25*(3), 231–242.

Williams, A.L. (2006). A systemic perspective for assessment and intervention: A case study. *Advances in Speech-Language Pathology*, *8*(3), 245–256.

REFERENCES

Bishop, D.V.M., & Adams, C. (1990). A prospective study of the relationship between specific language impairment, phonological disorders, and reading retardation. *Journal of Child Psychology and Psychiatry*, *31*(7), 1027–1050.

Bleile, K.M. (1995). *Manual of articulation and phonological disorders: Infancy through adulthood*. Clifton Park, NY: Thompson Delmar Learning.

Blockcolsky, V.D., Frazer, J.M., & Frazer, D.H. (1987). *40,000 selected words*. San Antonio, TX: Communication Skill Builders.

Cathell, V., & Ruscello, D. (2004). *Sound system disorders: Teaching broad versus deep*. Paper presented at the American Speech-Language-Hearing Association, Philadelphia.

Culatta, B., & Horn, D. (1982). A program for achieving generalization of grammatical rules to spontaneous discourse. *Journal of Speech and Hearing Disorders,* *47,* 174–180.

Dinnsen, D.A., & Elbert, M. (1984). On the relationship between phonology and learning. In M. Elbert, D.A. Dinnsen, & G. Weismer (Eds.)., *Phonological theory and the misarticulating child* (pp. 59–68). ASHA Monographs No. 22, Rockville, MD: American Speech-Language-Hearing Association.

Dollaghan, C.A. (2007). *The handbook for evidence-based practice in communication disorders.* Baltimore: Paul H. Brookes Publishing Co.

Donehew, C., & Williams, A.L. (2005). *The effects of receptive language deficits on phonological treatment outcomes.* Poster session presented at the annual convention of the Tennessee Association of Audiologists and Speech-Language Pathologists, Knoxville, TN.

Dunn, L.M., & Dunn, L.M. (1981). *Peabody Picture Vocabulary Test-Revised.* Circle Pines, MN: American Guidance System.

Elbert, M., Powell, T.W., & Swartzlander, P. (1991). Toward a technology of generalization: How many exemplars are sufficient? *Journal of Speech and Hearing Research, 34,* 81–87.

Fey, M.E. (1986). *Language intervention with young children.* Boston: Allyn & Bacon.

Fey, M.E. (2002, March). *Intervention research in child language disorders: Some problems and solutions.* Paper presented at the 32nd annual Mid-South conference on Communicative Disorders, Memphis, TN.

Fey, M.E. (2006). Commentary on "Making evidence-based decisions about child language intervention in schools" by Gillam and Gillam. *Language, Speech, and Hearing Services in Schools, 37,* 316–319.

Flipsen, P., Jr., Hammer, J.B., & Yost, K.M. (2005). Measuring severity of involvement in speech delay: Segmental and whole-word measures. *American Journal of Speech-Language Pathology, 14,* 298–312.

Forrest, K. (2002). Are oral-motor exercises useful in the treatment of phonological/articulatory disorders? *Seminars in Speech and Language, 23*(1), 15–25.

Forrest, K., & Morrisette, M.L. (1999). Feature analysis of segmental errors in children with phonological disorders. *Journal of Speech and Hearing Research, 42,* 187–194.

Gierut, J.A. (1989). Maximal opposition approach to phonological treatment. *Journal of Speech and Hearing Disorders, 54,* 9–19.

Gierut, J.A. (1990a). Differential learning of phonological oppositions. *Journal of Speech and Hearing Research, 33,* 540–549.

Gierut, J.A. (1990b). Linguistic foundations of language teaching: Phonology. *Journal of Speech Language Pathology Audiology/Revue d'orthophonie et d'audiologie, 14*(4), 5–16.

Gierut, J.A. (1991). Homonymy in phonological change. *Clinical Linguistics and Phonetics, 5,* 119–137.

Gierut, J.A. (1992). The conditions and course of clinically induced phonological change. *Journal of Speech and Hearing Research, 35,* 1049–1063.

Gierut, J.A. (1998). Treatment efficacy: Functional phonological disorders in children. *Journal of Speech, Language, and Hearing Research, 41,* S85–S100.

Gierut, J.A., Elbert, M., & Dinnsen, D.A. (1987). A functional analysis of phonological knowledge and generalization learning in misarticulating children. *Journal of Speech and Hearing Research, 30,* 462–479.

Gierut, J.A., Morrisette, M.L., Hughes, M.T., & Rowland, S. (1996). Phonological treatment efficacy and developmental norms. *Language, Speech, and Hearing Services in Schools, 27,* 215–230.

Goldman, R., & Fristoe, M. (2000). *Goldman-Fristoe Test of Articulation-2.* Circle Pines, MN: American Guidance Service.

Grunwell, P. (1997). Developmental phonological disability: Order in disorder. In B.W. Hodson & M.L. Edwards (Eds.), *Perspectives in applied phonology* (pp. 61–103). Gaithersburg, MD: Aspen Publications.

Kamhi, A.G. (2006). Treatment decisions for children with speech-sound disorders. *Language, Speech, and Hearing Services in Schools, 37,* 271–279.

Liles, T., & Williams, A.L. (2006). *A multiple oppositions approach with a mixed phonetic-phonemic speech disorder.* Poster session presented at the annual convention of the American Speech-Language-Hearing Association, Miami, FL.

Marcum, K., & Williams, A.L. (2005). *Treatment outcomes using multiple oppositions to treat unintelligible speech.* Poster session presented at the annual convention of the Tennessee Association of Audiologists and Speech-Language Pathologists, Knoxville, TN.

McCauley, R.J., & Fey, M.E. (Vol. Eds.). (2006). Introduction to *Treatment of Language Disorders in Children.* In S.F. Warren & M.E. Fey (Series Eds.), *Communication and language intervention series: Treatment of language disorders in children* (pp. 1–17). Baltimore: Paul H. Brookes Publishing Co.

McLeod, S., & Threats, T.T. (2008). The ICF-CY and children with communication disabilities. *International Journal of Speech-Language Pathology, 10*(1), 92–109.

Miccio, A.W. (2002). Clinical problem solving: Assessment of phonological disorders. *American Journal of Speech-Language Pathology, 11,* 221–229.

Pagliarin, K.C. (2009). *Analysis of therapeutic efficacy in three phonological models of contrastive approach.* Unpublished dissertation, Federal University of Santa Maria, Santa Maria, Brazil.

Powell, T.W., & Miccio, A.W. (1996). Stimulability: A useful clinical tool. *Journal of Communication Disorders, 29,* 237–254.

Rvachew, S., & Nowak, M. (2001). The effect of target-selection strategy on phonological learning. *Journal* of Speech, Language, and Hearing Research, 44, 610–623.

Scruggs, T.E., & Mastropieri, M.A. (1998). Synthesizing single subject research: Issues and applications. Behavior Modification, 22, 221–242.

Shriberg, L.D. (1994). Five subtypes of developmental phonological disorders. Clinics in Communication Disorders, 4(1), 38–53.

Shriberg, L.D., Austin, D., Lewis, B.A., McSweeny, J.L., & Wilson, D.L. (1997). The percentage of consonants correct (PCC) metric: Extensions and reliability data. Journal of Speech, Language, and Hearing Research, 40, 708–722.

Shriberg, L.D., & Kwiatkowski, J. (1982). Phonological disorders III: A procedure for assessing severity of involvement. Journal of Speech and Hearing Disorders, 47, 256–270.

Shriberg, L.D., Lewis, B.A., Tomblin, B., McSweeny, J.L., Karlsson, H.B., & Scheer, A.R. (2005). Toward diagnostic and phenotype markers for genetically transmitted speech delay. Journal of Speech, Language, and Hearing Research, 48, 834–852.

Weiner, F. (1981). Treatment of phonological disability using the methods of meaningful minimal contrast: Two case studies. Journal of Speech and Hearing Disorders, 46, 97–103.

Williams, A.L. (1991). Generalization patterns associated with training least phonological knowledge. Journal of Speech and Hearing Research, 34, 722–733.

Williams, A.L. (1993). Phonological reorganization: A qualitative measure of phonological improvement. American Journal of Speech-Language Pathology, 2, 44–51.

Williams, A.L. (2000a). Multiple oppositions: Case studies of variables in phonological intervention. American Journal of Speech-Language Pathology, 9, 289–299.

Williams, A.L. (2000b). Multiple oppositions: Theoretical foundations for an alternative contrastive intervention approach. American Journal of Speech-Language Pathology, 9, 282–288.

Williams, A.L. (2003). Speech disorders resource guide for preschool children. Clifton Park, NY: Thomson Delmar Learning.

Williams, A.L. (2004). A multiple oppositions intervention approach. In K.M. Bleile (Ed.), Manual of articulation and phonological disorders (pp. 331–335). Clifton Park, NY: Thomson Delmar Learning.

Williams, A.L. (2005a). A model and structure for phonological intervention. In S.F. Warren & M.E. Fey (Series Eds.), & A.G Kamhi & K.E. Pollock (Vol. Eds.), Communication and language intervention series: Phonological disorders in children—Clinical decision making in assessment and intervention (pp. 189–199). Baltimore: Paul H. Brookes Publishing Co.

Williams, A.L. (2005b). Assessment, target selection, and intervention: Dynamic interactions within a systemic perspective. Topics in Language Disorders, 25(3), 231–242.

Williams, A.L. (2006a). A systemic perspective for assessment and intervention: A case study. Advances in Speech-Language Pathology, 8(3), 245–256.

Williams, A.L. (2006b). SCIP: Sound Contrasts in Phonology [version 1]. Greenville, SC: Thinking Publications.

Williams, A.L. (2006c). Teachability in phonological intervention: Comparison of two homonymous approaches. Poster presented at the International Child Language Seminar, Newcastle-upon-Tyne, England.

Williams, A.L., Epperly, R., Rodgers, J.R., & Feltes, L. (1999). Treatment efficacy in phonological intervention: Clinical case studies. Paper presented at the American Speech-Language-Hearing Association, San Francisco.

Williams, A.L., & Kalbfleisch, J. (2001, August). Phonological intervention using multiple oppositions. Poster session presented at the 25th World Congress of the International Association of Logopedics and Phoniatrics, Montreal, Canada.

World Health Organization. (2001). International Classification of functioning, disability and health. Geneva: Author.

Appendix 3A

Example of a Multiple Oppositions Data Sheet

° = segmented

Multiple Oppositions Data Sheet

Name ___Adam R.___ Semester/Term ___Fall/2009___

Goal ___g~ d, f, tʃ, st / #___ Clinician ___

Contrast 1	Date 10/29		Date 10/29		Date 11/5		Date 11/5		Date 11/12		Date 11/12	
gear												
deer	—	—	—	—	+°	+°	+°	+°	+°	+°	+	+
fear	—	—	—	—	+°	+°	+°	+°	+°	+°	+°	+°
cheer	—	—	—	—	—	+°	+°	+°	+°	+°	+	+
steer	—	—	—	—	+°	+°	+°	+°	+°	+°	+°	+°
Contrast 2												
go												
doe	—	—	—	—	+°	+°	+°	+°	+°	+°	+	+
foe	—	—	—	—	+°	+°	+°	+°	+°	+°	+°	+°
tʃou	—	+	+	+	+°	+°	+°	+°	+°	+°	+	—
stow	—	—	—	—	—	+°	—	+°	+°	+°	+°	+°
Contrast 3												
goo												
dew	—	—	—	—	+°	+°	+°	+°	+°	+°	+	—
foo	—	—	—	—	+°	+°	+°	+°	+°	+°	+°	+°
chew	+	—	—	—	—	+°	+°	+°	+°	+°	+°	—
stew	—	—	—	—	+°	—	+°	+°	+°	+°	+°	+°
Contrast 4												
gill												
dill	—	—	—	—	—	+°	+°	+°	+°	+°	+	+
fill	—	—	—	—	+°	+°	+°	+°	+°	—	+°	+°
chill	+	+	+	+	—	+°	+°	+°	+°	+°	+	+
still	—	—	—	—	—	—	+°	+°	+°	+°	+°	+°
Contrast 5												
gain												
Dane	—	—	—	—	—	+°	+°	+°	+°	+°	+	+
feign	—	—	—	—	+°	+°	+°	+°	+°	+°	+°	+°
chain	+	—	+	+	—	+°	+°	+°	+°	+°	+	+
stain	—	—	—	—	—	+°	+°	—	+°	+°	+°	+°

Target	Percent Correct	Response Level	Percent Correct	Response Level	Percent Correct	Response Level	Percent Correct	Response Level	Percent Correct	Response Level	Percent Correct	Response Level
d	0 %	Ⓘ S	0 %	Ⓘ S	80 %	Ⓘ S	100 %	Ⓘ S	100 %	I Ⓢ	90 %	I Ⓢ
f	0 %	Ⓘ S	0 %	Ⓘ S	100 %	Ⓘ S	100 %	Ⓘ S	90 %	I Ⓢ	100 %	I Ⓢ
tʃ	50 %	Ⓘ S	60 %	Ⓘ S	60 %	Ⓘ S	100 %	Ⓘ S	100 %	Ⓘ S	80 %	I Ⓢ
st	0 %	Ⓘ S	0 %	Ⓘ S	50 %	Ⓘ S	80 %	Ⓘ S	100 %	Ⓘ S	100 %	I Ⓢ

Complexity Approaches to Intervention

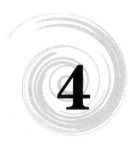

Elise Baker and A. Lynn Williams

ABSTRACT

The complexity approach has a unique focus in that *what* is targeted in intervention may be as important as *how* it is targeted (Gierut, 2005). Attention is given to analyzing children's phonological systems in order to understand what children know about the adult phonological system and what they need to learn. Research findings from the past 20 years guide the careful selection of complex targets. Selected targets expose children to complex aspects of the phonological system, which in turn is predicted to facilitate generalization learning: the efficient widespread change in children's phonological knowledge. Although the efficacy of the approach has been established internationally across 22 published intervention studies, the clinical effectiveness of the approach remains to be examined.

INTRODUCTION

The complexity approach to intervention is based on linguistic principles that govern human languages and the structure and function of phonemes within a language (Barlow & Gierut, 2002). The approach emerged out of a series of studies exploring the role of children's pretreatment knowledge of the phonological system on generalization learning (e.g., Elbert, Dinnsen, & Powell, 1984; Gierut, 1985; Gierut, Elbert, & Dinnsen, 1987; Williams, 1991). The repeated finding across much of the research has been that more complex linguistic input promotes greater learning or change on untreated related targets throughout children's phonological systems (Gierut, 2008b). As the merits of complexity in phonological learning have evolved, the approach has evolved and diversified. During the later 1980s and early 1990s, complexity research focused on the effect of nonhomonymous contrast approaches to intervention (maximal oppositions and treatment of the empty set) containing targets that encompassed global distinctions among multiple dimensions of place, voice, and manner. Research during the late 1990s and 2000s has built on this foundation to consider the impact of various linguistic, psycholinguistic, articulatory-phonetic, and conventional clinical characteristics of intervention targets within a noncontrast format. This chapter addresses these two aspects of the complexity approach: principally intervention targets, and secondarily, intervention approaches.

TARGET POPULATIONS

Primary Populations

The complexity approach was primarily designed for children with a functional phono-logical impairment. That is, children who have a linguistic basis for their speech sound disorder (SSD) that cannot be attributed to a physical difficulty involving oral structures or musculature. Across a number of investigations, children have ranged in age from 2;8 to 7;11, with most children being around 4;0 years of age. They have typically been mono-lingual speakers of English with normal hearing, typical oral and speech motor abilities, and typical intelligence (e.g., Gierut, 1990, 1999; Gierut, Morrisette, Hughes, & Rowland, 1996). Although most of the children have typical receptive and expressive language, Rvachew and Nowak (2001) included a small number of participants who had expressive syntax skills more than 1 standard deviation (*SD*) below the mean. Finally, the children have typically excluded six or more sounds from their phonetic and/or phonemic inven-tories across three manner classes (e.g, Gierut, 1990, 1999) and have scored at least 1 *SD* below the mean on the Goldman-Fristoe Test of Articulation (Goldman & Fristoe, 1986). Overall, the children could be described as having a moderate or severe phonological im-pairment of unknown origin.

Secondary Populations

Whereas the majority of the research on the complexity approach to intervention has fo-cused on preschool-age children with a functional phonological impairment only, Gierut suggested that intervention based on principles of complexity and language learnability "may assist a range of populations and disorder types" (2005, p. 208).

ASSESSMENT METHODS FOR DETERMINING INTERVENTION RELEVANCE

Assessment methods for the complexity approach are appropriate for children who pri-marily have difficulties with phonological content (e.g., limited phonetic inventory) rather than difficulties with phonological frame (e.g., limited word length or stress pat-tern inventory). Thus, assessment for a complexity approach warrants both adequate speech sampling of all segments across word positions, and a comprehensive independ-ent and relational phonological analysis.

A number of word lists have been developed for the purpose of sampling and analyz-ing children's speech so that appropriate complex targets can be identified. Gierut (2008b) included a list of 293 words, known as the Phonological Knowledge Protocol (PKP), which samples "all ambient English consonants in each relevant word position in a minimum of five different exemplars" (Gierut, 1999, p. 712) and "also elicits morpho-phonemically related forms by adding present progressive and diminutive suffixes to base forms so as to probe for the occurrence of systematic alternations" (Gierut, 2008b, p. 44). The majority of the words are mono- or disyllables, with a smaller portion (10 words) constituting three syllables. Another readily available word list is the Onset Cluster Probe (OCP; found in the appendix of Gierut, 1998). The OCP is a 146-item list designed to sample all American English two- and three-element word-initial clusters across a minimum of five different exemplars, including the full range of minimal sonority differences.

Productive Phonological Knowledge

Based on the extensive word list, children's productive phonological knowledge (PPK) is assessed. Gierut (1985) proposed that children can have six types of PPK, ranging on a continuum from most knowledge (accurate across all positions, in all morphemes) to least knowledge (inventory constraints). An important step in the selection of a complex target is ranking a child's PPK along this continuum, as described by Gierut (1985) and Gierut et al. (1987).

The Gierut et al. (1987) approach for ranking PPK has typically been applied to singleton consonants. Additional research has offered an alternative approach for examining a child's PPK of consonant clusters. This approach relies on an understanding of sonority, which is described in the following section.

Sonority

Speech segments have been ranked according to the relative amount of sound, or sonority, they contain, on a numerical sonority hierarchy (Steriade, 1990). Vowels are considered to be the most sonorous with a ranking score of 0, whereas voiceless plosives are considered least sonorous, with a ranking score of 7. Words are composed of sequences of speech segments, most typically (in English) containing a vowel, with or without an onset and/or a coda (e.g., *team:* onset /t/, vowel /i/, coda /m/). The sequencing of speech sounds is believed to follow an order: rising from least sonority through most sonority (the peak, being the vowel) then falling in sonority. This rise and fall in sonority is known as the sonority sequence principle (SSP). Consonant clusters typically conform to the SSP. For example, the word *plant* has a sequence of sonority hierarchy ranks of $7 > 2 > 0 > 3 > 7$. The difference in the ranked score between the two elements in a cluster creates a sonority difference score (e.g., /pl/: 7 ($-$ 2 = 5). Gierut (1999) considered whether consonant clusters have a relative markedness status according to their sonority difference score. She reported that intervention targeting clusters with small sonority difference scores, such as /fl/, facilitated greater widespread generalization to other clusters with the same as well as larger sonority difference scores compared with targeting clusters with small sonority difference scores, such as /tw/. The /s/ + stop clusters /sp, st, sk/ do not abide by the sonority sequencing principle and have been considered to be adjuncts rather than true clusters, and so are not part of such implicational relationships. See Gierut (1999) and Morrisette, Farris, and Gierut (2006) for further discussion of this issue.

Stimulability

One final, yet important, component of a comprehensive assessment is stimulability testing. According to Powell, a "stimulability assessment seeks to determine whether production of an erred sound is enhanced when elicitation conditions are modified (i.e., simplified)" (2003, p. 3). Erred sounds are typically those associated with Type 6 PPK—sounds never produced by a child despite sufficient speech sampling. A child is stimulable for a sound if the sound is produced in isolation or in CV, VCV, VC syllables with at least 20% accuracy after being given auditory and visual cues (Powell, 2003). Stimulability is important to assess because it is thought to reflect some degree of PPK (Dinnsen & Elbert, 1984). If a child is stimulable for a particular speech sound, he or she is thought to have more knowledge than a child who is not stimulable. Studies on the role of stimulability and intervention progress have suggested that greater widespread change is associated with targeting nonstimulable rather than stimulable sounds (Powell, Elbert, & Dinnsen, 1991). Thus, a thorough assessment of a child's speech sound stimulability provides insight into the articulatory phonetic complexity status of a potential intervention target—information that contributes to the ultimate selection of a complex target.

THEORETICAL BASIS

Dominant Theoretical Rationale for the Intervention Approach

The complexity approach draws on three different theoretical perspectives: linguistics, complexity, and learnability theory. A brief overview of each of these theoretical perspectives provides an accumulative theoretical rationale for the complexity approach.

Linguistic Theoretical Framework

Two major constructs within the linguistic framework are important to the complexity approach: 1) distinctive features; and 2) linguistic universals.

Distinctive Features

Distinctive features underlie the concept of a phonological contrast or distinctive opposition (Gierut, 1990). An example helps to illustrate this point. The words *Sue* and *zoo* have different meanings, because the phonemes /s/ and /z/ are distinguished by the feature +/− voice. Furthermore, just as phoneme pairs can be distinguished by a single distinctive feature, phonemes can be grouped into a class, on the basis of their shared features. The natural classes of English consonants include nasals, glides, liquids, stops, fricatives, and affricates. Consonants can also be classified into one of two groups, based on the presence or absence of the major class distinctive feature [+/− sonorant]. Sounds produced with little or no obstruction and with spontaneous voicing are categorized as [+ sonorant] and include nasals, liquids, and glides, whereas sounds that are categorized as [− sonorant] are produced with some level of obstruction, called "obstruents," and include the classes of stops, fricatives, and affricates.

If we look more closely at a range of minimal pair words and the phonemes that serve to contrast the pairs, phonemes can not only be distinguished based on the *nature* of their distinctive feature differences (major/nonmajor class distinctions) but also by the *number* of feature differences. Minimal pairs such as *tip* and *rip* contain a major class distinction because the phonemes /t/ and /ɹ/ represent a distinction between the major classes of obstruent and sonorant. These phonemes also have many other features that differ between them and hence may be described as having maximal feature differences, and as such, a maximal opposition pair.

The clinical application of distinctive feature theory (e.g., Blache, Parsons, & Humphreys, 1981; Dinnsen, Chin, & Elbert, 1992), studies of phonological acquisition (e.g., Menyuk, 1968; Yavaş, 1997), and studies of the world's languages (e.g., Jakobson, Fant, & Halle, 1952; Mielke, 2008) have suggested that not all features are equal. Features seem to be hierarchically organized such that some features (and therefore phonemes) are more or less complex. It is at this point where the concepts of linguistic universals, markedness, and implicational relationships are important to understand.

Linguistic Universals, Markedness, and Implicational Relationships

A linguistic universal is a phonological characteristic or trait across (nearly) all languages. A universal may either be absolute in nature, such as all languages have stops, or a tendency across many languages, such as most languages have at least one phonemic liquid (O'Grady, Archibald, Aronoff, & Rees-Miller, 2005). Extending this idea, the traits or features that are universally rarer (uncommon) across languages are considered to be marked (O'Grady et al.). Marked traits have been reported to be later developing and have been described as more complex. This idea that children gradually acquire features to create increasingly marked phonological contrasts was exemplified by Dinnsen et al. (1990). They reported that a five-level distinctive feature hierarchy (Levels A through E) accounted for the increasing complexity of children's phonetic inventories. It was also apparent that the existence of a more marked feature at a higher level *implied* the existence of a less marked feature at a lower level. An implicational law or relationship is therefore one in which two traits or features are in relationship with one another. Their relationship is hierarchically organized such that the existence of one implies the existence of the other, but not vice versa. Examples of implicational laws include consonants imply vowels, true clusters imply affricates, affricates imply fricatives, fricatives imply stops, liquids imply nasals, and voice obstruents imply voiceless obstruents (Gierut, 2007). In each case the former category is more complex than the latter. This is an important concept to understand as it underlies much of the complexity approach to intervention. Intervention targeting more complex traits or features is thought to facilitate widespread change in children's phonological systems because the existence of the more complex or marked traits implies the existence of the implicationally related less complex trait(s) through phonological generalization. So, what are complex targets? An answer to this question requires an understanding of the concept of complexity.

Complexity

Complexity is a useful, yet somewhat abstract concept for studying systems, the constituent parts of systems, and the way in which parts interrelate with one another (Baker, 2009). Rescher (1998) provided three perspectives for conceptualizing complexity: the epistemic perspective (descriptors that define a system), the ontological perspective (the parts and hierarchical organization of the parts within a system), and the functional perspective (the principles and rules that regulate or govern the working of the system). Consider a speech sound or segment. It is an integral constituent of a hierarchically organized phonological system. It can be described as being made up of a unique set of distinctive features, and it has a function within the system abiding by laws or rules about how it is to relate to other sounds and structures within the system.

In a helpful review of complexity as it relates to phonological learning, Gierut (2007) suggested that Rescher's (1998) epistemic perspective captures the description of a child's phonological system based on a comprehensive assessment and a description of the broad components of intervention required to treat the system. Gierut proposed that the ontological perspective reflects the phonological constituents (e.g., features, segments, syllables) and hierarchical organization of those constituents, whereas the functional perspective reflects lawful phonological principles "that permit variability but maintain systematicity" (2007, p. 7). It is this latter functional perspective of complexity underlying much of Gierut and colleagues' study of the selection of complex targets for inducing change in children's phonological systems. From this functional perspective, a phonological constituent, such as a speech sound, is part of a system—it has a complexity status relative to the other constituents of the phonological system and it abides by lawful relationships (Baker, 2009).

A metaphor for a phonological system may be helpful at this point in understanding the importance of selecting intervention targets. Consider the ranking system of an army—a well-organized hierarchy. If you needed to quickly find out as much as you could about the army, you would talk with the General. You would start with the person at the top who has a rich understanding about many aspects of the organization. You would not necessarily start with a Private at the bottom and work your way up. For a child with a phonological impairment, intervention research suggests that by prioritizing a complex target for intervention, you can help the child learn a lot about the phonological system more efficiently. In other words, if you teach children about the "General" of the phonology system from the outset, you help them learn the system more efficiently. This idea of teaching a child a complex part of a bigger system in order to learn the system is not limited to child phonology (Baker, 2009). The benefit of prioritizing complex targets over simpler targets has been demonstrated in other areas of linguistics such as syntax and semantics (Thompson, 2007).

In the area of child phonology, Gierut proposed four general categories of complexity: "linguistic structure, psycholinguistic structure, articulatory phonetic factors, and conventional clinical factors" (2001, p. 230). A brief summary of the intervention research evidence associated with each of these categories is provided later in this chapter. More detailed overviews have been provided by Gierut (2001, 2007).

Learnability Theory

How do complex targets facilitate change in children's phonological systems? This is where learnability theory (e.g., Pinker, 1984) becomes relevant. According to Gierut, learnability theory "aims to logically and mathematically formulate the possible ways that language can be learned from the input of the surrounding speech community" (2007, p. 7). In simple terms, what a child knows about a phonological system is a subset of what an accomplished speaker of the language knows. The child's task is to learn more and more about the phonological system and the complexities of the system (e.g., the parts and rules governing the relationships among the parts) so that the child's subset grows to match that of the accomplished speaker. Using this basic tenet of learnability, Gierut (2007) suggested that more complex input beyond or outside a child's existing knowledge facilitates phonological learning. The more complex the input *beyond* a child's existing knowledge, the greater the phonological learning. Another metaphor is helpful at this point. Consider a game show in which two contestants are competing to describe a picture on a puzzle. The picture is the face of a celebrity. We could assume that both contestants have one blank corner piece—a subset of the puzzle. Some of the puzzle pieces contain more information about the bigger picture. These pieces are in the middle of the puzzle, beyond their corner subset. The middle pieces might be thought of as the more difficult pieces to start with. If one contestant is given another easy piece that fits next to their current piece (that is, close to his or her current subset of knowledge about the puzzle), they certainly are one step closer to finishing the puzzle, but are not necessarily better informed about the bigger picture on the puzzle. If the second contestant is given the most informative (or complex) puzzle piece (e.g., a picture of the celebrity's eyes), he or she is now much closer to solving the picture. As an added bonus, this contestant also receives the puzzle pieces that fit between his or her current subset and the most informative piece. The second contestant is clearly closer to solving the picture and completing the puzzle. Gierut (2007) would suggest that children with limited phonetic repertoires need to be treated like the second contestant and given more complex input about the phonological system from the outset of intervention, rather than be given targets closer to their current knowledge subset. Indeed, Gierut points out that "it has been shown that simpler input actually makes language learning more difficult because the child is provided with only partial information about linguistic structure" (p. 8). Learnability theory is considerably more involved than this simplistic metaphor suggests. Readers are encouraged to source Gierut (2007) and selected references therein to gain a greater theoretical understanding of how complex inputs facilitate widespread change in children's phonological systems, and how the concepts of complexity, linguistics, and language learnability fit together, much like the pieces of a puzzle, to explain and guide the management of phonological impairment in children.

Levels of Consequences Being Addressed

Complexity approaches to intervention primarily focus on the International Classification of Functioning, Disability and Health for Children and Youth (ICF-CY; World Health Organization [WHO], 2007) component of Body Function and the ICF-CY domain of Articulation Function (b320; McLeod & Threats, 2008). The Children's Activities and Participation domains are not directly targeted in the complexity approach. Notably, some commentators have suggested that complex targets may be less suitable for children who have difficulties with other Body Functions (e.g., perceptual impairments, oral mechanism constraints, language or cognitive impairments), or other Personal Factors (e.g., low motivation or poor self-confidence), and may be more suitable for children who present as confident risk takers (Bernhardt, Stemberger, & Major, 2006; Bleile, 1996). These suggestions require empirical investigation.

Target Areas of Intervention

The majority of the published complexity research to date has targeted children's speech production skills. Broader domains such as speech perception, literacy, or morphosyntax have not been included. Moreover, the majority of the investigations have focused on children's production of singleton consonants (e.g., Gierut, 1989, 1990, 1991, 1992; Gierut et al., 1987; Mota, Begetti, Keske-Sozres, & Pereira, 2005; Mota, Keske-Sozres, Bagetti, Ceron, & Melo Filha, 2007) or word-initial consonant clusters (e.g., Gierut, 1998, 1999; Gierut & Champion, 2001). The clinical application of a complexity account of phonolog-

Table 4.1. Levels of evidence for studies of treatment efficacy for a complexity approach to intervention

Level	Description	References
Ia	Meta-analysis of > 1 randomized controlled trial	—
Ib	Randomized controlled study	Dodd et al. (2008); Rvachew & Nowak (2001)
IIa	Controlled study without randomization	Mota et al. (2007)
IIb	Quasi-experimental study	Dinnsen et al. (1992); Gierut (1989, 1990, 1991, 1992, 1998, 1999); Gierut & Champion (2001); Gierut et al. (1987); Gierut et al. (1999); Gierut et al. (1996); Gierut & Neumann (1992); Morrisette & Gierut (2002); Powell & Elbert (1984); Powell et al. (1991); Tyler & Figurski (1994); Williams (1991)
III	Nonexperimental studies, i.e., correlational and case studies	Morrisette (1999); Mota et al. (2005)
IV	Expert committee report, consensus conference, clinical experience of respected authorities	—

Adapted from the Scottish Intercollegiate Guidelines Network (http://www.sign.ac.uk).

ical learning is yet to be applied to a wider range of phonological difficulties (e.g., syllable deletion, prosodic difficulties). The impact of prioritizing complex speech production targets on children's language and literacy abilities remains to be determined.

EMPIRICAL BASIS

Our review of the empirical support for the complexity approach includes peer-reviewed published intervention research written in English or translated into English on 1) the impact of complex target characteristics (linguistic structures, psycholinguistic structures, articulatory-phonetic factors, conventional clinical factors) on children's phonological systems, and 2) unique intervention approaches associated with complex targets (maximal oppositions, treatment of the empty set). Most of the published intervention research comes from the Learnability Project (http://www.indiana.edu/~sndlrng) conducted by Judith Gierut and colleagues. Twenty-two studies were identified (see Table 4.1).

Complex Target Characteristics Research Outcomes

Complex Linguistic Structures: Singletons and Consonant Clusters

Dinnsen, Chin, and Elbert (1992) reported that minimal pair intervention targeting more complex feature distinctions, such as [strident] or [lateral], was associated with acquisition of less complex distinctions (e.g., [nasal]) in children's phonetic inventories. Tyler and Figurski (1994) prioritized /l/ (i.e., Level E [lateral] distinction) for a child age 2;8. Preintervention the child had nine sounds in his phonetic inventory reflecting Level A and B distinctions only. Postintervention the child added 12 sounds to his phonetic inventory, including the feature distinctions of [continuant], [delayed release], [nasal], and [strident].

Regarding consonant clusters, Powell and Elbert (1984) reported that intervention targeting fricative-liquid clusters implied stop-liquid clusters. Participants' patterns of generalization were also influenced by their prior PPK (Elbert et al., 1984; Powell & Elbert, 1984). In a study of six children, Gierut (1998) reported that the children who received intervention targeting consonant clusters, or consonant clusters in alternation with singleton consonants, evidenced more widespread change compared with the children who received intervention targeting singletons only. Gierut (1999) examined patterns of phonological generalization across 11 children given intervention targeting clusters reflecting different sonority difference scores. She reported that clusters with small sonority differences (e.g., /fl, sl/) implied clusters with larger sonority difference scores (e.g., /kw, tw/). For example, one child (3;8) from Gierut (1999), as further discussed in Gierut (2007), produced no clusters prior to intervention. The intervention target was /bl/ with a sonority difference score of 4. The child learned /tw, kw, pl, bl, sw, fl, sm, sn, sp, st/ in addition to /f, v, θ, ð, s, z, tʃ, h, l, ɹ/, with varying levels of accuracy in response to the intervention. Another child (4;2) was taught /kw/, with a sonority difference score of 6 (relatively less marked/less complex). Although this child did not acquire clusters, he did acquire /ʃ, dʒ/. Gierut and Champion (2001) examined the impact of targeting three-element consonant clusters (e.g., /stɹ, spl/). Using a multiple baseline design across eight participants, Gierut and Champion reported that although all the participants learned the treated three-element cluster, they did not all show generalized acquisition of other related three-element clusters. Notably, however, all the children increased the size of their singleton inventory following intervention and acquired varying combinations of two-element consonant clusters. Gierut and Champion recommended that if three-element clusters are to be targeted, then children should have some phonemic knowledge of a subset of the cluster constituents, ideally, the second and third consonants from a three-element cluster (e.g., spl, str).

In contrast to the findings of Gierut and colleagues, Williams (1991) examined cluster targets in a study of the generalization patterns associated with least PPK in nine children with a phonological impairment. In a multiple baseline design across behaviors with a counterbalanced training order, children received training on word-initial /st/ and /tr/ clusters. Study findings revealed differences in intervention outcomes that were related to phonotactic sequence constraints and minimal production of the singletons /s/ or /r/ on the PKP. Specifically, children who produced at least two correct productions of the singletons /s/ or /ɹ/ and/or who produced two sequential consonants demonstrated greater intervention gains than children who never produced the singletons correctly or did not produce sequential consonants. This suggested that PKP was not a dichotomous category of knowledge/no knowledge, but that children could possess partial knowledge. Furthermore, partial knowledge was related to greater intervention gains than no knowledge, which was contrary to the predictions based on training least knowledge. Thus, although most of the evidence points toward prioritizing two- and three-element consonant clusters over singleton consonants for inducing widespread phonological change (Gierut, 2005), evidence-based guidelines regarding the selection of complex consonant clusters for individual children requires further empirical investigation.

Complex Psycholinguistic Structures

Gierut (2001) proposed that the characteristics of the words used during intervention can have a complexity status. Two characteristics investigated to date include *word frequency* and *neighborhood density*. According to Morrisette and Gierut, "word frequency refers to the number of times a given word occurs in a language" whereas neighborhood density refers to "the number of words that minimally differ in phonetic structure from a given word as based on a one-phoneme substitution, deletion, or addition" (2002, p. 144). Of the relatively limited body of evidence on this issue to date, high-frequency words have been shown to facilitate more widespread improvements in children's phonological systems compared with low-frequency words (Gierut, Morrisette, & Champion, 1999; Morrisette, 1999; Morrisette & Gierut, 2002). By contrast, dense neighborhoods (i.e., words with a high-density count) have been associated with limited or restricted learning. Indeed, Morrisette and Gierut noted that "words from high-density neighborhoods may need to be avoided altogether if an end goal is generalization of any sort" (2002, p. 153). What remains to be well understood is the relative benefit of nonsense word (NSW) stimuli over real word stimuli targeting equally complex targets on phonological generalization. As described later in the chapter, NSWs have been an integral procedure component of much of the intervention research by Gierut and colleagues.

Complex Articulatory Phonetic Factors

Stimulability is presumed to reflect an individual's capacity for articulatory complexity. As noted earlier in the section on assessment, nonstimulable sounds are considered to be more complex and worth priortizing over stimulable sounds, if greater systemwide improvements are to be made (Powell, 2003). Powell, Elbert, and Dinnsen (1991) provide supporting evidence whereas Rvachew and Nowak (2001) provide evidence to the contrary.

Conventional Clinical Factors

In an extensive review of the evidence associated with complex clinical factors, Gierut (2001) identified three key issues to consider: the developmental status of a potential target, the consistency of a particular error, and the number of sounds to be targeted at one point in time.

The Developmental Status of a Target

Using SCED methodology with nine children, Gierut et al. (1996) reported that later acquired sounds facilitated more widespread phonological change compared with earlier developing sounds. They concluded that "a non-developmental approach may be more efficacious in promoting the most widespread and immediate phonological change" (p. 227). In an RCT involving 48 children, Rvachew and Nowak did not unequivocally support this finding. Specifically, Rvachew and Nowak found that the "children made significantly greater progress in therapy when their treatment targets were relatively early developing and associated with relatively greater productive phonological knowledge" (2001, p. 621). They further noted that "there were no between-group differences on our measures of generalization learning or child enjoyment of therapy sessions" (p. 621). In an editorial follow up of this investigation, Morrisette and Gierut (2003) disagreed with Rvachew and Nowak's (2001) findings, suggesting that Rvachew and Nowak's research in fact provided support for later developing, complex targets. In a rebuttal, Rvachew and Nowak refuted this claim stating that "the traditional target selection strategy resulted in superior outcomes, in comparison with the non-developmental strategy, even after controlling for between-group differences in pretreatment productive phonological knowledge" (2003, p. 386). As Rvachew and Nowak noted, "further research is required in order to determine the best means of promoting generalization from treated to untreated phonemes, and this research must employ research designs that include adequate controls for participant and maturation effects" (2003, p. 389).

Consistency of Sounds in Error

In a minimal pair study, Gierut et al. (1987) reported that sounds consistently in error, underpinned by least PPK, facilitated more widespread change compared with sounds of which a child had more PPK. Gierut et al. recommended that intervention prioritize sounds associated with least PPK over those associated with most PPK. The findings from Rvachew and Nowak (2001) and Williams (1991) did not provide unequivocal support for this recommendation.

Number of Sounds Targeted

Intervention targeting two maximally distinct sounds associated with least PPK (i.e., treatment of the empty set) was reported to facilitate greater systemwide changes compared with targeting one sound in a maximal opposition contrast (Gierut, 1991, 1992). These studies also contribute to the nonhomonymous contrast approaches.

Nonhomonymous Contrast Approaches: Maximal Oppositions and Treatment of the Empty Set Research Outcomes

Five published investigations were identified as providing evidence for the maximal opposition approach (Gierut, 1989, 1990, 1992; Mota et al., 2005, 2007) with one study reporting a modified version of maximal oppositions (Dodd et al., 2008). Treatment of the empty set evolved out of the maximal opposition approach. Three studies were identified as providing evidence for this approach (Gierut, 1991, 1992; Gierut & Neumann, 1992). A brief summary of the findings follows.

The first maximal oppositions investigation by Gierut (1989) reported on a boy, "J" (4;7), who was described as having unintelligible speech. For J, the maximal opposition approach involved pairing already known sounds (e.g., /m, b, w/) with a maximally opposing sound /s/ (voiceless, produced in a more posterior place of articulation and reflecting a manner not used by J in word initial position). Real word pairs contrasting these sounds (*sad:mad, sat:mat, see:bee, suit:boot, sail:whale*) were used in twice-weekly 30-minute sessions. After 3 months (23 intervention sessions), J was reported to have learned "16 word-initial consonants following treatment of only three sets of maximal opposition contrasts" (Gierut, 1989, p. 9).

Gierut (1990) extended this first study by comparing minimal oppositions with maximal oppositions in a study of three children with a functional phonological impairment. Using NSWs as treatment words, Gierut reported that "treatment of maximal oppositions led to greater improvement in the children's production of treated sounds, more additions of untreated sounds to the posttreatment inventory, and fewer changes in known sounds than treatment of minimal oppositions" (1990, p. 540).

Gierut (1991) explored the comparative benefits of minimal pairs versus treatment of the empty set in a study of three children. In this study, a more traditional minimal pair approach was used for the minimal opposition condition, in that homonymous word pairs were used (pairing the child's error with the target sound). The later developing sound /θ/ was targeted for all three participants for this condition. The empty set condition paired two sounds unknown to a child, typically an affricate with a fricative. Gierut reported that the empty set condition "resulted in greater accuracies of treated sounds and in more new untreated sounds being added to the phonological system" (1991, p. 127) compared with the homonymous minimal pair condition. She speculated that perhaps children do not need to be exposed to the functional impact of the homonymy in their speech, but to the structural differences between maximal opposition word pairs, to facilitate phonological change.

The potentially confounding variable of targeting /θ/ in the homonymous condition was addressed by Gierut and Neumann (1992) in a single case study. Using an alternating treatments design, a child with a functional phonological impairment received conventional minimal pairs intervention alternating with treatment of the empty set. Gierut and Neumann reported that "regardless of the specific sounds being treated in this or the previous study, it was always the case that the non-homonymous teaching condition was as good as or better than the homonymous condition in inducing sound change" (p. 196).

Gierut (1992) further extended the research on the maximal oppositions and empty set approaches by experimentally manipulating the number and nature of the feature distinctions. Four children served as the participants in this investigation. Using an alternating treatments design, the children received varying combinations of one or two new phonemes (i.e., maximal oppositions or treatment of the empty set) varying according to the nature of the feature distinctions (major class versus nonmajor class). Gierut (1992) reported that the best context for motivating the greater amount of change involved the empty set context in which two unknown phonemes were paired that differed by maximal and major class distinctive features.

The empirical evidence for the maximal opposition and empty set approaches is not limited to Gierut and colleagues. In a study of four children with a mild-to-moderate phonological disorder, Mota et al. (2005) reported that a maximal oppositions approach was effective. Using a between-subjects group design with 21 children, Mota et al. (2007) compared a maximal opposition approach with the Hodson (2007) cycles approach and an intervention targeting a complex target (described as "ABAB-withdrawal and multiple probe"). Mota et al. (2007) reported that the three intervention approaches were equally effective. Notably, the children in the modified cycles group had a less severe impairment relative to the children in the other two groups.

Collectively, the positive empirical evidence for the maximal oppositions and empty set approaches has identified three factors important for facilitating change: 1) the number of feature differences, 2) the nature of the feature differences (major class versus nonmajor class), and 3) the relationship of the selected targets to a child's pretreatment grammar (known versus unknown; Gierut, 1992). In line with notions of complexity and language learnability, it would seem that the more complex each of these factors, the greater the change.

In contrast with the positive findings, Dodd et al. (2008) raised questions about the purported advantage of maximal oppositions over minimal pairs. Dodd et al. randomly assigned 19 children with a moderate-to-severe phonological delay or disorder to one of two intervention conditions: homonymous and nonhomonymous word pairs (referred to as *minimal* and *nonminimal pair* approaches). The intervention was delivered by speech-language pathologists (SLPs) in community clinics under the direction of the Dodd et al. university-based research team. The minimal pair approach contrasted the child's error production with the target. One of the targets common across eight of the nine participants in this group was /s/ consonant clusters in contrastive pairs (e.g., /sp/ and /p/). In the nonminimal pair approach, word pairs contrasted a target with a maximally opposing contrast (typically known or produced by the child). The targets for 5 of the 10 participants in this group included consonant clusters (e.g., /st/ with /m/). Dodd et al. reported that although all participants evidenced considerable progress (based on a variety of measures, including percent consonants correct), there was no difference in the outcomes between the groups. Dodd et al. noted that "the small amount of intervention provided [6 hours], irrespective of whether it used minimal or non-minimal contrasts, resulted in improvement that seems to exceed that usually reported for maximal contrasts therapy, particularly when number of therapy hours is considered" (p. 343). It is important to underscore that the Dodd et al. nonminimal pair approach differed theoretically and procedurally from Gierut's (1992) maximal opposition approach. For instance, the theoretical approach for analyzing and identifying suitable intervention targets differed. All targets prioritized for intervention across both groups in the Dodd et al. study were stimulable. The Dodd et al. approach used real words, as opposed to NSWs, and they also included consonant clusters as intervention targets, which have not traditionally been a feature of maximal opposition research. If meaningful comparisons are to be made, then different research teams need to adopt a uniform method for conducting, measuring, and reporting outcomes.

Summary of Levels of Evidence

Using the American Speech-Language-Hearing Association (2004) guidelines regarding the levels of evidence, adapted from the Scottish Intercollegiate Guideline Network, two of the 22 studies identified could be classified as randomized controlled trials (RCTs), one as a controlled study without randomization, 17 as quasi-experimental investigations, and two as case studies. All of the quasi-experimental investigations used single-case experimental design (SCED) methodology. Across the studies, the majority could be described as efficacy studies (experimentally controlled studies typically conducted within university clinics), with a smaller portion of exploratory case studies (e.g., Mota et al., 2005) and one effectiveness study (Dodd et al., 2008).

PRACTICAL REQUIREMENTS

Nature of Sessions

Based on a review of the literature listed in Table 4.1, the complexity-based intervention approaches have typically been delivered by SLPs in one-to-one/individual session format in university speech and hearing clinics. Intervention sessions have typically been conducted for 30 or 60 minutes, three times per week. In the study by Dodd et al. (2008), sessions were conducted for 30 minutes once per week. As Dodd et al. noted, many SLP services cannot provide 1-hour intervention sessions three times per week. A challenge remains to determine the most efficient intervention session frequency and duration.

Personnel

The literature on complexity-based approaches to intervention has typically reported outcomes delivered by qualified SLPs who work in university clinics. Community-based SLPs conducted the intervention in the Dodd et al. (2008) study, under the guidance of a university-based research team. Parents and/or caregivers have typically been involved informally, in the form of carrying out homework (e.g., Gierut et al., 1996). The efficacy and effectiveness of complexity-based intervention delivered by personnel other than qualified SLPs remains to be determined.

Dosage

Across the literature, experimental investigations of complexity have typically been conducted for predetermined periods of time. For example, much of the research to emerge from Gierut and colleagues' Learnability Project has used a predetermined duration of up to 19 hours (based on 1-hour intervention sessions conducted three times per week). In the study by Dodd et al. (2008), 6 hours of intervention was provided. Such differences raise important issues for SLPs. How long should intervention persist on a complex intervention target? How much change can typically be expected within a prescribed number of SLP hours? The dosage required to achieve intelligible speech from the point of referral to the point of dismissal requires further investigation.

KEY COMPONENTS

Nature of Goals

The intervention goals are one of the defining traits of the complexity approach. Indeed, Gierut (2005) suggested that the goal or what is targeted may be more important than how targets are taught. The centrality of the target within this approach was noted previously in the theoretical section. In summary, intervention targets are typically consonants or consonant clusters that are linguistically complex, nonstimulable, later developing, consistently in error, and reflect least PPK for an individual child (Gierut, 2001, 2007). For a maximal opposition approach, a known consonant is paired with an unknown maximally contrastive consonant (differing by as many distinctive features as possible, including major class distinctions). For treatment of the empty set, two sounds reflecting least PPK for a child are selected. The two sounds need to be maximally contrastive with respect to the number of feature differences and the nature of those differences (major class distinctions). See Gierut (1992) for a helpful discussion and evidence-based examples.

For intervention targeting consonant clusters, the clusters ideally have relatively small sonority difference scores. Based on Gierut (1999), these consonant clusters might be /fl, sl, fr, θr, ʃr/. As discussed earlier, Gierut and Champion (2001) recommended that children have knowledge of the second and third consonant cluster constituents when prioritizing three-element consonant clusters. See Morrisette, Farris, and Gierut (2006) for a helpful, case-based discussion. Gierut (2004) also provides a helpful step-by-step case-based account for selecting and prioritizing complex intervention targets.

Goal Attack Strategies

A complexity-based approach to intervention generally uses a sequential goal attack strategy to induce widespread change in children's phonological systems. This means that typically one or two carefully selected singleton consonants or clusters are targeted for a period of time until predetermined performance criteria have been met. Elbert and Gierut (1986) proposed that a sequential strategy provides children with the opportunity for massed practice so that individual targets are given the opportunity to be learned and the accuracy of their production stabilized.

Description of Activities

For the nonhomonymous contrast approaches, eight NSW *pairs* are developed in accordance with individual children's needs and abilities. In Gierut's study, the "phonetic composition of the NSW pairs was consistent with English phonotactics and contrasting phonemes were always presented in the word-initial position" (1992, p. 1052). For example, if contrasting /l/ with /m/, word pairs could be [lib~mib], [lɛm~mɛm], and [lænu~mænu]. The NSW pairs are subsequently assigned lexical meaning via stories. According to Gierut, the "nonwords correspond to characters' names or unusual objects or actions that take place in the stories" (2008a, p. 105).

Intervention is conducted in two phases: imitation followed by spontaneous production. During the imitation phase, a child is instructed to repeat the clinician's production of each word. The clinician provides feedback regarding the accuracy of the child's production, including corrective models. The imitation phase continues until the child achieves 75% accuracy over two consecutive sessions, or until seven sessions have been completed (Gierut, 2008a). During the spontaneous phase, the child is instructed to produce the same treatment words independently without a model. Within experimental investigations, this phase continues until the child reaches 90% accuracy over 3 consecutive sessions, or until a further 12 sessions have been completed (Gierut, 2008a). Clinically, SLPs would need to devise a predetermined performance criteria, such as 50% accuracy in conversational speech, before stopping intervention on a selected target (e.g., Williams, 2000). Intervention activities during the imitation and spontaneous phases have included "a variety of conceptually based activities: sorting, matching, informal story telling, and disambiguation of word pairs" (Gierut, 1992, pp. 1052–1053).

Protocols similar to those used for nonhomonymous contrast approaches have been used in noncontrast studies targeting consonant clusters (e.g., Gierut, 1999; Gierut & Champion, 2001). Up to 16 NSWs serve as the treatment word stimuli, containing strategically selected word-initial consonant clusters. In the Gierut (1999) study, the words were phonotactically permissible, balanced for canonical structure, phonetic environment, and syntactic category (eight nouns and seven verbs). A variety of word shapes may be used, such as CCVC, CCVCV, and CCVCVC. In keeping with the maximal opposition procedure, the NSWs are assigned lexical meaning via a story. The picture stimuli for the NSWs can be displayed on flash cards and may be used during production practice activities (Gierut, 1999). Two phases are used: imitation followed by spontaneous production. The criteria for progressing from one phase to the next are identical to the criteria outlined in the maximal oppositions/empty set procedure.

Materials and Equipment Required

A complexity approach to intervention requires picture stimuli in conjunction with materials for conducting drill-play style activities. As noted previously, NSW stimuli are an integral component of most published procedures. SLPs would consequently need to create or source suitable picture stimuli using existing card files, Internet clip art, or Boardmaker (Mayer-Johnson, Pittsburgh, PA). Sound Contrasts in Phonology (SCIP; Williams, 2006) is a commercially available resource containing 100 different nonsense illustrations, designed to suit maximal oppositions, treatment of the empty set, or intervention targeting consonant clusters.

ASSESSMENT AND PROGRESS MONITORING TO SUPPORT DECISION MAKING

According to Gierut (2008a), evaluation of an intervention program is integral to the delivery of an intervention program. Conclusions regarding the effectiveness of the approach can therefore not be made without the regular collection and evaluation of phonological generalization data. Indeed, changes in a child's system may be observed in generalization data prior to observing improvements on a target consonant or cluster (Gierut, 2007). Identifying important changes in generalization data may persuade SLPs to continue with intervention rather than conclude that intervention was not working and/or modifying clinical decisions.

Generalization probes need to be developed for each child to monitor and detect changes in an individual child's system. Ideally, probes should be administered in accordance with a predetermined scheduled. According to Gierut (2008a), the schedule may be fixed (e.g., every third session) or variable (e.g., sessions 1, 2, then 6, being on average, every third session). The probe stimuli needs to consider both within- and across-class generalization, taking into account expected changes based on implicational relationships. Gierut suggested that "multiple renditions of each relevant sound and cluster are elicited to prevent lexical binding, and multiple copies of the probes are used longitudinally to prevent stimulus binding" (2008a, p. 107). Probes also need to consider generalization across word positions and generalization from single words to conversational speech. It may also be helpful to monitor the effect of intervention on children's speech intelligibility. This could be done through a child's parent/caregiver regularly completing a 5-point intelligibility rating scale. Qualitative evaluation of positive changes in a child's activity or participation may also add to an evaluation of the effects of complexity-based intervention. Readers are encouraged to review Gierut (2008a) for helpful guidelines on developing, administering, and evaluating children's performance on individualized generalization probes.

CONSIDERATIONS FOR CHILDREN FROM CULTURALLY AND LINGUISTICALLY DIVERSE BACKGROUNDS

Internationally, the complexity approach to intervention has been reported to be used in Brazil and across a number of English-speaking countries. Of the different procedural approaches associated with complex targets, maximal oppositions would have to be the most widely used approach. Specifically, the maximal opposition approach has been used with children who speak General American English (Gierut, 1990), British English (Joffe & Pring, 2008), Australian English (McLeod & Baker, 2004), and Brazilian Portuguese (Mota et al., 2005, 2007).

Intervention targeting complex clusters for the express purpose of facilitating widespread phonological change has also been reported to be used with children who speak General American English (Gierut, 1999; Gierut & Champion, 2001; Powell & Elbert, 1984; Williams, 1991), Australian English (Baker, 2007), and Spanish (Anderson, 2002). Theoretically, there are no limits to the languages to which a complexity approach could be applied. Implicational relationships apply across languages. The clinical application of the principles of complexity would, however, need to be guided by the phonological characteristics of an individual child, the characteristics of his or her language, and the relevant implicational relationships.

CASE STUDY

Barlow and Gierut (2002) presented the clinical case of Joseph (age 4;1) who exhibited a functional phonological impairment with normal hearing, intelligence, receptive and expressive language skills, and oral-motor structure and function. His phonetic inventory was limited to stops, nasals, glides, and the fricatives /f, v/, which reflected a phonotactic inventory constraint that restricted the presence of affricates, liquids, and fricatives, with the noted exception of labiodental fricatives. These inventory constraints formed the pool from which a potential treatment target would be selected. Based on findings from Gierut (1990, 1991, 1992), it was predicted that the greatest generalization would occur when two unrelated sound targets were chosen from the set of inventory constraints that involve both maximal feature differences and a major class distinction. Given Joseph's phonetic inventory, it was predicted that the most effective intervention would involve treatment of the empty set contrasting /s/ ~ /ɹ/ word-initially. These two sounds represent maximal feature differences with regard to all three dimensions of place, voice, and manner of production. They also represent a major class distinction with /s/ being an obstruent ([−sonorant]) and /ɹ/ being a sonorant ([+sonorant]). Treatment of the empty set approach could contrast /s/ ~ /ɹ/ in NSWs (Gierut, 1992) or real words, as used in the video demonstration with Noah (see accompanying DVD). Using real words, contrastive word pairs might include *sun~run, sew~row, sigh~rye, sight~write,* and *sip~rip.* Because /s/ and /ɹ/ represent unrelated error patterns, the contrastive word pairs would not be produced as homonyms by Joseph. For example, Joseph's production of *sip~rip* would be [tɪp]~[wɪp]. As a consequence, intervention would not be directed at disambiguating the homonymous productions or incorporate semantic confusion as the basis for motivating the sound change in Joseph's phonology. Rather, the phonemic distinctiveness of the two new sounds being contrasted was considered to be the critical agent for change; and homonymy, as hypothesized by Barlow and Gierut, "may not be a necessary component in phonological change" (2002, p. 63). An alternate goal for Joseph might have been the consonant cluster /sl/, which represents a small sonority difference score of 3. It is predicted that clusters, such as /sl/, will facilitate greater widespread generalization to other clusters of equal, as well as, greater sonority difference scores. Based on Gierut (1999), NSWs could be used for the treatment exemplars, such as [slɪb], [slɛm], [slæd], [slɛk], [slʌn], [slɔt], [slup], [slog], [slɪmɔ], [slʌgu], [slɔbi], [slɛdu], [sludəm], [slænɛk], and [slikog] in a noncontrastive format.

STUDY QUESTIONS

1. Describe a plan for monitoring Joseph's progress in response to empty set intervention.

2. Explain why consonant clusters with small sonority differences rather than large sonority differences have been associated with more widespread phonological change. Use the data from Subjects 2, 5, and 6 in Gierut (1999) to exemplify your answer.

3. Why is the concept of implicational relationships important to an understanding of the complexity approach?

FUTURE DIRECTIONS

The complexity approach to intervention has a relatively long history in the field of speech-language pathology. Grounded in the innovative work of linguistic pioneers such as Jakobson, Chomsky, and Halle, experimental investigations have discovered a theoretically motivated, yet clinically counterintuitive phenomenon: More complex input rather than less complex input seems to promote the greatest change in children's phonological systems (Gierut, 2008b). If past investigations are an indication of the future, the complexity approach will continue to evolve as theoretical insights transpire. Dinnsen and Gierut's (2008) publication *Optimality Theory, Phonological Acquisition and Disorders* provides an interesting window into this future. Gierut notes that "in future research, it may be fruitful to reconsider the available findings on complexity, from the view of optimality theory and the ranking of constraints" (2008b, p. 117). Future research may also consider the benefit of targeting more complex word lengths or stress patterns for children who have difficulties with the frame rather than content.

As such theoretically innovative discoveries are made, the clinical implications and application of the complexity approach merit investigation. Based on surveys of SLPs' methods of practicing when working with children with SSD, some SLPs would seem to be reluctant to apply the findings from the complexity approach, preferring to make clinical decisions in keeping with experience and tradition (McLeod & Baker, 2004) and preferring to select easier targets for children who are shy or have concomitant difficulties (Murray, 2006).

If the apparent gap between complexity intervention research and clinical practice is to be narrowed, future research on the approach could examine the role of individual children's personal-social and cognitive-linguistic factors on intervention outcomes, both as experimentally controlled efficacy investigations and as less controlled effectiveness studies of SLPs' clinical practice. Such investigations could include children with varying clinical profiles from more linguistically diverse backgrounds. Future research could also explore the role of clinical expertise on complex-based intervention outcomes. According to Kamhi, "clinical expertise in speech-language pathology is defined not only by technical, procedural and knowledge-based (intellectual) qualities, but by interpersonal and attitudinal qualities as well" (1994, p. 117). In light of the work of Chall (1967), it could be that SLPs not only need to know and understand the empirical basis for the approach, but have an instinctive belief (as opposed to counterintuitive belief) in the approach for positive outcomes to be achieved. Given the reports on the literacy outcomes for children with a history of SSD (Nathan, Stackhouse, Goulandris, & Snowling, 2004), it would also be important to consider the relative benefits of the complexity approach with and without evidence-based emergent literacy activities.

Finally, future research on the complexity approach could investigate the impact of prioritizing complex targets on the whole child—including functional measures of speech intelligibility and changes in a child's activity and participation. Although the approach may not initially lead to immediate success, it would be important to capture the relative efficiency with which significant and positive changes occur in the everyday lives of children.

SUGGESTED READINGS

Barlow, J.A., & Gierut, J.A. (2002). Minimal pair approaches to phonological remediation. *Seminars in Speech and Language, 23*(1), 57–67.

Gierut, J.A. (1992). The conditions and course of clinically induced phonological change. *Journal of Speech and Hearing Research, 35*, 1049–1063.

Gierut, J.A. (1999). Syllable onsets: Clusters and adjuncts in acquisition. *Journal of Speech, Language, and Hearing Research, 42*, 708–726.

Gierut, J. (2001). Complexity in phonological treatment: Clinical Factors. *Language, Speech, and Hearing Services in Schools, 32*, 229–241.

Gierut, J.A. (2004, Summer). Clinical application of phonological complexity. *CSHA Magazine*, 6–7, 16.

Gierut, J. (2005). Phonological intervention: The how or the what? In M.E. Fey & S.F. Warren (Series Eds.) & A.G. Kamhi & K.E. Pollock (Vol. Eds.), *Communication and language intervention series: Phonological disorders in children—Clinical decision making in assessment and intervention* (pp. 201–210). Baltimore: Paul H. Brookes Publishing Co.

Gierut, J. (2007). Phonological complexity and language learnability. *American Journal of Speech-Language Pathology, 16*(1), 6–17.

Gierut, J.A. (2008a). Fundamentals of experimental design and treatment. In D.A. Dinnsen & J.A. Gierut (Eds.), *Optimality theory, phonological acquisition and disorders* (pp. 93–118). London: Equinox.

Gierut, J.A., & Champion, A.H. (2001). Syllable onsets II: Three-element clusters in phonological treatment. *Journal of Speech, Language, and Hearing Research, 44*, 886–904.

Morrisette, M.L., Farris, A.W., & Gierut, J.A. (2006). Applications of learnability theory to clinical phonology. *Advances in Speech-Language Pathology, 8*(3), 207–219.

REFERENCES

American Speech-Language-Hearing Association. (2004). *Evidence-based practice in communication disorders: An introduction* [Technical Report]. Retrieved March 4, 2009, from http://www.asha.org/docs/html/TR2004-00001.html

Anderson, R.T. (2002). Onset clusters and the sonority sequencing principle in Spanish: A treatment efficacy study. In F. Windsor, M.L. Kelly, & N. Hewitt (Eds.), *Investigation in clinical phonetics and linguistics* (pp. 213–224). Mahwah, NJ: Lawrence Erlbaum Associates.

Baker, E. (2007, May). *Using sonority to explore patterns of generalization in children with phonological impairment*. Paper presented at the Speech Pathology Australia National Conference, Sydney, Australia.

Baker, E. (2009). The why and how of prioritizing complex targets for intervention. In C. Bowen (Ed.), *Children's speech sound disorders* (pp. 72–77). Oxford, England: Wiley-Blackwell.

Barlow, J.A., & Gierut, J.A. (2002). Minimal pair approaches to phonological remediation. *Seminars in Speech and Language, 23*(1), 57–67.

Bernhardt, B.H., Stemberger, J.P., & Major, E. (2006). General and nonlinear phonological intervention perspectives for a child with a resistant phonological impairment. *Advances in Speech-Language Pathology, 8*(3), 190–206.

Blache, S.E., Parsons, C.L., & Humphreys, J.M. (1981). A minimal-word-pair model for teaching the linguistic significance of distinctive feature properties. *Journal of Speech and Hearing Disorders, 46,* 291–296.

Bleile, K.M. (1996). *Articulation and phonological disorders: A book of exercises* (2nd ed.). San Diego: Singular Publishing.

Chall, J. (1967). *Learning to read: The great debate.* New York: McGraw-Hill.

Dinnsen, D.A., Chin, S.B., & Elbert, M. (1992). On the lawfullness of change in phonetic inventories. *Lingua, 86,* 207–222.

Dinnsen, D.A., Chin, S.B., Elbert, M., & Powell, T.W. (1990). Some constraints on functionally disordered phonologies: Phonetic inventories and phonotactics. *Journal of Speech and Hearing Research, 33,* 28–37.

Dinnsen, D.A., & Elbert, M.A. (1984). On the relationship between phonology and learning. In D.A. Dinnsen, M.A. Elbert, & G. Weismer (Eds.), *Phonological theory and the misarticulating child* (pp. 59–68). Rockville, MD: American Speech-Language-Hearing Association.

Dinnsen, D.A., & Gierut, J.A. (Eds.). (2008). *Optimality theory, phonological acquisition and disorders.* London: Equinox Publishing.

Dodd, B., Crosbie, S., McIntosh, B., Holm, A., Harvey, C., Liddy, M., et al. (2008). The impact of selecting different contrasts in phonological therapy. *International Journal of Speech-Language Pathology, 10*(5), 334–345.

Elbert, M., Dinnsen, D., & Powell, T. (1984). On the prediction of phonological generalization learning patterns. *Journal of Speech and Hearing Disorders, 49,* 309–317.

Elbert, M., & Gierut, J.A. (1986). *Handbook of clinical phonology: Approaches to assessment and treatment.* San Diego: College-Hill Press.

Gierut, J.A. (1985). *On the relationship between phonological knowledge and generalization learning in misarticulating children.* Unpublished doctoral dissertation, Indiana University, Bloomington, IL.

Gierut, J.A. (1989). Maximal opposition approach to phonological treatment. *Journal of Speech and Hearing Disorders, 54,* 9–19.

Gierut, J.A. (1990). Differential learning of phonological oppositions. *Journal of Speech and Hearing Research, 33,* 540–549.

Gierut, J.A. (1991). Homonymy in phonological change. *Clinical Linguistics and Phonetics, 5,* 119–137.

Gierut, J.A. (1992). The conditions and course of clinically induced phonological change. *Journal of Speech and Hearing Research, 35,* 1049–1063.

Gierut, J.A. (1998). Natural domains of cyclicity in phonological acquisition. *Clinical Linguistics and Phonetics, 12*(6), 481–499.

Gierut, J.A. (1999). Syllable onsets: Clusters and adjuncts in acquisition. *Journal of Speech, Language, and Hearing Research, 42,* 708–726.

Gierut, J. (2001). Complexity in phonological treatment: Clinical factors. *Language, Speech, and Hearing Services in Schools, 32,* 229–241.

Gierut, J.A. (2004, Summer). Clinical application of phonological complexity. *CSHA Magazine, 6–7,* 16.

Gierut, J. (2005). Phonological intervention: The how or the what? In S.F. Warren & M.E. Fey (Series Eds.), & A.G. Kamhi & K.E. Pollock (Vol. Eds.), *Communication and language intervention series: Phonological disorders in children—Clinical decision making in assessment and intervention* (pp. 201–210). Baltimore: Paul H. Brookes Publishing, Co.

Gierut, J. (2007). Phonological complexity and language learnability. *American Journal of Speech-Language Pathology, 16*(1), 6–17.

Gierut, J.A. (2008a). Fundamentals of experimental design and treatment. In D.A. Dinnsen & J.A. Gierut (Eds.), *Optimality theory, phonological acquisition and disorders* (pp. 93–118). London: Equinox.

Gierut, J.A. (2008b). Phonological disorders and the developmental archive. In D.A. Dinnsen & J.A. Gierut (Eds.), *Optimality theory, phonological acquisition and disorders* (pp. 37–92). London: Equinox.

Gierut, J.A., & Champion, A.H. (2001). Syllable onsets II: Three-element clusters in phonological treatment. *Journal of Speech, Language, and Hearing Research, 44,* 886–904.

Gierut, J., Elbert, M., & Dinnsen, D. (1987). A functional analysis of phonological knowledge and generalisation learning in misarticulating children. *Journal of Speech and Hearing Research, 30,* 462–479.

Gierut, J.A., Morrisette, M.L., & Champion, A.H. (1999). Lexical constraints in phonological acquisition. *Journal of Child Language, 26,* 261–294.

Gierut, J.A., Morrisette, M.L., Hughes, M.T., & Rowland, S. (1996). Phonological treatment efficacy and developmental norms. *Language, Speech, and Hearing Services in Schools, 27,* 215–230.

Gierut, J.A., & Neumann, H.J. (1992). Teaching and learning /th/: A non-confound. *Clinical Linguistics and Phonetics, 6*(3), 191–200.

Goldman, R., & Fristoe, M. (1986). *Goldman-Fristoe Test of Articulation–Revised.* Circle Pines, MN: American Guidance Service.

Hodson, B.W. (2007). *Evaluation and enhancing children's phonological systems: Research and theory to practice.* Greenville, SC: Thinking Publications.

Jakobson, R., Fant, G., & Halle, M. (1952). *Preliminaries to speech analysis: The distinctive features and their correlates (MIT Acoustics Laboratory Technical Report 13).* Cambridge, MA: The MIT Press.

Joffe, V., & Pring, T. (2008). Children with phonological problems: A survey of clinical practice. *International Journal of Language and Communication Disorders, 43*(2), 154–164.

Kamhi, A.G. (1994). Research to practice: Toward a theory of clinical expertise in speech-language pathology. *Language, Speech, and Hearing Services in Schools*, *25*, 115–118.

McLeod, S., & Baker, E. (2004). Current clinical practice for children with speech impairment. In B.E. Murdoch, J. Goozee, B.M. Whelan, & K. Docking (Eds.), *Proceedings of the 26th World Congress of the International Association of Logopedics and Phoniatrics*. Brisbane: The University of Queensland.

McLeod, S., & Threats, T.T. (2008). The ICF-CY and children with communication disabilities. *International Journal of Speech-Language Pathology*, *10*(1), 92–109.

Menyuk, P. (1968). The role of distinctive features in children's acquisition of phonology. *Journal of Speech and Hearing Research*, *11*(1), 138–146.

Mielke, J. (2008). *The emergence of distinctive features*. Oxford, England: Oxford University Press.

Morrisette, M.L. (1999). Lexical characteristics of sound change. *Clinical Linguistics and Phonetics*, *13*(3), 219–238.

Morrisette, M.L., Farris, A.W., & Gierut, J.A. (2006). Applications of learnability theory to clinical phonology. *Advances in Speech-Language Pathology*, *8*(3), 207–219.

Morrisette, M.L., & Gierut, J. (2002). Lexical organization and phonological change in treatment. *Journal of Speech, Language, and Hearing Research*, *45*, 143–159.

Morrisette, M.L., & Gierut, J.A. (2003). Unified treatment recommendations: A response to Rvachew and Nowak. *Journal of Speech, Language, and Hearing Research*, *46*(2), 382–385.

Mota, H.B., Begetti, T., Keske-Sozres, M., & Pereira, L.F. (2005). Generalization based on implicational relationships in subjects treated with phonological therapy. *Pro-Fono Revista de Atualizacao Cientifica, Barucri (SP)*, *17*(1), 99–110.

Mota, H.B., Keske-Sozres, M., Bagetti, T., Ceron, M.I., & Melo Filha, M.G.C. (2007). Comparative analyses of the effectiveness of three different phonological therapy models. *Pro-Fono Revista de Atualizacao Cientifica, Barucri (SP)*, *19*(1), 67–74.

Murray, E. (2006). *The impact of interactive EBP workshops on speech-language pathologists' selection of treatment targets*. Unpublished honours thesis, The University of Sydney.

Nathan, L., Stackhouse, J., Goulandris, N., & Snowling, M.J. (2004). The development of early literacy skills among children with speech difficulties: A test of the 'Critical age hypothesis.' *Journal of Speech, Language, and Hearing Research*, *27*(2), 377–391.

O'Grady, W., Archibald, J., Aronoff, M., & Rees-Miller, J. (2005). *Contemporary linguistics: An introduction* (5th ed.). Boston: Bedford/St. Martin's.

Pinker, S. (1984). *Language learnability and language development*. Cambridge, MA: Harvard University Press.

Powell, T.W. (2003). Stimulability and treatment outcomes. *Perspectives on Language Learning and Education*, *10*(1), 3–6.

Powell, T.W., & Elbert, M. (1984). Generalization following the remediation of early-and later-developing consonant clusters. *Journal of Speech and Hearing Disorders*, *49*, 211–218.

Powell, T.W., Elbert, M., & Dinnsen, D.A. (1991). Stimulability as a factor in the phonological generalization of misarticulating preschool children. *Journal of Speech and Hearing Research*, *34*, 1318–1328.

Rescher, N. (1998). *Complexity: A philosophical overview*. New Brunswick, NJ: Transaction.

Rvachew, S., & Nowak, M. (2001). The effect of target-selection strategy of phonological learning. *Journal of Speech, Language, and Hearing Research*, *44*, 610–623.

Rvachew, S., & Nowak, M. (2003). Clinical outcomes as a function of target selection strategy: A response to Morrisette and Gierut. *Journal of Speech, Language, and Hearing Research*, *46*(2), 386–389.

Steriade, D. (1990). *Greek prosodies and the nature of syllabification (Doctoral dissertation, Massachusetts Institute of Technology, 1982)*. New York: Garland Press.

Thompson, C.K. (2007). Complexity in language learning and treatment. *American Journal of Speech-Language Pathology*, *16*(1), 3–5.

Tyler, A.A., & Figurski, G.R. (1994). Phonetic inventory changes after treating distinctions along an implicational hierarchy. *Clinical Linguistics and Phonetics*, *8*(2), 91–107.

Williams, A.L. (1991). Generalization patterns associated with training least phonological knowledge. *Journal of Speech and Hearing Research*, *34*, 722–733.

Williams, A.L. (2000). Multiple oppositions: Case studies of variables in phonological intervention. *American Journal of Speech-Language Pathology*, *9*, 289–299.

Williams, A.L. (2006). *SCIP: Sound Contrasts in Phonology—Evidence-Based Treatment Program*. Greenville, SC: Super Duper Publications.

World Health Organization. (2007). *International classification of functioning, disability and health: Children and youth version (ICF-CY)*. Geneva: Author.

Yavaş, M. (1997). The effects of vowel height and place of articulation in interlanguage final stop devoicing. *International Review of Applied Linguistics*, *35*, 115–125.

Core Vocabulary Intervention

Barbara Dodd, Alison Holm,
Sharon Crosbie, and Beth McIntosh

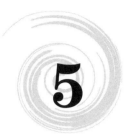

5

ABSTRACT

Core vocabulary intervention establishes consistent word production for functional speech sound disorders (SSD) characterized by inconsistent pronunciation of the same lexical item, in the absence of childhood apraxia of speech (CAS). The intervention is suitable for children 2 years of age and older, including those from bilingual backgrounds and those with a cognitive disability. Children are seen twice weekly for 30 minutes, for about 8 weeks. Daily practice, requiring support from caregivers, focuses on a specifically selected vocabulary of around 70 functionally powerful words. Each week, children learn to produce their best pronunciation of up to 10 of these words consistently, in isolation and connected speech. Nontreated probes measure generalization of consistency. Efficacy studies reveal gains in consistency and accuracy of speech production.

INTRODUCTION

Children with SSD differ in severity, the types of errors they make, and their response to specific intervention approaches. Given the complexity of speech processing, it is not surprising that impairments to different abilities cause differences in speech output (Duggirala & Dodd, 1991). The three interactive domains include input processing (sensation, perception), cognitive-linguistic abilities (phonological representation, derivation of language-specific phonological constraints), and output processing (assembly of phonological plans or templates, phonetic planning and articulation). This chapter focuses on intervention for children who have an impairment in phonological assembly: an impaired ability to plan the sequence of phonemes that make up a word, in the absence of any oro-motor signs of CAS. The impairment results in inconsistent pronunciation of the same word.

TARGET POPULATIONS

Primary Populations

The primary population for core vocabulary is children with inconsistent SSD. Inconsistency characterized by multiple error types (unpredictable variation among a relatively large number of phones) indicates pervasive speech processing difficulties (Grunwell,

1982) and is a potential indicator of persistent SSD (Forrest, Elbert, & Dinnsen, 2000). Children who make inconsistent speech errors pronounce the same words and phonological features differently not only from context to context, but also within the same context (Holm & Dodd, 1999; McCormack & Dodd, 1996). For example, one 7-year-old boy (Dodd, Holm, Crosbie, & McIntosh, 2006) was likely to pronounce the same word differently each time he said it (e.g., *tongue* [bʌns], [dʌn], [bʌʔm]; *witch* [bw:: ætʃ], [bwæ], [bwɛʔt]; *zebra* [dʒeuwa], [jeiʊa] [jeʔdwʌ]).

Approximately 10% of children with SSD make inconsistent errors. For example, Broomfield and Dodd (2004) assessed 320 English-speaking children with SSD, finding that 30 (9.4%) pronounced at least 40% of 25 words differently when they were asked to name the same pictures on three separate trials in one assessment session, each trial separated by a different activity. Cross-linguistic evaluations have identified about the same percentage of children with inconsistent speech in a range of languages, indicating that the impairment in the speech processing chain is not dependent on the phonology being learned (see Holm, Crosbie, & Dodd, 2005, for review).

Differential Diagnosis: Inconsistent Speech Sound Disorders and Childhood Apraxia of Speech

Table 5.1 summarizes clinical opinion (Forrest, 2003) and research (reviewed by Ozanne, 2005) concerning criteria for the diagnosis of CAS. The characteristics of errors made by children with inconsistent SSD are drawn from Holm et al. (2005). Two symptoms are shared among children with CAS and children with inconsistent SSD: inconsistent errors and increasing errors with increased word length. The two groups are discriminated, however, by two important differences. Children with CAS have oro-motor problems that result in inappropriate oral movements during speech (e.g., groping) and affect speech prosody, rate, and fluency. Children with inconsistent SSD do not show these symptoms. Children with CAS make more errors in imitation than they do in spontaneous production. The opposite is true of children with inconsistent SSD: They make fewer errors in imitation than in spontaneous production.

Table 5.1.   Differential diagnosis of childhood apraxia of speech and inconsistent speech disorder

CAS	Inconsistent speech disorder
Inconsistent errors	Inconsistent errors
Increasing errors with increasing length	Increasing errors with increasing length
Poor sequencing of sounds (e.g., metathesis)	Wrong choice of phoneme rather than order errors as in metathesis
Inability to imitate sounds, better spontaneously than in imitation	Better in imitation than in spontaneous production
General oro-motor difficulties	Oro-motor skills within normal limits
Groping, silent posturing	No groping, no silent posturing
Prolongations and repetitions of speech sounds	No prolongations and repetitions of speech sounds
Slow speech and DDK rates	Normal speech and DDK rates

Key: CAS, childhood apraxia of speech; DDK, diadochokinetic.

Secondary Populations

Core vocabulary has been trialed with children as young as 2 years as well as with preschool and school-age children with a functional SSD who make inconsistent errors. The approach has also been successfully used with a bilingual child (Holm & Dodd, 1999) and children who have Down syndrome (Dodd, McCormack, & Woodyatt, 1994). Broomfield and Dodd's (2005) randomized controlled trial (RCT) indicated that children with inconsistent SSD made most progress if core vocabulary intervention occurred when they were 3 years old. Early intervention is possible for children who make inconsistent errors because their low intelligibility means that they tend to be referred early (Broomfield & Dodd, 2004). Identification of inconsistent SSD requires assessment of multiple productions of the same words in the same phonetic context.

ASSESSMENT METHODS FOR DETERMINING INTERVENTION RELEVANCE

Research indicates that children who score 40% or higher on the Inconsistency subtest of the Diagnostic Evaluation of Articulation and Phonology (DEAP; Dodd, Crosbie, Zhu, Holm, & Ozanne, 2002) benefit from core vocabulary intervention. In this assessment children are asked to name 25 pictures (e.g., *girl, dinosaur, elephant*) on three trials within one session. Each trial is separated by another activity. A word produced identically (regardless of accuracy) on all three trials receives a score of 0 for that word. A word produced differently on at least one of the trials receives a score of 1 for that word. The child's score, for all words produced three times, is converted to a percentage, with a score of 40% being the criterion for diagnosis. The 40% criterion is justified by consistency of production data from typically developing children and children with SSD (Holm, Crosbie, & Dodd, 2007; McCormack & Dodd, 1998). More detailed information regarding describing inconsistency is outlined in Holm et al. (2005).

For these children, describing and analyzing inconsistent speech errors in terms of error patterns is not possible, and deciding what to target in intervention is difficult (Dodd & Bradford, 2000). Forrest et al. stated that intervening with children who make inconsistent errors is problematic because

> One may not know the appropriate sound to use in contrast to the error. This may mean that children with a variable substitution will fare worse in treatment than other children because the available protocols for this population are not as effective as other procedures. (2000, p. 529)

An alternative intervention, core vocabulary, has been developed to target consistency (rather than accuracy) of whole-word production (Dodd & Iacono, 1989).

THEORETICAL BASIS

Dominant Theoretical Rationale for the Intervention Approach

When children begin to produce recognizable words, at around 12 months, their phonology is idiosyncratic. It is characterized by a great deal of individual variation in the phones used, phonetic variability of production, and inconsistency of error types

(Grunwell, 1982). Ferguson and Farwell (1975) concluded that children's initial phonology is whole-word based. They argued that "a phonic core of remembered lexical items and articulations which produce them is the foundation of an individual's phonology" (p. 437).

Ingram (1976) claimed that once children's vocabularies begin to expand past 50 words, phonological error patterns (e.g., stopping, fronting) begin to occur across lexical items, suggesting reorganization from a whole-word to a segmental phonological system. Similarly Velleman and Vihman (2002) argued that although initially there are no consistent error patterns, this is followed by a stage characterized by dominant production patterns attributed to the development of word templates. The templates are abstract phonetic production patterns that integrate the adult target with the child's most common vocal patterns, resulting in explicit word learning.

Reorganization of their phonological system from whole words to phonemic segments seems to occur by most children's second birthday. By 3 years mean inconsistency of word production is 13% and by 4 years it is 6% (Holm, Crosbie, & Dodd, 2007). About 10% of those referred for assessment of suspected SSD, however, continue to make inconsistent errors while showing no oro-motor signs of CAS. Their speech is often unintelligible, even to adults interacting with them daily. Caregivers cannot learn how children say particular words because their productions are inconsistent. What type of impairment in speech processing underlies inconsistent speech errors? A series of experiments compared groups of children who make inconsistent errors but have no symptoms of CAS with typically developing children and those who make consistent speech errors (for a summary of published results, see Dodd, Holm, Crosbie, & McCormack, 2005).

Case History Factors

Fox, Howard, and Dodd (2002) examined parental reports of risk factors for 66 children with SSD according to types of surface speech errors and for 48 controls. Positive family history was statistically higher for the SSD group than controls but did not discriminate among subgroups. A reported family history of communication difficulty, however, was the only risk factor for children who consistently made atypical errors (e.g., backing, bilabial fricatives for clusters). According to parental reports, children with delayed phonological development were more likely than other groups to have a history of multiple middle ear infections. Children who made inconsistent errors were more likely to have a reported history of prenatal or perinatal complications (e.g., resuscitation, maternal infections, preterm birth). This finding is intriguing given the literature on phonological disorder in aphasia. An impairment in phonological planning (termed *phonological assembly* in Berndt & Mitchum, 1994) is reported to underlie inconsistent speech errors in adults with acquired speech difficulties that cannot be attributed to dyspraxia.

Input Processing

Studies of auditory processing abilities on children with SSD have yielded contradictory results (Bird & Bishop, 1992), probably due to the assessment of heterogeneous populations. One study (Thyer & Dodd, 1996) investigated the auditory processing skills of 30 children with SSD (10 phonologically delayed, 10 consistently using atypical error patterns, and 10 making inconsistent errors) and 30 typically developing controls. None of the SSD groups performed differently from the matched controls on standard auditory-processing assessments of speech discrimination, auditory figure–ground separation, or binaural integration. The findings indicate that auditory processing difficulties are unlikely to be a general explanation for SSD.

Cognitive Linguistic Processing

Lexical Impairment

The relationship between phonology and the size of the lexicon is important given that consistent production of words occurs once the lexicon reaches a critical size, and that children with larger lexicons produce a wider range of speech sounds and speech sound sequences (Storkel & Morrisette, 2002). One experiment (Dodd et al., 2005) compared the expressive vocabulary performance of subgroups of SSD on the Hundred Pictures Naming Test (Fisher & Glenister, 1992). Children with an inconsistent disorder performed more poorly than all the other subgroups. No other differences among the subgroups were significant. This finding might reflect a word-finding difficulty. Qualitative analysis of errors indicated that 46% of the inconsistent children's errors were semantically related to the target word, compared with 28% of the controls' errors, 33% of the delayed children's errors, and 33% of the consistent children's errors. That is, the children who made inconsistent errors often seemed to know what the picture was, but couldn't access the phonological shape of the word. An impaired ability to access full phonological specifications of words might contribute to inconsistent word production.

Linguistic Knowledge

An experiment tested the preference for phonological legality in subgroups of children with SSD and controls (Dodd, Leahy, & Hambly, 1989). Children had to choose between two nonsense words to give names to pictures of animals. The 12 nonsense word pairs differed by one phoneme that made one of the words phonologically legal and the other phonologically illegal. For example, /slætʃi/ is legal, whereas /svætʃi/ is illegal because /sv/ does not occur in Australian English. Only the children who consistently made atypical errors showed no preference for legal nonsense words. There were no significant differences among the other three groups.

Another experiment (Holm, Farrier, & Dodd, 2007) measured the syllable segmentation, rhyme awareness, and alliteration awareness of 61 preschool children: 46 with SSD and 15 typically developing controls. Children who made inconsistent errors performed poorly on the syllable segmentation task but no differently from controls on the other two tasks. In contrast, the children who made consistent atypical errors showed poor performance on rhyme and alliteration but appropriate performance on syllable segmentation.

The findings of these two experiments indicate that children who made inconsistent errors had relatively strong phonological awareness skills. In contrast, children who consistently made atypical errors had phonological awareness impairments that were associated with reading difficulties. The children who made inconsistent errors, however, had specific difficulty with syllable segmentation. If their underlying impairment was one of phonological planning, they would have difficulty assembling words for subvocal rehearsal. Subvocal rehearsal is an essential step in a number of phonological awareness tasks. For example, it allows the counting of how many syllables there are in *statistical.*

Output Processing

Bradford and Dodd (1996) compared their subgroups' abilities to establish motor plans for words to investigate the nature of the impairment underlying the inconsistent subgroup's variable production of words. A nonsense word learning task was used to assess children's ability to generate and execute motor plans. An attractively illustrated book, depicting the story of the *Three Little Pigs* was used. Each pig was given a legal disyllabic nonsense name (i.e., [paɪzi], [ʃɪlæk], and [neɪdæl]) that was modified to allow accurate production for each child. To differentiate visually between the pigs, who were portrayed 10 times throughout the book, one wore glasses, one wore a tie, and one wore a hat. The children learned the names of the three pigs. The story was told and children were encouraged to imitate the nonsense names. The children then had to tell the story. Spontaneous production of each test word was elicited five times. Children's comprehension of the names was assessed by asking them to point to named characters.

The inconsistent group performed more poorly than the other three groups on the expressive naming task. The control, delayed, and consistent groups performed equally well. Comparison of the four subgroups' performance on the receptive task showed that the groups performed equally well, although there was a trend for the inconsistent group to perform more poorly. The finding that children who made inconsistent errors had a more general motor-planning problem raises the question about the nature of their impairment.

Interpretation

Velleman and Vihman (2002) argued for a word "template" that contains the phonological specifications for word production—a phonological plan. The phonological plan, assembled when children have derived the wrong phonological constraints, results in a pronunciation that differs from both the target adult form and the developmental error form of a typically developing child of the same age. Nevertheless, the errors made, and therefore the phonological plan assembled, are the same when children pronounce the same word on different occasions and when the same phonological feature is produced in different words (e.g., using a bilabial fricative to mark consonant clusters).

In contrast, the evidence reviewed in this section leads to the conclusion that children whose speech is characterized by inconsistent errors may have difficulty selecting and sequencing phonemes (i.e., in assembling a phonological template or plan for production of an utterance). Their phonological knowledge seems intact: It is unlikely that they have an input or cognitive linguistic difficulty. They do not have oro-motor difficulties: It is unlikely that they have phonetic planning or implementation difficulties. Their impairment appears to be at the level of phonological planning.

Levels of Consequences Being Addressed

The World Health Organization (2001) classification of functioning, disability and health is relevant for speech-language pathology and specifies the need for clinicians to address impairment of Body Functions, Activities and Participation (McLeod & McCormack, 2007). Core vocabulary intervention focuses on the impairment underlying the functional limitation of unintelligible speech. Targeting the underlying impairment leads to improved intelligibility that enhances children's communication (Activity) and their academic and social skills (Participation).

Target Areas of Intervention

Core vocabulary intervention targets an underlying impairment in the speech processing chain: the ability to generate consistent phonological plans for words. The long-term goal of intervention for children who make inconsistent errors is to establish consistent (as opposed to correct) production of words in spontaneous speech. Unlike phonological contrast therapy, it does not target surface error patterns. Learning to consistently say a set of high-frequency, functionally powerful words targets the phonological planning impairment. The ability to create a phonological plan (i.e., to assemble a specific sequence of phonemes for a particular word that can be used in different utterance contexts) is improved by provision of detailed specific information about a limited number of words and drilling the use of that information with systematic practice.

EMPIRICAL BASIS

The primary reason for targeting inconsistency is the impact it has on intelligibility. Children who make inconsistent speech errors usually have a high degree of unintelligibility, even to family members. Consequently they are more likely to be referred for assessment of an SSD by their parents rather than another referral agent, and they are more likely to be referred at 3, rather than 4, years (Broomfield & Dodd, 2005). Intervention target selection is very difficult. A child with inconsistent SSD may use a range of sound substitutions that differ in manner of production, place of production, or voicing. For example, one young girl marked /s/ with a [b, f, v, t, d, s] or deleted the sound (see the case study described later in this chapter). It was impossible to select the appropriate error to contrast given the range of substitutions. Furthermore, it would not be effective to take an articulatory approach that targets a single sound when a child has adequate oro-motor control and sometimes produces the target accurately or, if not, is stimulable for the sound.

Intervention Research Outcomes

Children with inconsistent SSD are resistant to phonological contrast or articulation therapy. Forrest, Dinnsen, and Elbert (1997) conducted a retrospective post hoc analysis of 14 children with SSD. The children were divided into three groups: those who made consistent sound substitutions for sounds not present in their inventories (e.g., /k/ always produced as [t]), those who had inconsistent sound substitutions across word positions (e.g., /v/ substituted by [b] word initially, but [f] word finally), and those that used a different sound substitution within (e.g., word initial /s/ being substituted by /v, f, d, b/) and across word positions. The three groups were matched for severity of phonological impairment, and all groups received phonological contrast therapy targeting a single error in a single word position. The children with consistent sound substitutions learned the sound and generalized it to other word positions. The children with inconsistent sound substitutions across word positions learned the sound but only in the treated position.

The children with variable sound substitutions within and across word positions did not learn the sound in the treated or untreated word position.

Another intervention study (Forrest et al., 2000) compared two groups of children: those with consistent sound substitutions and those with variable sound substitutions. The children with variable substitutions did not respond to traditional articulation therapy. The children with consistent substitutions learned and generalized the taught sound. Forrest et al. acknowledged the limitation of these approaches to intervention in children with inconsistent SSD, concluding that "the challenge is to develop treatment protocols that instill learning and generalization, despite the complex pattern of errors that these children demonstrate" (2000, p. 530).

One plausible intervention approach would be to target whole words, rather than segments. Ingram and Ingram (2001) advocated a whole-word approach to phonological analysis and described how that approach would translate into a set of intervention goals. No intervention study was reported, however.

The core vocabulary approach for inconsistent SSD has included intervention case studies that explored the appropriateness of the approach; a group efficacy study comparing different interventions using an alternating treatments design; and an effectiveness study that was part of an RCT carried out in a speech and language therapy service in northeast England (see Table 5.2).

Case Studies

To date there have been three case studies of core vocabulary (Dodd & Bradford, 2000; Dodd & Iacono, 1989; McIntosh & Dodd, 2008).

Developing a Novel Therapy: Case Studies

MW, a boy age $4\frac{1}{2}$ who was part of a clinical research study evaluating phonological contrast intervention for phonological disorders (Dodd & Iacono,1989), made no progress despite weekly therapy for 8 months. The other six children in the study had improved and been discharged. MW differed from them in that he made inconsistent errors (e.g., he pronounced *tomato* as [mʌgʌg] and [tʌnawɔ] and *TV* as [pikɛg] and [titɪŋ]). He showed no oro-motor signs of CAS. To establish consistency of production of specific lexical

Table 5.2.   Levels of evidence for studies of treatment efficacy for core vocabulary

Level	Description	References
Ia	Meta-analysis of <1 randomized controlled trial	—
Ib	Randomized controlled study	Broomfield & Dodd (2005)
IIa	Controlled study without randomization	—
IIb	Quasi-experimental study	Crosbie et al. (2005)
III	Nonexperimental studies, i.e., correlational and case studies	Bradford-Heit (1996); Dodd & Bradford (2000); Dodd & Iacono (1989); McIntosh & Dodd (2008)
IV	Expert committee report, consensus conference, clinical experience of respected authorities	—

Adapted from the Scottish Intercollegiate Guidelines Network (http://www.sign.ac.uk).

items, a novel therapy approach was developed. The approach focused on whole words to establish a vocabulary of highly functional, powerful words that were produced consistently, although not necessarily correctly. After 2 months of weekly therapy establishing a consistent vocabulary of 70 words, consistency generalized, and a phonological contrast approach was successfully reintroduced.

Comparing Different Intervention Approaches for Different Types of Speech Sound Disorders

Bradford-Heit (1996) reported six intervention case studies that compared three therapy methods for children with different types of SSD (consistent atypical errors, inconsistent errors, and CAS). Two children in the study (see Dodd & Bradford, 2000) presented with SSD characterized by inconsistent productions. A multiple baseline with alternating treatments evaluated the effect of phonological contrast therapy (targeting error patterns), core vocabulary therapy (targeting consistency), and PROMPT system therapy (targeting articulatory gestures). Children were seen individually, twice weekly for twelve 30-minute sessions in each treatment block, with a 3-week withdrawal period between treatment blocks. The order of treatments was randomized across the six children in the study.

MC, age 4;3, received core vocabulary therapy first. Consistency of word production was established and generalized to untreated words (31% preintervention to 69% postintervention). He also benefited from the second block of therapy that targeted a phonological process (liquid and glide contrast), although generalization to untreated words was limited. MC did not benefit from the PROMPT therapy approach. TN, age 3;7, received core vocabulary followed by PROMPT and then phonological therapy. The results indicated that TN benefited from core vocabulary (consistency 36% preintervention, 75% postintervention). The other two blocks of therapy did not result in improvement. These findings suggest that once consistency is established, it may be possible to immediately target phonological contrasts effectively, as was done with MW (discussed in the previous section), if accuracy is still at unacceptable levels.

Core Vocabulary Intervention with Special Children

Three preschool boys who were referred to an efficacy study focusing on phonological contrast intervention did not meet the inclusion criteria because they made inconsistent speech errors. All three had additional complicating factors. Intervention case studies were undertaken to examine the effect of these complicating factors on core vocabulary intervention. The three factors were the nature of previous intervention, the use of default preferred word plans, and behavior difficulties (McIntosh & Dodd, 2008). Andrew had a history of previous intervention that had focused on the articulation of /s/, which had overgeneralized. Ben had behavior difficulties and limited attention. Cameron appeared to have a number of pervasive default plans for his word production. He most often began words with /w/, used a velar plosive syllable finally, and used default syllables (with variable vowels) /wak/ or /pɪk/ word-finally or as whole-word substitutes (e.g., [wʌɡuə] *apple*, [wɒkwɔ] *orange*, [wawak] *lighthouse*, [wɒɡ] *watch*, [pɪk] *swing*, [bɪkwak] *giraffe*).

The intelligibility, accuracy, and consistency of word production improved for all three boys. Their individual differences, however, required clinical adaptation of the ap-

Table 5.3. Case studies: Percent consistency and accuracy before and after core vocabulary intervention

Children	Consistency		Accuracy (PCC, PVC)	
	Preintervention	Postintervention	Preintervention	Postintervention
Andrew, age 3;8	44	90	46, 88	94, 99
Cameron, age 4;2	36	90	34, 78	69, 95
Ben, age 3;9	36	60	22, 53	52, 86

Key: PCC, percentage of consonants correct; PVC, percentage of vowels correct.

proach (see Table 5.3). Whereas Andrew received only 6 hours of intervention, Ben received 13.5 hours, and Cameron received 19 hours. It proved difficult to suppress preferred word shapes, but progress was achieved by an intermediary step of accepting a consistent production that included an aspect of his default word plan (e.g., accept [wɪg] for *swing*) before that was modified to [wɪŋ] and then [swɪŋ]. The case studies indicated that previous intervention focusing on articulation did not affect the outcome of core vocabulary intervention. It did, however, make differential diagnosis difficult: The inconsistent use of an intrusive /s/ might have reflected previous therapy rather than inconsistency. The children with behavioral difficulties and default templates for words required more intervention hours than had previously been found necessary for positive outcome.

Group Efficacy Study: Alternating Treatments Design

Crosbie, Holm, and Dodd (2005) evaluated the effect of two different types of intervention on the speech accuracy and consistency of word production of children with consistent ($N = 8$) and inconsistent ($N = 10$) SSD. The 18 children (ages 4;8 to 6;5) with severe SSD participated in an intervention study comparing phonological contrast and core vocabulary intervention. All children received two 8-week blocks of each intervention, receiving twice weekly, 30-minute sessions. A multiple baseline design with alternating treatments was used. Two pretherapy baseline measures were taken 3 weeks apart and showed no spontaneous change in number or type of speech errors. Once eligibility was confirmed children were allocated to one of the two therapies by order of referral. Treatment 1 was implemented after the baseline period, followed by a 4-week withdrawal period, then followed by treatment 2. The method of allocation to intervention ensured children in both subgroups of SSD received the blocks of therapy in both possible orders (core vocabulary followed by phonological contrast; phonological contrast followed by core vocabulary).

All of the children increased their consonant accuracy during intervention (see Table 5.4). Core vocabulary therapy resulted in greater change in children with inconsistent SSD, and phonological contrast therapy resulted in greater change in children with consistent SSD. The results of this study provide strong evidence that intervention targeting the speech-processing impairment underlying a child's SSD will result in efficient system-wide change. Differential response to intervention across subgroups provides evidence supporting theoretical perspectives regarding the nature of SSD: Different underlying impairments result in different types of speech errors requiring different types of therapy. Multiple baseline alternating treatments research design has been argued to have greater power than RCTs (e.g., Dodd, 2007) because all participants receive the same amount of

Table 5.4. Group summary of change in inconsistency score and percentage of consonants correct following each intervention

Group	Inconsistency (% mean, *SD*)		PCC (% mean, *SD*)	
	Core vocabulary	Phonological contrast	Core vocabulary	Phonological contrast
Consistent (*N* = 8)	5.00 (7.63)	9.50 (12.99)	6.75 (3.01)	24.62 (12.88)
Inconsistent (*N* = 10)	24.6 (9.14)	4.20 (7.57)	15.80 (9.05)	9.70 (6.57)
Overall	15.89 (12.99)	6.56 (10.35)	11.78 (8.28)	16.33 (12.22)

Key: PCC, percentage of consonants correct; *SD,* standard deviation.

intervention and children act as their own controls. This highly controlled research design allows stronger conclusions to be drawn about the relative benefit of a particular therapeutic approach using a constant service delivery model.

Randomized Controlled Trial: Effectiveness Study

Broomfield and Dodd (2005) reported an RCT that included 320 children with SSD who were referred to the pediatric speech and language therapy service in Middleborough, United Kingdom between January 1999 and April 2000. The study differentially diagnosed subtypes of SSD, specified the content of the therapeutic approaches implemented with each subgroup, and described the clinical pathway (including service delivery). Statistical analyses investigated treatment versus no treatment outcome. In addition, the effect of a range of factors on outcome was reported: dosage, age for cost-effective intervention for specific impairments, gender, case history factors, and comorbidity with other language disorders. Only data relevant to children with inconsistent SSD are discussed here.

The type and duration of the intervention offered were determined by the nature and severity of each child's SSD. Thirty children had inconsistent SSD, twenty of them classed as having a severe or profound level of unintelligibility. Core vocabulary therapy was the specified intervention for a diagnosis of inconsistency, and all clinicians (*N* = 12) employed by the service used the intervention approach when it was indicated by diagnosis. After assessment, children typically attended up to six diagnostic group sessions focusing on attention, listening, speech sound awareness, language concepts and categories, and oro-motor and speech skills to ensure all difficulties that a child was having had been identified by the standardized assessments routinely administered. These initial sessions also allowed children to become familiar with the clinicians and confident in the clinic environment. Children receiving core vocabulary intervention then received six individual, weekly, 30- to 45-minute intervention sessions. After a break from intervention (a consolidation period), children were reassessed and, if their consistency remained atypical, received a second episode of core vocabulary intervention.

So that a standard measure was available for comparison, assessment findings were converted to *z* scores. Each change in (accuracy) performance was measured in comparison with an age change, with 6 months passing between each randomized controlled trial assessment. Consequently, when a difference in *z* scores showed improvement, the child had progressed more than would have been expected for his or her change in age. Two of the children moved away and did not complete intervention.

The 18 children with inconsistent disorder who received intervention performed better ($z = 0.37$) than the 10 children who received no intervention ($z = 0.10$). Evidence, then, supports the theory that a core vocabulary approach is effective for inconsistent SSD at a clinical service level. The result suggests, however, that children who made inconsistent errors made less progress in intervention than other subgroups of SSD (e.g., treated consistent atypical disorders, $z = 0.59$; untreated, $z = 0.03$). A number of factors may contribute to this finding. Children who make inconsistent errors often have a severe, pervasive disorder that may need to be addressed by more intervention sessions. An alternative explanation is that many of the children in this group were younger (around 3 years old) than children in the other subgroups. Consequently, some children may have had poorer attention or less motivation to comply with intervention tasks. In addition, unlike other evaluations, intervention occurred once per week rather then twice. Furthermore, clinicians had been trained in the use of core vocabulary for only a short while and may have been less confident in its implementation than for other intervention approaches. Finally, for comparison with other children with SSD, the outcome measure focused on accuracy rather than consistency. Although not assessing the primary target of therapy, the findings demonstrate that improved accuracy is a by-product of intervention targeting consistency.

PRACTICAL REQUIREMENTS

Nature of Sessions

The service delivery model recommended for core vocabulary intervention is individual, twice-weekly sessions lasting around 30 minutes. In the first session each week, approximately 10 target words are randomly selected from a set of 70 target words chosen by the child, parents, and teachers to be the focus of intervention in an episode of care. The best production of these 10 words is taught by the clinician. Production is drilled sound by sound to elicit best production of each word, the words are then practiced in games for the remainder of the session and then targeted consistently by the child's parents and teacher until the next session. In the second session with the clinician, the words are revised and then children have a test in which the 10 words must be produced three times, the three trials separated by another activity. Untreated probes (a set of 10 untreated words) are also elicited three times to monitor generalization every 14 days.

Personnel

Roles of Parent and Teachers

The intervention approach depends on the child's family and teacher to reinforce use of the core vocabulary and carry out daily practice. Both must be involved from the outset of intervention. For example, after assessment and diagnosis, but before the first intervention session, the child, family, and teacher are asked to contribute to a list of 70 words that are frequently part of the child's functional vocabulary. These words are used as the basis for the intervention sessions. Parents and teachers must focus on the consistency of the child's production of the target words, in practice and spontaneously. It must be emphasized to caregivers that the primary target of the intervention is to make sure the child says a word in exactly the same way each time he or she attempts to say it, not necessarily an error-free production.

The Clinician's Role

The first session each week is devoted to eliciting the child's best production of up to 12 selected words and establishing their production. The number of words targeted depends on the child's ability to achieve a word's best possible production. The second weekly session focuses on drilling the newly learned words in order to monitor production, providing appropriate feedback when the best production is not produced. Parents and teachers must be encouraged to perceive the child's productions accurately and learn how to provide appropriate feedback. Clinicians need to be sensitive to parent and teacher feedback that could influence the content of the therapy session (e.g., words or phrases needing additional teaching, new words to target). Clinicians also need to customize the intervention approach for each child to take into account factors such as behavior and individual speech production limitations. Finally, an essential clinical role is to regularly monitor generalization of consistency to untreated probes.

Dosage

Core vocabulary intervention usually involves individual, twice-weekly, 30-minute sessions. Although the number of sessions varies according to severity and teacher and caregiver input, a clinician should not expect to exceed 16 half-hour sessions to attain consistency of production, as well as enhanced percentage of consonants correct (PCC), which generalizes to untreated words. Some studies of older children have held one session per week at school and the other at the speech-language pathology health-based clinic to ensure liaison with both the child's teacher and parents (Crosbie et al., 2005).

KEY COMPONENTS

The core vocabulary intervention approach should only be used for children who make inconsistent errors but have no oro-motor signs of CAS. The ultimate goal of intervention is intelligible speech. The long-term goal for a block of core vocabulary intervention is for the child to produce at least 70 target words consistently, that is, to produce a word exactly the same way each time it is produced. Generalization of consistency is expected once the child has mastered the consistent production of 70 words. The short-term goals are target specific; however, two general goals can be applied to each set of target words. The first goal is for the child to achieve an appropriate productive realization of each target based on the child's phonological system and phonetic inventory. This best production may be correct or contain a developmental error. The second goal is for the child to consistently use the established best production.

Nature of Goals

The aim of core vocabulary therapy is to teach children how to assemble phonology. That is, to plan the sequence of phonemes for a specific lexical item so that the word is produced consistently every time the child pronounces the word. Although correct production of words is the primary aim, if that is not achievable, then developmental errors are accepted. Once a word is produced consistently in isolation, its consistency of production is extended to sentence frames and spontaneous speech. Target words are words chosen by the child, caregivers, and teachers to be functionally powerful and to maximize motivation for learning. Some targets may be chosen by the clinician to illustrate a phonological contrast, but this is done to encourage implicit learning. Any intervention focus on phonological contrasts awaits the generalization of the consistent production of words.

Goal Attack Strategies

A core vocabulary of up to 70 functionally powerful target words is selected by the child, parents, and teacher. The types of words commonly included on children's lists are names (e.g., *teacher*, *friends*, *pet*), places (e.g., *address*, *toilet*), function words (e.g., *please*, *sorry*), foods (e.g., *cornflakes*, *juice*, *chips*), and the child's favorite things (e.g., *Nintendo*, *Polly Pocket*, *Spiderman*). The words are not selected according to word shape or segments. They are chosen because the child frequently uses these words in his or her functional communication. The child's intelligible use of the functionally powerful words selected motivates the use of consistent productions.

Description of Activities

Establishing Best Production

In the first session each week, the clinician teaches the child up to 10 target words, selected at random from a bag containing the vocabulary chosen. Words are taught sound-by-sound, using cues such as syllable segmentation, imitation, and cued articulation as outlined in Passy (1990). For example: To teach Joseph, the clinician would explain that the name *Joseph* has two syllables, [dʒoʊ] and [sɛf]. The first syllable [dʒoʊ] has two sounds, /dʒ/ and /oʊ/, and the second syllable [sɛf] has three sounds /s/, /ɛ/, and /f/. The child attempts the first syllable, receives feedback, and makes further attempts after being given models and receiving feedback about each attempt. When the child's best production of the first syllable has been established, the second is targeted, and then the two syllables are combined. For some children it is effective to link sounds to letters. Children with inconsistent SSD are usually able to imitate all sounds. If it is not possible to elicit a correct production, then the best production may include developmental errors (e.g., *Joseph* [doʊsɛf], *camera* [tæmɹa]).

Drill

It is important that the child practices the target words daily and receives feedback on those words in everyday communication situations. The second session each week with the clinician involves practice of the target words. Games are used to elicit a high number of repetitions. Any game that the child is highly motivated to participate in can be used to elicit productions. Initial picture naming games (e.g., stepping stones—with more than one picture on each stepping stone) can be followed by those requiring the target in a carrier phrase (e.g., picture lotto) and finally by story generation (asking for one, two, or three of the target words). Elbert, Powell, and Swartzlander (1991) suggested a child should produce about 100 responses in 30 minutes. Although this number may sound like a high rate of response, it is not difficult to elicit 150–170 responses in a 30-minute session of core vocabulary intervention.

Treatment on Error

It is important to provide children with feedback when their best production is not uttered. Leahy (2004) reported that children do not always understand why they attend intervention or what they are required to do. Consequently it is important to be explicit about the purpose of intervention, the nature of the error made, and how it can be corrected. If a child produces a target that deviates from the best production, the clinician can imitate the production and explicitly explain that the word differed and how it differed. For example if the child's target word was *sun* and he produced [gʌn], the clinician would say, "[gʌn], that's different from how we say it. That had a [g] sound at the start, but we need to make it an [s], [sʌn]. Have another try at telling me what this picture is." Clinicians should avoid simply asking for an imitation of the target word that provides a phonological plan. Instead, clinicians should provide information about the plan, requiring children to generate their own plan for the word.

Monitoring Consistent Production

Toward the end of the second session each week, the child is asked to produce, three times, the set of target words that have been the focus of therapy for the past week. Any word that the child can produce consistently is removed from the list of words to be learned. Words produced inconsistently remain on the list. Even though there are 70 target words that form a core vocabulary for the child's 8 weeks of intervention, monitoring allows for words that have not been mastered to be readdressed in another week.

Materials and Equipment Required

Equipment is minimal: pictures of the target words (with the written name beneath the picture), a box or bag for the vocabulary pictures, a wall chart where words produced consistently can be displayed, and games that elicit multiple productions of target words rapidly. A CD of text resources (e.g., teacher and parent information sheets, probe word lists) is available from the authors.

ASSESSMENT AND PROGRESS MONITORING TO SUPPORT DECISION MAKING

Generalization

Core vocabulary intervention aims to stabilize a child's system leading to consistent word production. The therapy would not be beneficial if the effect of therapy was limited to the treated target items. To monitor generalization, a set of untreated items (10 words) should be elicited three times, once every 14 days, in one therapy session to monitor system change (i.e., determine when consistency has generalized). Once untreated probes become consistent, the DEAP Inconsistency subtest (Dodd et al., 2002) should be read-ministered to ensure generalization has occurred.

What to Do When the Child's Speech Is Consistent

Core vocabulary intervention will increase the consistency of a child's speech produc-tion. The effect this has on the child' speech system can vary. Case studies suggest that most children's speech became both more consistent and more accurate, and that the children's speech was characterized by developmental, not atypical, error patterns. For some children, however, more than one intervention approach may be necessary to achieve age-appropriate speech. For example, Dodd and Bradford (2000) reported a case study of a boy with inconsistent speech production. Once consistency was established he benefited from phonological contrast therapy that targeted his remaining developmental error patterns. Assessment on a standardized phonological assessment, preferably after a consolidation break from intervention, would allow decisions about the need for fur-ther, different intervention.

CONSIDERATIONS FOR CHILDREN FROM CULTURALLY AND LINGUISTICALLY DIVERSE BACKGROUNDS

Core vocabulary intervention is suitable to use with children from all backgrounds. The child and family select the vocabulary, which helps to ensure that the target words are ap-propriate. Some evidence suggests that working in only one of an inconsistent bilingual child's languages will also generalize to their other language without specific intervention in that language (Holm & Dodd, 1999).

Hafis, a bilingual Punjabi-English–speaking child, had speech that was characterized by inconsistent errors (Holm & Dodd, 1999). Hafis was successfully treated using a core vocabulary approach, in English, which targeted consistency of production. Hafis re-ceived 16 (30 minutes) sessions over an 8-week period. His consistency of production in-creased. On untreated items, his inconsistency in English fell from 56% to 21% and in Pun-jabi from 45% to 30%. His accuracy, measured by PCC, increased significantly in Punjabi by 16% and in English by 26%. The significance of the generalization of intervention across languages is that it highlights the effect of targeting the underlying impairment rather than the surface speech error patterns.

CASE STUDY

Amy was assessed mid-way through her preschool year when she was age 4;8. She was monolingual, an only child, living with both parents. Her speech had always been difficult to understand. Amy's birth, medical, and developmental histories were normal. She had no hearing problems. Amy was reported to be conscious of her SSD, having difficulty establishing friendships at preschool, and upset and frustrated when she was not understood (Crosbie et al., 2005).

Standardized assessment indicated age-appropriate receptive language and nonverbal intelligence. The DEAP Articulation, Inconsistency, and Phonology Assessments (Dodd et al., 2002) indicated that Amy could produce all speech sounds in imitated simple syllables or in isolation. Her oro-motor skills were age-appropriate. The Inconsistency Assessment indicated that her speech was 56% inconsistent (a standard score of 3). The Phonology Assessment indicated that Amy's preintervention PCC was 50% and her percent vowels correct was 92%, which indicated performance at the 1st percentile. Reassessment 3 weeks after initial assessment showed no spontaneous change.

Intervention

Intervention with the clinician occurred individually, twice weekly. Therapy sessions were alternately conducted in Amy's home and preschool to allow liaison with both her teacher and parents. There were 16 (30 minutes) sessions over an 8-week period. Prior to intervention, Amy, her parents, and her teacher collaborated to produce a list of 50 words that were functionally powerful for her. The clinician explained the principles of core vocabulary therapy to Amy's parents and teacher. Each week 10 words were drawn randomly from the set of 50 target words. Amy was taught the 10 words by the clinician, and then those words were targeted consistently by her parents and teacher throughout the week and revised in the second session with the clinician. Some of the taught words were correct. For others, developmental errors were accepted. Production was drilled sound by sound. After the initial session in which Amy learned the target words, her parents and teacher consistently required her to produce those 10 words in the same way throughout the week. Practice of the 10 words occurred three times each day, as well as being reinforced when they occurred in everyday communication situations. Her parents and teacher used the same teaching strategies as the clinician. During the second weekly session with the clinician, the words were drilled, and then Amy had a test in which she had to produce the 10 words three times in three trials, each separated by another activity. Untreated probes (a set of 10 untreated words) were also elicited three times to monitor generalization every 14 days. Amy's progress was drawn on to her chart, and her parents implemented a reward scheme linked to her progress on the weekly words.

Amy found the intervention program difficult at times, particularly when learning the new words each week. She was well supported at home and school, however, and regularly did her practice. The intervention period was for a predetermined 8-week period so that everyone involved was able to commit to it knowing when it was going to end.

Progress

Amy learned to produce 57 words consistently in 8 weeks. When she was reassessed on the consistency tasks used in the initial and baseline assessments, her inconsistency had decreased from 56% to 32%. Her consonant accuracy increased by 10%. In addition she was more consistent in her substitution patterns following intervention. Instead of the almost free variation among up to six phonemes evident in her preintervention assessments, Amy generally only used either the correct phoneme or one other phoneme. Her speech was still affected by developmental phonological error patterns, but there was no evidence of atypical error patterns in her speech at the final assessment.

STUDY QUESTIONS

1. What type of impairment in speech processing underlies inconsistent SSD?

2. How might a clinician make the differential diagnosis between inconsistent SSD and CAS?

3. On the DEAP, a boy age 4;3 had a PCC score of 38% and an inconsistency score of 52%. Draw up a plan to manage his intervention that includes intervention goal, service delivery, and summary of intervention approach.

4. Describe how you would monitor progress and evaluate effectiveness of an episode of care that used a core vocabulary approach to intervention.

FUTURE DIRECTIONS

For core vocabulary intervention to be accepted as a useful treatment approach, clinical efficacy and effectiveness studies need to be carried out by other groups of clinical researchers to validate the findings already made. Although the use of the approach has been anecdotally reported to be successful by clinicians, it still needs to be rigorously tested. Future research could address some issues needing clarification. For example

- Does client choice of the vocabulary lead to better outcome than clinician choice that would manipulate word shape or phoneme contrast?

- How many words have to be taught before consistency generalizes?

- Does accepting best production rather than correct production result in differences in outcome of therapy for accuracy of production?

In addition, only one case study of a bilingual child with inconsistent SSD has shown generalization of core vocabulary intervention gains from the treated to the untreated language. This finding has important theoretical and clinical implications and needs repeating with other language pairs.

SUGGESTED READINGS

Crosbie, S., Holm, A., & Dodd, B. (2005). Intervention for children with severe speech disorder: A comparison of two approaches. *International Journal of Language and Communication Disorders, 40,* 467–491.

Dodd, B., Holm, A., Crosbie, S., & McCormack, P. (2005). Differential diagnosis of phonological disorder. In B. Dodd (Ed.), *Differential diagnosis and treatment of children with speech disorder* (2nd ed., pp. 44–70). London: Whurr.

Dodd, B., Holm, A., Crosbie, S., & McIntosh, B. (2006). A core vocabulary approach for management of inconsis-

tent speech disorder. *Advances in Speech-Language Pathology, 8,* 220–230.

Forrest, K., Elbert, M., & Dinnsen, D. (2000). The effect of substitution patterns on phonological treatment outcomes. *Clinical Linguistics and Phonetics, 14,* 519–531.

Holm, A., Crosbie, S., & Dodd, B. (2007). Differentiating normal variability from inconsistency in children's speech: Normative data. *International Journal of Language and Communication Disorders, 42,* 467–486.

REFERENCES

Berndt, R., & Mitchum, C. (1994). Approaches to the rehabilitation of 'phonological assembly.' In G. Humphreys & M. Riddoch (Eds.), *Cognitive neuropsychology and cognitive rehabilitation* (pp. 503–526). London: Lawrence Erlbaum Associates.

Bird, J., & Bishop, D. (1992). Perception and awareness of phonemes in phonologically impaired children. *European Journal of Disorders of Communication, 27*, 289–311.

Bradford, A., & Dodd, B. (1996). Do all speech disordered children have motor deficits? *Clinical Linguistics and Phonetics, 10*, 77–101.

Bradford-Heit, A. (1996). *Subgroups of children with developmental speech disorder: Identification and remediation.* Unpublished doctoral thesis, University of Queensland, Brisbane, Australia.

Broomfield, J., & Dodd, B. (2004). The nature of referred subtypes of primary speech disability. *Child Language Teaching and Therapy, 20*, 135–151.

Broomfield, J., & Dodd, B. (2005). Clinical effectiveness. In B. Dodd (Ed.), *Differential diagnosis and treatment of children with speech disorder* (pp. 211–230). London: Whurr.

Crosbie, S., Holm, A., & Dodd, B. (2005). Intervention for children with severe speech disorder: A comparison of two approaches. *International Journal of Language and Communication Disorders, 40*, 467–491.

Dodd, B. (2007). Evidence-based practice and speech-language pathology. *Folia Phoniatrica Logopedia, 59*, 118–129.

Dodd, B., & Bradford, A. (2000). A comparison of three therapy methods for children with different types of developmental phonological disorders. *International Journal of Language and Communication Disorders, 35*, 189–209.

Dodd, B., Crosbie, S., Zhu, H., Holm, A., & Ozanne, A. (2002). *The diagnostic evaluation of articulation and phonology.* London: Pearson PsychCorp.

Dodd, B., Holm, A., Crosbie, S., & McCormack, P. (2005). Differential diagnosis of phonological disorders. In B. Dodd (Ed.), *Differential diagnosis and treatment of children with speech disorder* (pp. 44–70). London: Whurr.

Dodd, B., Holm, A., Crosbie, S., & McIntosh, B. (2006). A core vocabulary approach for management of inconsistent speech disorder. *Advances in Speech-Language Pathology, 8*, 220–230.

Dodd, B., & Iacono, T. (1989). Phonological disorders in children: Changes in phonological process use during treatment. *British Journal of Communication Disorders, 24*, 333–351.

Dodd, B., Leahy, J., & Hambly, G. (1989). Phonological disorders in children: Underlying cognitive deficits. *British Journal of Developmental Psychology, 7*, 55–71.

Dodd, B., McCormack, P., & Woodyatt, G. (1994). An evaluation of an intervention program: The relationship between children's phonology and parents' communicative behavior. *American Journal of Mental Retardation, 98*, 632–645.

Duggirala, V., & Dodd, B. (1991). A psycholinguistic assessment model for disordered phonology. In *Congress for phonetic sciences* (pp. 342–345). Aix-en-Provence, Université de Provence.

Elbert, M., Powell, T., & Swartzlander, P. (1991). Toward a technology of generalization: How many exemplars are sufficient? *Journal of Speech and Hearing Research, 34*, 81–87.

Ferguson, C., & Farwell, C. (1975). Words and sounds in early language acquisition. *Language, 51*, 39–49.

Fisher, J., & Glenister, J. (1992). *The Hundred Pictures Naming Test (HPNT).* Camberwell, Victoria, Australia: Australian Council for Educational Research.

Forrest, K. (2003). Diagnostic criteria of developmental apraxia of speech used by clinical speech-language pathologists. *American Journal of Speech-Language Pathology, 12*, 376–380.

Forrest, K., Dinnsen, A., & Elbert, M. (1997). Impact of substitution patterns on phonological learning by misarticulating children. *Clinical Linguistics and Phonetics, 11*, 63–76.

Forrest, K., Elbert, M., & Dinnsen, D. (2000). The effect of substitution patterns on phonological treatment outcomes. *Clinical Linguistics and Phonetics, 14*, 519–531.

Fox, A., Howard, D., & Dodd, B. (2002). Risk factors in speech disorder. *International Journal of Language and Communication Disorders, 37*, 117–132.

Grunwell, P. (1982). *Clinical phonology.* London: Croom-Helm.

Holm, A., Crosbie, S., & Dodd, B. (2005). Treating inconsistent speech disorders. In B. Dodd (Ed.), *Differential diagnosis and treatment of children with speech disorder* (pp. 182–201). London: Whurr.

Holm, A., Crosbie, S., & Dodd, B. (2007). Differentiating normal variability from inconsistency in children's speech: Normative data. *International Journal of Language and Communication Disorders, 42*, 467–486.

Holm, A., & Dodd, B. (1999). An intervention case study of a bilingual child with phonological disorder. *Child Language Teaching and Therapy, 15*, 139–158.

Holm, A., Farrier, F., & Dodd, B. (2007). The phonological awareness, reading accuracy and spelling ability of children with inconsistent phonological disorder. *International Journal of Language and Communication Disorders, 42*, 1–23.

Ingram, D. (1976). *Phonological disability in children.* New York: Elsevier.

Ingram, D., & Ingram, K. (2001). A whole-word approach to phonological analysis and intervention. *Language, Speech, and Hearing Services in Schools, 32*, 271–283.

Leahy, M.M. (2004). Therapy talk: Analyzing therapeutic discourse. *Language, Speech, and Hearing Services in Schools, 35*, 70–81.

McCormack, P., & Dodd, B. (1996). A feature analysis of speech errors in subgroups of speech disordered children. In P. McCormack & A. Russell (Eds.), *Proceedings of the Sixth Australian International Conference on Speech Science and Technology* (pp. 217–222). Canberra, Australia: Australian Speech Science and Technology Association.

McCormack, P.F., & Dodd, B. (1998, September). *Is inconsistency in word production an artefact of severity in developmental speech disorders?* Poster Presented at Child Language Seminar, 1998, Sheffield, England.

McIntosh, B., & Dodd, B. (2008). Evaluation of core vocabulary intervention for treatment of inconsistent phonological disorder: Three case studies. *Child Language Teaching and Therapy, 24*, 305–327.

McLeod, S., & McCormack, J. (2007). Application of the ICF and ICF-Children and Youth in children with speech impairment. *Seminars in Speech and Language, 28*, 254–264.

Ozanne, A. (2005). Childhood apraxia of speech. In B. Dodd (Ed.), *Differential diagnosis and treatment of children with speech disorder* (pp. 71–82). London: Whurr.

Passy, J. (1990). *Cued articulation.* Camberwell, Victoria, Australia: Australian Council for Educational Research.

Storkel, H., & Morrisette, M. (2002). The lexicon and phonology: Interaction in language acquisition. *Language, Speech, and Hearing Services in Schools, 27*, 215–230.

Thyer, N., & Dodd, B. (1996). Auditory processing and phonologic disorder. *Audiology, 35*, 37–44.

Velleman, S., & Vihman, M. (2002). Whole-word phonology and templates: Trap, bootstrap, or some of each. *Language, Speech, and Hearing Services in Schools, 33*, 9–23.

World Health Organization. (2001). *International classification of functioning, disability and health.* Retrieved March 11, 2008, from http://www.who.int/classifications/icf/en/

The Cycles Phonological Remediation Approach

Raúl F. Prezas and Barbara Williams Hodson

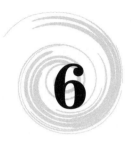

6

ABSTRACT

The cycles approach has evolved based on more than 30 years of clinical practice and research. It was designed explicitly for children with highly unintelligible speech but also has been used to treat clients with special etiologies (e.g., children with the label of childhood apraxia of speech [CAS]). Rather than following a traditional phoneme-oriented model (e.g., 85% criterion for mastery of each sound), practitioners identify phonological patterns (e.g., /s/ clusters) that are deficient, but stimulable, and present them in a cyclical fashion to expedite intelligibility gains. This chapter provides information regarding implementing the cycles approach and discusses theoretical underpinnings, selection of optimal target patterns, and evidence-based practices.

INTRODUCTION

The cycles approach was designed to facilitate the development of intelligible speech patterns in children with severe-to-profound expressive phonological impairments (intelligibility percentage typically less than 20%). A *cycle* (i.e., period of time, typically 10–15 weeks) is completed after each of the *phonological patterns* (e.g., /s/ clusters, velars) that need to be targeted during a cycle has been facilitated. In addition, each phoneme per pattern (e.g., postvocalic /k/, prevocalic /k/ [for velars]) has been presented for approximately 60 minutes per cycle. The duration of each cycle depends on two major factors: 1) the number of deficient patterns a child needs to target and 2) the number of deficient sounds in each pattern that are *stimulable* (i.e., consonants that are not being produced by the child but that can be imitated or produced with assistance; Hodson, 2007a). Stimulable sounds are a central tenet in the cycles approach because children have been found to demonstrate greater gains when stimulable (rather than nonstimulable) sounds are targeted (e.g., Rvachew & Nowak, 2001). Nonstimulable sounds (e.g., velars) are stimulated during each session but not targeted until the child can produce the sound. Practicing nonstimulable sounds is counterproductive because practicing an error sound reinforces the inaccurate kinesthetic image.

TARGET POPULATIONS

Primary Populations

The cycles approach has evolved from formulating and testing clinical research hypotheses while working with several hundred children between the ages of 2½ and 14 years (Hodson, 2007a). It was designed primarily for children with multiple speech errors and highly unintelligible speech who have major *phonological deviations* (e.g., cluster reduction). This population includes children who have been labeled as having CAS (Hodson & Paden, 1983, 1991; Velleman, 2003). Speech-language pathologists (SLP) generally have classified children with highly unintelligible speech differently from school-age children with mild speech disorders and minimal intelligibility concerns (e.g., Pascoe, Stackhouse, & Wells, 2006). Although a phoneme-oriented approach is adequate for children with mild speech disorders who demonstrate only a few misarticulations (e.g., lisps, substitutions of /f/ for *th*), children with severe-to-profound speech sound disorders (SSD) are ideal candidates for the cycles approach (Hodson, 2007a) in which the critical need is to expedite intelligibility gains so that children can be intelligible in time to succeed in school (see Critical Age Hypothesis in Bishop & Adams, 1990).

Secondary Populations

One of the key strengths of the cycles approach is its adaptability. This approach has been effectively modified for group treatment (e.g., Montgomery & Bonderman, 1989). The cycles approach also has been adapted for children with various etiological factors. Implementation of the cycles approach, for example, has been successful for children with recurrent otitis media, the most common etiological factor reported in case histories of children with severe SSD (Churchill, Hodson, Jones, & Novak, 1988). This intervention approach also has been used successfully for children with cochlear implants (Hodson, 2001), children with repaired cleft palate (Hodson, Chin, Redmond, & Simpson, 1983), children with mild-to-moderate (Gordon-Brannan, Hodson, & Wynne, 1992) and severe hearing losses (Garrett, 1986), and individuals with cognitive delays (e.g., Berman, 2001).

It is important to mention that phonological intervention procedures may need modification for children with additional etiological factors. Children with severe-to-profound hearing losses, for example, often require targeting suprasegmental aspects (e.g., phrasing, intonation) and morphophonological rules (e.g., pronunciations of *ed*) in addition to specific phonological pattern targets (e.g., /s/ clusters) in treatment (Hodson, 2007a). Cycle durations for children with cognitive delays typically are double in length (i.e., phonemes per pattern targeted for 2 hours, rather than 1 hour). Moreover, 3 or more years may be required before comparable intelligibility gains are observed by children with lower cognitive abilities (Hodson, 2007a).

ASSESSMENT METHODS FOR DETERMINING INTERVENTION RELEVANCE

Speech intelligibility is an important prognostic indicator in the diagnostic process of children with potential speech sound disorders (SSD). As such, the primary goal of the evaluation is the determination of an individual child's phonological system. Five major goals of the diagnostic process for phonological assessment include determining: 1) a child's *phonological strengths and weaknesses,* 2) the *severity* level, 3) *stimulability* information, 4), an optimal *direction for intervention,* and 5) baseline measures in order to *document change* following intervention (Prezas & Hodson, 2007).

The primary method for assessing children with potential SSD involves the elicitation of single words by naming pictures (e.g., Goldman Fristoe Test of Articulation-2 [GFTA-2]; Goldman & Fristoe, 2000) or objects (Hodson Assessment of Phonological Patterns, Third Edition [HAPP-3]; Hodson, 2004). Another widely used method for assessing speech sounds is to obtain a continuous speech sample and compute a percentage of consonants correct (PCC; Shriberg & Kwiatkowski, 1982). Although some assessments are pattern-oriented and designed for children with highly unintelligible speech who require phonological intervention (e.g., HAPP-3), most assessment measures are phoneme-oriented and are more appropriate for children with mild SSD who demonstrate only a few misarticulations.

Children with highly unintelligible speech often have extensive *omissions* and many *substitutions* (Hodson, 2007a). With most assessments (e.g., GFTA-2, PCC), omissions, substitutions, and *distortions* are not differentiated in the overall scoring process (Prezas & Hodson, 2007). In most assessment tools, distortions, for example, are given the same weight as omissions in the final score, regardless of the fact that omissions have a more adverse effect on intelligibility. Consequently, children with very different phonological systems often receive the same scores on these assessments. Posttreatment gains, therefore, may not be measured appropriately for a highly unintelligible child who has, through the course of treatment, replaced omissions with substitutions or distortions (e.g., Velleman, 2005). In addition, distortions (e.g., lisps) can occur with all children across the severity continuum of SSD (i.e., mild, moderate, severe, profound), but their impact on intelligibility is much less than deviations such as omissions. It is critical, therefore, that differentiations be made among substitutions, omissions, and distortions in the scoring process through the use of assessments that differentiate deviation types in final scores (e.g., HAPP-3).

THEORETICAL BASIS

Dominant Theoretical Rationale for the Intervention Approach

Several theoretical frameworks and models have contributed to the development of the cycles approach. This approach is based on developmental phonology theories (e.g., Browman & Goldstein, 1986; Stampe, 1972), cognitive psychology principles (e.g., Hunt, 1961; Vygotsky, 1962), phonological acquisition research (e.g., Dyson & Paden, 1983; Grunwell, 1987; Hodson & Paden, 1981; Porter & Hodson, 2001; Preisser, Hodson, & Paden, 1988), and ongoing clinical phonology research (Hodson, 2007a). *Gestural phonology,* which aligns most closely with the cycles approach, is a theory in which phonological representation serves as a foundation for speech perception and speech production physical constraints (Browman & Goldstein, 1986; Kent, 1997). The term *gesture* refers to a class of articulatory movements. One of the important tenets of gestural phonology is that it includes implications/applications for metaphonological awareness and literacy, as well as for phonological production. According to Mody, literacy acquisition appears to be related to the "integration of recurrent gestural patterns into segmental units" (2003,

p. 33). Incorporating metaphonological skill enhancement tasks along with production-practice tasks during intervention is a core component of the cycles approach.

Underlying Concepts for the Cycles Phonological Remediation Approach

Seven underlying concepts and recommendations serve as the basis for intervention decision making when implementing a cycles approach and are summarized in Table 6.1.

1. *Much of what is known regarding phonological acquisition comes from research on typically developing children.* Such children do not learn phonemes "one at a time" (e.g., /f/) to a specific criterion (e.g., 90%; Dyson & Paden, 1983; Hodson, 2007a). Instead, as David Ingram pointed out in his 1976 book, *Phonological Disability in Children*, phonological acquisition is a *gradual process* (emphasis added). Typically developing children continually explore and experiment with their speech sounds and learn to acquire the correct productions over time. The cycles approach more closely approximates how typical phonological development occurs (Ingram, 1976). Rather than aiming for a specific criterion of mastery for individual phonemes, it is recommended that practitioners introduce carefully selected targets and present them in a cyclical manner, recy-

Table 6.1. Underlying concepts of the cycles phonological approach and some recommendations

Underlying concept	Recommendation
1. Phonological acquisition is a gradual process (Ingram, 1976).	Allow children to practice phonological patterns (a carefully designed sequence) of primary targets that are stimulable early in treatment.
2. Children with normal hearing typically acquire the adult sound system primarily by listening (Van Riper, 1939).	Incorporate slight amplification with targets at the beginning and ending of each treatment session and also as needed when a child is experiencing a great deal of difficulty producing a particular target/word.
3. Children associate kinesthetic and auditory sensations as they acquire new patterns, enabling later self-monitoring (Fairbanks, 1954).	Production practice in treatment should be structured in a way that promotes successful responses, rather than a charting of errors, which allows reinforcement of incorrect kinesthetic images.
4. Phonetic environment can facilitate (or inhibit) correct sound productions (Kent, 1982).	Choose production-practice words wisely so that children will experience greater success during treatment sessions (e.g., avoid using a word with an alveolar consonant in it when the child demonstrates extensive velar fronting).
5. Children are actively involved in their treatment.	Create an enjoyable, spontaneous atmosphere for children filled with experiential play production-practice activities (e.g., bowling).
6. Children tend to generalize new speech production skills to other targets (McReynolds & Bennett, 1972).	Target /s/ clusters before singleton stridents for two major reasons: 1) Highly unintelligible children tend to say *stun* initially when asked to say *sun*. 2) The English language is "loaded" with /s/ consonant sequences. Success in producing /s/ clusters increases intelligibility substantially and also leads to productions of other stridents (e.g., /z/).
7. An optimal match facilitates a child's learning (Hunt, 1961).	Identify optimal target patterns based on phonological assessment results and choose targets for treatment that are stimulable so that a child can be challenged but also successful and not continue practicing the error production, which would reinforce the inaccurate kinesthetic image.

Source: Hodson & Paden (1991), pp. 76–85.

cling the patterns while adding complexity in later cycles until the patterns generalize to spontaneous speech.

2. Speech perception forms the basis for another critical underlying concept. *Children with normal hearing typically acquire the adult sound system primarily by listening.* Most parents do not teach their children tongue placement for speech sounds. It is important to incorporate auditory stimulation (see Van Riper, 1939) with slight amplification so that children become aware of the acoustic characteristics of sounds they are not yet producing and also how their own error productions sound. Theoretical support for auditory stimulation comes from cross-linguistic research. Ingram (1986) found that phonemes that have had the most frequent exposure in a child's phonetic environment are acquired first. Providing auditory stimulation for a deficient phoneme/pattern, therefore, increases the likelihood of its being acquired.

3. *Children associate kinesthetic and auditory sensations as they acquire new patterns, enabling later self-monitoring.* During production practice, focus is placed on developing new accurate kinesthetic images (Fairbanks, 1954) and adequate articulatory gestures (Kent, 1997) to match with new auditory images. This will, in turn, lead to better self-monitoring later. The goal is to provide production-practice words with an optimal phonetic environment initially so that a child is able to achieve 100% accuracy on target sound productions in order to develop new, accurate kinesthetic images. Practitioners are encouraged to initially select production-practice words that yield correct responses (moving away from "charting" errors), and then to add complexity gradually so that the child will be optimally challenged as well as successful.

4. *Phonetic environment can facilitate (or inhibit) correct sound production.* Production-practice words with facilitative phonetic environments (e.g., *cow* rather than *cat* for a child who demonstrates velar fronting; see Buteau & Hodson, 1989; Kent, 1982) must be selected, particularly during the beginning cycles. Monosyllabic production-practice words are recommended for beginning cycles. In addition, it is optimal to choose words in which the only potential error is the target.

5. *Children are actively involved in their treatment.* Results from child psychology and brain research studies indicate that children learn best when they are actively involved. It is no surprise that children also are actively involved in their phonological acquisition. A child's interactive participation (mental and physical) is a critical component of the cycles approach. It is important to create a clinical environment where the child enjoys the activity he or she is engaging in and maintains interest. Such an environment promotes active participation in the learning of new targets. Experiential-play activities (e.g., craft activities), which provide motivation for young children, are recommended.

6. *Children tend to generalize new speech production skills to other targets* (McReynolds & Bennett, 1972). In most cases, it is not necessary to target every deficient sound. What is necessary, however, is to choose target phonemes/patterns that will trigger the most extensive generalization. Targeting /s/ clusters before singleton stridents, for example, is recommended. Most preschool children generalize to other singleton stridents after /s/ clusters begin to emerge in conversation.

7. In order to facilitate a child's learning, *it is critical to identify the optimal "match"* (Hunt, 1961) and "zone of proximal development" (Vygotsky, 1962) based on phonological assessment results. It is important to determine at what level the child's phonological system is breaking down so that intervention can be initiated one step above the child's current level of functioning. This allows the child to be optimally challenged and yet experience immediate success.

Levels of Consequences Being Addressed

The enhancement of phonological patterns and metaphonological skills leads to rapid gains in productions of appropriate phonological patterns, which, in turn, helps young children become intelligible by the "critical age" (Bishop & Adams, 1990). Children who are still highly unintelligible when they begin school typically have excessive difficulties acquiring reading and spelling skills, leading to a downward spiral referred to as "Matthew Effects" (Stanovich, 1986). Thus, the cycles approach targets functional limitations (Body Function) and promotes Activities and Participation in society (World Health Organization, 2001).

Target Areas of Intervention

Multiple domains are introduced in a cycles approach. Although speech output is the primary concern, the cycles approach includes other factors related to auditory awareness, speech perception, language, and literacy. The purpose of production practice during intervention is not to establish a motor pattern of speech, but rather to develop new accurate kinesthetic images and provide a means for integrative rehearsal. During this process, the development of auditory awareness is a critical element. In most cases, unintelligible children do not seem to hear their own errors. If, for example, an adult repeats a word that a child with highly unintelligible speech said, the child will usually respond to the adult's production by saying "no" and then repeat the word with the identical error (Berko & Brown, 1960).

The cycles approach integrates auditory stimulation with slight amplification (upon the introduction of the target pattern and also whenever needed in each treatment session). Auditory stimulation is used to enhance speech perception and is particularly important during the first few cycles. Pragmatically appropriate activities are recommended whenever possible (e.g., camera used for the production-practice word *smile*). These activities also may include vocabulary words from a child's classroom list, as well as stories from the student's classroom (which ties into collaboration). In addition, the cycles approach includes a metaphonological awareness component (Hodson, 1994b; Hodson & Strattman, 2004). Children with highly unintelligible speech often have concomitant difficulties in *metaphonological awareness* and literacy (Bird, Bishop & Freeman, 1995; Clarke-Klein & Hodson, 1995; Larrivee & Catts, 1999; Raitano, Pennington, Tunick, Boada, & Shriberg, 2004; Rvachew & Grawberg, 2006; Rvachew, Ohberg, Grawburg, & Heyding, 2003). Metaphonological awareness activities (e.g., rhyming, syllable segmentation) are built into the cycles approach and are incorporated for a few minutes during each session. These activities function as a means to assist children in developing primary literacy skills (e.g., targeting underlying representation deficiencies; Mody, 2003; Stackhouse, 1997). Moreover, a metaphonological awareness assessment instrument (see Hodson, Scherz, & Strattman, 2002) often is administered to help identify any areas that may need facilitation.

EMPIRICAL BASIS

The efficacy of a modified cycles approach has been investigated by researchers who have implemented a group design (e.g., Almost & Rosenbaum, 1998). In addition, documentation of the effectiveness of the cycles approach exists in a number of refereed/peer-reviewed case studies (e.g., Hodson, 1994a. Moreover, videos are available in which dramatic changes in the intelligibility of children are observed after approximately 40–50 contact hours of cycles in less than 2 years (Hodson, 2005). Kamhi stated that the cycles approach combines an "efficient goal attack strategy with traditional speech therapy and metaphonological activities" (2006, p. 275) and appears to be "effective" but noted that more research is needed to investigate efficiency aspects.

Efficacy Studies

In a randomized controlled intervention study, Almost and Rosenbaum (1998) assigned 26 children who had received a phonological assessment rating of severe (based on Hodson, 1986) either to an immediate intervention group or to a controlled/delayed group. The first group received 4 months of intervention followed by 4 months of no intervention; the second group did not receive intervention the first 4 months, but then received 4 months of treatment. Four to six phonological patterns based on individual systems were presented in a modified cycles format (Hodson & Paden, 1991). At the end of the first 4 months, the first group received significantly higher scores than the delayed group on three measures (Assessment of Phonological Processes–Revised [Hodson, 1986]; Goldman-Fristoe Test of Articulation [Goldman & Fristoe, 1969]; and PCC [Shriberg & Kwiatkowski, 1982]). Scores of the first group continued to be significantly better at the end of 8 months.

Rvachew, Rafaat, and Martin (1999) examined stimulability and speech perception skills in the treatment of phonological disorders in children. In the first study, 10 children received nine group treatment sessions targeting three phonological processes using the cycles approach. Treatment progress was not observed for sounds that were nonstimulable before treatment. Given stimulability, treatment progress was greater for sounds that were well perceived before treatment in contrast with sounds that were poorly perceived before treatment. In the second study, 13 children received a modified cycles approach. In the modified version, each child received three brief, individual treatment sessions followed by six group treatment sessions. Phonetic placement was used to facilitate stimulability of target sounds. Perception of target sounds was treated using the Speech Assessment and Interactive Learning System (SAILS; AVAAZ Innovations, Inc.). In the second study, good progress was observed for most target phonemes, including those that were nonstimulable or poorly perceived before treatment. The researchers determined that increased speech perception is needed for sounds that are nonstimulable. Moreover, nonstimulable sounds often emerge after treatment using stimulable sounds (i.e., children tend to generalize sounds [McReynolds & Bennett, 1972]).

In an independent review of a number of studies involving the cycles approach, Baker, Carrigg, and Linich (2007) concluded that there seems to be evidence to support the efficacy of cycles. They noted the need for more studies comparing phonological intervention approaches.

Studies of Effectiveness

There have been a number of published, refereed/peer-reviewed case studies providing pre- and postintervention data (Gordon-Brannan, Hodson, & Wynne, 1992; Hodson, 1983, 1994a, 1998, 2005, 2007a; Hodson et al., 1983; Hodson, Nonomura, & Zappia, 1989; Hodson & Paden, 1983, 1991). The case studies presented in this section highlight not only the clinical application of the cycles approach, but also the variety of populations that benefit from the approach. Although case studies do not provide efficacy evidence, they do yield a measure of feasibility and also often provide an impetus for large-scale efficacy studies (Fey, 2004).

Two case studies have been published in refereed journals of the American Speech-Language-Hearing Association (ASHA). Hodson et al. (1983) reported treatment and results for a child with a repaired cleft palate. Gordon-Brannan et al. (1992) detailed treatment and results for a child with an unusual hearing loss. A report of a 3-year-old with highly unintelligible speech and possible CAS was published in an ASHA Monograph (Hodson, 1994a), and another report of a child with similar issues was published in an ASHA continuing education Master Clinician series (Hodson, 2005). In addition, a case study was published in *Topics in Language Disorders* (Hodson, 1983) and another study involving a child with more global issues and some literacy concerns was published in *Seminars in Speech and Language* (Hodson et al., 1989). Moreover, Hodson and Paden published a total of 10 case reports for clients with highly unintelligible speech between the ages of 3 and 14 years in their 1983 and 1991 editions of *Targeting Intelligible Speech: A Phonological Approach to Remediation.*

Studies of Feasibility

One of the strengths of the cycles approach is its efficiency (Hodson, 1982, 1997; Hodson & Paden, 1991). Many preschool children have required less than 1 year (1 hour per week) of phonological intervention to become intelligible (Hodson, 2007a).

Summary of Levels of Evidence

Two efficacy investigations and several peer-reviewed case studies noted previously provide evidence for the use of the cycles approach with children who have highly unintelligible speech. In addition, the cycles approach has been found to be feasible in individual and group treatment settings, as well as with children with other impairments (e.g., cleft palate). Researchers of a randomized controlled intervention study reported significant results with the use of the cycles approach. Other researchers of one efficacious study reported that stimulable, rather than nonstimulable, sounds were easier to produce (Rvachew & Nowak, 2001). Pre- and postintervention data, as well as treatment outlines, are reported in case study results. Table 6.2 lists major studies involving the cycles approach.

Table 6.2. Levels of evidence for studies of treatment efficacy for the cycles approach

Level	Description	References
Ia	Meta-analysis of $>$ 1 randomized controlled trial	—
Ib	Randomized controlled study	Almost & Rosenbaum (1998)
IIa	Controlled study without randomization	Tyler, Edwards, & Saxman (1987)
IIb	Quasi-experimental study	—
III	Nonexperimental studies (i.e., correlational and case studies)	Gordon-Brannan et al. (1992); Hodson, (1983, 1994a, 2005); Hodson et al. (1983); Hodson et al. (1989)
IV	Expert committee report, consensus conference, clinical experience of respected authorities	Hodson (2007b); Hodson & Paden (1991)

Adapted from the Scottish Intercollegiate Guidelines Network (http://www.sign.ac.uk).

PRACTICAL REQUIREMENTS

The cycles approach begins with target patterns that are lacking in the child's speech but that are stimulable. The majority of sounds/patterns of a child's phonological inventory that are in error are presented in a carefully planned succession to represent one cycle of treatment (e.g., /s/ clusters before singleton /s/ and liquids at the end of each cycle). Deficient phonological patterns from prior cycles are recycled as many times as needed until the targeted patterns begin to emerge in the child's spontaneous conversational utterances. In addition, the complexity of production-practice words increases with subsequent cycles to ensure an optimal match for treatment targets (Hunt, 1961). Table 6.3 provides the format for the cycles approach, which has been used in university clinics and has been modified and used effectively in schools, clinics, and hospitals.

One of the advantages of the cycles approach is that it can be modified to work in group (e.g., Montgomery & Bonderman, 1989) as well as individual sessions. Practitioners in various clinical settings (e.g., schools) have used cycles with a great deal of success (personal communications). Moreover, a homework component is incorporated in which caregivers (or paraprofessionals) actively participate in a 2-minutes-per-day home program.

Nature of Sessions

In the cycles approach, phonological patterns are presented and recycled as needed. Each phoneme (e.g., final /k/) within a pattern (e.g., velars) is targeted for 60 minutes a week (i.e., one 60-minute session, two 30-minute sessions, or three 20-minute sessions per week). Patterns are recycled as needed until they emerge in conversation. Children with highly unintelligible speech are usually seen individually but can be paired with another child when appropriate. Group sessions are appropriate after children progress from severe/profound levels of severity to mild/moderate levels.

Another part of the cycles approach includes a focused auditory input cycle that is used for children younger than 3 years for the initial cycle. These sessions are typically 30–45 minutes long. Target patterns are identified (e.g., final consonants), and a phoneme

Table 6.3. Session-structure model for the cycles approach

1. Review production-practice words from prior session.
2. Provide auditory stimulation (with slight amplification).
3. Have child name prospective picture word cards to determine appropriateness of each for production practice.
4. Incorporate motivational experiential play production-practice activities.
5. Probe for stimulability to determine next session's target.
6. Include metaphonological awareness activities (e.g., a folder with a four-line rhyme, syllable segmentation).
    a. Clinician reads rhyme to child, and child takes rhyme folder home (parents read rhyme to child pausing after a few readings for the child to fill in the rhyme word).
    b. The amount of intervention session time devoted to enhancing metaphonological awareness skills often is increased during the final cycles.
7. Repeat listening activity at the end of the session (with slight amplification).
8. Incorporate a home program in which caregivers (or paraprofessionals) participate in 2-minutes-per-day home (or school) activities. The week's listening list is read to the child each day, and the child is asked to name the picture cards that contain the week's production-practice words.

Source: Hodson & Paden (1991), pp. 116–121.

within the pattern (e.g., final /p/) is presented/facilitated for a session via activities/ materials containing the target (e.g., *up*, *hop*, *cup*). The child participates in parallel play activities but is not required to say anything during these sessions. After this focused auditory input cycle, the child moves into a regular cycle involving production practice.

Personnel

The goal of any treatment approach for children with highly unintelligible speech should be to expedite intelligibility gains in an optimal and efficient manner and to develop accurate underlying phonological representations. Speech sounds/patterns that are in error must first be identified through assessment, then followed by careful selection of targets and production practice words for treatment. The systematic process of speech assessment and phonological remediation should be implemented by a certified SLP.

The cycles approach is relatively easy to implement. One of the important components of the cycles approach is the home program. Caregivers can contribute greatly to a child's overall success with treatment (e.g., reading the listening list and having the child name the carefully selected production-practice words at home). In some cases, the home program can be implemented each day in a school setting by a member of the school staff (e.g., paraprofessional).

Dosage

It is recommended that each target phoneme within a target pattern be presented for 60 minutes a week. Children in our university phonology clinics participate in 1-hour sessions once a week. School clinicians who use shorter sessions present the target phoneme an equivalent amount of time (e.g., three 20-minute sessions or two 30-minute sessions). The goal in the cycles approach is 100% accuracy for all target productions so that the child can develop a new accurate kinesthetic image. Typically, the child must say the target (but not necessarily the whole word) correctly before taking a turn in an activity.

Typically, three or four cycles (requiring approximately 30–40 hours of an SLP's contact time) are required for children with severe expressive phonological impairments to become intelligible. The longest amount of treatment time (on record) required for clients with extremely disordered phonological systems (within normal limits cognitively, neurologically, and auditorily) to become intelligible (not perfect) has been 65 contact hours over a period of approximately 2 years (Hodson, 2007a).

KEY COMPONENTS

The ordering of phonological patterns within cycles is based on developmental and clinical phonology research findings and on each individual child's phonological abilities (Hodson, 2007a). Targets for which a child demonstrates readiness and stimulability should be selected based on the client's severity level (e.g., profound) as well as the sounds/patterns in error. A major goal for phonological remediation in cycles is for the child to experience immediate and tangible success (Hodson, 2007a; Hunt, 1961).

The recommended order for treatment targets for cycles (i.e., primary and secondary target patterns) is a result of formulating and testing clinical research hypotheses in a university clinic since 1975 to determine which patterns would increase intelligibility most expeditiously. Table 6.4 provides potential primary and secondary target patterns based on these clinical research findings.

Table 6.4.   Primary and secondary target patterns for the cycles approach

Potential Optimal Primary Target Patterns* for Beginning Cycles

*Target *only* those that are *consistent* deviations. Targets must be *stimulable* (otherwise would reinforce inaccurate kinesthetic image)

Stimulate nonstimulable sounds (e.g., /k/) for a few minutes during sessions until they become stimulable. (*Exception:* Facilitate liquids even if not stimulable.)

Word/syllable structures (omitted segments)
- "Syllableness" (i.e., number of vowels/diphthongs)
  - Compound words (e.g., *cowboy, baseball*)
  - Three-syllable/word combinations (e.g., *cowboy hat, baseball bat*)
- Singleton consonants (syllable/word structures)
  - C̲V (word-initial /p, b, m, w/ if lacking)
  - VC̲ (voiceless final stops /p, t, k/; final /m, n/ if lacking; also these depend on child's word-initial phonetic repertoire [e.g., if child produces prevocalic /t/ or /d/, then word-final /t/ can be targeted])
  - VC̲V (e.g., *apple*)

/s/ clusters (for omissions, not substitutions/distortions)
  - Word-initial (e.g., /sp/, /st/, /sm/*)
  - Word-final (e.g., /ts/, /ps/)

*Note: Add /s/ to consonant child already produces (e.g., if child produces /b/ or /p/, can target /sp/)

Incorporate phrase "It's a [/s/ cluster word]" after child demonstrates facility producing /s/ clusters in production-practice words (typically by third cycle).

Reminder: Model soft, short, precise /s/

Anterior/Posterior Contrasts (when stimulable)
- Velars (if fronter)
  - Word-final /k/ (before prevocalic velars; never final /g/)
  - Word-initial /k, g/
- Alveolars/labials [if backer]

Facilitation of Liquids (even if not stimulable)
- Word-initial /l/ (preceded by week of tongue-tip clicking)
- Word-initial /ɹ/ (suppress gliding initially)
  Exaggerate and prolong the vowel (rather than /ɹ/)
  Do not blend initially

Incorporate /kɹ/, /gɹ/ (when child has velars [typically by third cycle])

General Comments Regarding Targets
- Spend approximately 60 minutes per PHONEME target.
- Target at least two phonemes per target PATTERN.
- Reassess phonology between cycles.
- Recycle primary patterns as needed (until they begin to emerge in conversation)

Proceed to SECONDARY Patterns after
- Early developing patterns are established
- /s/ clusters are in conversation
- Contrastive use of velars and alveolars
- Practice words for liquids—produced without glide

Potential Optimal Secondary Targets

Target any of the following secondary patterns/phonemes that are still consistently lacking/deficient. Incorporate minimal pairs for production practice when possible.

Palatals
  Glide /j/ and glide clusters (e.g., /kj/)
  Palatal sibilants
  Medial and vocalic (ɹ); other /ɹ/ clusters

Singleton stridents (e.g., /f/, /s/)

All other consonant clusters (e.g., three consonants)

Source: Hodson, B. (2007a).

Potential Optimal Primary Phonological Target Patterns

Word/syllable structures (omissions) are the first targets (if lacking) for children with highly unintelligible speech. Most 2-year-olds, for example, commonly produce utterances that contain two or three syllables, as well as word-initial and word-final consonants. In addition, typically developing 2-year-olds produce word-initial singleton stops, nasals, and glides (particularly labials) and some word-final nasals and voiceless obstruents (Preisser et al., 1988; Stoel-Gammon & Dunn, 1985). Children with expressive phonological impairments, however, vary greatly in their abilities to produce these early developing patterns.

Syllableness (omission of syllable nuclei: vowels, diphthongs, vocalic/syllabic consonants) is a target for children who speak in monosyllables. Preschool children are generally able to produce at least two syllables. Two- and three-syllable compound words (e.g., *cowboy, ice-cream cone*) are optimal early targets for children who have not yet learned to produce syllables in sequences. For these early targets, an emphasis on the appropriate number of syllables, rather than on the accuracy of specific consonants, is recommended.

Singleton consonants (when consistently omitted in a word position (e.g., **CV, VC**) are appropriate early intervention targets. Although word-initial singleton consonants rarely need to be targeted, the consistent omission of word-initial consonants seems to have a particularly adverse effect on intelligibility. When a child lacks word-initial consonants, the labial stops /p, b/, nasal /m/, and glide /w/ (for 2 or 3 hours) are ideal targets to help the client learn to produce prevocalic consonants. Word-final singleton consonants are frequent targets for children with highly unintelligible speech. Targeting voiceless word-final stops (e.g., /p/, /t/, and/or /k/, depending on whether the child has velars or alveolars in his or her word-initial consonant repertoire) for 2 or 3 hours helps children become aware of word closings.

The most frequent targets for all children with severe-to-profound phonological impairments are /s/ clusters/sequences. Virtually every young child with highly unintelligible speech has demonstrated difficulty with /s/ clusters. For example, at the University of Illinois Phonology clinic (i.e., 1975–1977), /s/ and /f/ singletons were targeted initially. When words such as *sun* and *soap* were presented, children typically said *stun* and *stoap*. Then after they learned to say /s/ singleton appropriately in words, they lost the stop in clusters and would say *say* for *stay*, thus requiring considerable additional time to teach the children to say /s/ clusters. It was hypothesized that starting with /s/ clusters might be easier for children rather than requiring deletion of the stop and putting on the /s/. This finding has passed the test of time during the last 30 years with hundreds of children. Moreover, because the English language is loaded with /s/ consonant sequences in connected speech, the incorporation of /s/ clusters in a child's speech truly expedites intelligibility gains. After children learn to produce /s/ clusters consistently, it is extremely easy for them to learn /s/ singleton productions.

Anterior/posterior contrasts are targeted for children who lack velars (either because of fronting or omissions) or alveolars or labials (either because of backing or omissions). Velars need to be targeted much more frequently than anterior consonants. Some children have an incredibly difficult time producing velars; thus, velars need to be stimulated until they are stimulable and then can be produced appropriately in production-practice words. Typically word-final /k/ is targeted before word-initial /k/ or /g/. For backers, typical targets are /t/ and /d/.

Liquids typically are targeted at the end of each of the beginning cycles even if they are not stimulable. This is another change from what was done the first few years at the Illinois Phonology Clinic. It has been found that facilitating liquids at the end of each cycle lays a foundation for later productions. Typically, /l/ is fairly easy to elicit after the child has been taught to click his or her tongue independent of jaw movement. When targeting /ɹ/, the initial emphasis is on suppressing the /w/ substitution. The /ɹ/ is modeled for the child, followed by wide open mouth position and an exaggeration of the vowel. For some children, this is an easy procedure; for others it is very difficult. Also, after the child produces velars, the /kɹ/ and /gɹ/ clusters are incorporated because these have a facilitative phonetic environment.

Beginning cycles typically last from 10 to 15 weeks depending on the number of patterns/phonemes needing to be targeted. The HAPP-3 is readministered at the end of each cycle to document progress and to determine what needs to be recycled.

Potential Secondary Target Patterns

Secondary patterns are not targeted until the following criteria have been achieved in spontaneous utterances: 1) appropriate syllableness, 2) productions of singleton consonants, 3) some emergence of /s/ clusters and velars, and 4) productions of practice words for /l/ and /ɹ/ without inserting the glide.

Many of the secondary patterns that had been noted on the original HAPP-3 will no longer need to be targeted. The most common targets at this time are 1) palatals (glide /j/, sibilants, /ɹ/), 2) all other consonant clusters/sequences (e.g., /j/ clusters, medial /s/ clusters, 3-consonant clusters), and 3) other singleton stridents (e.g., /f/, /s/, /z/). If there are any remaining vowel/diphthong or prevocalic voicing/devoicing difficulties, these would be targeted at this time.

Inappropriate Targets for Preschoolers

Some phonemes/patterns have been identified as being inappropriate targets for preschoolers because many, if not most, of their typically developing peers do not fully produce these. These include 1) voiced final obstruents (e.g., /b/, /d/); 2) the velar nasal (a common substitution by American adults as well as children, especially in bisyllabic words, is the alveolar nasal *singin* for *singing*); 3) postvocalic /l/ (children and adults often simply alter their pitch more than placing the tongue tip to the alveolar ridge); 4) unstressed weak syllables (e.g., *pro<u>bab</u>ly*), which are commonly omitted by adults as well as typical peers; and 5) "th" sounds, which generally are considered to be among the last sounds acquired and not optimal targets for preschoolers. It seems inappropriate to ask preschoolers to produce sounds that their typically developing peers (and sometimes even adults) are not fully producing.

Advanced Target Patterns for Older Children with Intelligibility Issues

Some older elementary school (and also middle school and high school) children demonstrate difficulties with productions of multisyllabic words (e.g., *extinguisher*, *aluminum*). These students usually will score well on a traditional articulation test. The HAPP-3 Multisyllabic Word Screening instrument is administered first. Then typically a list of troublesome words is obtained with the help of parents and teachers. The students are first taught how to break the words into syllables. Then phonic writing is used for each syllable. After the student can produce all the sounds of each syllable, syllables are put together two at a time, then three at a time, and so forth. After the student can say the multisyllabic words with automaticity, sentences using the words are generated.

Materials and Equipment Required

Few materials and equipment are required for proper implementation of the cycles approach. Although practitioners adapt the approach for individual client needs, the following materials are recommended: an amplification device, 5 × 8-inch index cards, and motivational experiential play items. An amplifier is recommended for slight amplification of the listening list at the beginning and ending of the session. The child does not repeat words from the listening list. The amplifier also can be used so that children hear their own productions of targets and contrast error productions with target productions. Some practitioners have used audio recording devices (e.g., a tape recorder or iPod with microphone) to set up listening stations. Large cards are recommended for production-practice activities for targeting patterns during treatment sessions. Experiential play items (games/toys) vary (depending on the child's interests). A manila folder commonly is used to include a metaphonological awareness rhyme. Moreover, a listening list is sent home with caregivers for the home program along with the production-practice cards containing pictures of the practice words for the week.

ASSESSMENT AND PROGRESS
MONITORING TO SUPPORT DECISION MAKING

The HAPP-3 (Hodson, 2004), which is a standardized norm-referenced as well as criterion-referenced test, is administered prior to intervention to determine 1) severity level (based on total occurrences of major phonological deviations; TOMPD), 2) major phonological deficiencies (e.g., omissions and consonant category deficiencies) to determine optimal target patterns, and 3) baseline data to be used for comparisons to document treatment effects over time. The HAPP-3 is also administered after each cycle in order to evaluate changes in a child's phonological system and also to determine what needs to be recycled. Graphs are made to illustrate changes in phonological patterns and TOMPD over time. After optimal target patterns are identified, probing occurs at the end of each session to determine the optimal phoneme/pattern target for the next session.

CONSIDERATIONS FOR CHILDREN FROM
CULTURALLY AND LINGUISTICALLY DIVERSE BACKGROUNDS

The seven underlying concepts that serve as the foundation for the cycles approach are highly universal. Considerations related to amplification, development of accurate kinesthetic images, and facilitative phonetic environments of production-practice words, for example, are critical and applicable to children from all backgrounds. Children (regardless of language) are actively involved in their phonological acquisition. The main structure and model of the cycles approach, therefore, is transferrable to other populations.

Although recommendations for primary and secondary targets were chosen with extreme care and ordered with consideration for the English language, more research is needed to determine appropriate targets (i.e., phonemes/patterns) for cycles approaches in other languages. Investigations of phonological development in Vietnamese (e.g., Hwa-Froehlich, Hodson, & Edwards, 2001) and Spanish (e.g., Lozano, Hodson, & Prezas, 2009; Mann & Hodson, 1994; Prezas, 2008) have provided preliminary data for further exploration of target selection and use. In bilingual (Spanish-English) children, for example, the most frequent phonological deviations that are shared in both languages are consonant sequence reduction, postvocalic singleton omissions, velar deficiencies, and liquid deficiencies (Mann & Hodson, 1994; Prezas, 2008).

Although more data are needed to examine the efficacy of a cyclical intervention model for bilingual children, the cycles approach can be adapted to fit the governing phonological rules of a language. Efforts are underway (i.e., case studies) to evaluate effectiveness of the cycles approach for bilingual (Spanish-English) children in the United States. In addition, a revised phonological assessment instrument, Assessment of Phonological Patterns in Spanish, 2nd Edition (Hodson & Prezas, 2009), is in development.

CASE STUDY

Joey (pseudonym) was age 3;5 when he was referred to our university phonology clinic. Video clips of his speech over time (from 3;6 to 5;7) are available from the American Speech-Language-Hearing Association in *Enhancing Phonological and Metaphonological Skills of Children with Highly Unintelligible Speech* (Hodson, 2005).

At the time of his initial evaluation, Joey produced the following consonants: /p, b, t, d, m, n, w, j/. His utterances were lengthy with the appropriate number of syllables, but no final consonants or consonant clusters were evidenced. The only word that could be identified by unfamiliar listeners in a connected-speech sample at the time of his initial evaluation was *Daddy*. Many characteristics of his speech were identical to those commonly reported for children with CAS. Table 6.5 provides pretreatment phonological assessment scores (Hodson, 2003, 2004).

Joey's parents were well-educated professionals, and he had one younger sibling. His medical history was unremarkable except for chronic upper respiratory infections and recurrent otitis media. Four months after treatment began, pressure-equalizing tubes were inserted in his tympanic membranes, and his adenoids were removed.

Joey attended 60-minute treatment sessions once a week during the university semesters. In addition, his parents provided a 2-minute home program on a daily basis. Targets during his first cycle of treatment included 1) word-final consonants (/p/ and /t/), 2) /s/ clusters (word-initial and word-final), 3) velars (word-final /k/, word-initial /k/, and word-initial /g/), and 4) facilitation of prevocalic liquids. By the end of the first cycle, Joey was producing velars and word endings in spontaneous speech, although there were some substitutions for word-final consonants. In addition, he readily produced /s/ clusters in his production-practice words, but carryover into conversation had not yet begun to occur.

Table 6.5. Pretreatment phonological assessment scores for Joey at age 3;6, based on the Hodson Assessment of Phonological Patterns–Third Edition (HAPP-3; Hodson, 2004)

Major phonological deviations	Occurrence percentages
Omissions	
Syllables	0%
Consonant clusters/sequences*	118%*
Consonant singletons	
Prevocalic	0%
Intervocalic	7%
Postvocalic	100%
Consonant category deficiencies	
Sonorants	
Liquids	100%
Nasals	76%
Glides	60%
Obstruents	
Stridents	100%
Velars	100%
Other (Anterior Nonstridents/Backing)	33%
Substitutions and other major strategies	
Other phonological deviations	Occurrences
Vowel alterations (phonemic)	31
Stopping	16
Fronting	12
Gliding	12
Reduplication	10
Labial assimilation	8
Total occurrences of major phonological deviations**	195
Severity interval level—high profound	

*The percentage for consonant sequence omissions exceeds 100% if all consonants of any cluster/sequence are omitted (rather than being reduced with at least one consonant remaining).

**For severity intervals, 0–50 = mild; 51–100 = moderate; 101–150 = severe; >151 = profound. In addition, the top 10 points per interval are designated "high" and the bottom 10 points are "low."

From Hodson, B.W. (2005). *Enhancing phonological and metaphonological skills of children with highly unintelligible speech* (p. 28). Rockville, MD: American Speech-Language-Hearing Association; reprinted by permission.

During the second cycle of phonological treatment, /s/ clusters were recycled and then were incorporated into "It's a _____" phrases (e.g., "It's a spoon"). Liquids were also recycled with /kɹ/ and /gɹ/ being added. In addition, other consonant clusters were targeted including medial and final /st/ (e.g., *toast, toaster*) and glide clusters /kw/ and /kj/ (e.g., *queen, cue*).

For cycles three and four, liquids were recycled. In addition, palatal sibilants and other consonant clusters (e.g., three-consonant clusters) were presented. Table 6.6 provides pretreatment, interim, and posttreatment phonological assessment scores (ages 3;6, 4;7, and 5;7) for the patterns that were targeted. Figure 6.1 shows TOMPD for the five assessment sessions based on his results from

Table 6.6. Pretreatment, interim, and posttreatment Hodson Assessment of Phonological Patterns–Third Edition (HAPP-3; Hodson, 2004) phonological assessment results for targeted phonological patterns

Phonological deviation	Chronological age		
	3;6	4;7	5;7
Omissions			
Consonant sequences	118%*	62%	18%
Postvocalic singletons	100%	0%	0%
Consonant category deficiencies			
Stridents	100%	10%	5%
Velars	100%	50%	5%
Liquids	100%	100%	95%
TOMPD	195	65	30
Severity level	High profound	Moderate	Mild

*The percentage for consonant sequence omissions exceeds 100% if all consonants of any cluster/sequence are omitted (rather than being reduced with at least one consonant remaining).

Key: TOMPD, total occurrences of major phonological deviations.

From Hodson, B.W. (2005). *Enhancing phonological and metaphonological skills of children with highly unintelligible speech* (p. 28). Rockville, MD: American Speech-Language-Hearing Association; reprinted by permission.

the Hodson Computerized Analysis of Phonological Patterns–Third Edition (Hodson, 2003).

Joey was dismissed from the phonology clinic after 52 contact hours of treatment over a period of 2 years and 1 month. His speech was not perfect, but he was essentially intelligible. When he entered kindergarten in the fall, he did not qualify for speech services in the school because the only consistent deviation at that time was liquids. By the time he entered second grade, he produced liquids appropriately and reportedly was an excellent reader.

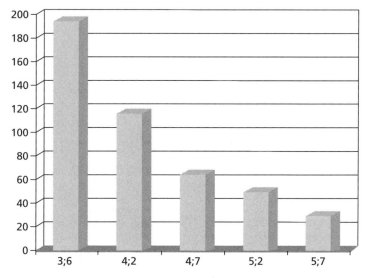

Figure 6.1. Total occurrences of major phonological deviations (TOMPD) for Joey, ages 3;6–5;7.

STUDY QUESTIONS

1. What is the *major goal* of the cycles approach?

2. What is the *critical age hypothesis* and why is it important?

3. Why is the emphasis of the cycles approach on targeting phonological *patterns* in a cyclical manner rather than mastering (e.g., 90%) individual sounds in all positions, one at a time?

4. Why do sounds need to be *stimulable* before being targeted in production-practice words?

5. Why should assessment instruments for speech sounds/patterns *differentiate* among types of deviations (e.g., omissions vs. distortions) in final scores?

6. What evidence is available regarding effectiveness of the cycles approach?

FUTURE DIRECTIONS

A large, randomized, well-designed, controlled study comparing results of approaches (e.g., oral motor, contrasts, patterns, phoneme mastery) for highly unintelligible children by independent investigators is needed—with the proponents of the respective methods being involved for fidelity. Moreover, children in the various groups would need to be matched as well as possible at the onset of treatment.

In addition, more research is needed to determine how the cycles approach can be adapted for use with children who speak languages other than English. Optimal intervention modifications and implementations for specific languages are needed.

SUGGESTED READINGS

Hodson, B.W. (2005). *Enhancing phonological and meta-phonological skills of children with highly unintelligible speech.* Rockville, MD: American Speech-Language-Hearing Association. [Master clinician DVD that includes case study and client videos along with presentation.]

Hodson, B.W. (2007). *Evaluating and enhancing children's phonological systems: Research and theory to practice.* Greenville, SC: Thinking Publications University.

REFERENCES

Almost, D., & Rosenbaum, P. (1998). Effectiveness of speech intervention for phonological disorders: A randomized controlled trial. *Developmental Medicine and Child Neurology, 40,* 319–325.

Baker, E., Carrigg, B., & Linich, A. (2007). What's the evidence for . . .? The cycles approach to phonological intervention. *ACQuiring Knowledge in Speech, Language, and Hearing, 9,* 29–30.

Berko, J., & Brown, R. (1960). Psycholinguistic research methods. In P. Mussen (Ed.), *Handbook of research methods in child development* (pp. 517–557). New York: Wiley.

Berman, S. (2001). *Speech intelligibility and the Down syndrome child.* Poster session presented at the annual convention of the American Speech-Language-Hearing Association, New Orleans, LA.

Bird, J., Bishop, D.V.M., & Freeman, N.H. (1995). Phonological awareness and literacy development in children with expressive phonological impairments. *Journal of Speech, Language, and Hearing Research, 38,* 446–462.

Bishop, D., & Adams, C. (1990). A prospective study of the relationship between specific language impairment, phonological disorders, and reading retardation. *Journal of Child Psychology and Psychiatry, 31,* 1027–1050.

Browman, C., & Goldstein, L. (1986). Towards an articulatory phonology. *Phonology Yearbook, 3,* 219–252.

Buteau, C., & Hodson, B.W. (1989). *Phonological remediation targets: Words and primary pictures for highly unintelligible children.* Austin, TX: PRO-ED.

Churchill, J., Hodson, B.W., Jones, B., & Novak, R. (1988). Phonological systems of speech-disordered clients with positive/negative histories of otitis media. *Language, Speech, and Hearing Services in Schools, 19,* 100–107.

Clarke-Klein, S., & Hodson, B.W. (1995). A phonologically based analysis of misspellings by third graders with disordered-phonology histories. *Journal of Speech and Hearing Research, 38,* 839–849.

Dyson, A., & Paden, E. (1983). Some phonological acquisition strategies used by 2-year-olds. *Journal of Childhood Communication Disorders, 7,* 6–18.

Fairbanks, G. (1954). Systematic research in experimental phonetics: A theory of the speech mechanism as a servosystem. *Journal of Speech and Hearing Disorders, 19,* 133–139.

Fey, M. (2004, May). *EBP in child language intervention: Some background and some food for thought.* Paper presented at the conference of the Working Group on EBP in Child Language Disorders, Austin, TX.

Garrett, R. (1986). *A phonologically based speech improvement classroom program for hearing impaired students.* Unpublished manuscript, San Diego State University, San Diego.

Goldman, R., & Fristoe, M. (1969). *Goldman-Fristoe Test of Articulation.* Circle Pines, MN: American Guidance Service.

Goldman, R., & Fristoe, M. (2000). *Goldman-Fristoe Test of Articulation-2.* Circle Pines, MN: American Guidance Service.

Gordon-Brannan, M., Hodson, B.W., & Wynne, M. (1992). Remediating unintelligible utterances of a child with a mild hearing loss. *American Journal of Speech-Language Pathology, 1,* 28–38.

Grunwell, P. (1987). *Clinical phonology* (2nd ed.). Baltimore: Williams & Wilkins.

Hodson, B.W. (1982). Remediation of speech patterns associated with low levels of phonological performance. In M. Crary (Ed.), *Phonological intervention: Concepts and procedures* (pp. 91–115). San Diego: College-Hill.

Hodson, B.W. (1983). A facilitative approach for remediation of a child's profoundly unintelligible phonological system. *Topics in Language Disorders, 3,* 24–34.

Hodson, B.W. (1986). *Assessment of Phonological Processes–Revised.* Danville, IL: Interstate.

Hodson, B.W. (1994a). Determining intervention priorities for preschoolers with disordered phonologies: Expediting intelligibility gains. In E.J. Williams & J. Langsam (Eds.), *Children's phonology disorders: Pathways and patterns* (pp. 65–87). Rockville, MD: American Speech-Language-Hearing Association.

Hodson, B.W. (1994b). Helping individuals become intelligible, literate, and articulate: The role of phonology. *Topics in Language Disorders, 14,* 1–16.

Hodson, B.W. (1997). Disordered phonologies: What have we learned about assessment and treatment? In B.W. Hodson & M. Edwards (Eds.), *Perspectives in applied phonology* (pp. 197–224). Gaithersburg, MD: Aspen.

Hodson, B.W. (1998). Research and practice: Applied phonology. *Topics in Language Disorders, 18,* 58–70.

Hodson, B.W. (2001). *Phonological cycles approach adapted for a child with a cochlear implant.* Proceedings of the International Association of Logopedics and Phoniatrics, Montreal, Quebec.

Hodson, B.W. (2003). *Hodson Computerized Analysis of Phonological Patterns* (HCAPP). Wichita, KS: Phonocomp Publishers..

Hodson, B.W. (2004). *Hodson Assessment of Phonological Patterns* (3rd ed.; HAPP-3). Austin, TX: PRO-ED.

Hodson, B.W. (2005). *Enhancing phonological and metaphonological skills of children with highly unintelligible speech.* Rockville, MD: American Speech-Language-Hearing Association.

Hodson, B.W. (2007a). *Evaluating and enhancing children's phonological systems: Research and theory to practice.* Wichita, KS: Phonocomp Publishers.

Hodson, B.W. (2007b). Identifying phonological patterns and projecting remediation cycles: Expediting intelligibility gains of a 7-year-old Australian child. *Advances in Speech-Language Pathology, 8*(3), 257–264.

Hodson, B.W., Chin, L., Redmond, B., & Simpson, R. (1983). Phonological evaluation and remediation of speech deviations of a child with a repaired cleft palate: A case study. *Journal of Speech and Hearing Disorders, 48,* 93–98.

Hodson, B.W., Nonomura, C., & Zappia, M. (1989). Phonological disorders: Impact on academic performance? *Seminars in Speech and Language, 10,* 252–259.

Hodson, B.W., & Paden, E.P. (1981). Phonological processes which characterize unintelligible and intelligible speech in early childhood. *Journal of Speech and Hearing Disorders, 46,* 369–373.

Hodson, B.W., & Paden, E. (1983). *Targeting intelligible speech: A phonological approach to remediation.* Austin, TX: PRO-ED.

Hodson, B.W., & Paden, E. (1991). *Targeting intelligible speech: A phonological approach to remediation* (2nd ed.). Austin, TX: PRO-ED.

Hodson, B.W., & Prezas, R.F (2009). *Assessment of Phonological Patterns in Spanish* (2nd ed.). Unpublished manuscript, Wichita State University, Wichita, KS.

Hodson, B.W., Scherz, J., & Strattman, K. (2002). Evaluating communicative abilities of a highly unintelligible child. *American Journal of Speech-Language Pathology*, *11*, 236–242.

Hodson, B.W., & Strattman, K.H. (2004). Phonological awareness intervention for children with expressive phonological impairments. In R. Kent (Ed.), *MIT encyclopedia of communicative disorders* (pp. 153–156). Cambridge, MA: The MIT Press.

Hunt, J. (1961). *Intelligence and experience*. New York: Ronald Press.

Hwa-Froehlich, D., Hodson, B.W., & Edwards, H.T. (2001). Characteristics of Vietnamese phonology. *American Journal of Speech-Language Pathology*, *11*, 236–242.

Ingram, D. (1976). *Phonological disability in children*. New York: Elsevier.

Ingram, D. (1986). Explanation and phonological remediation. *Child Language Teaching and Therapy*, *2*, 1–19.

Kamhi, A. (2006). Treatment decisions for children with speech-sound disorders. *Language, Speech, and Hearing Services in Schools*, *37*, 271–279.

Kent, R.D. (1982). Contextual facilitation of correct sound production. *Language, Speech, and Hearing Services in Schools*, *13*, 66–76.

Kent, R.D. (1997). Gestural phonology: Basic concepts and applications in speech-language pathology. In M. Ball & R. Kent (Eds.), *The new phonologies: Developments in clinical linguistics* (pp. 247–265). San Diego: Singular Publishing.

Larrivee, L.S., & Catts, H.W. (1999). Early reading achievement in children with expressive phonological disorders. *American Journal of Speech-Language Pathology*, *8*, 118–128.

Lozano, V., Hodson, B.W., & Prezas, R.F. (2009, November). *Adapting phonological pattern approach for highly unintelligible bilingual (Spanish/English) client*. Poster presented at the Annual Convention of the American Speech-Language-Hearing Association, New Orleans.

Mann, D., & Hodson, B.W. (1994). Spanish-speaking children's phonologies: Assessment and remediation. *Seminars in Speech and Language*, *15*, 137–148.

McReynolds, L.V., & Bennett, S. (1972). Distinctive feature generalization in articulation training. *Journal of Speech and Hearing Disorders*, *37*, 462–470.

Mody, M. (2003). Phonological basis in reading disability: A review and analysis of the evidence. *Reading and Writing: An Interdisciplinary Journal*, *16*, 21–39.

Montgomery, J., & Bonderman, R. (1989). Serving preschool children with severe phonological disorders. *Language, Speech, and Hearing Services in Schools*, *20*, 76–83.

Pascoe, M., Stackhouse, J., & Wells, B. (2006). *Persisting speech difficulties in children's speech and literacy difficulties: Book 3*. West Sussex, England: Whurr.

Porter, J., & Hodson, B.W. (2001). Collaborating to obtain phonological acquisition data for local schools. *Language, Speech, and Hearing Services in Schools*, *32*, 165–161.

Preisser, D., Hodson, B.W., & Paden, E. (1988). Developmental phonology: 18–29 months. *Journal of Speech and Hearing Disorders*, *53*, 125–130.

Prezas, R.F. (2008). *An investigation of bilingual preschool children's intelligibility in Spanish and English: Comparing measures of performance with listener ratings in both languages*. Unpublished doctoral dissertation, Wichita State University, Wichita, KS.

Prezas, R.F., & Hodson, B.W. (2007). Diagnostic evaluation of children with speech sound disorders. *In Encyclopedia of language and literacy development* (pp. 1–8). London, Ontario, Canada: Canadian Language and Literacy Research Network. Retrieved March, 3, 2009, from http://www.literacyencyclopedia.ca/pdfs/topic.php?topId=21

Raitano, N.A., Pennington, B.F., Tunick, B.F., Boada, R., & Shriberg, L.D. (2004). Pre-literacy skills of subgroups of children with speech sound disorders. *Journal of Child Psychology and Psychiatry*, *45*, 821–835.

Rvachew, S., & Grawberg, M. (2006). Correlates of phonological awareness in preschoolers with speech-sound disorders. *Journal of Speech, Language, and Hearing Research*, *49*, 74–87.

Rvachew, S., & Nowak, M. (2001). The effect of target selection strategy on phonological learning. *Language, Speech, and Hearing Services in Schools*, *44*, 610–623.

Rvachew, S., Ohberg, A., Grawburg, M., & Heyding, J. (2003). Phonological awareness and phonemic perception in 4-year-old children with delayed expressive phonology skills. *Language, Speech, and Hearing Services in Schools*, *12*, 463–471.

Rvachew, S., Rafaat, S., & Martin, M. (1999). Stimulability, speech perception skills, and the treatment of phonological disorders. *American Journal of Speech-Language Pathology*, *8*, 33–43.

Shriberg, L., & Kwiatkowski, J. (1982). Phonological disorders III: A procedure for assessing severity of involvement. *Journal of Speech and Hearing Disorders*, *47*, 256–270.

Stackhouse, J. (1997). Phonological awareness: Connecting speech and literacy problems. In B.W. Hodson & M. Edwards (Eds.), *Perspectives in applied phonology* (pp. 157–196). Gaithersburg, MD: Aspen.

Stampe, D. (1972). *A dissertation on natural phonology*. Unpublished doctoral dissertation, University of Chicago.

Stanovich, K. (1986). Matthew effects in reading: Some consequences of individual differences in the acquisition of literacy. *Reading Research Quarterly*, *21*, 360–407.

Stoel-Gammon, C., & Dunn, C. (1985). *Normal and disordered phonology in children*. Austin, TX: PRO-ED.

Tyler, A.A., Edwards, M.L., & Saxman, J.H. (1987). Clinical application of two phonologically based treatment procedures. *Journal of Speech and Hearing Disorders*, *52*, 393–409.

Van Riper, C. (1939). *Speech correction: Principles and methods* (2nd ed.). Upper Saddle River, NJ: Prentice Hall.

Velleman, S. (2003). *Childhood apraxia of speech resource guide.* Clifton Park, NY: Delmar Learning.

Velleman, S. (2005). Perspectives in assessment. In S.F. Warren & M.E. Fey (Series Eds.) & A.G. Kamhi & K.E. Pollock (Vol. Eds.), *Phonological disorders in children: Clinical decision making in assessment and intervention* (pp. 23–34). Baltimore: Paul H. Brookes Publishing Co.

Vygotsky, L. (1962). *Thought and language.* Cambridge, MA: The MIT Press.

World Health Organization. (2001). *International classification of functioning, disability and health.* Geneva: Author.

The Nuffield Centre Dyspraxia Programme

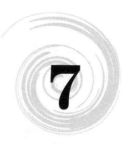

Pam Williams and Hilary Stephens

ABSTRACT

The Nuffield Centre Dyspraxia Programme (NDP) is an intervention package for children 3 years and older with severe speech sound disorders (SSDs) including childhood apraxia of speech (CAS). This resource, which is popular in the United Kingdom, comprises a detailed therapy manual, an assessment procedure, and a set of picture-based therapy materials. The NDP treatment approach is based on motor learning theory and aims to build speech skills from single sounds to word and sentence levels. In addition, it addresses linguistic issues by creating a contrastive system at each syllable-structure level. The current edition—the NDP3 (Williams & Stephens, 2004)—is set within the psycholinguistic model of Stackhouse and Wells (1997). Empirical case study evidence of the effectiveness of the NDP3 approach is beginning to emerge.

INTRODUCTION

NDP is a published intervention package for children 3–7 years of age with severe SSD, particularly CAS. It was designed to address these children's typical presenting difficulties, such as articulating individual consonants, vowels, and diphthongs; sequencing sounds together in simple and complex words; and maintaining segmental and suprasegmental (prosodic) accuracy when words are connected together into phrases and sentences.

The NDP3 (Williams & Stephens, 2004) resulted from extensive revisions of two earlier editions (Connery, 1985, 1992). It comprises a detailed therapy manual, an assessment procedure, and 550 pages of pictorial therapy materials. Target test and intervention stimuli are represented using simple black and white line drawings, divided into three sections: 1) single sounds (consonants, vowels, and diphthongs); 2) words of different phonotactic structures—CV, VC, CVCV, CVC, CCV (in which C = consonant and V = vowel)—and polysyllabic words ; and 3) combinations of words in phrases, clauses, and sentences. The single consonants, vowels, and diphthongs are represented by picture cues (e.g., /t/ is represented by a picture of a *tap;* /aɪ/ is represented by a picture of an *eye*). The majority of the depicted words occur with high frequency in the typical vocabulary of a young child.

TARGET POPULATIONS

Primary Populations

A clinician can use the NDP3 pictorial materials simply as a resource when designing therapy activities for a child with SSD. However, Williams and Stephens (2004) advocate a specific therapy approach for children with CAS that is primarily based on motor-learning theory. The underlying assumptions and principles behind the approach are explained in detail in the therapy manual along with guidance on treatment planning and step-by-step delivery.

Because NDP3 uses pictorial materials, it is best used with children with normal visual acuity and the ability to recognize the line-drawing pictures. Although adaptations can be made, the approach is ideally presented via table-top activities. Therefore, it is most suitable for children who can sit at a table and give focused attention to adult-directed tasks (for at least short periods of time). It is most effective when a good working relationship has been established between the speech-language pathologist (SLP) and child so that the child develops trust in the clinician and is willing to take risks to change his or her speech production (Weiss, 2004).

The approach also requires the child to have some symbolic skills; that is, he or she must understand that a picture is being used to represent a sound or a word. In addition, he or she must have, or be able to develop, some metalinguistic skills in order to understand how sounds or syllables can be blended together to create words and how words can be segmented into component parts. A developmental level of around 3 years of age is, therefore, recommended as an appropriate lower age level for using NDP3.

Older children with learning difficulties can use this approach, provided that they have reached this developmental level. Children with severe autistic spectrum disorders may have difficulties with the metalinguistic aspects of the approach. Although there is no upper age limit for using the approach, the materials may seem "childish" to children older than 8 years. Consequently, the materials may need to be adapted to be more acceptable for older children. (See Appendix 5 of the NDP3 therapy manual for ideas about ways to do this.)

ASSESSMENT METHODS FOR DETERMINING INTERVENTION RELEVANCE

No formal criteria exist for determining the appropriateness of the NDP3 approach for a particular child. However, it could be considered for a child presenting with typical features of CAS, such as those described previously; normal visual acuity; and in the developmental age range of 3–7 years. Although an SLP may derive this information from other assessment procedures, NDP3 has its own assessment procedure. The NDP3 assessment provides information on the child's ability to produce individual speech sounds, words of increasing phonotactic complexity, and combinations of words in phrases and sentences.

THEORETICAL BASIS

Dominant Theoretical Rationale for the Intervention Approach

The original NDP resource (Connery, 1985) was designed as a clinical tool to meet the needs of children presenting with severe speech difficulties. As an intervention approach, it was primarily influenced by the motor impairment theory of developmental verbal dyspraxia (referred to as CAS), which was expressed in the literature at the time (Jaffe, 1984; Yoss & Darley, 1974). The author, therefore, advocated an intervention approach that would address motor programming and planning impairments using principles of motor-learning theory (Connery, 1994).

Reflecting more recent views in the NDP3 intervention manual, Williams and Stephens (2004) utilized the speech processing model incorporated in the psycholinguistic framework of Stackhouse and Wells (1997; also see Chapter 9) to explain where breakdown(s) in speech processing may be occurring for a child with CAS. Although multiple levels of breakdown may occur across the speech processing chain, Williams and Stephens highlighted that children with CAS typically have significant difficulty with motor programs, motor programming, and motor planning. Motor programs are part of the stored lexical representations and consist of a series of gestural targets for the articulators, designed to achieve an acceptable pronunciation of the word. For example, accurate production of the word *tea* would require the following instructions: initiate airstream, close velopharyngeal sphincter, make closure with margins of tongue at the alveolar ridge, release closure, assume raised front tongue body posture, spread lips, and initiate voicing. Motor programming is considered to be an online output process through which new motor programs can be created. It is thought to include a store of phonological units, which can be combined to create new motor programs for unfamiliar words. For example, motor programming is required when a child is asked to blend /s/ with /i/ to create the new motor program *sea* (for a child who can articulate /s/ as a single sound, but usually replaces /s/ with /t/ in words). Once the new motor program for *sea* is created, it may take a good deal of repetitive practice to establish it in the stored representations in place of *tea*. In the Stackhouse and Wells (1997) model, motor planning is considered to be the stage at which a plan for the whole utterance is formed, for example, *I want a cup of tea*. It involves retrieving motor programs for individual words, then assembling the different gestural targets in the correct sequence and incorporating appropriate grammatical structures and prosodic features.

Support for the idea that children with CAS have motor impairments has been provided by the American Speech-Language-Hearing Association (ASHA; 2007) in its position statement and technical report on CAS, documents that were prepared following detailed review of the literature. Those documents described the core impairment of CAS to be in "planning and/or programming spatiotemporal parameters of movement sequences" that "results in errors in speech sound production and prosody" (ASHA, 2007, p.1). However, those documents also suggested that it is hard to account for some of the difficulties typically seen in CAS using a motor impairment theory alone. In particular, clinical and research findings with regard to difficulties with speech perception, phonological awareness, phonological patterns, and expressive language indicate that a linguistic impairment is also likely to be involved.

Developing Motor Skills

Williams and Stephens (2004) described speech production as a complex, hierarchical motor skill, which they analogize as a brick wall consisting of a number of layers of bricks (see Figure 7.1). The bottom layer consists of single speech sounds, the next layer is CV words, followed by CVCV words, CVC words, multisyllabic words, consonant cluster words, phrases, and sentences. Finally, the top layer is connected speech. The overall aim of intervention using NDP3 is to build accurate speech from the bottom up using core

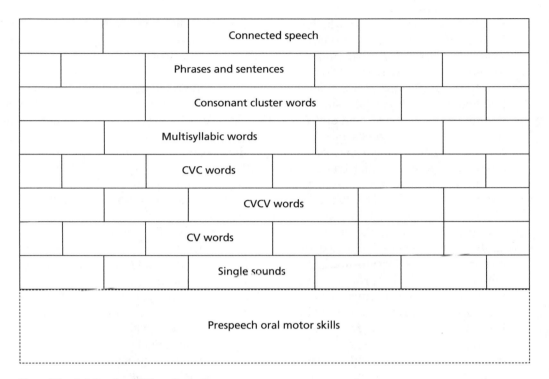

Figure 7.1. Building the wall from the bottom up.

units of consonants, vowels, and CV syllables. When faulty speech patterns have been developed, the aim is to break these down to the basic level of single sounds and CV syllables, then rebuild them again accurately. The focus of intervention is on establishing as
full a set as possible of accurate motor programs at each layer or level of the wall. The
starting point is generally with single sounds (consonants and vowels) and CV words, but
in some cases, prespeech oral motor skills need to be practiced first to support accurate
production of individual consonant and vowel sounds. Therapy gradually moves on to
more complex phonotactic structures once a number of the core single sound and CV
units have been established.

At each level, skills are established in stages by means of frequent repetition, elicited
by cues and reinforced or modified with the support of specific feedback, in keeping with
a motor skills learning approach. SLPs are also advised to utilize a child's strengths by
starting with speech sounds and words the child can already make, then following a fine-
tuned graded intervention approach (Hall et al., 1993). In this approach, tasks are broken
into small achievable steps, with each step challenging the individual's learning a little
more.

Developing a Linguistic System

Although the main focus of the NDP3 therapy approach is on developing motor skills,
there is also a linguistic, and specifically a phonological, component to the approach. As
new sounds, syllables, and words are acquired, they need to be incorporated into the cur-

rent sets of sounds and words that the child can already produce, thereby allowing the development of a contrastive system at each phonotactic level (C, V, CV, VC, CVCV, CVC, and so forth). NDP3 is therefore both a motor and a linguistic approach.

Developing a Full Range of Psycholinguistic Processing Skills

The aim of the NDP3 approach is not only to establish as full a set as possible of motor programs at each layer/level of the "wall," or skill level, but also to support the development of a full range of psycholinguistic processing skills. With regard to output, motor *programming* skills are practiced while establishing motor programs for a wide range of vocabulary at each level and while practicing sequencing tasks. Motor *planning* skills are also practiced during sequencing and repetition tasks and specifically when working at more complex phrase and sentence levels.

Input skills are utilized initially, along with oro-motor exercises to facilitate the production of speech sounds that cannot be elicited by imitation. At word and word-combination levels, auditory discrimination should continue to be utilized, as necessary, to support production work, and the child is always encouraged to listen carefully to the SLP's model. Stored phonological representations are clarified while working on developing accurate motor programs for individual words, making the structure of the word explicit through the use of picture cues representing sounds, and developing phonological awareness. Therefore, the child should be developing a full range of psycholinguistic processes at each level, as therapy progresses. At each level, they should be able to do each of the following things:

- Discriminate between sounds

- Have accurate phonological representations and readily accessible motor programs for a wide range of sounds, syllables, and words

- Execute those motor programs as accurately as possible and incorporate them in contrastive sequences/phrases

- Imitate unfamiliar words and nonwords

- Follow instructions to modify productions

- Sort by onset and rime, or be working toward this

- Segment and blend sounds, or be working toward this

Because of these goals, NDP3 is not simply a motor-based therapy approach; rather, it involves a combination of motor, linguistic, and psycholinguistic approaches.

Level of Consequences Being Addressed

Children with CAS are often reported to be unintelligible to unfamiliar listeners and sometimes even to close family members. Because they have difficulties in making themselves understood, children with CAS can be socially isolated and have difficulties in forming peer relationships. Although the NDP3 treatment approach does not address social integration issues directly, the consequence of the approach is that the child's speech becomes increasingly intelligible, which in turn results in improved social interaction.

Target Areas of Intervention

The primary focus of NDP3 is on the development of speech output skills. However, in the development of these skills, activities for both production and discrimination of targets are recommended. The approach also supports the development of phonological awareness skills. It does this by using picture cues to represent sounds and by making explicit the phonological structure of words—for example, to help teach blending, NDP3 uses worksheets in which a consonant is joined with a vowel to create a CV word (e.g., /b/ + /i/ = *bee*). At an appropriate stage, segmentation tasks can also be included using the same materials. For example, on the same worksheet, the CV picture *bee* can be kept covered while the child produces the sequence of /b/ + /i/, to see if he or she can work out what the CV picture will be. CV words can also be sorted by initial consonant sound or vowel sound, either silently or following a verbal presentation. The clinician may well need to provide considerable support and modeling when such tasks are first introduced. Further information on using NDP3 to support the development of phonological awareness skills and literacy acquisition can be found in Chapter 6 of the NDP3 manual.

EMPIRICAL BASIS

Six descriptive case studies are included in Chapter 7 of the NDP3 manual (Williams & Stephens, 2004) to illustrate intervention planning and the NDP3 therapy approach in specific cases. The children in these case studies ranged in age from 4 to12 years, had a range of speech profiles and severities, and were seen under different models of service provision. All achieved intelligible speech after use of NDP3, but the duration of intervention varied from between 1 and 4 years and was delivered within different schedules by different SLPs.

Saunders (2006) reported a case study of 3-year-old Caelan, who had a diagnosis of autistic spectrum disorder and verbal dyspraxia (CAS). Caelan received once weekly therapy sessions from the author, supported by daily practice at home and in his nursery. Intervention methods utilized NDP3 resources and followed the principles of the NDP3 approach (Williams & Stephens, 2004). Following intervention, Caelan was reported to have made excellent progress with his speech sound development. In addition, his expressive language level had also improved considerably.

The effectiveness of the NDP3 therapy approach has also been explored in two student projects. Teal (2005) used two different treatment approaches, NDP3 (Williams & Stephens, 2004) and core vocabulary (Dodd, 2005), when working with Ruth, age 6;11, who had persisting speech difficulties. The study involved a detailed period of assessment, followed by 3 weeks of intervention, which comprised two 1-hour sessions per week. The sessions were split into two 30-minute periods that were spent on either NDP3 or core vocabulary. The order of the two approaches was alternated across the therapy sessions to control for Ruth tiring toward the end of a session.

The treatment target using NDP3 was to achieve the consonant /k/ in initial position in words. Twelve words of one and two syllables were selected from the index in the NDP3 manual to be targeted in intervention. All of them contained /k/ word-initially. In order to measure generalization, a matched set of untreated real words and nonwords were also selected. The intervention followed the principles of the NDP3 therapy approach, that is, linking the target sound /k/ to the symbol picture, creating CV syllables by combining /k/ + V = CV, practicing the newly formed CV words through repetitive and contrastive sequencing practice, and combining CV syllables to create longer words.

Ruth's production of the treated words, untreated words, and nonwords was assessed pre- and postintervention and compared using statistical analysis. Two-tailed paired sample t-tests showed a significant increase in the use of word-initial /k/ after intervention for the treated words. There was also a significant increase in the use of word-initial /k/ in the matched untreated words, but not in the nonwords, where only a slight nonsignificant increase occurred. A further pre-and postintervention measurement of percentage consonants correct (PCC) for each word showed a significant increase after intervention for both the treated and untreated real words, which was mainly due to the improved use of word initial /k/. Although acknowledging that this was only a small scale study, Teal (2005) concluded that both NDP3 and core vocabulary were effective in bringing about change in different aspects of Ruth's speech processing system. However, NDP3 also produced significant generalization to untreated words.

Belton (2006) investigated the effectiveness of intervention utilizing the NDP3 therapy resources and following the principles of the NDP3 therapy approach for four boys, ages 4–6 years. At the start of the study, they all scored below the 1st percentile on PCC on the Diagnostic Evaluation of Articulation and Phonology (DEAP; Dodd, Zhu, Crosbie, Holm, & Ozanne, 2002). They all had difficulties at a number of speech output levels and reduced phonetic inventories but were unimpaired on auditory discrimination tasks. The children received 20 hours of individual therapy (1 hour per week) delivered by two experienced SLPs in a real-life clinical setting, supported by practice sessions at home and in school. Assessments were carried out before and after each block of 10 therapy sessions and included measures closely related to the therapy targets (the NDP3 assessment), as well as more global speech production measures (the DEAP Oromotor, Phonology, and Inconsistency subtests and parent and clinician intelligibility ratings). Detailed analyses of the data were carried out, including PCC and process analysis on the DEAP (Dodd et al., 2002), an inconsistency analysis, and quantitative and qualitative analysis of the NDP3 data. The qualitative analysis involved the use of the probe scoring system (PSS; Hall, Adams, Hesketh, & Nightingale, 1998). The PSS has been used as an outcome measure in other therapy studies with children with severe speech disorders (Carter & Edwards, 2004; Hall et al., 1998) because it can detect subtle changes in the "right direction" after therapy, which may not show on formal tests. Belton (2006) used it to detect changes in each child's phonological system in terms of place, manner, and voicing for consonants, and length and tongue position (front/back, open/close) for vowels.

The results showed that all of the children increased their phonetic inventories, reduced the number and frequency of their phonological processes, and increased their intelligibility ratings following therapy. They also increased their accuracy at single word and phrase/sentence levels but to very different degrees, ranging from highly significant change at all levels of complexity to small changes in phonetic similarity to target phonemes. Of the four children, Callum made the greatest progress, showing significant change on all levels of the NDP3 assessment over the course of therapy. In addition, his PCC on the DEAP (Dodd et al., 2002) increased from 39% to 93% and progressed from the 1st to the 25th percentile, indicating that he had changed from having a severe speech disorder at the start of the study to having speech within the normal range by the end. In contrast, Daniel made the least progress of the four children. His PCC only increased from 58% to 61% and remained at the 1st percentile at the end of the study. Despite this, the PSS indicated that some encouraging changes had occurred in his consonant scores at single sound, cluster words, and multisyllabic words, as well as vowel scores in multisyllabic words by the end of the study.

Gareth's scores increased on all levels of the NDP3 assessment, except cluster words, with considerable change being made at single consonant, CVC, and phrase/sentence levels. However, on the DEAP test, Gareth only progressed from 36% to 54% PCC and remained at the 1st percentile at the end of the study. Simon's scores increased over therapy on the NDP3 measures to an important degree for single consonants, CVC words, and phrases/sentences. In addition, the PSS revealed that Simon's realizations became more phonetically similar to the target consonants at all levels, with the exception of CV words that were almost at ceiling at the start of the study. On the DEAP, Simon's PCC progressed from 70% to 87%, which was above the rate expected from age, but this only amounted to change from the 1st to the 5th percentile at the end of the study.

The study highlighted the variability in response to therapy and the complexity of the factors involved in treating children with severe speech disorders. Daniel demonstrated emotional and behavioral difficulties in the treatment sessions, a barrier to the therapeutic process (Weiss, 2004). Simon and Gareth also had additional difficulties, when compared with Callum. Both were significantly inconsistent in their speech production and had oro-motor difficulties, as measured on the DEAP (Dodd et al., 2002). Moreover, Gareth also had delayed expressive language development. These factors were considered to have contributed to their poorer outcomes.

Pagnamenta and Williams (2009) evaluated the effectiveness of NDP3 in treating Callum and Gareth. They examined the results just described in detail to see whether the changes reported could be specifically attributed to the NDP3 therapy targets. Overall, they reported that some changes were clearly related to the therapy targets; for example, Gareth's scores on single vowels increased in the first therapy block, when they were targeted in therapy, and Callum's scores on the cluster words made most change in the second block, when clusters were targeted. However, for both children, the authors noted evidence of generalization to some untreated areas. For example, gains in scores at the levels of single sounds and CV and VC words had a positive effect on CVC words, despite the latter not being targeted in therapy. Similarly, gains in CVCV words had a positive effect on phrases and sentences when these were not included in the therapy targets. Although there were some methodological shortcomings of this study, Pagnamenta and Williams proposed that these findings indicate that a "bottom up" therapy approach, such as NDP3, which focuses on addressing accuracy and consistency of production in single sounds and simple CV/VC word structures in the early stages of therapy, can have a more widespread effect on a child's overall speech profile than interventions without these components.

Summary of Levels of Evidence

As indicated in Table 7.1, the evidence in support of NDP3 is limited to case studies at this point.

PRACTICAL REQUIREMENTS

Nature of Sessions

NDP3 requires ongoing regular therapy sessions, with daily practice carried out at home by a parent or caregiver or in school by a teacher or teaching assistant. For most children, once weekly therapy sessions of 30–60 minutes are recommended. Children with more severe CAS may require twice weekly or even daily therapy sessions.

Table 7.1. Levels of evidence for studies of treatment efficacy for the Nuffield Centre Dyspraxia Programme

Level	Description	References
Ia	Meta-analysis of > 1 randomized controlled trial	—
Ib	Randomized controlled study	—
IIa	Controlled study without randomization	—
IIb	Quasi-experimental study	—
III	Nonexperimental studies, i.e., correlational and case studies	Belton (2006); Teal (2005)
IV	Expert committee report, consensus conference, clinical experience of respected authorities	—

Adapted from the Scottish Intercollegiate Guidelines Network (http://www.sign.ac.uk).

Therapy sessions can be delivered in a range of settings, such as clinics, hospital outpatient departments, schools, and sometimes in the home. They are generally delivered one to one, but paired or group sessions can be effective provided that children are working on similar targets.

Clinical experience indicates that most children with CAS and/or other severe SSD require intervention over a period of at least 12 months. Those with the most severe disorders may require intervention for 3 to 4 years.

Personnel

Therapy sessions should be delivered by a qualified SLP, with postqualification training or experience with this client group, or under the guidance of a specialist SLP. Parents, caregivers, or assistants who are carrying out daily practice with the child should observe therapy sessions and, ideally, demonstrate activities modeled by the SLP. SLPs should select targets for home or school practice that are readily elicited but require consolidation. Less stable targets should only be included if it is possible to give the parent or assistant sufficient instruction to avoid reinforcing unhelpful patterns or contributing to a loss of confidence. New skills and difficult areas require the expertise of the SLP. If a child becomes stuck at a particular stage, a period of more intensive therapy may be required to allow the SLP to build the next set of skills to the point where they can be elicited readily.

We recommend 20–30 minutes of home or school practice, 5–6 days per week. Practice time can be arranged as appropriate to the child and the setting. When possible, two to three short practice sessions are recommended rather than one longer session. The NDP3 provides worksheets and materials that can easily be used for home- or school-based practice. However, repetitive practice can also be integrated into a range of everyday home and school activities, such as repeating syllables while walking up- and downstairs, or babbling in the bath.

KEY COMPONENTS

Nature of Goals

The overall goal of the NDP3 therapy approach is to build speech processing skills, from the bottom up, starting from isolated speech sounds (and sometimes individual articulatory features) and progressing from simple to more complex syllables structures, then to sentences and connected speech. The primary focus is on establishing accurate motor programs, programming, and planning skills.

Goal Attack Strategies

At the outset of therapy, a baseline of the child's current speech skills is obtained by using the NDP3 assessment and evaluating the results. Individual intervention goals are established based on this information. Although these are specific to the child, they usually involve goals to develop the child's phonetic inventory at the single-sound level and to increase the number of CV words the child can produce. They might also include production of simple reduplicated CVCV words, using sounds the child can already produce at the CV level. For example, a child's initial goals may be to establish simultaneously 1) vowels and diphthongs requiring an intermediate jaw posture /ɛə/, /ɔ/, /ɜ/; 2) velar consonants /k/ and /g/ at the single-sound level; 3) extend his range of CV words and syllables with /b, d, m, n/ at the CV level; and 4) attempt simple CVCV words such as *baby*, *mommy*, *daddy*, and *nanny* at the CVCV level. At a later stage, he might be working on production of the consonants /ʃ/, /tʃ/, and /dʒ/ in isolation at the single-sound level, production of multisyllabic words and consonant clusters at the word level, and incorporating CVCV and CVC words at sentence level. Thus, in the NDP3 approach, multiple targets are worked on simultaneously, but at different levels of speech production.

Description of Activities

Motor Programs for Single Sounds

The first aim of therapy is to increase the inventory of motor programs for single sounds that the child can produce accurately so that it includes a full range of standard English vowels and a basic range of consonants, usually consisting of /p, b, m, t, d, n, k, g, f, s, h, w, j, l/. To address this aim, the SLP starts by teaching the child to associate sounds already within his or her phonetic repertoire with the NDP3 picture cues. Then the SLP attempts to elicit sounds the child cannot currently articulate through the use of teaching strategies such as modeling; imitation; verbal, tactile, and manual cues; auditory discrimination; and nonspeech oral motor tasks.

Typically the clinician starts by introducing four to six NDP3 picture cues to the child, ideally including both vowels and consonant sounds from different phoneme classes and/or involving maximal contrasts. Then, the SLP utilizes procedures and activities provided in the NDP3 manual to check auditory discrimination and reinforce production, thereby establishing and consolidating the child's ability to associate the sounds with the related pictures. Once the child learns this first set of sounds and associated picture cues, the SLP can gradually introduce more from the child's current phonetic inventory.

Next, the clinician teaches one or more sounds that the child can neither currently produce spontaneously nor imitate. Often a trial and error approach is required to find the best nonstimulable sounds to target. Imitation may be attempted first, but often other techniques are necessary. These can include utilizing features present in other sounds supported by tactile cues. For example, a child who can imitate /m/ but not /b/ would be helped to produce /b/ by saying /m/ while the SLP gently blocked his nostrils. In addition, the SLP could use one or more of a variety of cues, including verbal cues such as "this sound needs to come out through your mouth," manual cues such as those in Cued Artic-ulation (Passy, 1990), diagrammatic cues such as articulograms (Stephens & Elton, 1986) to represent features of a particular sound, and orthographic cues such as written letters.

Specific nonspeech oral motor exercises may also be used to develop missing artic-ulatory features, which are then linked with other features to create a sound through the use of verbal, visual, or tactile cues. For example, accurate tongue tip placement for alve-olar sounds may be facilitated by developing awareness and control of tongue move-ments through nonspeech licking activities, followed by practicing placement of the tongue behind, or initially between, the teeth. This placement is then linked to visual feed-back from a mirror, the diagrammatic articulogram "tongue on teeth," and the verbal cue "put your tongue up behind your teeth," as the child attempts to say /t/ or /d/. Further de-tails for eliciting individual sounds are included in Appendix 4 of the NDP3 manual.

Individual children learn at different rates, depending on such factors as their age, severity of difficulty, general cognitive abilities, motivation, and amount of practice. Nonetheless, in the first few sessions, the clinician should aim for the child to be able to produce 10–15 single sounds accurately (or almost accurately) in response to the NDP3 picture symbols. Ideally, these will include a combination of some well-established sounds and some recently learned sounds.

Both in the intervention and homework sessions, frequent repetitive practice of each newly elicited sound is required in order to establish the new motor program. NDP3 pro-vides materials such as sets of therapy cards and lotto worksheets, which the clinician can select to enable the child to practice sequences involving up to eight repetitions of the same sound (e.g., /p, p, p, p, p, p, p, p/). The next stage is to introduce contrastive se-quencing (e.g., /p, t, p, t, p, t, p, t/) using the NDP3 worksheets. This task challenges the child to retrieve two different motor programs and use motor planning skills to maintain accurate production of the individual sounds throughout the sequence. Many children with CAS find this activity very difficult, and for this reason the starting point should in-volve two or more distinctive feature changes and a slow production rate. Closer feature contrasts should be controlled carefully by the SLP and introduced gradually, with each step challenging the child a little more. For example, for a child who replaces /k/ with /t/, but has now learned to say /k/ as a single sound, contrastive sequencing might start with /m-k/, then /b-k/, /p-k/, and finally /t-k/. Speed of production can gradually be increased, with rhythmic and stress patterning incorporated.

Motor Programs for CV Words

In addition to the single sound targets, CV targets are introduced from the outset, start-ing with pictures of CV words that the child can already say. As at the single-sound level, the clinician uses tasks, games, and activities to elicit discrimination and production to help the child learn to recognize the pictures, select them correctly on request, and name them accurately.

Motor Programming

Next, the SLP begins to teach CV words that the child cannot produce accurately, in a staged manner similar to that used at the single-sound level. In many cases, a child with CAS is unable to imitate the clinician's spoken model and, therefore, new CV words have to be developed by combining two existing established motor programs involving one consonant and one vowel (C + V = CV). The child is faced with the challenge of learning to modify the two existing motor programs so that they join smoothly, without the gap in production left in sequencing tasks. This is frequently a difficult stage for the child because it involves motor programming, a core impairment in CAS (ASHA, 2007). NDP3 includes many blending worksheets that have been specifically designed for this purpose by presenting the sequence of a consonant and a vowel, followed by the CV word created when they join (e.g., /m/ + /u/ = *moo;* /p/ + /aɪ/ = *pie*). The clinician needs to provide careful modeling during these tasks and give verbal instruction regarding the articulatory modifications the child needs to achieve, for example, "You need to put a 'puff of air' after the /p/."

Establishing a Contrastive System at Single-Sound and CV Levels

At the outset of therapy, most children will have at least a small number of single consonants, vowels, and diphthongs they can already produce accurately. As intervention progresses the child adds to this set as new motor programs are mastered. Once this has occurred, intervention tasks should include sounds that the child can produce easily, as well as newer acquisitions. This enables the child to practice retrieval of the correct motor program, as well as consistency and accuracy of production. So, for example, for a child who has recently learned to say /b/, having previously produced it as /m/, the first step would be to practice single and repetitive productions of /m/ and /b/ separately. Once this is easily achieved, activities can be attempted involving both /m/ and /b/ sounds, with the child's task to select and say each phoneme correctly.

Although the main focus of therapy is on speech production, tasks focusing on auditory discrimination may also be included to support production. For example, before attempting the /m-b/ contrastive production activity just described, an input task involving selection of the correct target in response to a spoken model might be introduced using the same materials.

As was done when single sounds were the production focus, newly created CV words also need to be incorporated into the set of CV words the child can already produce, thereby creating a contrastive phonological system at the CV level. This may be achieved through minimal pair activities incorporating discrimination and production and utilizing the therapy cards or worksheets provided in NDP3. The SLP carefully selects worksheets to ensure the child achieves success but is increasingly challenged, in small graded steps, by the phonetic demands of the individual words in the sequence. For example, for a child who has recently learned to produce the word *sea* accurately, having previously produced it as *tea*, staged sequencing practice might move from a vowel change (e.g., *sea, saw, sea, saw*) to an easy placement change (e.g., *sea, bee, sea, bee*) to a harder placement change (e.g., *sea, tea, sea, tea*). Visual prompts using the NDP3 picture cues (e.g., a small picture of a snake to represent /s/ placed next to the picture of the sea) and/or written letters and verbal cues (e.g., "Remember this one starts with an /s/") make the structure of words explicit, thereby clarifying phonological representations, as well as establishing motor programs. Basic vocal control involving changes in length, loudness, and pitch contours should also be incorporated when producing word sequences.

Motor Programs Beyond CV Words

Once the child can produce a range of consonants, vowels, and CV syllables and words, he or she has the building blocks to create words of increasing phonotactic complexity, such as CVCV, CVC, CCV, CVCVC, and multisyllabic words. Again, the child is required to utilize motor programming skills to modify two or more existing motor programs and join them together smoothly to create a new motor program. The NDP3 materials facilitate this process by providing pictures and blending worksheets for various levels such as CV + CV = CVCV (e.g., *bay* + *bee* = *baby*), CV + C = CVC (e.g., *bow* + /t/ = *boat*), and C + CV(C) = CCV(C) (e.g., /s/ + *tar* = *star*). The manual provides strategies for dealing with typical problems (e.g., sound additions or insertions) that may occur at specific levels and provides advice on achieving appropriate stress patterning.

As already described at the single-sound and CV levels, the aim within each phonotactic level is to develop accurate motor programs for as wide a range of words as possible and to develop a contrastive system. For this reason, contrastive sequencing worksheets are also included for CVC and CCV(C) levels (e.g., *pie:pipe*, *tea:tree*, *car:scar*). At the same time, other psycholinguistic processes should be facilitated, including phonological representations and phonological awareness skills.

Younger children and those with more severe difficulties who cannot achieve full accuracy at more complex levels are encouraged to extend their range of CV syllables and their functional communication by using modified targets for meaningful words (e.g., /gɑ/ for *car*, /bəʊ/ for *boat*, /neɪ/ for *snake*).

Motor Planning: Phrases and Clauses to Connected Speech

The transfer of skills from the word level to connected speech requires the integration of speech skills and language formulation, as well as the ability to sustain articulatory control over longer sequences, incorporate prosodic features (stress, intonation, rate, rhythm), and use word joining strategies. Early in intervention, the development of motor planning skills starts with sequencing tasks as well as simple two-word phrases and clauses involving CV words (e.g., *no bee*, *car go*) and CVCV words (e.g., *daddy('s) car key*, *kitten eating dinner*). At this stage, each word can be supported by a familiar picture from the NDP3 materials so that language formulation is minimal. Once this is easily achieved, intervention moves on to a more demanding stage in which the child is required to formulate language and retrieve motor programs internally (e.g., *chocolate milkshake*, *The hippopotamus is playing the tambourine*). Numerous additional suggestions are provided in Chapter 5 of the therapy manual. These include tips for working on the articulation of grammatical morphemes, strategies for joining words smoothly, and activities for working on intonation and vocal control, as well as activities for monitoring and pacing of connected speech.

Materials and Equipment Required

The NDP3 intervention approach is supported by a set of pictorial therapy materials. In addition to a therapy manual, there are two large boxes of 1,800 picture cards involving four sets of 450 different images and 550 line-drawn worksheets, which can be photocopied for use with clients. The worksheets are divided into sections: oro-motor/voice, single sounds (consonants and vowels), C + V and V + C transitions, words of increasing phonotactic levels (CV, VC, CVCV, CVC, CCV, complex and multisyllabic words), and word combinations. The materials include a set of picture cues to represent single consonants, vowels, and diphthongs; sets of pictures of words at each of the phonotactic levels; transition worksheets to support joining of sounds or syllables to create a word; and sequencing worksheets, which provide repetitive and contrastive practice at all levels.

Guided by the manual, the SLP uses these materials to elicit the targets set for the treatment sessions. Typically, they are presented to the child through table-top games, such as lotto, posting cards in a letterbox, card games, or "fishing" for cards. The SLP also typically facilitates the therapeutic process through the use of simple rewards. For example, "You can put a monkey on the tree after you have done this worksheet." See Appendix 6 of the NDP3 therapy manual for suggestions of tasks, activities, and games.

ASSESSMENT AND PROGRESS MONITORING TO SUPPORT DECISION MAKING

NDP3 includes an assessment procedure, which is closely linked to the therapy program. The oro-motor assessment includes separate sections on lips and jaw, tongue, airstream, and voice and palate, as well as a diadochokinetic (DDK) assessment. The speech assessment samples production of 1) all the single consonants, vowels, and diphthongs through imitation; 2) a set of 20 single words at each phonotactic structure (CV/VC, CVCV, CVC, CCV, and multisyllabics) assessed through picture naming; and 3) phrases and sentences, which are assessed through imitation, with pictures for support. In addition, there is a connected speech checklist, which can be used as a severity rating scale.

For the speech assessments, the majority of items are scored as correct (1 point) or incorrect (0 point), according to the local adult model. However for the phrases and sentences, a score of 2, 1, or 0 points is awarded, as advised in the manual. In addition, a series of questions are asked on the assessment forms to guide the SLP in analyzing the assessment data qualitatively. For example, at the CVC level, questions such as the following are asked: What consonants does the child use in initial position? What vowels are used accurately? Are sounds joined smoothly? Are there any voice/prosodic features of note? To facilitate the evaluation, a list of possible syntagmatic and paradigmatic processes are provided under consonants along with a list of processes that might affect vowels.

The assessment can be used to provide a baseline before starting treatment and can then be re-administered at intervals (after a block of therapy or after a 6-month period) to record progress by examining results in relation to the baseline on the individual subtests. Although the NDP3 assessment is not standardized, data from 4-year-old children indicated that a typically developing child of this age should perform at 90% or higher on most subtests. However, for the multisyllabic words and phrases and sentences subtests, a score of 80% can be expected. These figures can be useful in evaluating a child's progress relative to his or her age and in deciding whether treatment is still required.

For children with very severe difficulties, the NDP3 scoring system may be too gross to demonstrate progress in the short term. Belton (2006) successfully used a fine-tuned level of scoring to supplement the NDP3 standard scoring in order to detect small changes in the child's phonological system in terms of place, manner, and voicing for consonants and length and tongue position (front/back, open/close) for vowels. See a description of how this might be used by examining the description of a study by Belton (2006) in the Empirical Basis section of this chapter.

CONSIDERATIONS FOR CHILDREN FROM CULTURALLY AND LINGUISTICALLY DIVERSE BACKGROUNDS

NDP3 was designed in London, United Kingdom for children with a typical British Southern English accent. It uses the consonant and vowel inventories of this accent and the typical phonotactic structures of British English. For other English accents, the vowel picture cues will need to be adapted to match the local vowel inventory.

Because NDP3 is a language-specific tool, it cannot simply be translated into another language. Although the principles of the approach can be applied to any language, careful adaptation needs to be made to reflect phoneme inventories and phonotactic structures of the specific language. In addition, the pictures need to be presented in a style familiar and acceptable to young children in a particular country. To date, such adaptation has been carried out successfully in Dutch and Swedish, and work is in progress on Danish and Greek adaptations.

Although many children in the United Kingdom are from culturally and linguistically diverse backgrounds, most attend English-speaking nurseries or schools and generally receive speech and language therapy from English-speaking therapists. NDP3 would be used with these children without modification, although in certain cases adaptations to the picture materials or word stimuli may be recommended by professionals who advise on issues related to bilingual children.

CASE STUDY

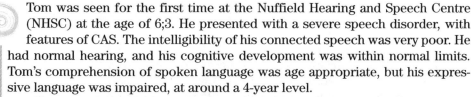

Tom was seen for the first time at the Nuffield Hearing and Speech Centre (NHSC) at the age of 6;3. He presented with a severe speech disorder, with features of CAS. The intelligibility of his connected speech was very poor. He had normal hearing, and his cognitive development was within normal limits. Tom's comprehension of spoken language was age appropriate, but his expressive language was impaired, at around a 4-year level.

Tom attended ten 1-hour sessions of weekly therapy at the NHSC. His parents were asked to practice specific targets, demonstrated by the SLP in the treatment sessions, on a daily basis.

Assessment

Data from Tom's initial NDP assessment are shown in Table 7.2. After more detailed investigation of specific targets during therapy, it became apparent that, in addition to his difficulties with motor aspects of speech production, Tom's awareness of the target sound sequence for particular words was poor. Therefore, input work on treatment targets was included alongside output practice at all levels.

Table 7.2.   Data from Tom's Nuffield Centre Dyspraxia Programme assessment

Single consonants imitated correctly	Single vowels imitated correctly
p b m t̪ d̪ n̪ k g h w j f s	i ɑ ɜ ɛə aɪ ɑʊ ɪ æ ʊ ʌ

Oromotor skills

Lips: difficulty with lip shaping, resulting in poor lip rounding for speech sounds
Tongue: difficulty with tongue tip differentiation and elevation, resulting in dental placement of alveolar consonants

CV and VC	CVCV	CVC	Complex words
moo – mum	Mummy – mʌmɪ	cake – kaɪ	banana – ənʌnʌ
door – d̪ʌː	baby – bʌjɪ	boat – bəʊ	helicopter – hæʔəkəʔt
bee – bi	teddy – t̪ɛd̪ɪ	bird – bʌːk	computer – put̪ə
go – gʌː/gɑʊ	cooker – kʊʔə	down – d̪ʌm	hospital – hɒʔkɪwəl
knee – n̪i	dirty – d̪ʌʔɪ	moon – mum	pocket – pʌʔɪʔ
deer – d̪i	dinner – d̪ɪn̪ə	dog – d̪ʌg	dinosaur – t̪aɪn̪əsʌː
boy – baɪ	party – pʌjɪ	girl – gɑʊ	television – t̪ʌjɪvɪdən̪
car – kɑ	table – t̪ˀʌjəl	tap – t̪æ	swing – fɪn̪
cow – kɑʊ	picking – pɪʔɪn̪	pig – pɪt̪	blue – bu
two – t̪u	cowboy – kʌʔbaɪ	cat – kæ	tree – t̪i
pay – pi/paɪ/baɪ	kettle – kæʔʊl	duck – d̪ʌʔ	hand – hæn̪
four – fʌː	garden – gʌːɪn̪	farm – fɑm	lift – jɪt̪
sea – si	tiger – t̪ʌjə	horse – hʌʔts	monkey – mʌmʔi
shoe – su	water – wɔt̪ə	leaf – jit	Christmas – kɪʔt̪ɪːn̪t̪
chair – t̪ɛə	fire – fɑjə	sum – sʌm	
lie – jaɪ	jelly – d̪ʌjɪ	fish – fɪt̪	
out – ɑʊ	kitchen – kɪʔɪn̪	light – jaɪ	
up – ʌpˀ	coffee – kʌʔkɪ	watch – wʌʔtʃ	
arm – ɑm	tissue – t̪ɪʔʊ	jam – d̪æn	
ice – aɪt̪	sitting – sɪʔɪn̪	web – wɛt̪	

Treatment Planning

Treatment planning was based on the identification of which sounds (consonants and vowels) were used, and which were not used, at different levels of syllable structure. Tom worked concurrently on a range of targets at single-sound and CV levels over the 10 intervention sessions and also at CVCV level from session 6 onwards.

Single-Sound Level

At the single-sound level Tom could imitate a basic range of consonants, including all plosives and easier nasals, approximants, and fricatives, although alveolar consonants were imprecise. He was able to imitate a limited range of vowels. These included both open and close vowels, and even some vowels with an intermediate jaw posture. However, during therapy it became apparent that he had particular difficulty with jaw control for half-open vowels. He achieved lip spreading but rounding was poor. He was able to differentiate long and short vowels and move from one vowel shape (lip, jaw, and tongue posture) to another to produce diphthongs. Although Tom demonstrated many of the articulatory features required for a complete vowel system (with the exception of lip rounding and intermediate jaw posture), he had not established all the necessary combinations of features.

Early intervention targets included linking existing consonants and vowels to picture cues and practicing until sounds were produced consistently and accurately (using contrasting and sequencing activities).

A further major area involved developing a full vowel system at single-sound level. Verbal, visual, and tactile cues were used to improve lip rounding. New long and short vowels and diphthongs were introduced using lip, jaw, and tongue postures demonstrated in Tom's existing vowel inventory. Work on half-open vowels was introduced with auditory discrimination and nonspeech oro-motor work. Half-open jaw posture was then combined with spread, rounded, and neutral lip postures to produce long vowels, short vowels, and diphthongs. Nonspeech oro-motor work was also used to improve placement for alveolar consonants and elicit appropriate placement for /l/ and /ʃ/.

CV Level

At the CV level, Tom was already using all the sounds in his single-sound inventory. Tom's existing CV syllables were linked to pictures and consolidated using repetition, contrasting, and sequencing activities. New CV words were added by combining existing consonants with new vowels (e.g., /f/ + /ɔ/ = *four*), once these were established at the single-sound level. CV nonsense syllables with short vowels were also practiced. In addition, auditory discrimination tasks and segmentation and blending were used to develop Tom's phonological representations for CV words.

CVCV Level

Tom was able to use his inventory of consonants in initial position in CVCV words. However, in medial position, consonants were frequently replaced by a glottal stop or /j/. Vowels were also less accurate at this level. It was decided that CVCV words would not be targeted until a wider range of vowels was established at the CV level. CVCV targets were therefore only introduced in session six. Initially this involved using transition sheets (e.g., *cow* + *boy* = *cowboy*). Tom then built up a set of CVCV words that he could produce accurately, starting with the same initial and medial consonant (e.g., *paper*), and later adding those with different consonants (e.g., *table*).

CVC Level

CVC targets were not included in Tom's 10 sessions. These would be introduced once a range of CVCV words were established.

Outcome

After 10 sessions (over 3–4 months), Tom had established all vowels at the single-sound level, except /eɪ/, which remained inconsistent. /l/ and /ʃ/ were also established. At CV level, /l/ was established, and Tom was beginning to achieve the half-open vowels, but these remained inconsistent. He was beginning to use /ʃ/, but /s/ and /ʃ/ were confused. At the CVCV level, Tom had learned motor programs for a limited range of target words.

Tom was subsequently placed in a language unit within a mainstream school, where he had access to continued regular therapy and daily practice of skills. He was not followed up at the NHSC but was expected to achieve intelligible speech within the following 2 years.

FUTURE DIRECTIONS

Intervention Studies

At NHSC, the team of SLPs follows the principles of the NDP3 intervention approach and utilizes its therapy materials on a daily basis in their work with children who have severe speech disorders. This group is committed to demonstrating the effectiveness of the approach through further research on this intervention. Morgan and Vogel (2008) as well as ASHA (2007) identified a critical need for more treatment studies in CAS. Morgan and Vogel also advised that given the state of the evidence base in CAS, well-controlled single case studies were the way forward. In response, the team at the NHSC is carrying out a further series of case studies to study the effectiveness of the NDP3 approach while addressing some of the methodological shortcomings from Belton (2006). Additional independent investigation of the effectiveness of the NDP3 therapy approach for children with CAS or other severe speech disorders could also add considerably to our preliminary demonstrations of its effectiveness.

Standardization of the NDP3 Assessment

As reported in this chapter, the NDP3 assessment is not yet standardized. Normative data are being collected for 4-year-old children, with subsequent data collection planned for children 3 and 5 years old. These data will enable SLPs to compare the performance of a child suspected of having a severe speech disorder to same-age peers who have normal speech development, thereby strengthening the validity of this test procedure for use in the identification of severe speech problems.

Developments Beyond NDP3

Building on the considerable revisions that were made in the 2004 edition of NDP3, another project is to develop a computerized version (NDP3i) to supplement the current hard copy of the NDP3 resource. This will allow clinicians the flexibility and convenience of creating worksheets and other therapy materials that are specific to the needs of each individual child.

In addition, we are committed to supporting adaptations of NDP3 for other languages. Typically, this involves collaboration between the clinicians at the Nuffield Centre; our publisher, Anthony Allison from the Miracle Factory; and the team of SLPs from the country involved. To date, adaptation of NDP3 has been carried out successfully in Dutch and Swedish and work is in progress on Danish and Greek adaptations. Further information with regard to the development of NDP3 can be obtained from our web site (http//:www.ndp3.org).

SUGGESTED READINGS

Belton, E. (2006). *Evaluation of the effectiveness of the Nuffield Dyspraxia Programme as a treatment approach for children with severe speech disorders.* Unpublished master's dissertation, University College London, Department of Human Communication Science.

Saunders, H. (2006, Summer). How I (2): Phonology: Never too soon to start. *Speech and Language Therapy in Practice, 27–28.*

Williams, P., & Stephens, H. (Eds.). (2004). NDP3 therapy manual from *The Nuffield Centre Dyspraxia Programme* (3rd ed.). Windsor, England: The Miracle Factory.

REFERENCES

American Speech-Language-Hearing Association. (2007). *Childhood apraxia of speech.* Retrieved September 23, 2009, from http://www.asha.org/policy

Belton, E. (2006). *Evaluation of the effectiveness of the Nuffield Dyspraxia Programme as a treatment approach for children with severe speech disorders.* Unpublished master's dissertation, University College London, Department of Human Communication Science.

Carter, P., & Edwards, S. (2004). EPG for children with long-standing speech disorders: Predictors and outcomes. *Clinical Linguistics and Phonetics, 18,* 359–372.

Connery, V.M. (1985). *The Nuffield Centre Dyspraxia Programme.* London: Royal National Throat, Nose and Ear Hospital.

Connery, V.M. (1992). *The Nuffield Centre Dyspraxia Programme* (2nd ed.). London: The Miracle Factory.

Connery, V.M. (1994). The Nuffield Dyspraxia Programme: Working on the motor programming of speech. In J. Law (Ed.), *Before school: A handbook of approaches to intervention with preschool language impaired children* (pp. 125–141). London: Afasic.

Dodd, B. (Ed.). (2005). *Differential diagnosis and treatment of children with speech disorder* (2nd ed.). London: Whurr.

Dodd, B., Zhu, H., Crosbie, S., Holm, A., & Ozanne, A. (2002). *Diagnostic evaluation of articulation and phonology.* London: Pearson PsychCorp.

Hall, P.K., Jordan, L.S., & Robin, D.A. (1993). *Developmental apraxia of speech: Theory and clinical practice.* Austin, TX: PRO-ED.

Hall, R., Adams, C., Hesketh, A., & Nightingale, K. (1998). The measurement of intervention effects in developmental phonological disorders. *International Journal of Language and Communication Disorders, 33* (Suppl.), 445–450.

Jaffe, M. (1984). Neurological impairment in speech production: Assessment and treatment. In J. Costello (Ed.), *Speech disorders in children: Recent advances* (pp. 157–186). Baltimore: College Hill Press.

Morgan, A., & Vogel, A. (2008). Intervention for childhood apraxia of speech. *Cochrane Database of Systematic Reviews 2008, Issue 3.* Art. No. CD006278.

Pagnamenta, E., & Williams, P. (2009). *Evaluation of the effectiveness of the Nuffield Dyspraxia Programme in treating two children with severe speech disorders.* Paper presented at the Royal College of Speech and Language Therapy Conference, London.

Passy, J. (1990). *Cued articulation.* Ponteland, Northumberland: STASS Publications.

Saunders, H. (2006, Summer). How I (2): Phonology: Never too soon to start. *Speech and Language Therapy in Practice, 27–28.*

Stackhouse, J., & Wells, B. (1997). *Children's speech and literacy difficulties: A psycholinguistic framework.* London: Whurr.

Stephens, H., & Elton, M. (1986, December). Description of systematic use of articulograms. *College of Speech and Language Therapists Bulletin,* 8–10.

Teal, J. (2005). *An investigation into classification approaches and therapy outcomes for a child with a severe persisting speech difficulty.* Unpublished master's dissertation, University of Sheffield, Department of Human Communication Sciences.

Weiss, A.L. (2004). The child as agent for change in therapy for phonological disorders. *Child Language Teaching and Therapy, 20,* 221–244.

Williams, P., & Stephens, H. (Eds.). (2004). *The Nuffield Centre Dyspraxia Programme* (3rd ed.). Windsor, England: The Miracle Factory.

Yoss, K., & Darley, F. (1974). Developmental apraxia of speech in children with defective articulation. *Journal of Speech and Hearing Research, 17,* 399–416.

Stimulability Intervention

Adele W. Miccio and A. Lynn Williams*

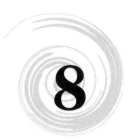

8

ABSTRACT

Stimulability has a long clinical history beginning with research that examined general speech stimulability as a prognostic indicator of intervention outcomes to research that has investigated sound-specific stimulability and generalization. Following research findings that suggest nonstimulable sounds should be targeted in intervention, as well as the emphasis on earlier identification of younger children with phonological disorders, Miccio and Elbert (1996) and Miccio (2005) developed an intervention program to enhance stimulability skills in very young children who have restricted phonetic inventories. The stimulability approach is based on the intervention research literature and encompasses seven important components, including the pairing of consonants with alliterative characters and hand/body motions for all consonants (both stimulable and nonstimulable) within turn-taking activities that are designed to maintain joint focus between the clinician and child and result in early communicative success that encourages vocal practice.

INTRODUCTION

Stimulability is the ability of an individual to correctly imitate a sound that was previously produced in error when provided with auditory and visual cues by the clinician (cf., Miccio, 2002; Rvachew, 2005). Given that differences can occur in children's production abilities with the aid of auditory and visual cues, stimulability has long been a component of assessment of speech sound disorders (SSD; Carter & Buck, 1958; Miccio, 2005; Milisen, 1954; Powell & Miccio, 1996) and an important factor in determining target selection (cf., Miccio, Elbert, & Forrest, 1999; Powell, Elbert, & Dinnsen, 1991; Rvachew & Nowak, 2001).

Typically, stimulability is assessed by having the child imitate the target sound in isolation, syllables, words, and sometimes phrases and sentences. If the child can correctly imitate the target sound, then he or she is considered to be stimulable for that sound. In early studies of stimulability, a global measure of a child's general imitative abilities was calculated as a stimulability score, which was based on an error difference score between spontaneous and imitative error productions divided by the number of spontaneous error productions (Powell & Miccio, 1996). This correction score reflected the child's general level of stimulability and was used as a prognostic indicator of the child's success in in-

Note: This chapter was completed after Dr. Adele W. Miccio's death by Dr. A. Lynn Williams, who wishes to acknowledge that although the work is solely that of Dr. Miccio, any misrepresentations of that work are Dr. Williams's responsibility.

tervention (Sommers, 1987; Sommers et al., 1967). That is, a child judged to have good stimulability skills would be predicted to do well in intervention.

Since the 1990s, stimulability has been defined as a sound-specific measure rather than as a general ability that a child possesses. In this regard, a child might be stimulable for one sound but not another. Stimulability, then, for a particular sound is examined with regard to learning outcomes for that sound and used as a basis for target selection. Stimulable sounds have traditionally been targeted in intervention because they are assumed to be more efficiently remediated and easier for the child to acquire, which will reduce frustration and increase early success (Bleile, 2002; Hodson, Scherz, & Strattman, 2002; Secord, 1989). This view has been challenged in the past two decades with evidence indicating that targeting nonstimulable sounds will likely result in acquisition of both treated and nontreated sounds (Miccio, 2002; Miccio, Elbert, et al., 1999; Powell, 1991; Powell et al., 1991). Choosing a nonstimulable sound for intervention, however, is somewhat counterintuitive and has not been widely embraced by speech-language pathologists (SLPs; McLeod & Baker, 2004). Concerns about time involved in instruction, difficulty teaching a nonstimulable sound, and increased frustration for the child are reasons expressed for this reluctance in selecting nonstimulable sounds for intervention (Fey & Stalker, 1986; Miccio, 2009; Rvachew, 2005).

Consequently, a natural extension of the construct of stimulability resulted in the development of intervention methods to stimulate children's production of errored sounds that have been assessed to be nonstimulable. In this way, concerns about selecting nonstimulable sounds for intervention are allayed while providing a means to address the more difficult targets that potentially will lead to more efficient and greater systemwide change. This chapter describes an intervention program developed by Miccio and Elbert (1996) and Miccio (2005, 2009) to enhance stimulability for young children with limited sound inventories who are not stimulable for the missing sounds from their phonetic inventories.

TARGET POPULATIONS

Primary Populations

The stimulability treatment program was designed for very young children, ages 2–4, who have very small phonetic inventories and are not stimulable for production of many or all of the absent sounds (Miccio, 2005; Miccio & Elbert, 1996). For these children, their restricted inventories limit the phonological contrasts that they can produce, which leads to homonymy and highly unintelligible speech. This, in turn, limits the number of different utterances they can produce. Typically, the stimulability treatment approach has been used with young children who have nonorganic speech delays. In stimulability intervention studies, children have been described as scoring between the 1st and 10th percentiles on the Goldman-Fristoe Test of Articulation (Goldman & Fristoe, 1986), representing a moderate or severe delay in phonological development, and as exhibiting normal oral-motor structure, hearing, and expressive and receptive language skills (Miccio & Elbert, 1996; Rvachew, Rafaat, & Martin, 1999), with the exception of morphosyntactic delays, which were attributed to phonological constraints (Rvachew et al., 1999), or exhibiting expressive syntax skills that were below normal limits (Rvachew & Nowak, 2001).

Secondary Populations

Powell (1996) described a stimulability approach for a slightly older child (5;1) with persistent SSD who exhibited speech behaviors that were consistent with childhood apraxia of speech (CAS) in order to increase his phonetic inventory as an early intervention goal. Although the research on stimulability treatment programs has been limited to functional SSD in children, the intervention principles and methods provide a foundation that would have theoretical support for application to other populations of children with SSD, such as children with hearing impairments or those with Down syndrome or cleft palate.

ASSESSMENT METHODS FOR DETERMINING INTERVENTION RELEVANCE

Stimulability has long been a major component of assessment and is most pertinent for those sounds that are never produced correctly in any position. A variety of methods have been used to assess a child's stimulability skills, including subtests of standardized tests of articulation (e.g., the Stimulability Subtest of the Goldman-Fristoe Test of Articulation-2 [GFTA-2; Goldman & Fristoe, 2000]) and stimulability probes that have been developed to evaluate stimulability in isolation, syllables, and words. A variety of cues across different linguistic contexts has been used to determine if a child is stimulable for a particular sound. Cues have included placement instructions (Rvachew et al., 1999), verbal and/or visual models (Carter & Buck, 1958), or tactile cues (Bain, 1994). However, most often the cues have been auditory and visual in which the child is instructed to watch the clinician's face while a verbal model is provided (Lof, 1996). Similarly, different linguistic environments have been used to assess stimulability. Rvachew et al. (1999) assessed stimulability at the isolation/syllable level and in syllable-initial position of words and sentences using an imitative model. Flint and Costello Ingham (2005) assessed stimulability in the releasing and arresting positions of words using visual and auditory models.

The different cue and linguistic levels are systematically manipulated in the Scaffolding Scale of Stimulability developed by Glaspey (2006) and described by Glaspey and Stoel-Gammon (2007). This stimulability assessment encompasses the model of dynamic assessment by methodically moving through a hierarchy of four cue levels and seven linguistic environments. All English consonants are examined in the word-initial and word-final positions, as well as five consonant clusters. The child's imitative response for each phoneme or cluster is scored from 1 (representing stimulable with minimal support provided) to 21 (representing not stimulable with the maximum level of support).

Powell and Miccio (1996) and Miccio (2002) used a modification of the Carter and Buck (1958) Nonsense Syllable Test to assess sound stimulability. This stimulability probe elicits production of the target sound in isolation and in three positions of syllables (initial, medial, and final) across three different vowel contexts (e.g., [/i, u, ɑ/]; some research has used [æ] rather than [u].) For example, /s/ would be modeled by the clinician in isolation and in the following syllable and vowel contexts: [si], [isi], [is]; [su], [usu], [us]; [sɑ], [ɑsɑ], [ɑs] for a total of 10 opportunities. A percentage of correct productions is then computed for each sound (i.e., correct imitation of [s] two times is calculated as 20% accuracy). A copy of this stimulability probe is included in Appendix 8A.

THEORETICAL BASIS

Dominant Theoretical Rationale for the Intervention Approach

Stimulability, though a relatively simple concept, reflects a complex task. At a basic level, stimulability has been considered to reflect an intact speech mechanism. Researchers have questioned whether stimulability reflects information at other levels as well. For instance, if a child is stimulable for production of an errored sound, does that indicate that he or she has *knowledge* of that sound at an underlying representation level? Does it also suggest that the child's *perception* of that sound is intact? Although there is no definitive answer to these long-asked questions, a number of theories have been advanced. One theory that integrates all three levels (production, linguistic, and perception) is that stimulability represents a cognitive-motor skill, which suggests that the child's sensory, linguistic, and motor systems are intact (cf., Shelton & McReynolds, 1979). This theory suggests a close relationship between perception and production abilities. A number of studies have examined this relationship, largely through intervention studies that investigated the effects of perception training on production of stimulable and nonstimulable target sounds. If there is a relationship between perception and stimulability skills, intervention targeted at one skill should improve the other without direct intervention. Converging evidence across studies indicates that perception training was effective only if the target sound was stimulable (Rvachew, 1994; Saben & Costello Ingham, 1991). For nonstimulable target sounds, the combination of perception and production training was required (Rvachew, 1994; Rvachew et al., 1999). Taken together, these studies support the notion that perception and stimulability are independent skills.

Another theory suggests that stimulability reflects a level of underlying phonological knowledge (Dinnsen & Elbert, 1984). Based on this theory, a child's ability to imitate production of a sound that is absent from his or her phonetic inventory suggests that the child has a correct underlying representation that is conceptualized as a distinct linguistic entity from the errored production (Powell & Miccio, 1996). It is likely that underlying phonological knowledge incorporates stimulability as well as perceptual skills. Lof (1996) investigated the relationship between stimulability and phonological knowledge. Based on children's underlying phonological knowledge, which was determined by their phonemic perception, stimulability was not found to be associated with speech perception abilities. Therefore, the correct underlying representation was not required for stimulability. These findings, along with those from Rvachew et al. (1999) provide additional support for the independence of perception and stimulability.

Collectively, these studies demonstrate that perception and stimulability represent independent abilities, which likely reflect different underlying phonological knowledge. The independence of perception and stimulability is consistent with a two-lexicon model of phonological development (Baker, Croot, McLeod, & Paul, 2001; Locke, 1988; Menn, 1978). According to this model, a perceptual representation serves as the input lexicon while an articulatory representation (stimulability) serves as the output lexicon. Support for this model was provided by McGregor and Schwartz (1992) who found that both stimulability (output lexicon) and perception (input lexicon) were required to account for the phonological errors exhibited by their case study participant. Further support for the two-lexicon model was provided in intervention studies in which perception training improved production (Jamieson & Rvachew, 1992; Saben & Costello Ingham, 1991). Conversely, in a pilot study, Wolfe, Presley, and Mesaris (2003) found that production training may improve perceptual abilities. These studies also support the independence of stimulability and perception. Although there is stronger evidence in support of perception training improving production of stimulable sounds, there is some evidence that supports the opposite direction; that is, production training on stimulable sounds improves perceptual skills.

A theory that incorporates the interaction between perception and stimulability is a neural network model called DIVA (*Directions in* auditory space to *Velocities in Articulator* space; Guenther, 1995). According to this model, articulation is assumed to represent the achievement of an acoustic-phonetic product. Auditory feedback of the acoustic-phonetic product of speech movements allows the child to map the phoneme, the appropriate articulatory gestures, and the acoustic-phonetic outcome of the gestures (Rvachew, 2005). The DIVA model, therefore, suggests that a combination of perception and stimulability training will enhance intervention outcomes.

Finally, Bain (1994) linked the theoretical construct of dynamic assessment with stimulability (Glaspey & Stoel-Gammon, 2007). Dynamic assessment encompasses Vygotsky's cognitive model of development (Bain & Olswang, 1995; Vygotsky, 1978) that suggests there are actual and potential levels of development. Stimulability represents the difference between a child's actual level of performance and his or her potential level of performance within a highly supportive context. The region between the actual and potential levels of development is referred to as the *zone of proximal development*, or ZPD (Vygotsky, 1978). The importance of stimulability is highlighted within this theoretical framework as a critical component in determining the child's articulatory abilities, as well as for planning intervention.

Levels of Consequences Being Addressed

The stimulability approach directly stimulates a child's production of errored sounds; consequently this approach targets a functional limitation that underlies the speech sound disorder. With improvement in speech production, a secondary benefit is an increase in the child's activities and participation involving communication and social life.

Target Areas of Intervention

The primary focus in intervention is on stimulating the correct production of nonstimulable errored sounds; as such, speech output is the primary concern in intervention. However, as noted earlier, stimulability and perception are related skills. Consequently, although stimulability training focuses on production, there is some evidence that perceptual skills may improve as a result of the production training (Wolfe et al., 2003). Another aim of this approach is to encourage more verbalization in young children who are reticent to interact given their severely limited phonetic inventories. The incorporation of stimulable and nonstimulable sounds that are associated with alliterative characters and hand motions and are practiced within turn-taking activities ensures successful communicative attempts, which encourages more verbalization. The alliterative characters are of high interest to young children, and the hand and body motions that are paired with the speech sounds motivate the child to attend and participate in the therapy activities, with the goal of encouraging vocal practice, which is "a crucial element for the acquisition of new sounds" (Miccio, 2005, p. 166).

EMPIRICAL BASIS

In order to fully understand the research conducted on the stimulability intervention approach, it is useful to have a summary of the studies that have examined stimulability as an articulatory skill related to intervention outcomes. Although a number of studies have been conducted on the relationship between stimulability and intervention outcomes, there are only a few studies that have examined stimulability as an intervention approach. This section provides a review of the studies in each of these two categories.

Studies Examining the Relationship Between Stimulability and Learning

Stimulability, as an articulatory construct, has a long history of study. Although this review will focus on sound-specific stimulability studies, the earliest studies focused on general stimulability skills as a prognostic indicator (Carter & Buck, 1958; Farquhar, 1961; Irwin, West, & Trombetta, 1966; Snow & Milisen, 1954; Sommers et al., 1967). The general finding across the studies was that children with stronger stimulability skills were likely to achieve greater gains in intervention than children with poorer stimulability skills. Further, without intervention, children with high stimulability tended to perform better than children with low stimulability. Accordingly, intervention was required for children who were not stimulable.

Of the sound-specific stimulability studies, there are four experimental and four case studies. In an early study, Powell et al. (1991) used a multiple baseline across behaviors design with six children (ages 4;11 to 5;6) to examine intervention outcomes for stimulable and nonstimulable targets. Each child received therapy on [ɹ] plus one other sound that was absent from their phonetic inventory. For two of the children, both targets were stimulable sounds; for two other children, both targets were nonstimulable sounds; and for the last two children, one target was a stimulable sound and the other target was a nonstimulable sound. Minimal pair therapy was implemented in 30-minute individual sessions three times weekly. Across all children, 28 sounds that were characterized as inventory constraints were monitored (14 were stimulable and 14 were nonstimulable). A moderately high relationship between stimulability and generalization was obtained in which 12 of the 14 stimulable sounds met generalization criterion, whereas only 2 of the 14 nonstimulable sounds generalized. From these findings, the authors concluded that intervention could be enhanced by addressing nonstimulable sounds rather than stimulable sounds.

In a hypothesis-testing case study, Powell (1991) applied findings from intervention efficacy research in the target selection for one child (age 5;8). Specifically, a nonstimulable and linguistically marked sound, /z/, was chosen for intervention in the word-final position. Intervention outcomes were consistent with predictions that generalization occurred to the expected final voiced and voiceless fricatives, as well as to final voiced stops. By targeting the more complex (nonstimulable and marked) sound, the child demonstrated significant improvement on the targeted sound, as well as within and across class generalization to untrained sounds.

Powell (1993) continued the examination of the relationship between sound learning and selection of intervention targets with six children (ages 4;9 to 5;5) who had participated in the previous Powell et al. (1991) study. Recall that all children were trained on [ɹ] plus a second sound that was stimulable for three of the children and nonstimulable for the remaining three children. The introduction of sounds into the children's phonetic inventories that were previously excluded was examined with regard to their stimulability status. A total of 28 sounds were monitored across the children; half were stimulable and half were nonstimulable. When the stimulability status of the newly added sounds was examined, Powell found that stimulable sounds (13 of 14 sounds) were almost always added to the children's phonetic inventories regardless of the intervention target. Conversely, examination of sounds that were *not* added to the children's sound inventories revealed that almost all were nonstimulable sounds (6 of 7 sounds). These results provided further experimental validation of the importance of stimulability in sound acquisition, which suggests that nonstimulable sounds will not be acquired without direct intervention.

Miccio, Elbert, et al. (1999) extended this line of investigation of stimulability and phonological acquisition with eight children, four of whom had phonological disorders (ages 3;10 to 5;7) and formed the intervention group, and four children with typically developing sound systems (ages 3;6 to 4;1), who served as the control group. In a multiple baseline across subjects design, children in the intervention group received intervention on a fricative that was missing from their phonetic inventory. A stimulability probe that was an adaptation of the Carter and Buck (1958) Nonsense Syllable Task was administered to the children in both groups to evaluate their stimulability of singleton consonants in isolation and in consonant-vowel syllables. Their results supported the earlier Powell studies that stimulable sounds are likely to change without intervention. They found that children in the intervention group acquired the stimulable sounds that were missing from their phonetic inventories without direct intervention. Similarly, children with typically developing sound systems acquired stimulable sounds within 5 months. Miccio et al. suggest that stimulability for production of a sound is likely an indication that the sound is being acquired naturally. Consequently, they concluded that nonstimulable sounds should be given priority in intervention because they are least likely to change.

Rvachew et al. (1999) expanded the study of the relationship between stimulability and phonological learning with the inclusion of another related skill, speech perception. Within a capability-focus paradigm (Lof, 1996; Kwiatkowski & Shriberg, 1998), they examined children's stimulability and speech perception skills as a reflection of both capability (i.e., underlying phonological knowledge) and focus (i.e., ability to focus, attend, and respond). In two descriptive studies, they assessed stimulability and speech perception as two variables that reflect a child's capability and focus, and therefore serve as intervention and client variables that could influence intervention outcomes. In the first study, they included 10 children (mean age of 4;6) in a pre-post treatment design that included pretreatment assessment, nine group intervention sessions, and posttreatment assessment. Using a modified cycles approach (Hodson & Paden, 1991), children were assigned to one of three intervention groups based on scheduling, age, and similarity of error patterns. Each group received intervention on three common phonological processes that were addressed in cycles of three sessions each. A target sound was chosen from each phonological process that was common to all group members and was developmentally appropriate. Their findings showed that no progress was made on any of the unstimulable sounds (i.e., score of 0 on the stimulability measure), and limited intervention gains (0.5 point difference between posttreatment and pretreatment production scores) were observed on poorly perceived sounds (i.e., less than 70% score on the speech perception task). The authors noted that some gain in production performance was most likely to occur if the child demonstrated both stimulability and good perception skills prior to intervention, though only modest improvements were achieved (mean posttreatment accuracy on production probe was only 36%). Consequently, the authors modified the intervention program in a second study to provide three individual sessions to train stimulability and speech perception for each of the three target sounds before the initiation of the group intervention. Thirteen children (mean age of 4;7) were assigned to one of four groups. Following the three individual training sessions on stimulability and perception, each target received two cycles of production training in the six group intervention sessions. Greater gains in production accuracy were achieved as a result of the children's improved stimulability and perception abilities. With regard to pretreatment stimulability status, stimulable and unstimulable sounds achieved mean difference scores of 4.56 and 3.00, respectively. Similarly, sounds with good pretreatment perceptual ability demonstrated a mean gain of 4.19 points, with a 3.90 mean gain for poorly perceived pretreatment sounds. As in the first study, the probability for greater intervention gains was associated with sounds for which children demonstrated good pretreatment stimulability and perception. These findings support those of the previous studies; specifically, unstimulable sounds are not likely to change without direct intervention.

Finally, additional support for the relationship between stimulability and phonological learning was provided in a study by Flint and Costello Ingham (2005). In a descriptive study, seven children (ages 4;0 to 5;7) participated in individual intervention on either stimulable or nonstimulable sounds. Using a traditional articulation approach that initiated intervention in isolation and progressed to spontaneous production of the target sound in words in sentences, three children received training on stimulable sounds whereas four children were trained on nonstimulable sounds. Across all seven children, a total of 132 untreated and misarticulated sounds were monitored, 24 of which were stimulable and 108 were nonstimulable. The percentage of untreated sounds that exhibited generalization was only 12% for the nonstimulable sounds as compared with 83% for the stimulable sounds. These findings further corroborate earlier findings that nonstimulable speech sounds are unlikely to show generalization without direct intervention.

Additional support for this relationship is also found in two studies that did not directly examine stimulability. In an early study to explain differences in learning patterns, Elbert and McReynolds (1978) found that generalization to [s] in different vowel contexts only occurred when the children learned to imitate the sound. Rvachew and Nowak (2001) looked at the effect of phonological knowledge and developmental status of target sounds on phonological learning. Although they did not directly assess the children's stimulability abilities, they assumed that sounds characterized as "least knowledge" represented unstimulable sounds while sounds characterized as "most knowledge" represented stimulable sounds. Their results indicated that greater progress was demonstrated by children who received intervention for early developing sounds that were associated with greater phonological knowledge than children who received intervention for later developing, least knowledge sounds.

Collectively, these studies suggest that there is a strong relationship between stimulability and phonological learning that support the prognostic indicators of the earliest studies on general speech stimulability skills. Specifically, stimulable sounds are likely to be acquired even without direct intervention. Conversely, the prognosis for short-term sound normalization of nonstimulable sounds is much poorer (Powell, 2003). This body of research, then, was the impetus for developing specific intervention procedures that focus on training nonstimulable sounds, which is the focus of the next section.

Studies on Stimulability Intervention Approaches

Limited data are available on stimulability as an intervention approach. Rvachew et al. briefly described the short three-session stimulability training that was provided in their second study as including "phonetic placement, mirrors, verbal instruction, and auditory-visual models" (1999, p. 37) for imitation in isolation/syllables and progressing to words and sentences. Only three published case studies in the literature describe intervention outcomes of an intervention approach that focuses specifically on enhancing stimulability skills. Powell (1996) reported on a case study involving a child, Zachary (age 5), who exhibited a persistent SSD. The goal of intervention was to increase the child's consonant inventory through the development of stimulability skills for unknown sounds. Powell used brief 5-minute sound stimulation activities as warm-up and cool-down play activities to facilitate the child's sound imitation skills. He used either objects (e.g., a car, toy musical instruments, or playdough) or picture cards while producing different consonant sounds, such as producing an elongated [ʃ:::] while moving a car quickly across the floor to represent the continuant fricative or producing repeated strings of [gʌgʌgʌ] with a picture for drinking water. As the child became amenable to the activity, placement and visual cues were occasionally introduced. Following the sound stimulation activity at the beginning of the intervention session, different modules were incorporated within the session to evoke, stabilize, generalize, and maintain the sound production skills. Although the emphasis was on the sounds missing from Zachary's phonetic inventory, inconsistently produced sounds were also stimulated. Following an intensive 3-month summer intervention program of four 1-hour sessions per week, Zachary's phonetic inventory increased in both size (from 11 consonants to 17 consonants) and complexity (progressed from Level C with fricatives and affricates to Level D that included a liquid, based on Dinnsen, Chin, Elbert, and Powell's [1990] typology for complexity of phonetic inventories).

Although the Rvachew et al. (1999) and Powell (1996) studies incorporated brief intervention activities within a session to facilitate stimulability skills, Miccio and Elbert (1996) and Miccio (2009) described stimulability as an intervention approach that is solely focused on enhancing a child's stimulability skills. The first case study reported with the stimulability intervention approach was Stacy (age 3;4), whose phonetic inventory was severely limited to production of labial and alveolar stops, nasals, and glides. In an A-B case study design, three baseline sessions were conducted prior to the initiation of the stimulability approach. Stacy was taught to produce all consonant sounds, stimulable and nonstimulable, with the exception of the liquids [l, r], which served as control sounds. A total of 12 intervention sessions were completed during twice-weekly 45-minute sessions. Character cards representing each of the consonant sounds were introduced along with associated hand/body movements that accompanied the sound production for each consonant in isolation (e.g., [s:::::::] while moving the index finger up the arm for "Silly Snake") or in a CV context (e.g., [pʌ] while gliding hands in a skating motion for "Putt-Putt Pig"). Multimodal cues (auditory, visual, and tactile) were provided during a variety of games and activities that involved turn taking between the clinician and the child. One third of the stimulability probe (Powell & Miccio, 1996) was administered at the beginning of each therapy session to measure generalization. No nonstimulable sounds were produced on the first baseline probe, but by the final probe, Stacy produced 26 of the treated sounds in probe items, as well as both of the untreated nonstimulable control sounds. Based on the final phonological analysis, Stacy added [v, ŋ] to her phonetic inventory, as well as [k, dʒ] as emerging phones. With regard to complexity, her pretreatment phonetic inventory was consistent with a Level B inventory (Dinnsen et al., 1990) with labial and alveolar stops, nasals, and glides. Following intervention, the two new phones plus the two emerging phones advanced her phonetic inventory to a Level C.

In another case study, Miccio (2009) reported the intervention outcomes for Fiona (age 4;3), whose phonetic inventory was limited to glides and anterior stops and nasals. Using intervention procedures identical to those described in Miccio and Elbert (1996), Fiona completed 50-minute intervention sessions that were held twice weekly for 12 weeks. Following the intervention program, Fiona added all fricatives, affricates, and [r] to her phonetic inventory, and she was stimulable for all targeted sounds and produced many of them in simple words.

Miccio, Yont, Landefeld, Nelson, and Stubblebine (1999) gave a presentation on a two-part intervention study involving six children (ages 2;10 to 5;2) that examined intervention outcomes aimed at enhancing stimulability skills (Study 1) and intervention outcomes aimed at enhancing generalization (Study 2). All children participated in intervention to enhance stimulability, using three sound-elicitation activities that involved turn taking and requesting, as described in Miccio and Elbert (1996). Three baseline sessions were conducted prior to the 12 intervention sessions that targeted all consonants with the exception of the control sounds, /l, ɹ/. In Study 2, three of the six children then participated in an additional 12 intervention sessions that targeted one maximal opposition to enhance generalization. Their findings indicated that intervention to enhance stimulability resulted in sounds becoming stimulable and generalizing across syllable positions, and that stimulable sounds generalized to correct production in words without further direct intervention. They found differences in generalization patterns for children who exhibited atypical phonetic inventories such that nonstimulable sounds were not acquired and newly stimulable sounds were used in words, but often incorrectly. Based on their results, Miccio, Yont, et al. (1999) suggested that intervention to enhance stimulability is appropriate for children with small, typical phonetic inventories, whereas intervention to enhance stimulability plus generalization is recommended for children with small, atypical inventories.

Summary of Levels of Evidence

This review of the research in stimulability included studies of the relationship between stimulability skills and phonological learning, as well as reports of intervention outcomes with a stimulability intervention approach. The level of evidence for studies across both categories of research is summarized in Table 8.1. With regard to the relationship between stimulability and learning, six empirical studies directly examined this relationship, and two additional studies that were not direct investigations of stimulability were summarized. These studies, conducted over 3 decades, encompassed 104 children ranging in age from 3;6 to 6;4 and included primarily single-subject research designs with one randomized control design and one pretest-posttest design. The results across the studies consistently reported that nonstimulable sounds are associated with poorer intervention outcomes and are unlikely to improve without direct intervention. These findings motivated the development of a stimulability intervention approach to enhance children's production of the more complex, nonstimulable sounds. This body of research is much smaller and limited to three case study reports that encompassed three children who ranged in age from 3;4 to 5;1 and one presentation involving six children (ages 2;10 to 5;2). Although the research is rather limited, the available evidence indicates that the stimula-

Table 8.1. Levels of evidence for studies of treatment efficacy for stimulability studies and intervention approach

Level	Description	References
Ia	Meta-analysis of > 1 randomized controlled trial	—
Ib	Randomized controlled study	Rvachew & Nowak (2001)
IIa	Controlled study without randomization	—
IIb	Quasi-experimental study	Elbert & McReynolds (1978); Flint & Costello Ingham (2005); Miccio, Elbert, et al. (1999); Miccio, Yont, et al. (1999); Powell (1993); Powell et al. (1991); Rvachew et al. (1999)
III	Nonexperimental studies, i.e., correlational and case studies	Miccio (2009); Miccio & Elbert (1996); Powell (1996)
IV	Expert committee report, consensus conference, clinical experience of respected authorities	—

Adapted from the Scottish Intercollegiate Guidelines Network (http://www.sign.ac.uk).

bility intervention approach is a promising intervention with probable efficacy for increasing a child's correct imitative production of sounds that are missing from the phonetic inventory across a wide range of manner, place, and voice characteristics.

PRACTICAL REQUIREMENTS

Nature of Sessions

Although all published reports using the stimulability intervention approach have incorporated individual intervention sessions, Miccio and Elbert (1996) reported that the intervention has been implemented in small groups, though usually with more than one clinician. Miccio (2005) again stated that the intervention program can be adapted to small groups and also suggested that the character cards could be used for sound awareness activities during classroom circle time.

Personnel

The stimulability approach is typically implemented by an SLP. Although no reports are available for parent training, Miccio and Elbert (1996) and Miccio (2005) stated that parents and siblings have participated in stimulability intervention. Miccio reported that anecdotal feedback from parents has been positive because they can easily use the associated hand/body motions to bring their children's attention to the target sounds at home to encourage speech production within a nonthreatening atmosphere.

Dosage

Stimulability intervention is intended to be a short-term approach with *stimulability*, not *acquisition*, being the intervention target (Miccio, 2005). Consequently, intervention has been reported as typically lasting for 12 sessions (Miccio & Elbert, 1996), but no longer than 12 weeks (Miccio, 2009). In both reports, intervention included twice weekly 45- or 50-minute sessions.

KEY COMPONENTS

Nature of Goals

Although the goal of the stimulability approach is to increase the number of stimulable sounds, Miccio and Elbert (1996) described a broad approach in which all consonants, both stimulable and nonstimulable, are addressed within each session. Incorporating stimulable sounds is done to achieve early success with very young children while targeting the more difficult nonstimulable sounds. The sounds are taught in isolation (e.g., [s:::::]) or CV contexts (e.g., [kʌkʌkʌ]) for stops and glides. A stimulability probe, as described previously, is administered to determine which sounds are stimulable and nonstimulable. A sound is considered stimulable if it is produced with at least 10% accuracy (Powell et al., 1991) or produced correctly at least twice (Miccio et al., 1999).

Goal Attack Strategies

According to Miccio (2005), a horizontal goal attack strategy (Fey, 1986; Williams, 2003) is incorporated with the stimulability intervention program, as all consonants are addressed within each therapy session.

Description of Activities

The stimulability intervention approach is based on a number of intervention studies that cover a diverse range of research. This research foundation provides the basis for the seven major components of the stimulability intervention approach (Miccio, 2005, 2009). A brief summary of each component is provided in the following sections, followed by a description of the stimulability activities.

Intervention Components to Enhance Stimulability

Directly Target Nonstimulable Sounds

Directly targeting nonstimulable sounds is based on two lines of research related to complexity and stimulability of intervention targets (Gierut, 2001; Miccio et al., 1999; Powell et al., 1991). Specifically, teaching nonstimulable sounds results in acquisition of both nonstimulable sounds as well as untreated stimulable sounds (Miccio et al., 1999; Powell et al., 1991). Similarly, teaching more complex sounds, which are often nonstimulable sounds, results in the addition of more sounds to the phonetic inventory (Gierut, 2001).

Make Targets the Joint Focus of Attention

Research on children's semantic development indicates that objects that are the focus of joint attention are associated with children spontaneously repeating words that were labeled by their parents (Baldwin & Markman, 1989; Baldwin et al., 1996). Based on this research, then, it is predicted that speech sounds will be easier for children to learn if they are associated with interesting objects that have been labeled by adults.

Associate Speech Sounds with Hand/Body Motions

Hand motions can serve as retrieval cues, as demonstrated by a study by Fazio (1997) of children with a specific language impairment who were able to recall a poem following a 2-day delay when the poem was learned with accompanying hand motions. In addition, Rauscher, Krauss, and Chen (1996) reported that multimodal input increased children's ability to retain newly learned speech sounds. Miccio and Elbert (1996) incorporated this research in the stimulability approach through pairing speech sounds with hand/body motions to facilitate children's retrieval of newly learned speech sounds. The motions are only elicited when paired with a speech sound, even if the sound is produced incorrectly.

Associate Speech Sounds with Alliterative Characters

A central component of the stimulability approach is the use of alliterative characters for each consonant sound. Similar to using hand/body motions as retrieval cues, pairing speech sounds with alliterative characters that are of interest to young children will encourage their participation in the intervention activities and help them recall the speech sounds. Moreover, the alliterative characters provide children with the phoneme-grapheme association that is an important element in acquiring alphabet knowledge, which has been identified as one of the strongest indicators of reading success (Ehri, 2004; Hulme, Goetz, Gooch, Adams, & Snowling, 2007). Readers can download the alliterative characters for the stimulability approach at no cost at http://www.brookespublishing.com /williams/miccio.htm. Large and small characters are included for the consonant sounds, which can be used for different intervention activities. A brief description of each sound character and its associated hand/body motion is provided in Table 8.2.

Encourage Vocal Practice

For very young children, drill activities are not likely to hold their attention and encourage vocal practice, which has been reported by earlier studies to be a critical component in the acquisition and generalization of new sounds (Powell, Elbert, Miccio, Strike-Roussos, & Brasseur, 1998; Saben & Costello Ingham, 1991). The stimulability approach includes a variety of interesting sound elicitation activities that encourage vocal practice through fun, play-based turn-taking and requesting activities.

Ensure Early Success

A common principle of intervention programs is that targets should not be so difficult that the child is easily frustrated. In fact, Edwards (1983) suggested that early success is important and therefore targets should be included that are produced correctly some of the time or are part of the child's phonetic inventory. This principle would appear to violate the first component of the stimulability intervention approach that recommends that nonstimulable sounds are directly targeted. To address this concern, Miccio and Elbert (1996) designed the intervention program to include stimulable sounds as well as the non-stimulable sounds. In this way, children will be ensured success on the stimulable sounds while also receiving intervention for the more difficult, nonstimulable sounds. Miccio (2005) stated that a child may not correctly imitate a nonstimulable sound in one instance, but can then request a character that is associated with a stimulable sound; for example, "Putt-Putt Pig," which might be a stimulable sound that is part of the child's phonetic inventory. The stimulable sounds not only provide the child with opportunities to

Table 8.2. Stimulus characters and associated motions

Consonant		Character	Associated motion
Stops	/p/	Putt-Putt Pig	Hands move in a skating motion
	/b/	Baby Bear	Pantomime rocking a baby
	/t/	Talkie Turkey	Hand at ear (telephone sign)
	/d/	Dirty Dog	Digging motion with hands
	/k/	Coughing Cow	Cough with hand at top of throat
	/g/	Goofy Goat	Roll eyes toward ceiling
Fricatives	/f/	Fussy Fish	Hand fussily pushes away from body
	/v/	Viney Violet	Move arm up as a winding vine
	/θ/	Thinking Thumb	Wiggle thumb
	/s/	Silly Snake	Slinkily move finger up arm
	/z/	Zippy Zebra	Zip jacket front
	/ʃ/	Shy Sheepy	Clutch hands together and slowly push down shyly
Affricates	/tʃ/	Cheeky Chick	Sassily tap hand towards cheek
	/dʒ/	Giant Giraffe	Make stair steps with hand
Nasals	/m/	Munchie Mouse	Push lips together and rub tummy
	/n/	Naughty Newt	Scold with finger
Liquids	/l/	Lazy Lion	Stretch arms in *L* shape
	/ɹ/	Rowdy Rooster	Rev motorcycle gears
Glides	/w/	Wiggly Worm	Shiver
	/j/	Yawning Yoyo	Yawn with hand tapping mouth
	/h/	Happy Hippo	Laugh and shake shoulders

Note: All motions for fricatives are continuous. All motions for stops are ballistic.

Readers can download the alliterative characters for the stimulability approach at no cost at http://www.brookespublishing.com/williams/miccio.htm

From *Journal of Communication Disorders, 29,* Miccio & Elbert, Enhancing Stimulability: A treatment program, pp. 335–351; copyright (c) 1996, with permission from Elsevier.

be successful, but the activities can also reinforce and stabilize stimulable sounds within the child's sound system. For instance, the clinician and child could talk about "Putt-Putt Pig" being *pink* and that she carries a *purple purse* and wears *purple* ribbons. In this way, the child has many opportunities to be successful and positively reinforced for producing [p] in connected speech. Although the child can choose any sound character (often the stimulable sounds), the clinician chooses the nonstimulable sounds in order to increase the child's imitative skills for those sounds. This is done by the clinician modeling the nonstimulable sounds during a request or turn. The child is encouraged, though not required, to imitate the sound with the clinician. Modeling and production are integral components of the stimulability approach.

Ensure Successful Communicative Attempts

This final intervention component is an extension of the previous two components that address encouragement and early success. Even though the child can choose any of the consonant sounds during the turn-taking and requesting intervention activities, the clinician will always choose a nonstimulable sound. To encourage risk taking for production of the nonstimulable sounds, the paired hand/body motions communicate the child's intent even if their production is incorrect. Based on research by Rescorla and Ratner (1996), the successful communication between child and clinician, in turn, encourages more verbalization, which maintains the child's interest and participation in the intervention activities. For example, Miccio (2005) described a scenario in which a child did not correctly produce [s:] but demonstrated the associated hand motion of zipping up a coat. Consequently, the clinician is able to respond to the child's intent and provide positive feedback while also modeling the correct production within a recast. The clinician might respond, "Do I have 'Silly Snake?' 'Silly Snake' says [s::::]. [The clinician might draw attention to his or her mouth to show how the sound is produced.] Here's the 'Silly Snake.' He says [s::::]." In this way there is no breakdown in communication, and the child is encouraged to continue his or her participation within a nonthreatening activity.

Taken together, these seven components of the stimulability approach work to increase a child's imitative production of nonstimulable sounds through the use of alliterative characters paired with hand/body motions in a variety of interesting turn-taking and requesting activities that encourage vocal practice of more difficult nonstimulable sounds while also guaranteeing early success on the easier stimulable sounds. Miccio and Elbert (1996) summarized the following hypotheses from intervention research that underlie the stimulability approach:

1. Facilitate systemwide generalization: Greater generalization will occur when unknown aspects are taught (Gierut, Elbert, & Dinnsen, 1987).

2. Increase phonetic inventory: More sounds will be added to a child's phonetic inventory when more complex sounds are taught (Powell, 1991).

3. Teach nonstimulable sounds: Acquisition of both trained and untrained stimulable sounds will occur when nonstimulable sounds are targeted (Powell et al., 1991).

In addition, Miccio and Elbert (1996) listed the following clinical considerations that the stimulability approach was designed to address:

1. Increase focused attention to targeted sounds through associations with interesting objects and movements that encourage full and engaged participation in the intervention activities.

2. Early success is achieved by incorporating stimulable sounds along with the nonstimulable sounds and by utilizing gestural movements that result in successful communication attempts even when productions are incorrect.

The following sections will describe a variety of stimulability activities and the format of a typical 50-minute individual intervention session.

Stimulability Intervention Activities

Miccio (2005, 2009) and Miccio and Elbert (1996) described a number of fun, play-based activities that can be used to enhance stimulability. For very young children who may be reticent to engage in structured, drill-like activities, these stimulability activities provide a fun and encouraging format to actively engage the children in highly motivating and interesting activities that will maintain their participation throughout the 45- to 50-minute intervention session. Miccio (2005) recommended using the larger 5 × 7-inch pictures of the characters for many of the turn-taking and requesting activities, whereas the smaller 2 × 3-inch pictures can be used with board game activities. Pasting the illustrations onto index cards or cardstock will make them more durable.

Miccio (2005) stated that any number of activities can be used to enhance a child's stimulability. Simple game-like activities that offer several opportunities to request or name the sounds of the characters are fun ways to stimulate production of the sounds. Some examples of activities listed by Miccio (2005) include

1. Go Fish: Clinician and child take turns requesting character cards from each other

2. Lotto boards with the alliterative characters

3. Sound character card games

4. Post office: Mail the character cards

5. Space: Send the character cards to space in a rocket

6. Guessing game: Place cards in a basket and take turns giving cues using hand motions and sound for the other player to guess the character. A demonstration of this activity is shown in the accompanying DVD video.

7. Fishing game: Clinician and child take turns fishing for character cards using a magnet tied to a pole to pick up cards with metal clips and then naming the character that was "caught." This activity is also demonstrated with Carter in the DVD video clip.

8. Spinner games: Clinician and child take turns producing the sound and associated motion of the character on which the spinner lands. These activities are well-liked by children who are a little older.

9. Board games: Clinician and child take turns playing board games using the character cards. These activities work well with slightly older children.

Miccio and Elbert (1996) suggested that many different experiential play activities can be used with the character cards, including activities suggested by Hodson and Paden (1991). The activities provide a supportive structure for facilitating children's imitative production of nonstimulable sounds. Correct productions are reinforced while modeling is provided early in intervention for incorrect productions; placement cues are provided to shape more precise articulations as the child becomes acclimated to the activities and comfortable imitating the clinician. At that point, the child is instructed to watch the clinician and listen while the clinician produces the sound and phonetic placement cues are given.

Typical Intervention Session

Miccio and Elbert (1996) and Miccio (2005) outlined a typical 50-minute individual intervention session. The intervention tasks/activities and corresponding times are described in the following list.

1. *Elicitation of one third of the stimulability probe* (see Appendix 8.1; 5 minutes): Each consonant is elicited within one of the three vowel contexts. For example, [f] is imitated in isolation and within the [i] vowel context ([fi], [ifi], [if]). In the second session, all consonants are imitated within the second vowel context ([ɑ]), such as [fɑ], [ɑfɑ], [ɑf]. Finally all consonants are elicited in the third vowel context ([u]) in the third session ([fu], [ufu], [uf]). In this way the entire stimulability probe is administered every third intervention session.

2. *Review character cards with their sounds and associated motions* (5 minutes): Following the probe, the clinician and client review the character cards. Using focused joint attention, the clinician presents each character card one at a time, naming the character, modeling the sound, and demonstrating the associated movement. The child is encouraged but not required to produce each target sound as the clinician reviews each character card.

3. *Engage child in play-based stimulability activities* (30 minutes): Three different 10-minute stimulability activities comprise the primary focus of the intervention session. As described previously, play-based activities that are developmentally appropriate are used with the character cards in turn-taking games in which the child hears the clinician model the sounds and the child attempts to imitate. For example, the clinician and child might play Go Fish (10 minutes), Guessing Game (10 minutes), and a Spinner Game (10 minutes). Direct imitation is not required, although vocal practice is encouraged through the turn-taking activities, using verbal requests during the various activities. As the child becomes more acclimated to the activities, the focus and intensity of the instruction can be increased as the clinician instructs the child to watch and listen as the sound is produced. Occasionally phonetic placement cues are used to shape the child's production of the target sound. As noted previously, the child can request any card during the activities; however, the clinician always selects a nonstimulable sound. This nonthreatening environment reduces frustration and encourages the child to be actively engaged in vocal practice. Thus, the intervention activities provide a supportive framework for increasing the child's successful imitation of nonstimulable sounds.

4. *Elicit the palindrome generalization probe* (5–8 minutes): To assess generalization to real words, a short palindrome probe is elicited at the end of each session. Generalization to words and across syllable positions is assessed in simple CVC words (see Appendix 8.2). The child is asked to imitate the clinician's productions.

In summary, these activities provide multiple opportunities for intensive modeling and vocal practice within a supportive and encouraging framework of fun, play-based activities. Thus, modeling and speech production are integral parts of the intervention approach. Motions are always paired with speech sounds and are never used as a replacement for speech. Miccio (2005) noted that this approach has been successful with children who have not responded to more conventional intervention approaches, such as the minimal pair or traditional articulation approaches. Miccio (2005) further noted that the stimulability approach can be characterized as a hybrid phonetic-phonological approach to intervention. The multimodality of the auditory, visual, and tactile cues facilitates the phonetic learning of the sounds, whereas the play-based interactive activities assist in the child's appropriate use of sounds to communicate. In addition, the sound-based activities encourage acquisition of critical phonological awareness skills, particularly knowledge of sound-letter relationships that form alphabet knowledge.

Materials and Equipment Required

The materials needed for the stimulability approach are 21 alliterative sound characters that are associated with each consonant sound. Miccio (2005) described these stimulus characters as interesting to young children to maintain their interest and participation during intervention activities. Hand/body motions are paired with each character to help as retrieval cues for children to learn the new speech sounds. As noted previously, the alliterative characters facilitate children's learning of the alphabetic principle. These stim-

ulus characters are available for free download at the Brookes web site (http://www
.brookespublishing.com/williams/miccio.htm). A list of the stimulus characters and associated motions is provided in Table 8.2.

ASSESSMENT AND PROGRESS
MONITORING TO SUPPORT DECISION MAKING

Assessment is based on the stimulability probe to determine the stimulability status of
each consonant sound. One third of the stimulability probe is elicited at the beginning of
each session to evaluate changes in the child's stimulability abilities. Progress monitoring for this short-term intervention is based on the brief palindrome probe that measures
generalization to real words and across syllable positions. The 17-item palindrome probe
is administered at the end of each session. Given that the stimulability approach is designed to be a short-term intervention aimed at enhancing a child's ability to imitate nonstimulable sounds, changes in the intervention plan are not required. In fact, the only intervention changes that Miccio (2005) described were related to increases in the intensity
of the clinician models with occasional phonetic placement cues provided when the children were more comfortable with speech production and imitating the clinician.

CONSIDERATIONS FOR CHILDREN FROM
CULTURALLY AND LINGUISTICALLY DIVERSE BACKGROUNDS

The only reports of the stimulability approach have been in the United States with American English-speaking children, although the activities and concepts can easily be used
within any language. The intervention research that provides the foundation on which the
activities of the stimulability approach are based would be similar regardless of the native language of the children.

CASE STUDY

Carter, who demonstrated the stimulability approach in the DVD, was 3;2 and
produced 42 errors on the GFTA-2. His phonetic inventory consisted of nasals
[m, n], stops [b, d, g], and glides [w, j, h]. Stimulability testing revealed that
Carter was stimulable for only 4 of the 15 sounds that were inventory constraints.
Three sessions were conducted prior to filming to introduce him to the sound
character cards and their associated movements. The sessions followed the general order that was described earlier; that is, one third of the stimulability probe
was administered at the beginning of each session, followed by a review of the
character cards and movements, three 10-minute stimulability activities were
completed, and the palindrome probe was administered at the end of the session.
In the video demonstration on the DVD, viewers can see that Carter had learned
the alliterative characters and their associated movements and was actively engaged and participating in each of the stimulability activities (review of cards,
fishing game, guessing game). Although posttesting was not completed after
these few sessions, it is interesting to note that Carter was correctly imitating six

nonstimulable sounds ([f, v, ʧ, ʤ, l, t]) during the final intervention session. His mother also commented that Carter was producing new sounds at home and was impressed with the progress he had made in the very short period of only three sessions plus the one recording session. It was recommended that Carter's clinician continue the stimulability approach for an additional eight sessions. It was anticipated that by the completion of the 12 sessions, Carter would have expanded his phonetic inventory, as well as increased his imitation of sounds that were outside his inventory. This would have established a broader repertoire of sounds, which would then prepare him for moving on toward a contrastive intervention approach. Carter would also be ready for direct phonetic placement training, if required (Miccio, 2009).

STUDY QUESTIONS

1. Describe the ways in which the stimulability approach is phonetic and phonological.

2. What are the seven key components of the stimulability approach?

3. For what children would the stimulability approach be most appropriate?

FUTURE DIRECTIONS

Powell (2003) outlined several areas that require further investigation. He suggested the following areas to direct future studies in understanding the relationship between stimulability and speech sound learning:

1. Refinement and standardization of stimulability assessment procedures, with particular emphasis on predictive validity studies.

2. Systematic replications with children of different ages, diagnoses, and backgrounds are needed to fully understand the relationship between stimulability and sound learning, particularly with children who have been diagnosed with CAS.

3. Stimulability assessment and the relationship between stimulability and phonological differences with bilingual children.

4. Additional research on stimulability as a measure for distinguishing dialectal differences from SSD in order to help define best practices.

Flint and Costello Ingham (2005) suggested that additional intervention studies are needed to empirically validate the efficiency of targeting nonstimulable sounds even though they commonly take longer to teach than stimulable sounds. Rvachew et al. (1999) also recommended additional intervention studies using an experimental design with random assignment of children to intervention groups to determine the best methods of facilitating stimulability skills. Finally, the specific stimulability enhancement approach described in this chapter is designed as a short-term primer to prepare the child for more conventional intervention approaches, such as contrastive phonological intervention. This premise requires empirical study to determine if this preparatory approach results in more efficient intervention later or if there is more benefit if the components of stimulability were encompassed within the contrastive approach from the outset.

SUGGESTED READINGS

Miccio, A.W. (2005). Components of phonological assessment. In S.F. Warren & M.E. Fey (Series Eds.), & A.G. Kamhi & K.E. Pollock (Vol. Eds.), *Communication and language intervention series: Phonological disorders in children—Clinical decision making in assessment and intervention* (pp. 163–173). Baltimore: Paul H. Brookes Publishing Co.

Miccio, A.W. (2009). First things first: Stimulability therapy for children with small phonetic repertoires. In

C. Bowen (Ed.), *Children's speech sound disorders* (pp. 96–101). Oxford: Wiley-Blackwell.

Miccio, A.W., & Elbert, M. (1996). Enhancing stimulability: A treatment program. *Journal of Communication Disorders, 29,* 335–351.

Powell, T.W. (2003). Stimulability and treatment outcomes. *Perspectives on Language Learning and Education, 10*(1), 3–6.

Rvachew, S. (2005). Stimulability and treatment success. *Topics in Language Disorders, 25*(3), 207–219.

REFERENCES

Bain, B.A. (1994). A framework for dynamic assessment in phonology: Stimulability revisited. *Clinics in Communication Disorders, 4,* 12–22.

Bain, B.A., & Olswang, L.B. (1995). Examining readiness for learning two-word utterances by children with specific expressive language impairment: Dynamic assessment validation. *American Journal of Speech-Language Pathology, 4,* 81–92.

Baker, E., Croot, K., McLeod, S., & Paul, R. (2001). Tutorial paper: Psycholinguistic models of speech development and their application to clinical practice. *Journal of Speech, Language, and Hearing Research, 44,* 685–702.

Baldwin, D.A., & Markman, E.M. (1989). Establishing word-object relations: A first step. *Child Development, 60,* 381–398.

Baldwin, D.A., Markman, E.M., Bill, B., Desjardins, R.N., Irwin, J.M., & Tidball, G. (1996). Infants' reliance on a social criterion for establishing word-object relations. *Child Development, 67,* 3135–3153.

Bleile, K. (2002). Evaluating articulation and phonological disorders when the clock is running. *American Journal of Speech-Language Pathology, 11,* 243–249.

Carter, E.T., & Buck, M. (1958). Prognostic testing for functional articulation disorders among children in the first grade. *Journal of Speech and Hearing Disorders, 23,* 124–133.

Dinnsen, D.A., Chin, S.B., Elbert, M., & Powell, T.W. (1990). Some constraints on functionally disordered phonologies: Phonetic inventories and phonotactics. *Journal of Speech and Hearing Research, 34,* 1318–1328.

Dinnsen, D.A., & Elbert, M. (1984). On the relationship between phonology and learning. In M. Elbert, D.A. Dinnsen, & G. Weismer (Eds.), *Phonological theory and the misarticulating child* (ASHA Monograph No. 22, pp. 59–68). Rockville, MD: American Speech-Language-Hearing Association.

Edwards, M.L. (1983). Selection criteria for developing therapy goals. *Journal of Childhood Communication Disorders, 7,* 36–45.

Ehri, L.C. (2004). Teaching phonemic awareness and phonics: An explanation of the National Reading Panel meta-analyses. In P. McCardle & V. Chhabra (Eds.), *The voice of evidence in reading research* (pp. 153–186). Baltimore: Paul H. Brookes Publishing Co.

Elbert, M., & McReynolds, L.V. (1978). An experimental analysis of misarticulating children's generalization. *Journal of Speech and Hearing Research, 21,* 136–150.

Farquhar, M.S. (1961). Prognostic value of imitative and auditory discrimination tests. *Journal of Speech and Hearing Disorders, 26,* 342–347.

Fazio, B.B. (1997). Learning a new poem: Memory for connected speech and phonological awareness in low-income children with and without specific language impairment. *Journal of Speech, Language, and Hearing Research, 40,* 1285–1297.

Fey, M.E. (1986). *Language intervention with young children.* San Diego: College-Hill Press.

Fey, M.E., & Stalker, C. (1986). A hypothesis testing approach to treatment of a child with an idiosyncratic (morpho)phonological system. *Journal of Speech and Hearing Disorders, 41,* 324–336.

Flint, C.B., & Costello Ingham, J. (2005). Pretreatment stimulability and percentage of consonants correct as predictors of across-phoneme generalization. *Contemporary Issues in Communication Science and Disorders, 32,* 53–63.

Gierut, J.A. (2001). Complexity in phonological treatment: Clinical factors. *Language, Speech, and Hearing Services in Schools, 32,* 229–241.

Gierut, J.A., Elbert, M., & Dinnsen, D.A. (1987). A functional analysis of phonological knowledge and generalization learning in misarticulating children. *Journal of Speech and Hearing Research, 30,* 462–479.

Glaspey, A.M. (2006). *Dynamic assessment in phonological disorders: The Scaffolding Scale of Stimulability.* Unpublished doctoral dissertation, University of Washington, Seattle, Washington.

Glaspey, A.M., & Stoel-Gammon, C. (2007). A dynamic approach to phonological assessment. *Advances in Speech-Language Pathology, 9*(4), 286–296.

Goldman, R., & Fristoe, M. (1986). *Goldman-Fristoe Test of Articulation.* Circle Pines, MN: American Guidance Service.

Goldman, R., & Fristoe, M. (2000). *Goldman-Fristoe Test of Articulation-2.* Circle Pines, MN: American Guidance Service.

Guenther, F.H. (1995). Speech sound acquisition, coarticulation, and rate effects in a neural network model of speech production. *Psychological Review, 102*(3), 594–621.

Hodson, B.W., & Paden, E.E. (1991). *Targeting intelligible speech: A phonological approach to remediation.* Austin, TX: PRO-ED.

Hodson, B.W., Scherz, J.A., & Strattman, R.H. (2002). Evaluating communicative abilities of a highly unintelligible preschooler. *American Journal of Speech-Language Pathology, 11*, 236–247.

Hulme, C., Goetz, K., Gooch, D., Adams, J., & Snowling, M.J. (2007). Paired-associate learning, phoneme awareness, and learning to read. *Journal of Experimental Child Psychology, 96*, 150–166.

Irwin, R.B., West, J.F., & Trombetta, M.A. (1966). Effectiveness of speech therapy for second grade children with misarticulations: Predictive factors. *Exceptional Children, 32*, 471–479.

Jamieson, D.G., & Rvachew, S. (1992). Remediation of speech production errors with sound identification training. *Journal of Speech-Language Pathology and Audiology, 16*, 201–210.

Kwiatkowski, J., & Shriberg, L.D. (1998). The capability-focus treatment framework for child speech disorders. *American Journal of Speech-Language Pathology, 7*, 27–38.

Locke, J.L. (1988). The sound shape of early lexical representations. In M.D. Smith & J.L. Locke (Eds.), *The emergent lexicon: The child's development of a linguistic vocabulary* (pp. 3–22). San Diego: Academic Press.

Lof, G.L. (1996). Factors associated with speech-sound stimulability. *Journal of Communication Disorders, 29*, 255–278.

McGregor, K.K., & Schwartz, R.G. (1992). Converging evidence for underlying phonological representation in a child who misarticulates. *Journal of Speech and Hearing Research, 35*, 596–603.

McLeod, S., & Baker, E. (2004). Current clinical practice for children with speech impairment. In B.E. Murdoch, J. Goozee, B.M. Whelan, & K. Docking (Eds.), *Proceedings of the 26th World Congress of the Inter-*

national Association of Logopedics and Phoniatrics. Brisbane: University of Queensland.

Menn, L. (1978). Phonological units in beginning speech. In A. Bell & J. Bybee (Eds.), *Syllables and segments* (pp. 157–171). Amsterdam: North-Holland.

Miccio, A.W. (2002). Clinical problem solving: Assessment of phonological disorders. *American Journal of Speech-Language Pathology, 11*, 221–229.

Miccio, A.W. (2005). Components of phonological assessment. In S.F. Warren & M.E. Fey (Series Eds.), & A.G. Kamhi & K.E. Pollock (Vol. Eds.), *Communication and language intervention series: Phonological disorders in children—Clinical decision making in assessment and intervention* (pp. 163–173). Baltimore: Paul H. Brookes Publishing Co.

Miccio, A.W. (2009). First things first: Stimulability therapy for children with small phonetic repertoires. In C. Bowen (Ed.), *Children's speech sound disorders* (pp. 96–101). Oxford: Wiley-Blackwell.

Miccio, A.W., & Elbert, M. (1996). Enhancing stimulability: A treatment program. *Journal of Communication Disorders, 29*, 335–351.

Miccio, A.W., Elbert, M., & Forrest, K. (1999). The relationship between stimulability and phonological acquisition in children with normally developing and disordered phonology. *American Journal of Speech-Language Pathology, 8*, 347–363.

Miccio, A.W., Yont, K.M., Landefeld, H., Nelson, C., & Stubblebine, J. (1999, May). *Generalization patterns following treatment to enhance stimulability for phonological acquisition.* Presentation at the International Clinical Phonetics and Linguistics Association, Montrèal, Quèbec, Canada.

Milisen, R. (1954). The disorder of articulation: A systematic clinical and experimental approach. *Journal of Speech and Hearing Disorders, Monograph Supplement 4.*

Powell, T.W. (1991). Planning for phonological generalization: An approach to treatment target selection. *American Journal of Speech-Language Pathology, 1*, 21–27.

Powell, T.W. (1993). Phonetic inventory constraints in young children: Factors affecting acquisition patterns during treatment. *Clinical Linguistics and Phonetics, 7*(1), 45–57.

Powell, T.W. (1996). Stimulability considerations in the phonological treatment of a child with a persistent disorder of speech-sound production. *Journal of Communication Disorders, 29*, 315–333.

Powell, T.W. (2003). Stimulability and treatment outcomes. *Perspectives on Language Learning and Education, 10*(1), 3–6.

Powell, T.W., Elbert, M., & Dinnsen, D.A. (1991). Stimulability as a factor in the phonological generalization of misarticulating preschool children. *Journal of Speech and Hearing Research, 34*, 1318–1328.

Powell, T.W., Elbert, M., Miccio, A.W., Strike-Roussos, C., & Brasseur, J. (1998). Facilitating [s] production in young children: An experimental evaluation of motoric and conceptual treatment approaches. *Clinical Linguistics and Phonetics, 12*, 127–146.

Powell, T.W., & Miccio, A.W. (1996). Stimulability: A useful clinical tool. *Journal of Communication Disorders, 29*, 237–253.

Rauscher, F., Krauss, R.M., & Chen, Y. (1996). Gesture, speech and lexical access: The role of lexical movements in speech production. *Psychological Science, 7*, 226–231.

Rescorla, L., & Ratner, N.B. (1996). Phonetic profiles of toddlers with specific expressive language impairment. *Journal of Speech and Hearing Research, 39*, 153–165.

Rvachew, S. (1994). Speech perception training can facilitate sound production learning. *Journal of Speech and Hearing Research, 37*, 347–357.

Rvachew, S. (2005). Stimulability and treatment success. *Topics in Language Disorders, 25*(3), 207–219.

Rvachew, S., & Nowak, M. (2001). The effect of target selection strategy on sound production learning. *Journal of Speech, Language, and Hearing Research, 44*, 610–623.

Rvachew, S., Rafaat, S., & Martin, M. (1999). Stimulability, speech perception skills, and the treatment of phonological disorders. *American Journal of Speech-Language Pathology, 8*, 33–43.

Saben, C.B., & Costello Ingham, J. (1991). The effects of minimal pairs treatment on the speech-sound production of two children with phonologic disorders. *Journal of Speech and Hearing Disorders, 34*, 1023–1040.

Secord, W. (1989). The traditional approach to treatment. In N.A. Creaghead, P.W. Newman, & W.A. Secord (Eds.), *Assessment and remediation of articulatory and phonological disorders* (2nd ed.; pp. 129–153). Columbus, OH: Merrill.

Shelton, R.L., & McReynolds, L.V. (1979). Functional articulation disorders: Preliminaries to treatment. In N.J. Lass (Ed.), *Speech and language: Advances in basic research and practice* (Vol. 2; pp. 1–111). New York: Academic Press.

Snow, K., & Milisen, R. (1954). Spontaneous improvement in articulation as related to differential responses to oral and picture tests. *Journal of Speech and Hearing Disorders, Monograph Supplement 4*, 46–49.

Sommers, R.K. (1987). *Stim-Com: A prognostic inventory for misarticulating kindergarten and first grade children.* Buffalo, NY: United Educational Services.

Sommers, R.K., Leiss, R.H., Delp, M., Gerber, A., Fundrella, D., Smith, R., et al. (1967). Factors related to the effectiveness of articulation therapy for kindergarten, first, and second grade children. *Journal of Speech and Hearing Research, 13*, 428–437.

Vygotsky, L.S. (1978). *Mind in society: The development of higher psychological processes.* Cambridge, MA: Harvard University Press.

Williams, A.L. (2003). *Speech disorders resource guide for preschool children.* Clifton Park, NY: Thomson Delmar Learning.

Wolfe, V., Presley, C., & Mesaris, J. (2003). The importance of sound identification training in phonological intervention. *American Journal of Speech-Language Pathology, 12*, 282–288.

Stimulability Probe

	Iso	#_i	i_i	i_#	#_ɑ	ɑ_ɑ	ɑ_#	#_u	u_u	u_#	Total
p											
b											
t											
d											
k											
g											
f											
v											
θ											
ð											
s											
z											
ʃ											
ʒ											
tʃ											
dʒ											
m											
n											
ŋ	▓		▓			▓				
w			▓			▓				▓
j			▓			▓				▓
h			▓			▓				▓
l											
r											

Note: Shaded boxes indicate that the sound does not occur in that position.

From Powell, T.W., & Miccio, A.W. (1996). Stimulability: A useful clinical tool. *Journal of Communication Disorders, 29,* 245; adapted by permission.

Palindrome
Generalization Probe

1. pop   _____
2. Bob   _____
3. tot   _____
4. dad   _____
5. Coke   _____
6. gag   _____
7. fife   _____
8. Viv   _____
9. sis   _____
10. zazz   _____
11. shush   _____
12. Cheech   _____
13. judge   _____
14. mom   _____
15. none   _____
16. Lil   _____
17. roar   _____

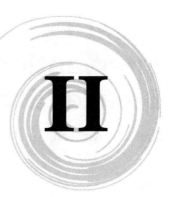

II

Speech Interventions in Broader Contexts

Speech Interventions in Broader Contexts

Sharynne McLeod, Rebecca J. McCauley, and A. Lynn Williams

S peech sound interventions target speech production and speech movements, or target these areas in conjunction with a focus on broader aspects of communication. Section II includes the following 12 interventions for speech sound disorders that target speech production within a broader context, such as language, literacy, the speech continuum (from perception to production), and the communicative context:

- Psycholinguistic intervention (Chapter 9)

- Metaphonological intervention (Chapter 10)

- Computer-based interventions (Chapter 11)

- Perceptual intervention (Chapter 12)

- Nonlinear phonological intervention (Chapter 13)

- Dynamic systems (whole language; Chapter 14)

- Morphosyntactic intervention (Chapter 15)

- Naturalistic speech intelligibility training (Chapter 16)

- Parents and Children Together (PACT; Chapter 17)

- Enhanced milieu teaching with phonological emphasis (EMT/PE; Chapter 18)

- Prompts for Restructuring Oral Muscular Phonetic Targets (PROMPT; Chapter 19)

- Family-focused interventions (Chapter 20)

As with the chapters in Section I, this overview provides comparisons among these 12 interventions with regard to the following 10 factors: client age, primary client populations, key intervention agents, key components, broad goals, basis of target selection, level of focus, session type, technology and/or materials required, and key codes from the *International Classification of Functioning, Disability and Health: Children and Youth Version* (ICF-CY; WHO, 2007). Table II.1 provides a comparative summary of these 10 factors across the 12 intervention approaches. Before discussing each of these factors, however, it is important to summarize each approach with regard to the available levels of evidence (LOE).

LEVELS OF EVIDENCE

As in Section I, the chapter authors in Section II used the Scottish Intercollegiate Guideline Network (SIGN; http://www.sign.ac.uk) as a common framework for characterizing the scientific evidence available for each intervention approach. Table II.2 provides a summary of the authors' findings. From the 12 interventions within Section II, Chapter 10 includes the only documented example of the highest LOE (Ia: meta-analysis of more than one randomized controlled trial). Over time it is anticipated that more meta-analyses will be available about interventions for children with speech sound disorders (SSD). As can be seen in Table II.2, the majority of research that has been undertaken about intervention techniques that target speech production within a broader context have been randomized controlled studies (Level Ib), controlled studies without randomization (Level IIa), quasi-experimental studies (Level IIb), and nonexperimental studies (Level III). Almost every intervention includes at least one quasi-experimental study—a popular research design within speech-language pathology for many years, possibly due to the heterogeneity of children with SSD. Within Table II.2 there are few examples of expert committee reports, consensus conferences, or clinical experience of respected authorities (Level IV). It is likely that there are more examples of Level IV evidence available for the interventions; however, these may not be published in peer-reviewed journals, so the authors chose to highlight examples of higher LOE. Readers are encouraged to examine each chapter's summary of evidence to understand the elements and contexts of each intervention approach that are supported or not supported by the documented evidence.

COMPARATIVE FACTORS

Client Age

The majority of the interventions in Section II are aimed at preschool-age children who are 3 years of age or older; that is, those who are at a rule-based stage of phonological acquisition (see Table II.1). However, there are exceptions. Naturalistic speech intelligibility training is primarily aimed at toddlers and preschoolers. Interventions targeting both speech and literacy are suitable for school-age children (e.g., metaphonological intervention). Some interventions have been described as appropriate for adults and children of all ages (e.g., psycholinguistic intervention, nonlinear phonological intervention).

Primary Client Populations

Children with SSD of unknown origin are the primary client population for the majority of techniques in Section II (see Table II.1). A number of the interventions target children with concomitant difficulties such as speech and language impairment (e.g., morphosyntactic intervention, whole language, EMT/PE), or speech and literacy impairment (e.g., psycholinguistic intervention, metaphonological intervention). Some interventions that target speech production within a broader context have been developed for children with known causes. For example, EMT/PE focuses on children with cleft lip and/or palate, and

Table II.1. Characteristics of speech interventions featured in Section II

Intervention approach (chapter)	Client age	Primary client populations	Key intervention agents	Key components	Broad goals
Psycholinguistic intervention (9)	Any age (from preschool children to adults); mostly school-age children	Children with delayed and/or disordered speech and literacy difficulties	SLPs supported by trained assistants or parents	Speech input (e.g., auditory discrimination), lexical representations (e.g., semantic, phonological, motor), speech output (e.g., programming and production of speech)	Improve intelligibility and literacy; work on strengths and weaknesses in the speech processing system as a whole
Metaphonological intervention (10)	All children with SSD; mostly school-age children	Children with delayed and/or disordered speech and literacy difficulties	SLPs supported by parents, teachers, or assistants	Phonological awareness including rhyming, syllable clapping, alliteration, and blending and segmenting games, followed by production of contrasting sounds and minimally paired words	Stimulate speech change via training phonological awareness
Computer-based interventions (11)	3+ years (i.e., at a rule-based stage of phonological acquisition)	Children with delayed and/or disordered speech	SLPs supported by teachers, parents, or assistants	Depending on program: ease and accessibility, efficiency, data management, report generation	Depending on program: phonological awareness, perception, speech sound production
Speech perception intervention (12)	Tested with 4- to 5-year-olds	Children with moderate to severe primary SSD	Planning by SLP, intervention by a communication disorders assistant, research assistant, or parent	Phonemic perception training	Develop specific acoustic-phonetic representations for phonemes misarticulated by the child

Basis of target selection	Level of focus	Session type	Technology and/or materials required	Key ICF-CY codes[a]
Level of breakdown from the speech processing profile	Speech perception, speech production, phonological awareness, and literacy	Flexible—individual and/or small-group sessions	None	b320: Articulation Functions; b2304: Speech Discrimination; d140: Learning to Read
Developmental and stimulable	Phoneme primarily at the word level	Individual and/or small-group sessions	None; but can use relevant computer programs	b320: Articulation Functions; d140: Learning to Read
Various depending on the program	Various depending on the program: includes focus on the phoneme at the word level	Individual and/or small-group sessions	Essential	b320: Articulation Functions; b2304: Speech Discrimination; d140: Learning to Read
Perception of misarticulated phonemes	Speech perception of misarticulated phonemes	Individual computer-based sessions	SAILS computer program	b320: Articulation Functions; b2304: Speech Discrimination

(continued)

Table II.1.   *(continued)*

Intervention approach (chapter)	Client age	Primary client populations	Key intervention agents	Key components	Broad goals
Nonlinear phonological intervention (13)	Adults and children	Adults and children with delayed and/or disordered speech and a range of etiologies	SLPs assisted by parents, caregivers, family, teachers, and speech assistants	Constraint-based nonlinear approach targeting prosodic structures and segments by considering individual phonological units and interactions between phonological units	Increase communicative competence; establish new elements, new features, new prosodic structures, new combination of features, and/or new locations for old elements
Dynamic systems and whole language intervention (14)	Children across a wide age range, particularly preschool children	Children with concomitant speech and language impairment	SLPs, parents, and teachers	Discourse structure, semantic, syntactic, morphological, and letter-sound knowledge	Multiple goals for integrated communication skills: macrostructure (discourse), connotative (complex syntax), denotative (phrases), referential (vocabulary and pronouns), canonical (syllable), categorical (phonemes), perceptual
Morphosyntax intervention (15)	Children ages 3;0–6;0 years	Children with phonological and morphological difficulties	SLPs, SLP students, and early childhood special educators	Cross-domain effects of morphosyntax and phonology	Cycles targeting speech sounds and grammatical morphemes

Basis of target selection	Level of focus	Session type	Technology and/or materials required	Key ICF-CY codes[a]
Presence and absence of structures and features in the child's phonological system	All levels of the phonological hierarchy; speech perception, phonological awareness, literacy	Individual and/or small-group sessions	None; however, CAPES can be used for assessment and analysis	b320: Articulation Functions; b2304: Speech Discrimination; b330: Fluency and Rhythm of Speech Functions; d330: Speaking
Developmental	Interaction among all levels of language processing at a narrative level	Individual and/or small-group sessions	None	b320: Articulation Functions; b2304: Speech Discrimination; b16710: Expression of Spoken Language; d330: Speaking; d140: Learning to Read
Low percentage of correct usage, finiteness, and target morpheme's relationship to child's speech errors	Grammatical morphemes marking tense and agreement plus complex morphophonemic forms (consonant clusters)	Weekly individual and group sessions	None	b320: Articulation Functions; b16710: Expression of Spoken Language

(continued)

Table II.1. *(continued)*

Intervention approach (chapter)	Client age	Primary client populations	Key intervention agents	Key components	Broad goals
Naturalistic intervention for speech intelligibility and speech accuracy (16)	Primarily toddlers and preschoolers	Children with severe SSD; Secondary populations include children with Down syndrome or autism spectrum disorders and children who stutter	Accuracy: SLPs or others trained in the procedure Intelligibility: untrained personnel, including teachers, parents, teachers' aides, and other family members	Recasts of child productions during naturalistic activities	Functional speech intelligibility and speech accuracy
Parents and Children Together (PACT) intervention (17)	Children 3–6 years	Children with delayed and/or disordered speech	SLPs and caregivers	Parent/family education, metalinguistic training, phonetic production training, multiple exemplar training (minimal contrasts therapy and auditory bombardment), homework	Speech perception and production; differentiated production of minimally contrastive words to promote phonological restructuring and intelligible speech
Enhanced milieu teaching with phonological emphasis (EMT/PE) (18)	Not specified	Children with cleft lip and/or palate who have difficulty acquiring vocabulary and speech	Experienced SLPs and parents	Phonetic awareness and phonological recasting	Vocabulary and speech sound production

Basis of target selection	Level of focus	Session type	Technology and/or materials required	Key ICF-CY codes[a]
Intelligibility and accuracy of speech sounds	Intelligibility and accuracy at conversation level	Individual sessions	None	b320: Articulation Functions; d330: Speaking
Developmental error patterns	The phoneme at word level or above to expand a child's consonant, vowel, syllable-shape, syllable-stress, phonotactic, and suprasegmental repertoires and accuracy	Individual sessions	None; however, the Quick Screener and other resources are available online	b320: Articulation Functions; b2304: Speech Discrimination; d350: Conversation
Target words are selected to reflect developmental vocabulary and phonological targets	Word	Individual sessions	None	b320: Articulation Functions; b16710: Expression of Spoken Language

(continued)

Table II.1. *(continued)*

Intervention approach (chapter)	Client age	Primary client populations	Key intervention agents	Key components	Broad goals
PROMPT: A tactually grounded model (19)	Children 2;0 and older	Children with mild-severe articulation, motor speech delay, or speech production disorder affecting execution, planning, fluency, or prosody	PROMPT-certified SLPs with support from family members and peers	Consideration of cognitive-linguistic, social-emotional, and physical-sensory domains; refinement of speech-motor actions through successive shaping	Motor-phonemes and lexicon priorities are selected to work on broad language-based, long-term communication goals
Family-friendly intervention (20)	Children across a wide age range	Children with SSD	SLPs and families	Involvement of parents in intervention via parent-as-therapist, family-centered, and/or family-friendly practices	Increase intelligibility and functional communication

Key: CAPES, Computerized Articulation and Phonology Evaluation System; SAILS, Speech Assessment and Interactive Learning Program; SLP, speech-language pathologist; SSD, speech sound disorders.
[a]Within the ICF-CY, Articulation Functions includes phonological functions.

naturalistic speech intelligibility training can be used with children with Down syndrome or autism spectrum disorders, or with children who stutter. A few of the interventions in Section II are appropriate for anyone. For example, psycholinguistic intervention is designed for "any population that has difficulty with spoken and/or written language."

Key Intervention Agents

For each of the interventions in Section II, a speech-language pathologist (SLP) is required to assess individual children, select the most appropriate intervention, determine intervention targets, identify specific intervention goals, and monitor the progress of the intervention (see Table II.1). PROMPT intervention can only be provided by PROMPT-certified SLPs. However, for the majority of the other approaches, intervention can also be facilitated by input from teachers, parents, assistants, and significant others. A few approaches specify that training is required for these additional personnel. Computer-based approaches use technology to support this training. Both PACT and family-focused interventions specify that family involvement is essential.

Basis of target selection	Level of focus	Session type	Technology and/or materials required	Key ICF-CY codes[a]
Motor-speech control	Motor-phonemes (via auditory-tactual input) and lexicon within the broader linguistic context	Individual sessions	None	b320: Articulation Functions; b176: Mental Function of Sequencing Complex Movements
Various depending on the approach	Various depending on the approach	Individual and/or small-group sessions	None	b320: Articulation Functions; d350 Conversation

Key Components

Key components of the interventions that target speech in Section II depend on their emphasis along the speech and language continuum. Some approaches target speech along the entire speech continuum from perception and storage to production (psycholinguistic intervention), and intervention comprises components from each stage. Some approaches only target one of the components of the speech continuum; for example, perceptual intervention specifically targets speech production via emphasizing speech perception. Many of the approaches within Section II simultaneously target speech and language; in this case key components are vocabulary (EMT/PE), morphology, syntax (morphosyntactic intervention), or discourse (dynamic systems). Interventions that target speech and literacy include phonological awareness components (e.g., metaphonological intervention).

Broad Goals

As with the majority of interventions within this book, the main goal of intervention for children with SSD is to increase intelligibility and communicative competence. Some in-

Table II.2. Number of published research studies pertaining to each level of evidence for speech interventions in broader contexts identified by chapter authors in Section II

Intervention approach (chapter)	Ia: Meta analysis of > 1 randomized controlled trial	Ib: Randomized controlled study	IIa: Controlled study without randomization	IIb: Quasi-experimental study	III: Non-experimental study	IV: Expert report, consensus conference, clinical experience of respected authorities
Psycholinguistic intervention (9)	0	0	0	4	8	9
Metaphonological intervention (10)	1	2	5	1	2	0
Computer-based interventions (11)	0	1	0	3	0	0
Speech perception intervention (12)	0	3	1	0	0	0
Nonlinear phonological intervention (13)	0	0	2	9	4	0
Dynamic systems and whole language intervention (14)	0	2	0	1	2	0
Morphosyntax intervention (15)	0	1	2	2	0	0
Naturalistic intervention for speech intelligibility and speech accuracy (16)	0	5	3	0	6	0
Parents and Children Together (PACT) intervention (17)	0	0	2	0	1	0
Enhanced milieu teaching with phonological emphasis (EMT/PE) (18)	0	0	2	0	1	1
PROMPT: A tactually grounded model (19)	0	0	3	1	1	0
Family-friendly intervention (20)	0	5	1	0	0	0
TOTAL	1	19	21	21	25	10

terventions holistically target intelligibility (e.g., naturalistic speech intelligibility training), whereas other approaches target intelligibility via speech sound production (nonlinear phonological intervention, PACT, PROMPT). For children with co-occurring speech and language impairment, some interventions target both speech and language goals (EMT/PE, morphosyntactic intervention, dynamic systems). An additional and interrelated goal of some interventions is to increase phonological awareness and literacy skills (psycholinguistic intervention, metaphonological intervention) due to the close association between speech production and phonemic awareness (Gillon, 2004).

Basis of Target Selection

Selection of targets for the majority of interventions within Section II typically occurs after a comprehensive speech and language (and literacy) assessment and analysis of assessment results. Strengths and weaknesses are described, and intervention goals are determined. Some intervention approaches use a developmental approach to target selection (e.g., EMT/PE), whereas other approaches use a target selection informed by the mismatch between speech perception and speech production (perceptual intervention) or morphology and speech production (morphosyntactic intervention).

Level of Focus

Many of the interventions in Section II focus on perception or production of phonemes within words and sentences (see Table II.1), for example, psycholinguistic intervention, nonlinear phonological intervention, morphosyntactic intervention, and PACT. Rarely are phonemes targeted outside of the context of the word; for example, sometimes phonetic awareness is taught to children with cleft lip and/or palate during EMT/PE. Often phonemes are targeted within connected speech during narratives or conversation (dynamic systems, naturalistic speech intelligibility training).

Session Type

The majority of interventions that target speech production within a broader context are conducted in individual and/or small-group sessions (see Table II.1). Morphosyntactic intervention specifies weekly individual *and* group sessions. A few intervention approaches are more suited to individual sessions (naturalistic speech intelligibility training, PACT, EMT/PE, PROMPT), with perceptual intervention being delivered in individual computer-based sessions. Many of the interventions are typically conducted more than once per week.

Technology and/or Materials Required

The majority of interventions featured in Section II make little use of technology. Most rely on the interaction between the child and other people, including the SLP. Interventions described in Chapter 11 specifically describe computer-based interventions. In addition, perceptual intervention requires the Speech Assessment and Interactive Learning (SAILS) computer program (AVAAZ Innovations, 1994). A few other interventions have computerized assessment and/or analysis software to facilitate decision making about appropriate intervention targets (e.g., nonlinear intervention, PACT).

Key Codes from the *International Classification of Functioning, Disability and Health for Children and Youth*

The ICF-CY (WHO, 2007) is a holistic framework emphasizing health and well-being for all people. The ICF-CY links Body Structure, Body Function, and Activities and Participation with Environmental Factors and Personal Factors. Table II.1 outlines the ICF-CY codes relating to each of the interventions in Section II. All of the interventions within Section II address Body Functions and Articulation Functions (b320: "Functions of the production of speech sounds"; WHO, 2007, p. 71).

Other aspects of Body Functions addressed by some of the interventions include

- Fluency and Rhythm of Speech Functions (b330: "Functions of the production of flow and tempo of speech"; WHO, 2007, p. 71)

- Speech Discrimination (b2304: "Sensory functions relating to determining spoken language and distinguishing it from other sounds"; WHO, 2007, p. 65)

- Mental Function of Sequencing Complex Movements (b176: "Specific mental functions of sequencing and coordinating complex, purposeful movements"; WHO, 2007, p. 60)

- Expression of Spoken Language (b16710: "Mental functions necessary to produce meaningful spoken messages"; WHO, 2007, p. 59)

Some interventions also emphasize Activities and Participation, specifically

- Learning to Read (d140: "Developing the competence to read written material . . . with fluency and accuracy, such as recognizing characters and alphabets, sounding out written words with correct pronunciation, and understanding words and phrases"; WHO, 2007, p. 134)

- Speaking (d330: "Producing words, phrases and longer passages in spoken messages . . . such as . . . telling a story in oral language"; WHO, 2007, p. 146)

- Conversation (d350: "Starting, sustaining and ending an interchange of thoughts and ideas, carried out by means of spoken. . . . language, with one or more persons one knows or who are strangers, in formal or casual settings"; WHO, 2007, p. 147)

REFERENCES

AVAAZ Innovations. (1994). *Speech assessment and interactive learning system* (Version 1.2). London, Ontario, Canada: Author.

Gillon, G.T. (2004). *Phonological awareness: From research to practice*. New York: Guilford Press.

World Health Organization. (2007). *International classification of functioning, disability and health: Children and youth version*. Geneva: Author.

Psycholinguistic Intervention

Joy Stackhouse and Michelle Pascoe

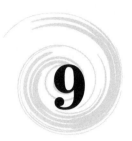

9

ABSTRACT

This chapter illustrates how a psycholinguistic approach can contribute to our understanding of the nature of speech sound disorders (SSDs) in children. It describes the psycholinguistic framework developed by Stackhouse and Wells (1997) and provides examples of how to 1) select investigations and interpret assessment data, 2) use this data for planning intervention and task design, 3) evaluate interventions. Service delivery issues are also raised. The approach is not tied to any particular clinical entity but can be used to develop hypotheses about children's speech and literacy difficulties as a basis for planning appropriate intervention. The principles of the approach can be applied to any age but specifically designed psycholinguistic tasks are most helpful for children older than 4 years of age, and the explicit links made in the framework between speech and literacy development make it ideal for working with school-age children with persisting SSDs. However, the framework is as much a training tool for the user as the client. Psycholinguistic reflection on popular assessment and intervention tasks enables speech-language pathologists (SLPs) and others to question why and how we do what we do and encourages a particular way of thinking about the treatment of children's speech and literacy difficulties.

INTRODUCTION

A psycholinguistic approach involves a particular way of thinking about the theoretical nature of speech sound disorders (SSD), the interpretation of assessment findings, and the planning and evaluation of intervention. It does not stand alone. Information derived from a psycholinguistic perspective needs to be mixed with that from other essential perspectives (e.g., linguistic, medical, educational, psychosocial) to ensure that a comprehensive management program is carried out.

This chapter presents an example of such a psycholinguistic approach. The psycholinguistic framework devised by Stackhouse and Wells (1997) is particularly useful for children with SSDs. Inherent in the design of this framework is that

1. SSDs arise from one or more points in a child's speech processing system comprising speech input, speech output, and storage of linguistic information.

2. Speech processing skills are not only the basis for intelligible speech production but also for phonological awareness and literacy development.

3. Intervention can be carried out individually or in groups by a range of people in various contexts but needs to be managed by an SLP who understands the principles involved.

4. Evaluation and monitoring are built in to the program from the start.

TARGET POPULATIONS

An advantage of the psycholinguistic approach is that it can be used with any age and with any population that has difficulty with spoken and/or written language. Although the administration of psycholinguistic tests is best reserved for school-age children and adults, the approach can still be used with preschool children through other means (e.g., observation, games, qualitative data analysis). Furthermore, the psycholinguistic approach is not tied to a diagnostic label. In fact, it specifically does not treat a diagnostic label; rather it pursues a child's speech processing strengths and weaknesses and uses this information to plan appropriate intervention. This is important given that children with the same diagnosis (e.g., childhood apraxia of speech [CAS], phonological impairment, dyslexia) can present with very different underlying processing strengths and weaknesses (Stackhouse & Snowling, 1992; Williams & Stackhouse, 1998). As a result the approach has been used with children with a wide range of difficulties. These include children with childhood apraxia of speech, phonological impairment, word-finding difficulties, dyslexia, cleft lip and palate, dysfluent speech, Down syndrome, hearing impairment, cerebral palsy, pragmatic difficulties, and acquired language impairment. The framework can also be used to study typical development in its own right (e.g., Vance, Stackhouse, & Wells, 2005) or as a basis for comparison with children with SSD (Stackhouse, Vance, Pascoe, & Wells, 2007).

ASSESSMENT METHODS FOR DETERMINING INTERVENTION RELEVANCE

Psycholinguistic assessment aims to find out exactly where, within a chosen model, a child's speech processing skills are breaking down, and how this might be affecting his or her speech, lexical, and literacy development. Such an assessment aims to identify two important components of a child's speech production difficulties. First, the "psycho-" aspect *uncovers* what is underlying a child's speech sound production difficulties. This includes tasks of speech input (e.g., auditory discrimination), speech output (e.g., naming, repetition), and lexical representation (e.g., mispronunciation detection tasks to check if there are clear or fuzzy representations of a target word in the word store). This information is essential for deciding what modalities and strategies to use in intervention. Second, the "-linguistic" aspect aims to *describe* a child's speech output using tools derived from phonetics and phonology. The aim is to present a child's phonetic repertoire and show how segments are used phonologically in syllables, words, and connected speech. This aspect does not explain why a child is making speech errors, but it is essential for knowing what segments, contrasts, and linguistic levels to target in intervention (i.e., what stimuli to design). Thus, combining these components examines the relationship between the two (e.g., Is a speech output error arising from a problem with auditory processing, or lexical storage, or articulatory skill, or a combination of all three?) and tells the practitioner *what* to target and *how* to work on those targets.

No specific or new assessment materials are needed to carry out a psycholinguistic assessment. This is because a psycholinguistic approach is a way of interpreting results from observations of behavior or from popular assessments. According to Stackhouse and Wells, it is "in the head of the user and not in a case of tests" (1997, p. 48).

For example, whatever test or speech assessment procedure you use to gather speech output data, it can be analyzed in a way to identify if the child is using a full phonetic range of segments for his or her language, how the child is contrasting these segments, if simplifying processes are being used, and if there are syllable or word boundary features that need to be targeted. Similarly, any test of auditory discrimination will identify some aspect of speech input skills. However, adopting a systematic approach to this investigation can ensure that important areas are not missed. To facilitate this, a *Compendium of Auditory and Speech Tasks* (Stackhouse et al., 2007) has been developed, which presents 30 tasks that can be used to identify a child's speech processing strengths and weaknesses. The compendium includes investigations of connected speech and formats for the practitioner and researcher to design assessments for investigating the origins of specific speech errors in individual children. Normative data from children between the ages of 4 and 7 years is provided for guidelines. The procedures include

Speech Input: Auditory discrimination of simple and complex real words and nonwords, words with and without clusters, and words in connected speech

Lexical Representations: Mispronunciation detection with and without pictures in words and connected speech; detection of legal (an acceptable word structure in English; e.g., *blick*) versus illegal (a nonpermissible word structure in English; e.g., *bnick*) nonwords

Speech Output: Naming; repetition of real and nonwords; connected speech; self-correction; speech rate, accuracy, and consistency on diadochokinetic tasks

Not all of these assessments need to be carried out to plan an intervention program—far from it; this is not recommended at all. In many cases no tests are done, but a child's behavior is interpreted psycholinguistically. This captures the essence of the psycholinguistic approach: It is a particular way of thinking about data collected rather than a prescribed battery of tests to administer and score.

Believing that a psycholinguistic assessment requires a lot of time and tests is missing the point of the approach. A comprehensive profile of a child's speech processing skills is not needed before starting therapy; this would be unrealistic in a busy practice where time might be limited to a set number of sessions per child. Indeed, hypotheses about a child's level(s) of difficulty are often best tested through therapy tasks rather than further assessments. Even better, sometimes a child will tell you where his or her level of difficulty is (e.g., Stackhouse et al., 2007, p. 126).

Assessment Principles

When using specific tasks to test out hypotheses about a child's SSDs, the following principles should be taken into account:

1. *No single task will answer your psycholinguistic questions.* Always try and administer a pair of investigations for comparison close in time.

2. *Include a task of nonword processing in any investigation* (e.g., auditory discrimination of nonwords or repetition of nonwords). This will reveal a child's ability to

deal with new words, because all real words are nonwords until a child learns their meanings. Dealing with new words is an essential skill for any child at school and home. Children with SSDs can have significant auditory discrimination difficulties on unfamiliar material (tested by using nonwords) but not necessarily on words that are familiar to them (Bridgeman & Snowling, 1988).

3. *Include an investigation of phonological awareness* at the appropriate level for the age of the child as another measure of a child's speech processing skills. It is a premise of the psycholinguistic approach that phonological awareness is a product of the speech processing system and not a separate entity as often presented. Thus, developing phonological awareness requires a child to have an intact speech processing system that allows them to listen, discriminate, access stored information, and produce appropriate utterances. Linking this with the first principle listed, a pair of matched phonological awareness tasks should be administered. For example, it is important to administer both an input and output rhyme task to differentiate those children who cannot perform rhyme tasks at all from those who can perform "silent" input rhyme tasks (e.g., pointing to pictures that rhyme), thus demonstrating they have a concept of rhyme, but cannot produce rhyme on output tasks (e.g., tell me as many words as you can that rhyme with *cat*) because of their speech difficulties.

4. *Collate the results from tasks and observations onto a single speech processing profile.* This records a child's input, output, representation, and phonological awareness performance (i.e., these areas are not treated as separate entities but examined together in a summary of a child's speech processing strengths and weaknesses). This profile forms the basis for planning and evaluating intervention.

5. *Do not plan intervention on psycholinguistic data alone.* It is also important to take on other perspectives. Collecting information about a child's developmental history, medical circumstances, educational performance, psychosocial development, and family background are all equally important in determining the nature of the child's SSDs and the subsequent intervention package. (See Stackhouse et al., 2007, for questionnaire formats.)

THEORETICAL BASIS

Dominant Theoretical Rationale for the Intervention Approach

A psycholinguistic approach explores how a child receives different types of information (e.g., spoken or written utterances), remembers and stores it within *lexical representations* (information about words) within the *lexicon* (a store of words), and how he or she selects and produces spoken and written words. Figure 9.1 illustrates the basic structure of a psycholinguistic model of speech processing.

On the left of the figure there is a channel for the auditory input of information via the ear and on the right a channel for the spoken output of information through the mouth. If we want to represent written language explicitly in this model an eye can be added to the input channel by the side of the ear to receive printed information and a hand to the output side of the model by the side of the mouth to mark writing or signing. However, both eye and hand will still be connected by a channel to the same word store

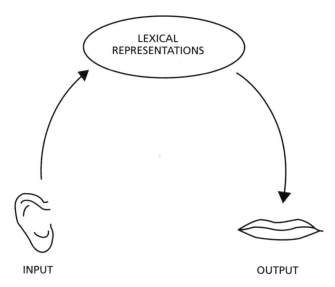

Figure 9.1. The basic structure of the speech processing system. (From Stackhouse, J., & Wells, B. [1997]. *Children's speech and literacy difficulties: Book 1. A psycholinguistic framework* [p. 9]. Chichester, England: Wiley; reproduced by permission of John Wiley & Sons Limited.)

at the top of the model as the ear and the mouth. The top is where the lexical representations of previously processed information are stored. Thinking about what you know about the word *cat* will reveal what type of information is stored in the lexical representations. For example

1. *Semantic representation*—information about what the word means, the attributes of the word, and what category it is in (e.g., a *cat* is a domestic or wild animal with fur and whiskers that makes a distinctive sound)

2. *Phonological representation*—information about how the word sounds, allowing for discrimination of the target word from other similar words (e.g., *cat:cap; cat:pat*)

3. *Motor program*—a stored set of instructions for how to say the word automatically (i.e., the pronunciation of the word *cat*)

4. *Grammatical representation*—information about the class of word (e.g., noun), how it can be used in a sentence, and whether there is a plural form that can be derived from a rule (e.g., *one cat, two cats*)

5. *Orthographic representation*—information about what the word looks like in its written form, thus enabling automatic recognition when reading the word *cat*.

Although this seems very straightforward for skilled adults told to think about a word such as *cat*, it is not necessarily so for children with speech and literacy difficulties. For example, children with SSDs may not be able to discriminate between minimal pair words such as *cat:cap* and will therefore store fuzzy representations for those lexical items in their word store. As this is an important basis not only for the motor program for speaking the word but also for spontaneous spelling, fuzzy representations have been suggested as a major contributing factor to children's speech and literacy difficulties (see Snowling, 2006, for a review). However, not all speech difficulties can be explained by a top-down speech processing difficulty like this. Some children have more difficulty with lower level articulatory production of sounds that affects not only their speech but also 1) their rehearsal of new words prior to storing them, and 2) their reflection on the structure of words prior to spelling them—more of a bottom-up speech processing difficulty. Children with persisting speech difficulties (beyond the age of 5 years) typically have both pervasive top-down and bottom-up speech processing difficulties; hence the strong association among speech, phonological awareness, and literacy difficulties.

Levels of Consequences Being Addressed

A number of models use the same basic structure of input/output and representations as depicted in Figure 9.1 (e.g., Chiat, 2000; Dodd, 1995/2005; Hewlett, Gibbon, & Cohen-McKenzie, 1998; Stackhouse & Wells, 1997). Although different in their presentations, these models share the premises that children's speech development is dependent on the normal functioning of this system and that children's speech difficulties arise at one or more points in a faulty speech processing system. (See Baker, Croot, McLeod, & Paul, 2001 for a review of psycholinguistic models.) The psycholinguistic framework developed by Stackhouse and Wells attempts to explain the origins of speech sound production errors and to incorporate the link between speech production skills and phonological awareness and literacy development. It comprises three components

1. Speech processing profile

2. Box-and-arrow model of speech processing

3. Developmental phase model

Speech Processing Profile

The speech processing profile is based on the simple speech processing model in Figure 9.1. It provides a structure for organizing information about a child's speech processing skills by posing questions to be addressed in order to understand the nature of a child's SSDs and arrive at a greater understanding of the intervention needs (see Figure 9.2). The left-hand side of the profile focuses on input skills; the right-hand side focuses on output skills. Information on the top half of the sheet involves some kind of top-down processing.

The speech processing profile allows space to indicate a child's performance at each level. This may be in the form of ticks or checkmarks for age-appropriate performance or above, and Xs for performance that is less than age appropriate. When the child's performance can be compared with normative data, the degree of severity can be marked in terms of distance from the mean by standard deviation (*SD*). For example, one X would indicate 1 *SD* below the mean, 2 Xs would indicate 2 *SD* below the mean, and so forth. When normative data is not available, a more subjective indication of degree can be given.

A Box-and-Arrow Model of Speech Processing

The conventional way of representing levels of processing and routes between them is through an information-processing model in the form of boxes (levels of processing) and arrows (flow of information). Figure 9.3 presents the box-and-arrow model of speech

SPEECH PROCESSING PROFILE

Name: _____   Comments: _____

Age: _____   DOB: _____   _____

Date: _____   _____

Profiler: _____   _____

INPUT	OUTPUT
F Is the child aware of the internal structure of phonological representations?	**G** Can the child access accurate motor programs?
E Are the child's phonological representations accurate?	**H** Can the child manipulate phonological units?
D Can the child discriminate between real words?	**I** Can the child articulate real words accurately?
C Does the child have language-specific representations of word structures?	**J** Can the child articulate speech without reference to lexical representations?
B Can the child discriminate speech sounds without reference to lexical representations?	**K** Does the child have adequate sound production skills?
A Does the child have adequate auditory perception?	

L Does the child reject his/her own erroneous forms?

Figure 9.2. Questions on the Speech Processing Profile. (From Stackhouse, J., & Wells, B. [1997]. *Children's speech and literacy difficulties: Book 1. A psycholinguistic framework* [p. 348]. Chichester, England: Wiley; reproduced by permission of John Wiley & Sons Limited.)

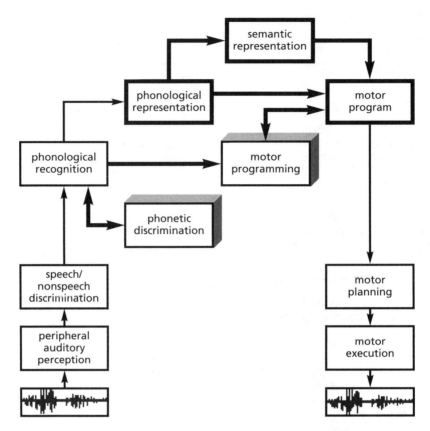

Figure 9.3. The box-and-arrow model from Stackhouse and Wells (1997). (From Stackhouse, J., & Wells, B. [1997]. *Children's speech and literacy difficulties: Book 1. A psycholinguistic framework* [p. 350]. Chichester, England: Wiley; reproduced by permission of John Wiley & Sons Limited.)

processing from Stackhouse and Wells (1997). It is also based on the simple model in Figure 9.1 (input on the left, output on the right, and storage at the top) but attempts to fill in the gaps between the ear and the mouth. Plain boxes represent levels of processing, boxes in bold represent stored knowledge, and shaded boxes represent offline processing. Arrows show the route of processing of spoken material, and the broad arrows show how information flows among boxes as part of the learning process (see Stackhouse et al., 2007, pp. 17–18, for a summary of the components of this model, and Stackhouse and Wells, 1997, for further discussion).

Such a model allows us to be more explicit about the levels of processing and processing routes that our assessment and intervention tasks are tapping. For example, tracking the route a specific task takes through this model illuminates the demands being made on the child and where any difficulties might be (see Stackhouse & Wells, 1997, pp. 173–187). Figure 9.4 compares the routes of three common speech tasks: word repetition, nonword repetition, and naming. When a child is asked to repeat a familiar word he or she has to hear the word and recognize it as a spoken legal word for the relevant language spoken. Because it is a familiar word, a stored phonological representation exists that allows the child to detect the target from similarly sounding words and then access a stored motor program for automatic production of that word. If the stored information

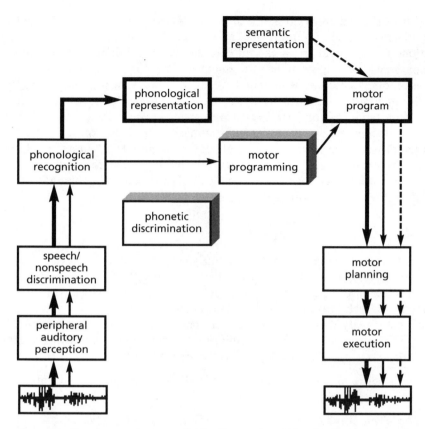

Figure 9.4. Speech processing routes for familiar word repetition, legal nonword repetition, and naming familiar pictures. *Key:* bold arrow, familiar word repetition; fine arrow, legal nonword repetition; dashed arrow, naming of familiar pictures.

is accurate and if the flow of information between each box is unimpaired, then the child will produce the word correctly. Consider how the route for naming a picture of a familiar word would be different from the route for repeating that word. This time there is no auditory input of the target as it is not presented verbally. Therefore, the child has to identify the target via the visual system (i.e., via the eye rather than the ear). As there is no direct link between the eye and what a word sounds like, the child has to access the semantic representation of the target (to know what it is) in order to access the stored motor program in order to say the word. Comparing a child's performance on real word repetition versus naming will therefore reveal if the child can perform both tasks perfectly well as in typical development (Vance et al., 2005), or if there is a specific difficulty with 1) input skills (if performance is poorer on repetition than naming), or 2) with lexical representations and retrieval (if performance is poorer on naming than repetition). Now, consider how the processing routes for legal nonword repetition might differ from real word repetition. The child hears the legal nonword (e.g., *blick*) but because it is new there is no stored information about it in terms of its meaning and phonology. As the child has never had to say the word before, there is no ready-made motor program to pronounce it either. The child therefore needs to activate motor programming skills to assemble the components of this new word in order to devise a new motor program that will instruct the articulators in how to pronounce it.

This exercise allows the practitioner/researcher to understand what is in a task is essential information for interpreting assessment results and designing appropriate intervention. The box-and-arrow model can also be used for recording points of difficulty compared with strengths in the processing system. For example, Waters (2001) presented the psycholinguistic assessment and management of Alan, a 5-year-old boy with a "severe developmental speech disorder in the absence of any identifiable causative factors and significant family history" (p. 165). Alan's speech processing performance is interpreted through the box-and-arrow model and summarized by using checkmarks (✓) for strengths and Xs for weaknesses on the model itself (see Figure 9.5). Waters concluded that Alan's internal representations were accurate, but that he had an inability to devise motor programs to reproduce either stored phonological representations or auditorily presented familiar or novel combinations of phonemes.

Developmental Phase Model

One criticism of using box-and-arrow models with children has been the failure to account for developmental change (Stackhouse & Wells, 1996). Thus, a developmental phase model is the third component of the psycholinguistic framework. This phase model summarizes research into the speech development of typically developing children and can be linked directly with phase models of children's literacy development (Stackhouse & Wells, 1997). It is particularly helpful in understanding both typical and atypical speech sound development. The developmental phase model comprises the following five phases:

1. *The Prelexical Phase* includes the pre–first words phase up to about 1 year of age (babbling period).

2. *The Whole Word Phase* captures the learning of first words as gestalts, up to about 2 years of age. Speech production has a limited sound and syllable structure repertoire and is typically inconsistent in this phase.

3. *The Systematic Simplification Phase* is characterized by the emergence of simplifying processes (e.g., fronting, stopping, cluster reduction) in speech output between the ages of 2;6 and 4;0. Speech is typically consistent in this phase.

4. *The Assembly Phase* describes the mastering of connected speech production at about 3–4 years of age. (See Newton & Wells, 1999, 2002, for further information about connected speech development, and see Stackhouse et al., 2007, for assessment procedures.)

5. *The Metaphonological Phase* relates to the breakthrough to phonological awareness by about 5 years of age. This phase builds on consistent speech production developed in the systematic simplification phase, which is necessary for the child to reflect on the structure of the word (e.g., what segment is at the beginning or end of a word).

It is proposed that typically developing children move through these phases smoothly and, as a consequence, develop the skills necessary for intelligible speech, phonological awareness, and literacy. In contrast, children with speech difficulties have trouble at one or more of these phases. Furthermore, the precise nature of their speech difficulties will depend on which particular phase (or phases) is troublesome for them. Children stuck at the whole word phase, who are not yet using phonological simplifying processes, present with inconsistent speech typical of CAS. Children with persisting phonological simplify-

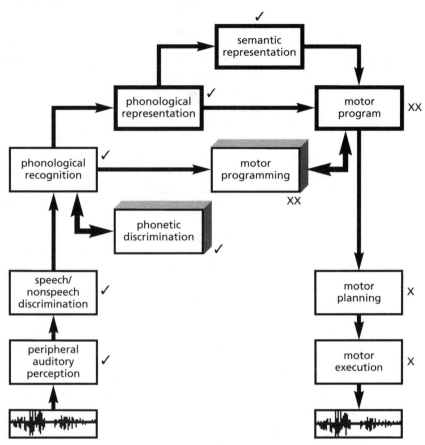

Figure 9.5. Speech processing model indicating Alan's strengths and weaknesses at age 5 years. (From Stackhouse, J., & Wells, B. [Eds.]. [2001]. *Children's speech and literacy difficulties: Book 2. Identification and intervention.* Chichester, England: Wiley; adapted from Figure 6.3, with permission of John Wiley & Sons Limited.)

ing processes are slower moving through the systematic simplification phase and may be described as having a phonological delay or impairment. A delay in moving on from the systematic simplification phase, in particular, affects the development of connected speech production (in the assembly phase) and phonological awareness, thus putting the child at risk for literacy problems. Children who have not moved through these five phases by the time they are 5;6 are seriously at risk for developing associated literacy problems (Bishop & Adams, 1990; Nathan, Stackhouse, Goulandris, & Snowling, 2004a).

The developmental phase model can also help conceptualize popular therapy approaches. For example the recommended core vocabulary approach for children with inconsistent speech production (see Chapter 5) targets whole-word production. It aims to stabilize the consistency of a child's speech production so that specific segments can be targeted in intervention if/as needed. This can be construed as moving the child through normal developmental phases: from the whole word to the systematic simplification process phase. Children who remain in the systematic simplification phase for longer than they should present with phonological delay, characterized by the persisting but consistent use of normal simplification processes, (e.g., fronting, stopping). Therapy for such children typically targets reducing the occurrence of simplifying processes in order to move the child on from the systematic simplification phase to intelligible connected speech (in the assembly phase) and to phonological awareness. In this metaphonological phase, children's previously tacit awareness of their speech sound production becomes more explicit. Children with difficulties at this phase of development may find it hard to self-correct their speech sound errors and to generalize skills learned in intervention tasks to new items and contexts. As explicit sound awareness is also necessary to understand the link between speech sounds and letters when reading and spelling, children stuck at this stage will also exhibit literacy difficulties. Children with persisting and complex SSDs struggle at each of these phases of development and may show features from more than one of them. For example, Jarrod, a 7-year-old boy with persisting speech difficulties, had inconsistent production of multisyllabic words, consistent but immature production of simple words, delayed phonological awareness, and literacy difficulties (Stackhouse, Pascoe, & Gardner, 2006).

This phase model does not explain why a child might be stuck at a particular phase or not progressing as quickly as he or she should; for that we need the information from the speech processing profile and/or box-and-arrow model discussed previously. However, it does enable a developmental perspective to be taken on a child's SSDs and a charting of any progress made in intervention to be based on the dominant speech production characteristics.

Target Areas of Intervention

Information derived from these three components of the psycholinguistic framework ensures that intervention is based on a child's strengths and is targeted appropriately. Intervention may target a child's speech output specifically but rarely does so in isolation. More often than not, it also includes other domains such as speech input and/or literacy, either because these need to be improved or because they are a strength that can be utilized.

EMPIRICAL BASIS

Summary of Levels of Evidence

The empirical basis for a psycholinguistic approach to intervention can be divided into two main groups of studies: 1) single case investigations of effectiveness, and 2) exploratory studies of potential treatment (see Table 9.1). Psycholinguistic intervention has been effective with children with language difficulties (e.g., Norbury & Chiat, 2000; Spooner, 2002; Stiegler & Hoffman, 2001), literacy difficulties (Broom & Doctor, 1995), and auditory processing difficulties (Crosbie & Dodd, 2001; Vance, 1997). However, this section focuses specifically on examples of studies that have used psycholinguistic interventions for children with SSDs.

Single Case Investigations of Effectiveness

Bryan and Howard (1992) carried out a detailed early single case study of psycholinguistic intervention for DF, a 5-year-old boy with "very deviant speech production" (p. 343). DF's speech processing difficulties were investigated through a series of psycholinguisti-

Table 9.1. Levels of evidence for studies of treatment efficacy for psycholinguistic intervention for speech sound difficulties

Level	Description	References
Ia	Meta-analysis of > 1 randomized controlled trial	—
Ib	Randomized controlled study	—
IIa	Controlled study without randomization	—
IIb	Quasi-experimental study	Bryan & Howard, 1992; Pascoe et al., 2005, 2006; Waters et al., 1998
III	Nonexperimental studies, i.e., correlational and case studies	Corrin, 2001a, 2001b; Crosbie & Dodd, 2001; Dent, 2001; Nathan & Simpson, 2001; Nathan et al., 2004a; Rees, 2008a; Stackhouse & Wells, 1993; Vance, 1997; Waters, 2001
IV	Expert committee report, consensus conference, clinical experience of respected authorities	Constable, 2001; Popple & Wellington, 1996, 2001; Rees, 2001; Stackhouse, 1992, 1993; Stackhouse, Pascoe, & Gardner, 2006; Stackhouse & Wells, 1997

Adapted from the Scottish Intercollegiate Guidelines Network (http://www.sign.ac.uk).

cally motivated tasks and interpreted in the light of models of speech and language processing (Smith, 1978; Spencer, 1988). The findings from these and from a phonological analysis of the child's surface speech errors were used to inform intervention planning. DF's speech production was better for nonwords (i.e., new words) compared with familiar ones, suggesting that he kept "frozen forms" of familiar words in his representations, perhaps from an earlier phase of development. The authors describe how phonological input tasks (e.g., same/different judgments) were used to update DF's underlying phonological representations. Outcome measures were single-word naming of pictures and repetition of single real words. There was significant improvement in both speech production and auditory discrimination skills.

Waters et al. (1998) also emphasized the need to integrate psycholinguistic information with phonological information in their account of intervention for Alan, a 5-year-old boy with unintelligible speech, who was introduced earlier in this chapter (see Figure 9.5). Through adopting the psycholinguistic framework, Waters et al. hypothesized that intervention should not focus directly on Alan's speech production difficulties but should exploit his strengths in input processing to help him discover how to modify his pronunciation patterns. By 6 years of age, there was significant improvement on both of the outcome measures: single-word picture naming and spontaneous speech. This study also highlighted the importance of other factors to take into account when planning intervention, such as children's attitudes, behaviors, and preferred learning styles.

Pascoe, Stackhouse, and Wells (2005) described a single-subject research design that was used with Katy, a girl age 6;5 with mild ataxic cerebral palsy and unintelligible speech. The psycholinguistic framework was used to guide the assessment process, develop hypotheses about the nature of Katy's difficulties, and understand the changes that arose as a result of intervention. Katy was in her second year at school and had significant SSDs (e.g., only 22% of her consonants were correct in a speech sample). Pre- and post- intervention assessments were carried out, focusing on two levels: 1) investigations of her phonetic, phonological, and speech processing skills (macro level); and 2) focus on targets in intervention and the matched control stimuli (micro level).

The macro assessment revealed that Katy had specific difficulties on the output side of the speech processing model, specifically with retrieval of stored motor programs, creation of online motor programs, and motor planning. Developmentally she had speech characteristics of the whole-word phase (e.g., simple CV syllable structures were a feature of her speech production). Expanding her syllable structures to include CVC would enable her to make a much greater range of lexical contrasts and facilitate her moving on to the systematic simplification stage. The intervention program therefore aimed to encourage Katy to produce exemplars of the CVC frame. Initially, any CVC attempt to produce a target word was accepted; for example, *goal* or *goad* or *goat* for the target word *goat* was acceptable but *go* was not. Stricter criteria were then applied as she became more comfortable with producing CVC structures, so that gradually only the correct production of *goat* was deemed to be correct.

A range of therapy approaches were used with Katy to achieve the goals (e.g., maximal and minimal pair therapy); whole-word phonological therapy (Velleman, 2002); and materials from the Nuffield Centre Dyspraxia Programme were particularly helpful (Williams & Stephens, 2004; see Chapter 7). Katy's relative strengths were incorporated into the therapy tasks to support her speech production. For example, meaningful stimuli were used in minimal contrast work, and auditory tasks were supported by pictures and written words. Katy received two sessions of therapy per week at her school for 15 weeks, a total of 30 hours in all. Intervention was divided into three phases that targeted the following:

1. A specific set of single words

2. A wider range of single words

3. Words in connected speech

The outcome measures chosen were Katy's speech production in single words and connected speech, auditory discrimination, and spelling abilities. The three phases of intervention significantly improved Katy's production of final consonants in single words. Furthermore, significant gains were made on percentage of consonants correct from pre- to postintervention. However, the significant improvement in her speech production of single CVC words did not generalize spontaneously to her connected speech following the first two phases of therapy. It was only following the third phase of the intervention, in which connected speech was targeted specifically through phonetically controlled sentences, that there was a significant main effect for intervention. The incidence of phonological simplifications in her speech also showed changes, with final consonant deletion, the process specifically addressed in intervention, showing the most significant change: reduced from 96% to 54%. These changes were maintained at follow up 7 months after intervention had ceased. Phonological analyses revealed that Katy had expanded her word-final phonetic inventory following intervention but that she was still not using a complete range of segments to realize appropriate contrasts.

Katy's intervention for CVC words was also reinforced in real communication contexts in which she was encouraged to speak with more confidence. As a result, she was perceived as being more intelligible by her family and teachers. Pascoe et al. (2006) presented in detail five other cases of children with persisting SSDs and demonstrated how targeted intervention can significantly improve children's speech sound production, clusters, connected speech, and literacy performance.

Exploratory Studies of Potential Treatment

In order to inform service delivery, Nathan et al. (2004a) used the psycholinguistic framework in a 4-year longitudinal study to discover predictors of speech and literacy outcome in children with SSD. Single case studies have also explored the nature of children's speech sound production difficulties and the relationship between these and literacy difficulties. Some of these studies offer suggestions for treatment and discuss the clinical and educational implications of the child's speech difficulties without systematically presenting or evaluating the intervention, because this was not the aim of the study.

Stackhouse and Wells (1993, 1997) describe the speech and literacy development of Zoe, a girl with significant SSDs, from the age of 2;10 to the age of 9;8. At the age of 5;11, psycholinguistic assessment revealed that her difficulties in making voiced/voiceless contrasts in her speech production were also evident in her spelling productions, and both were arising from problems on the input side and top of the model in Figure 9.1 (i.e., auditory discrimination difficulties and fuzzy phonological representations of these contrasts). Other aspects of her speech sound production difficulties were arising on the output side of the model, (e.g., her articulatory difficulty with producing clusters). Zoe's case study was important in highlighting that 1) there is not necessarily a single underlying cause of a child's SSD; 2) there can be a direct relationship between a child's SSDs and spelling errors; and 3) intervention should address not only the surface pattern of speech simplification but also the source of the individual types of speech errors, in speech processing terms. Intervention for Zoe at this time included

1. Auditory work on voice/voiceless contrasts (e.g., *pin:bin*) with visual support to strengthen phonological recognition and representation

2. Self-monitoring of her phonological retrieval errors and strengthening of her motor programs for words

3. Articulation of postalveolar fricatives and affricates

4. Phonological awareness activities at the syllable level (e.g., syllable segmentation and rhyme) directed primarily at the levels of phonological recognition and motor programming

5. New word learning activities to develop motor programming of unfamiliar multisyllabic words

6. Connected speech practice focusing on the junction between words

7. Breathing and voice production exercises to improve control, intonation, and phrasing of connected speech

At 9 years of age Zoe was not considered by her teachers and parents to have any speech difficulties. She was perfectly intelligible but still produced "jerky" speech across some syllables within words and between word boundaries in connected speech. Although no longer receiving regular intervention for her speech, she was receiving support at school for her literacy difficulties. A psycholinguistic investigation at 9;8 revealed that her underlying speech processing skills, as recorded on her speech processing profile, remained almost the same as at 5;11. Zoe's difficulties with nonword repetition tasks in particular suggested persisting motor programming difficulties that meant that she could not learn or pronounce new words as quickly as her peers. Phonological awareness skills had improved but were still not sufficiently strong to support her literacy development, particularly when speech output was involved. Spelling in particular remained a problem and still had traces of earlier speech difficulties (e.g., transcription errors on voice/voiceless contrasts and clusters).

PRACTICAL REQUIREMENTS

Nature of Sessions

The psycholinguistic framework presented in this chapter has been used flexibly in a range of contexts and can be adapted to meet the needs of individual children and their circumstances. It enables the user to understand the nature of a child's difficulties, the impact it is likely to have at home and school, and what is needed in an intervention program. However, it does not prescribe how such a service is delivered.

Individual Versus Group Therapy

Although some individual contact can be helpful when investigating a child's speech processing skills or if a child feels reticent in front of other children, it is not necessarily the best format for delivering intervention. There are many advantages to working with a pair of children or with a group, particularly when trying to practice taught skills and generalize training. For example, in the second phase of Katy's intervention (at chronological age [CA] = 6;5), described previously, when the focus was final consonants in a larger set of words, she was joined by another girl, Rachel (CA = 7;1), who also had SSD. Each session was structured around a theme (e.g., household items, holidays, animals). One activity involved Katy being the teacher (which she greatly enjoyed), with Rachel and the SLP playing the children in Katy's class. The task was for Katy to ask Rachel and the SLP to write down the names of target words that were within her speech production capabilities but not being used spontaneously. Katy had a set of picture cards representing these targets that she had to name (while keeping the picture concealed) for Rachel and the SLP to spell. This led to confusion if Katy did not pronounce the word correctly. Rachel on several occasions spontaneously asked for clarification from Katy (e.g., "Katy, is it *car* or *card* or *cart* we must write?").

Rachel's presence meant that Katy was obliged to repeat what she had said and make clear the target item to which she referred. This highlighted for Katy the communicative importance of the final consonants of words in a naturalistic way. This seemed more useful than earlier sessions when Katy was on her own and was less motivated to make repairs to her productions because she knew the SLP knew what she was saying given that the SLP had prepared the materials in the first place.

Personnel

Intervention based on psycholinguistic principles may need to be designed by an SLP but can be delivered by assistants or parents, either to individual children or to groups. However, these assistants need to be trained in the basic principles of the approach. The simple speech processing model presented in Figure 9.1 has been useful for this when explaining how children develop their speech skills, where a child might/might not be having difficulties, and what is involved in listening and speaking tasks to be practiced at home or at school. One father, for example, felt the explanation of the relationship between speech and literacy difficulties in children with dyslexia really made sense to him when it was related to a speech processing model because he was already familiar with computer models. Similarly, school-age children themselves can be interested in similar explanations, and many older children have terrific insights into their speech and literacy difficulties (Stackhouse, 1992). In fact, one of the strengths of the psycholinguistic framework is how it has provided a means of communication between professionals and their clients and caregivers.

However, training does not stop at the psycholinguistic principles derived from a two-dimensional model. Even the best designed tasks will not be successful if the interaction between the speaker and listener is not handled appropriately. Perhaps, along with their phonetics training, the way SLPs handle mispronunciations in intervention and in spontaneous conversation is what makes them unique. Such a skill is not automatically present in parents of children with SSDs (Gardner, 2004) or in assistants/teachers (Ridley, Radford, & Mahon, 2002). Gardner (2006) devised a training program to promote these interaction skills in assistants (e.g., classroom assistants, SLP assistants, student practitioners, parents) working with children with SSDs. Two aspects of interaction that form an important part of intervention are

1. Giving the child precise information about the target behavior

2. Moving the child toward self-correction

Both of these are central to delivering psycholinguistic-based intervention. How tasks should be presented is part of task design, and the development (or not) of self-correction is an important marker of progress. Level L on the speech processing profile in Figure 9.2 focuses on a child's self-monitoring and self-correction abilities. It aims to

1. Investigate children's ability to correct their own speech errors at the time they are made

2. Investigate a child's self-correction strategies on specific targets

3. Measure consistency of self-correction strategies

4. Establish a preintervention baseline of self-correction for comparison with postintervention

Training to do the steps described involves monitoring if and how the child self-corrects (e.g., on specific target words). The following questions can be used to facilitate this:

1. Is there spontaneous speech correction indicating not only self-monitoring skills but also an ability to change speech production?

2. Are there spontaneous attempts at speech correction but these are not always successful because of difficulties elsewhere noted on the speech processing profile?

3. Is any change to speech output only in response to the listener misunderstanding the child's speech output?

4. Can the child change their speech output only if directed to do so in therapy or a teaching situation?

5. Is there a difference between self-correction of single words and of connected speech?

6. Is there a mixture of responses? Is this related to the targets (e.g., certain sounds, position in words, lexical items, grammatical structures, and/or to the speaker-listener contexts; e.g., child with therapist/parent/sibling/friends/a group)?

(Stackhouse et al., 2007, p. 126; reproduced by permission of John Wiley & Sons Limited)

Training also involves what to do in order to promote self-correction and, most important, what is an acceptable response. For example, children may be rewarded for self-correcting because they have moved from item 3 to item 2 above, that is, they are now attempting to self-correct spontaneously, showing self-monitoring and awareness of speech output errors, but cannot yet get an accurate production.

In summary, the psycholinguistic framework can be used to demonstrate basic principles of speech processing in a very simple way to a range of professionals and caregivers as well as to the children themselves. A major strength is its effectiveness in training others and facilitating communication among the range of people involved with a child with SSDs (Popple & Wellington, 2001).

Dosage

The frequency and length of sessions varies across services (Lindsay, Dockrell, Letchford, & Mackie, 2002; Stackhouse et al., 2007) and may be determined more by time and resource constraints (Law & Conti-Ramsden, 2000) than research findings (Joffe & Pring, 2008). Ideally, however, the age of the child and the nature of his or her difficulties will determine the type and frequency of service delivery. For example, children with SSD normally benefit most from direct and intensive work that is managed by a speech specialist even if not delivered on a regular basis by that specialist. Data from the National Outcomes Measurement System (NOMS) organized by the American Speech-Language-Hearing Association (ASHA) revealed that 83.6% of children with severe SSD require more than 17 hours of treatment. The five children between ages 5;6 and 9;0 with severe and persisting speech difficulties presented by Pascoe et al. (2006) all received tailor-made one-to-one intervention that took place on a twice-weekly basis, for approximately 1 hour per session with a specialist SLP over the course of a school year. All made significant gains in their speech input and output processing and with their literacy. However, intensive intervention is costly and further research is needed into alternative methods of intensive delivery. Computer-based interventions can be useful in ensuring cost-effective intensive practice of relevant skills. The psycholinguistic framework has been used as a theoretical basis for a software application addressing *input* aspects of the model (Wren & Roulstone, 2001), and there is further scope for development of this mode of delivery (see Chapter 11).

KEY COMPONENTS

Moving from assessment to intervention is often the most daunting part of adopting a psycholinguistic framework in practice. However, by following simple principles and addressing prescribed questions, it can be a rewarding and fascinating journey (Corrin, 2001a, 2001b).

Nature of Goals

A basic principle when planning intervention within a psycholinguistic framework is that identifying a child's speech processing strengths is as important as discovering their weaknesses. A second principle is the setting of achievable and measurable aims.

Rees (2001a) outlined both long-term and short-term aims when planning intervention from a psycholinguistic perspective. Long-term aims are concerned with functional communication and are often quite general (e.g., to improve intelligibility or communicative competence in social situations). Short-term aims are more specific and should be based on hypotheses derived from a speech processing profile for an individual child, be integrated with aims and objectives set by other professionals, specify targets to be achieved in a given time, and be measurable.

Goal Attack Strategies

Rees (2001a) suggested the following principles for setting short-term intervention goals:

Work on the speech processing system as a whole: If targeting a weak aspect of the model (e.g., auditory discrimination of a specific contrast) then use lower-level articulatory skill if present for the child to feel the difference in sound production and match this with the auditory image received. Simultaneous feeling and hearing of targets is emphasized by Hodson and Paden (1991).

Strengthen links in the lexicon: Intervention should target the links among the different forms of representations at the top of the model (i.e., semantic, phonological, grammatical, orthographic, motor program). Meaningful minimal contrast therapy (e.g., Weiner, 1981) can be effective at doing this if the child has the prerequisite skills; that is, if the child has auditory discrimination of the contrasting sounds and sufficient articulatory skill to produce them. The Nuffield Centre Dyspraxia Programme (Williams & Stephens, 2004) is an excellent resource for working on the skills necessary to do this (see Chapter 7).

Familiarize: A child may need time to just listen to contrasting sounds without having to make any decisions about them as a prerequisite for more active auditory discrimination tasks. Another popular approach to familiarization is via auditory bombardment activities as advocated by Hodson and Paden (1991).

Include nonword stimuli: This is necessary for training motor programming skills for speech and new word learning. Some children with SSD can produce familiar words perfectly well but need extra help when dealing with novel stimuli that require assembling new motor programs. Using nonwords in intervention promotes a functional skill because children are exposed to new words every day of their lives, particularly within the curriculum at school.

Mirror normal phonological development: If a child's speech production is inconsistent (i.e., at the whole-word phase of development) then adopting a core vocabulary approach (see Chapter 5) plus appropriate phonological awareness activities can help to anchor speech and move him or her on to the next phase. If the child is systematically using simplifying processes, then these might be targeted in intervention, (e.g., stopping or fronting). However, an important contribution of the psycholinguistic approach is to underpin these normal stages of phonological development. Simplifying processes are often targeted in intervention for children with SSD. However, there is not necessarily a one-to-one match between a process and underlying skills.

Design stimuli that reflect patterns of errors: Stimuli design is a key factor in the success of an intervention program and is based on phonetic and phonological analysis of a child's speech production. Decisions need to be made about what syllable structure to target, (e.g., single, bi-, or multisyllabic words) as well as what segments to include or avoid. For example, if a child is fronting /k/ to /t/, stimuli used at the beginning of an intervention program to practice /k/ in words should not include /t/ (e.g., *kite, cat*) as the presence of the error sound (/t/) will trigger the fronting process. However these stimuli may be used later in the intervention program when the child is better able to produce /k/ in words with ease (see Stackhouse & Wells, 1997, and Pascoe et al., 2006, for further discussion and examples of stimuli design).

Confront the child with his or her own speech errors: This encourages self-monitoring and updating of motor programs. It is a necessary phase of intervention though cannot be introduced until a child has two basic prerequisites: 1) auditory discrimination between targets and errors, and 2) the ability to articulate the differences between them. Without these, a child cannot win a game involving minimal pair confrontation and likely will become demotivated.

Supplement weak auditory processing skills: For some children, the SLP can support auditory training with visual feedback. This may take the form of visual cuing, for example, as sounds may be represented by symbols (e.g., as included in the Nuffield Centre Dyspraxia Programme; see Chapter 7; Williams & Stephens, 2004) or hand signs (e.g., cued articulation; Passy, 1993). These visual cues can accompany auditory discrimination tasks in which a child has to decide if two words presented are the same or not. To begin with, the child can *see* that words must be different because the symbol or sign for the beginning of one (e.g., *key*) is different from that for the beginning of the other (e.g., *tea*). Gradually the cues can be phased out so that the child relies on the auditory modality alone. More technical support can also be used if available (e.g., the laryngograph; Abberton, Hu, & Fourcin, 1998).

Provide the child with experience of producing new speech patterns: Articulatory practice of new segments and patterns is as important as listening practice for many children with SSD. Articulatory ease in producing segments is necessary for those segments to be used in a phonological way in the child's language (i.e., to contrast words meaningfully). This practice should not stop at the single-word level but needs to continue into connected speech through specifically designed phrases and sentences and then in spontaneous utterances (as for Katy in Pascoe et al., 2005). Articulatory practice can be supported by verbal instructions, reflecting on tactile feedback and visual aids such as cued articulation (Passy, 1993) or, if the technology is available, electropalatography (see Dent, 2001, for how to use this technique within a psycholinguistic framework).

Promote generalization: A challenge for children with SSD is often using what they have learned in structured intervention tasks in real-life situations. Tackling the underlying speech processing system through working on the child's speech production helps to strengthen the child's chances of doing this. Generalization can be facilitated by activities that encourage the child to reflect on his or her listening and production skills, such as identification of mispronunciations, self-monitoring, and phonological awareness activities (e.g., see activities from Metaphon; Howell & Dean, 1994).

Make links with literacy explicit: Phonological awareness tasks are key here but will not promote literacy development unless they incorporate explicit links between sounds and letters (Hatcher, 2006). The Nuffield Centre Dyspraxia Programme (Williams & Stephens, 2004) links sound symbols and letters and allows for working on speech and literacy simultaneously (see further discussion in Gillon, 2004; Pascoe et al., 2006; and Chapters 7 and 10 in this volume).

Having presented some principles for how to move from assessment to aims, the next step in intervention planning is to move from aims to tasks.

Description of Activities

An activity or intervention task includes any materials used for intervention, the procedure followed (including any instructions), the feedback given to the child, and any technique used to support speech processing, (e.g., signs or symbols). This can be summarized by the following equation (Rees, 2001b, p. 67):

TASK = Materials + Procedure + Feedback +/− Technique

There are three levels for practitioners to achieve when working on task design within a psycholinguistic framework:

1. Design intervention tasks based on this equation.

2. Understand why altering any one of these four components, even minimally, can change the psycholinguistic nature of the tasks and therefore the demands made on the child.

3. Use this knowledge to manipulate tasks at the time of delivering them to meet the needs of the child (i.e., how to make a task easier or more challenging for the child).

To help achieve these levels, Rees (2001b) listed 7 key questions that need to be addressed when designing tasks from a psycholinguistic perspective and gave examples of appropriate tasks for individual children (p. 68):

1. Does the child have to use his or her lexical representations to complete the task? If not, how likely is it that representations may be accessed?

2. Does the task target the input channel, the output channel, or both?

3. Does the task target a specific level (or levels) of speech processing? If so, which levels are targeted?

4. Metaphonological Skills:

   a. Does the child have to reflect on his or her speech production?

   b. Does the child have to show awareness of the internal structure of phonological representations or of spoken stimuli?

    c.   If so, what kind of segmentation is required?

    d.   Does the child have to manipulate phonological units?

5.   What demands are made on the child's memory in order to make responses during the task?

6.   What are the instruction demands? Can all or parts of the task be demonstrated?

7.   Is any technique being used to support the child with the task? If so, how is the technique providing support?

Materials and Equipment Required

Adopting a psycholinguistic approach to intervention does not require any new or specific materials or equipment. Rather, all resources can be used in a psycholinguistic way because the approach is in the head and hands of the user and not within the materials themselves.

ASSESSMENT AND PROGRESS MONITORING TO SUPPORT DECISION MAKING

An attractive feature of adopting the psycholinguistic framework for intervention is its inbuilt assessment and monitoring procedure. Various baselines can be established before intervention begins and compared with measures during and after intervention has finished (see cases presented in Pascoe et al., 2006). Three examples of profiling, generalization, and self-monitoring and correction are presented in the following sections.

Profiling

Collating assessment results and/or observations on the speech processing profile can show if a child's speech processing skills have improved or not. Some children will improve both their sound production and their underlying speech processing skills. Others will have obvious speech production difficulties and underlying problems.

    Profiling children's speech processing skills and monitoring their language and alphabetic skills in this way provides a systematic record of speech and literacy skills over time and has been particularly useful in uncovering hidden speech difficulties such as in children with dyslexia who have subtle SSD (Stackhouse & Wells, 1991). The profile also reveals how children may appear to have resolved their SSDs but as underlying speech processing difficulties persist they are still at risk for underachieving at school (Nathan & Simpson, 2001; Nathan et al., 2004a, 2004b).

Generalization

Although the speech processing profile is useful to capture the nature of a child's persisting difficulties, it can be too blunt an instrument to chart small steps forward in intervention. For this, measures of how much the child has generalized teaching and learning in intervention is important. This can be considered at two levels:

1.   *Across-item generalization:* Has a child's speech production improved on words that have not actually been targeted in intervention? To measure this, matched control words are used.

2. *Across-task generalization:* Has a child's performance on a task not targeted in intervention improved (e.g., improvement in speech output following targeted speech input work; improvement in spelling following speech output or input work)?

Self-Monitoring and Correction

Stackhouse et al. (2007) included score sheets and formats for recording a child's performance on a wide range of tasks. These are not standardized tests but procedures that can be used flexibly to assess, monitor, and chart a child's progress. For example, one procedure useful in monitoring change in a child's speech production behavior is a checklist and scale for recording the development of self-correction and under what circumstances. This scale can be used to capture general progress or to track progress on the following specifically targeted items:

1. Corrects own speech error spontaneously.

2. Attempts to correct speech error and produces a response closer to the target, but not yet correct.

3. Attempts to correct speech error and produces a variable response, which may or may not be closer to the target.

4. Attempts to correct speech error, but response is the same as original error.

5. Only attempts to correct speech error if listener does not understand.

6. Makes no attempt to correct speech error.

CONSIDERATIONS FOR CHILDREN FROM CULTURALLY AND LINGUISTICALLY DIVERSE BACKGROUNDS

One of the tenets of the psycholinguistic approach is that practitioners should feel free to devise their own tasks for individual children and to compare results for a given child to a set of norms gathered from typically developing children from that child's speech community. Stackhouse et al. (2007) included an accent warning with their procedures for the psycholinguistic framework.

This is particularly important when presenting targets for a child to imitate or judge how many syllables are present. For example, the word *mirror* can have one long syllable for American English speakers rather than two as in some other accents of English; *balloon* has one or two syllables depending on the accent of the speaker, *strawberry* has two or three, and *rhinoceros* three or four. If the child is asked how many syllables are in the target *balloon*, which is pronounced "bloon" by the SLP or teacher, is the correct response 1) what the adult speaker said (one syllable), 2) what is expected from the orthography of the target (two syllables), 3) what the child has in their representation of the target (could be one or two syllables), or 4) what the child says in their production of the target that may or may not match their representations? In other words, presenters of assessment and intervention tasks need to be aware of how variation in accents between themselves and their clients can affect not only a child's interpretation of the task but also how performance on that task is scored. When scoring speech productions and judgments regional variations must be taken into account. Training in stimuli design heightens awareness of this issue and is an essential part of using the psycholinguistic framework.

The psycholinguistic framework has also been used to investigate children's ability to understand speakers from different speech communities where accents differ. It is often taken for granted that children can understand speakers in different accents. However, Nathan, Wells, and Donlan (1998) found that typically developing 7-year-old children in London were significantly better than 4-year-olds on a task that involved defining and repeating single words presented in a Scottish (Glaswegian) accent. Applying this work to children with SSD, Nathan and Wells (2001) investigated the accent processing skills of 6-year-old children who had speech output difficulties and compared them to typically developing controls. All the children were from London. The children with speech difficulties, but not the controls, had significantly greater difficulty in correctly identifying words spoken in a Glaswegian accent compared with words spoken in a London accent. In terms of the speech processing model, the results suggest that these children had impairments in phonological recognition and/or representation that impeded the mapping of unusual variants of a word (e.g., a Glaswegian pronunciation) onto their stored lexical representation. This finding has implications for the management of children with speech processing difficulties who will be exposed, like all children, to an increasing range of speech variability in their teachers, SLPs, and other key people in their lives. Experience of processing different accents may need to be included in intervention programs for some children with SSD.

The psycholinguistic framework can also be used to work with children with SSD who speak more than one language. Level C on the speech processing profile is particularly important here (see Stackhouse et al., 2007), as is phonological recognition and phonetic discrimination on the box-and-arrow model. The framework has also been translated and adapted for use in different languages and cultures, such as German (Fox, 2004; Fricke & Schaefer, 2008), Danish (Thompson, 2000), French (Wells, Stackhouse, & Vance, 1999), and Portuguese (Vance, 1996).

More recently the framework has been used in developing countries (e.g., South Africa) to understand the speech and literacy abilities of multilingual school-age children in linguistically complex classrooms (Cramb et al., 2008) and for training teachers and teaching assistants to promote new word learning in English-speaking children with delayed speech and language development associated with social disadvantage (Trott, Stackhouse, & Clegg, 2008).

CASE STUDY

Case studies have played a key role in understanding the nature of speech difficulties in children and how best to treat them. Jarrod, for example, reveals how developmentally complex persisting speech difficulties are, and Zoe highlights 1) how the different aspects of a child's speech difficulties can be mapped on to different points in the speech processing model, and 2) that auditory discrimination skills are not necessarily all-or-nothing phenomena but may be quite specific (e.g., voice/voiceless confusion) in the context of otherwise intact auditory skill. Katy reminds us that 1) intervention on segments in words may not generalize to connected speech without being targeted specifically, and 2) connected speech, if designed appropriately, may be a starting point in intervention rather than a goal for the end. All practicing SLPs have the opportunity to carry out case studies in some form within their workplace; by doing so we add experience, skills, and knowledge to our professional expertise in SSD.

STUDY QUESTIONS

1. What have you learned about a psycholinguistic approach from this chapter that might influence your practice?

2. Think of three children you know (or those presented in this chapter) with SSD. How have they contributed to your knowledge about the nature and/or treatment of SSD?

3. How do you link speech and literacy skills in your intervention programs?

4. What criteria do you use to select a child's speech targets?

5. What outcome measures do you use to evaluate your intervention?

6. In what ways do you take the child's, caregivers', and school's perspective into account in your intervention planning and collaborations?

FUTURE DIRECTIONS

The psycholinguistic approach is an active means of extending knowledge about intervention and contributing toward the theory of therapy. Adopting this approach can help to address important practical and theoretical issues. For example

1. Does intervention on output bring about changes in input processing (e.g., auditory discrimination)?

2. Does intervention on input support changes in output?

3. Will better motor planning affect other aspects of the speech processing system (e.g., upward into motor programs as measured by increased accuracy in single word production and downward into motor execution)?

4. Does working on consonant clusters improve segmental production?

5. Does work on letter knowledge and phonological awareness generalize to both speech and literacy development?

6. Can work on controlled connected speech be more efficient than working on single words?

7. Do underlying speech processing difficulties manifest in each language spoken by a child?

The approach can also be used to tackle important service delivery issues such as dosage, carryover, training, and who should be involved in the delivery of intervention and in what contexts (see Pascoe et al., 2006, for further discussion).

The specific psycholinguistic framework presented here aims to guide the practitioner in making decisions about the nature of a child's SSD, the impact on educational and social performance, appropriate intervention strategies and targets, and when to end intervention and discharge. The framework also provides a means of communication among professionals, caregivers, and clients and encourages active questioning about how and why we do what we do. It is a flexible tool and does not require any specific equipment. Neither does it prescribe one way of working with children with SSD. Rather, it is a way of thinking about the selection and design of intervention tasks and ensures that the intervention is based on continuing hypothesis testing, interpretation of data, appropriate feedback, and evaluation of outcomes.

SUGGESTED READINGS

Pascoe, M., Stackhouse, J., & Wells, B. (2006). *Children's speech and literacy difficulties: Book 3. Persisting speech difficulties in children.* Chichester, England: Wiley.

Stackhouse, J., Pascoe, M., & Gardner, H. (2006). Intervention for a child with persisting speech and literacy difficulties: A psycholinguistic approach. *Advances in Speech-Language Pathology, 8*(3), 231–244.

Stackhouse, J., & Wells, B. (1997). *Children's speech and literacy difficulties: Book 1. A psycholinguistic framework.* Chichester, England: Wiley.

Stackhouse, J., Vance, M., Pascoe, M., & Wells, B. (2007). *Compendium of auditory and speech tasks: Children's speech and literacy difficulties 4.* Chichester, England: Wiley.

Stackhouse, J., & Wells, B. (2001). *Children's speech and literacy difficulties: Book 2. Identification and intervention.* Chichester, England: Wiley.

REFERENCES

Abberton, E., Hu, X., & Fourcin, A. (1998). Real-time speech pattern element displays for interactive therapy. *International Journal of Language and Communication Disorders, 33,* 292–297.

Baker, E., Croot, K., McLeod, S., & Paul, R. (2001). Psycholinguistic models of speech development and their application to clinical practice. *Journal of Speech, Language, and Hearing Research, 44,* 685–702.

Bishop, D., & Adams, C. (1990). A prospective study of the relationship between specific language impairment, phonological disorders and reading retardation. *Journal of Child Psychology and Psychiatry, 31,* 1027–1050.

Bridgeman, E., & Snowling, M. (1988). The perception of phoneme sequence: A comparison of dyspraxic and normal children. *British Journal of Disorders of Communication, 23*(3), 245–252.

Broom, Y., & Doctor, E. (1995). Developmental phonological dyslexia: A case study of the efficacy of a remediation programme. *Cognitive Neuropsychology, 12,* 725–766.

Bryan, A., & Howard, D. (1992). Frozen phonology thawed: The analysis and remediation of a developmental disorder of real word phonology. *European Journal of Disorders of Communication, 27,* 343–365.

Chiat, S. (2000). *Understanding children with language problems.* Cambridge, MA: Cambridge University Press.

Constable, A. (2001). A psycholinguistic approach to word-finding difficulties. In J. Stackhouse & B. Wells (Eds.), *Children's speech and literacy difficulties: Book 2. Identification and intervention* (pp. 330–365). Chichester, England: Wiley.

Corrin, J. (2001a). From profile to programme: Steps 1–2. In J. Stackhouse & B. Wells (Eds.), *Children's speech and literacy difficulties: Book 2. Identification and intervention* (pp. 96–132). Chichester, England: Wiley.

Corrin, J. (2001b). From profile to programme: Steps 3–6. In J. Stackhouse & B. Wells (Eds.), *Children's speech and literacy difficulties: Book 2. Identification and intervention* (pp. 133–163). Chichester, England: Wiley.

Cramb, L., Diehl, C., Francis, C., Ismail, Y., Jonker, C., & Samuel, K. (2008). *Exploring literacy in linguistically complex intermediate phase classrooms: From developmental, biopsychosocial and psycholinguistic perspectives.* Unpublished honours thesis. Division of Communication Sciences and Disorders, University of Cape Town, South Africa.

Crosbie, S., & Dodd, B. (2001). Training auditory discrimination: A single case study. *Child Language Teaching and Therapy, 17*(3), 173–194.

Dent, H. (2001). Electropalatography: A tool for psycholinguistic therapy. In J. Stackhouse & B. Wells (Eds.), *Children's speech and literacy difficulties: Book 2. Identification and intervention* (pp. 204–248). Chichester, England: Wiley.

Dodd, B. (Ed.). (1995/2005). *Differential diagnosis and treatment of children with speech disorder.* London: Whurr.

Fox, A. (2004). *Kindliche aussprache-störungen* [Children's speech disorders]. Idstein, Germany: Schulz-Kirchner Verlag.

Fricke, S., & Schaefer, B. (2008). *Test für phonologische bewusstheitsfähigkeiten (TPB)* [Test for phonological awareness skills]. Idstein, Germany: Schulz-Kirchner Verlag.

Gardner, H. (2004). A comparison of a speech and language therapist and a mother working on speech. In P. Seedhouse & K. Richards (Eds.), *Applying conversation analysis* (pp. 56–74). Basingstoke, England: Palgrave Macmillan.

Gardner, H. (2006). Training others in the art of therapy for speech sound disorders: An interactional approach. *Child Language Teaching and Therapy, 22*(1), 27–46.

Gillon, G. (2004) *Phonological awareness: From research to practice.* New York: Guilford Press.

Hatcher, P. (2006). Phonological awareness and reading intervention. In M. Snowling & J. Stackhouse (Eds.), *Dyslexia speech and language: A practitioner's handbook* (2nd ed., pp. 167–197). London: Whurr.

Hewlett, N., Gibbon, F., & Cohen-McKenzie, W. (1998). When is a velar an alveolar? Evidence supporting a revised psycholinguistic model of speech production in children. *International Journal of Language and Communication Disorders, 33*, 161–176.

Hodson, B., & Paden, E. (1991). *Targeting intelligible speech: A phonological approach to remediation.* San Diego: College-Hill Press.

Howell, J., & Dean, E. (1994). *Treating phonological disorders in children: Metaphon—Theory to practice.* London: Whurr.

Joffe, V., & Pring, T. (2008). Children with phonological problems: A survey of clinical practice. *International Journal of Language and Communication Disorders, 43*(2), 154–164.

Law, J., & Conti-Ramsden, G. (2000). Treating children with speech and language impairments. *British Medical Journal, 321*, 908–909.

Lindsay, G., Dockrell, J., Letchford, B., & Mackie, C. (2002). Self esteem of children with specific speech and language difficulties. *Child Language Teaching and Therapy, 18*, 125–143.

Nathan, L., & Simpson, S. (2001). Designing a literacy programme for a child with a history of speech difficulties. In J. Stackhouse & B. Wells (Eds.), *Children's speech and literacy difficulties: Book 2. Identification and intervention* (pp. 249–298). Chichester, England: Wiley.

Nathan, L., Stackhouse, J., Goulandris, N., & Snowling, M. (2004a). The development of early literacy skills among children with speech difficulties: A test of the "critical age hypothesis." *Journal of Speech, Language, and Hearing Research, 47*, 377–391.

Nathan, L., Stackhouse, J., Goulandris, N., & Snowling, M. (2004b). Educational consequences of developmental speech disorder: Key Stage I National Curriculum assessment results in English and mathematics. *British Journal of Educational Psychology, 74*, 173–186.

Nathan, L., & Wells, B. (2001). Can children with speech difficulties process an unfamiliar accent? *Applied Psycholinguistics, 22*(3), 343–361.

Nathan, L., Wells, B., & Donlan, C. (1998). Children's comprehension of unfamiliar regional accents: A preliminary investigation. *Journal of Child Language, 25*, 343–365.

Newton, C., & Wells, B. (1999). The development of between-word processes in the connected speech of children aged between three and seven. In N. Maassen & P. Groenen (Eds.), *Pathologies of speech and language: Advances in clinical phonetics and linguistics* (pp. 67–75). London: Whurr.

Newton, C., & Wells, B. (2002). Between word junctures in early multiword speech. *Journal of Child Language, 29*, 275–299.

Norbury, C.F., & Chiat, S. (2000). Semantic intervention to support word recognition: A single-case study. *Child Language Teaching and Therapy, 16*(2), 141–163.

Pascoe, M., Stackhouse, J., & Wells, B. (2005). Phonological therapy within a psycholinguistic framework: Promoting change in a child with persisting speech difficulties. *International Journal of Language and Communication Disorders, 39*, 1–32.

Pascoe, M., Stackhouse, J., & Wells, B. (2006). *Children's speech and literacy difficulties: Book 3. Persisting speech difficulties in children.* Chichester, England: Wiley.

Passy, J. (1993). *Cued articulation.* Ponteland, Northumberland, England: STASS Publications.

Popple, J., & Wellington, W. (1996). Collaborative working within a psycholinguistic framework. *Child Language Teaching and Therapy, 12*, 60–70.

Popple, J., & Wellington, W. (2001). Working together: The psycholinguistic approach within a school setting. In J. Stackhouse & B. Wells (Eds.), *Children's speech and literacy difficulties Book 2: Identification and intervention* (pp. 299–329). Chichester, England: Wiley.

Rees, R. (2001a). Principles of psycholinguistic intervention. In J. Stackhouse & B. Wells (Eds.), *Children's speech and literacy difficulties: Book 2. Identification and intervention* (pp. 41–65). Chichester, England: Wiley.

Rees, R. (2001b). What do tasks really tap? In J. Stackhouse & B. Wells (Eds.), *Children's speech and literacy difficulties: Book 2. Identification and intervention* (pp. 66–95). Chichester, England: Wiley.

Rees, R. (2008). *Deaf children's acquisition of speech skills: A psycholinguistic perspective through intervention.* Unpublished doctoral thesis, University College, London.

Ridley, J., Radford, J., & Mahon, M. (2002). How do teachers manage topic and repair? *Child Language Teaching and Therapy, 18*(1), 43–58.

Smith, N. (1978). Lexical representation and the acquisition of phonology. *Studies in the Linguistic Sciences, 8*, 259–273.

Snowling, M. (2006). Language skills and learning to read: The dyslexia spectrum. In M. Snowling & J. Stackhouse (Eds.), *Dyslexia speech and language: A practitioner's handbook* (2nd ed., pp. 1–14). London: Whurr.

Spencer, A. (1988). A phonological theory of phonological development. In M. Ball (Ed.), *Theoretical linguistics and disordered language* (pp. 115–151). London: Croom-Helm.

Spooner, L. (2002). Addressing expressive language disorder in children who also have severe receptive language disorder: A psycholinguistic approach. *Child Language Teaching and Therapy, 18*(3), 289–313.

Stackhouse, J. (1992). Developmental verbal dyspraxia: A longitudinal case study. In R. Campbell (Ed.), *Mental lives: Case studies in cognition.* Oxford, England: Blackwell.

Stackhouse, J. (1993). Phonological disorder and lexical development: Two case studies. *Child Language Teaching and Therapy, 9*(2), 230–241.

Stackhouse, J. (2006). Speech and spelling difficulties: What to look for. In M. Snowling & J. Stackhouse (Eds.), *Dyslexia, speech and language: A practitioner's handbook.* London: Whurr.

Stackhouse, J., Pascoe, M., & Gardner, H. (2006). Intervention for a child with persisting speech and literacy difficulties: A psycholinguistic approach. *Advances in Speech Language Pathology, 8*(3), 231–244.

Stackhouse, J., & Snowling, M. (1992). Barriers to literacy development in two cases of developmental verbal dyspraxia. *Cognitive Neuropsychology, 9*, 272–299.

Stackhouse, J., Vance, M., Pascoe, M., & Wells, B. (2007). *Compendium of auditory and speech tasks: Children's speech and literacy difficulties 4.* Chichester, England: Wiley.

Stackhouse, J., & Wells, B. (1991). Dyslexia: The obvious and hidden speech and language disorder. In M. Snowling & M. Thomson (Eds.), *Dyslexia: Integrating theory and practice* (pp. 16–25). London: Whurr.

Stackhouse, J., & Wells, B. (1993). Psycholinguistic assessment of developmental speech disorders. *European Journal of Disorders of Communication, 28*, 331–348.

Stackhouse, J., & Wells, B. (1996). Developmental supermodels. *Bulletin of the Royal College of Speech and Language Therapists, 527*, 9–10.

Stackhouse, J., & Wells, B. (1997). *Children's speech and literacy difficulties: Book 1. A psycholinguistic framework.* Chichester, England: Wiley.

Stackhouse, J., & Wells, B. (Eds.). (2001). *Children's speech and literacy difficulties: Book 2. Identification and intervention.* Chichester, England: Wiley.

Stiegler, L.N., & Hoffman, P.R. (2001). Discourse-based intervention for word finding in children. *Journal of Communication Disorders, 34*, 277–303.

Thompson, I. (2000). *Børns taleog skriftsprologue varskeligher.* Herning: Special–Paedagogisk Forlag.

Trott, K., Stackhouse, J., & Clegg, J. (2008). *Supporting schools in developing children's vocabulary, attention, listening, and conversation* [Training folder]. Department of Human Communication Sciences, University of Sheffield, England. Manuscript in preparation.

Vance, M. (1996). Assessing speech processing skills in children: A task analysis. Portuguese translation. In M. Snowling & J. Stackhouse (Eds.), *Dislexia, fala e linguagem: Um manual do profissional.* São Paulo, Brazil: Artmet São Pablo .

Vance, M. (1997). Christopher Lumpship: Developing phonological representations in a child with an auditory processing deficit. In S. Chiat, J. Law, & J. Marshall (Eds.), *Language disorders in children and adults: Psycholinguistic approaches to therapy* (17–41). London: Whurr.

Vance, M., Stackhouse, J., & Wells, B. (2005). Speech production skills in children aged 3–7 years. *International Journal of Language and Communication Disorders, 40*(1), 29–48.

Velleman, S. (2002). Phonotactic therapy. *Seminars in Speech and Language, 23*, 1–18.

Waters, D. (2001). Using input processing strengths to overcome speech output difficulties. In J. Stackhouse & B. Wells (Eds.), *Children's speech and literacy difficulties: Book 2. Identification and intervention* (pp. 164–203). Chichester, England: Wiley.

Waters, D., Hawkes, C., & Burnett, E. (1998). Targeting speech processing strengths to facilitate pronunciation change. *International Journal of Language and Communication Disorders, 33*(Suppl.), 469–474.

Weiner, F. (1981). Treatment of phonological disability using the method of meaningful contrast: Two case studies. *Journal of Speech and Hearing Disorders, 46*, 97–103.

Wells, B., Stackhouse, J., & Vance, M. (1999). La conscience phonologique dans le cadre d'une evaluation psycholinguistique de l'enfant [Assessment of phonological awareness within a psycholinguistic framework]. *Re-education Orthophonique, 197*, 3–12.

Williams, P., & Stackhouse, J. (1998). Diadochokinetic skills: Normal and atypical performance in children aged 3–5 years. *International Journal of Language and Communication Disorders, 33*(Suppl.), 481–486.

Williams, P., & Stephens, H. (2004). *Nuffield Centre Dyspraxia Programme* (3rd ed.).Windsor, England: Miracle Factory.

Wren, Y., & Roulstone, S. (2001). *Hear IT–Sound IT Project.* Bristol, England: Speech and Language Therapy Research Unit.

Metaphonological Intervention

Phonological Awareness Therapy

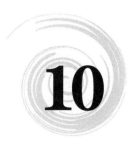

10

Anne Hesketh

ABSTRACT

Metaphonological intervention develops and uses a child's phonological awareness to support and drive speech change. Activities that require the child to think about speech and about the structure of words are tailored specifically to the current speech target and are integrated into therapy sessions alongside production practice. Improvement in phonological awareness, particularly when combined with letter knowledge, will also support early literacy development. Metaphonological intervention can be suitable for children with speech sound disorders (SSD) from around 4 years as long as they are ready to learn to reflect on their speech and the structure of words. It can fit into a variety of service delivery options but is particularly suitable for individual and small-group work.

INTRODUCTION

Phonological awareness (PA) is the ability to pay attention to the sound structure of language. It is an umbrella term, covering a range of skills from the ability to segment an utterance into its constituent words right up to the subtle and complex manipulation of phonemes involved in spoonerisms or "pig Latin." Children usually begin to be able to demonstrate some explicit, conscious meta-awareness of word structure in their fourth year, and more detailed awareness continues to develop well into the school years. PA is almost universally accepted as an important factor in early literacy development (Vellutino, Fletcher, Snowling, & Scanlon, 2004) and has been the subject of much interest in speech-language pathology, particularly for its role in intervention for children with SSD (Denne, Langdown, Pring, & Roy, 2005; Gillon, 2005). The term *phonemic* or *phoneme awareness* refers to the higher levels of PA involving awareness of individual phonemes within words.

PA is the general ability to attend to sound structure and is often assessed by children making judgments about words spoken aloud by the tester. This does not *require* access to their own lexical store (these tasks could also be carried out using nonwords). A separate, although related, issue is the status of a child's internal phonological representations for the words in their vocabulary. Phonological representations are described by Sutherland and Gillon (2005) as the repository in long-term memory of information about the sound structure of words. The detail and accuracy of these representations, as well as a child's metalinguistic ability to reflect on them, is beginning to be a focus of research and therapeutic interest for children with SSD.

During the past decade there has been a strong trend in the United Kingdom to include a specific emphasis on PA in intervention for children with SSD. PA in itself is not a useful everyday skill; it is included in the belief that it is necessary for speech development and/or as a prevention against difficulties in literacy acquisition. The relationship among PA, phonological representations, speech, and literacy will be discussed in the following sections. The clinical emphasis in this chapter will be the heightening of metaphonological awareness as a component *within* therapy, not as an intervention that targets PA alone.

TARGET POPULATIONS

Broadly, the inclusion of PA activities within speech sound work can be appropriate for all children with SSD who have the physical potential to improve their speech and who have the cognitive capacity to benefit from the metalinguistic tasks.

Much of the published evidence on PA has included school children older than 5 years (e.g., Gillon, 2000), although increasingly research is targeting younger participants 3 and 4 years old (e.g., Denne et al., 2005; Gillon, 2005). Most of the strong evidence for the benefits of PA work in the field of SSD has excluded children with broader language or cognitive difficulties. Attempts have been made to extend our knowledge of the populations for whom it is appropriate (Moriarty & Gillon, 2006; Munro et al., 2008), but most of the evidence suggests that cognitively able children will be able to take more immediate benefit from PA work. This is probably because speech-language pathology introduces PA early, at the boundary of children's competence to deal with the abstraction of speech sounds as word constituents.

ASSESSMENT METHODS FOR DETERMINING INTERVENTION RELEVANCE

Overall Assessment

A metaphonological approach to intervention requires an underlying knowledge of a child's audiological, motor, language, cognitive, educational, social, and speech status just as any other approach to therapy. The following discussion focuses on those issues of particular relevance to PA and assumes that overall assessment has indicated that the child's speech problem is the priority for intervention.

Language and cognitive assessment are necessary in order to judge whether a child will be able to benefit from metaphonological elements of therapy. Because phoneme awareness is challenging for most preschoolers, children with significant additional language or cognitive limitations may not be ready to acquire these skills. Vocabulary size is a likely influence on the development of PA and detailed lexical representations; therefore, children with a restricted receptive vocabulary may not respond as well to PA therapy. It is a matter of debate in all kinds of therapy for SSD whether working on established vocabulary or introducing new words will stimulate most change in the system, but in PA approaches, it is particularly essential to know whether a child already has an internal representation for a word. It is necessary to check understanding of relevant concepts such as same/different, right/wrong, and beginning/end and to be able to pitch explanations appropriately. Language assessment is also necessary as a prognostic indicator. Children with language delay, in addition to their speech problem, have a much poorer prognosis for literacy development, and it will be particularly important to plan for the integration of letter knowledge and to collaborate with teachers about literacy progress in such cases.

A detailed assessment of a child's speech is of course essential. One approach is to use a relatively short initial screening word list followed by a more detailed investigation of the problem areas. The detailed data will elicit multiple exemplars of specific sounds and contexts, check for variability of production, and allow reliable analysis of the patterns and processes used by the child. Analysis of a short sample of connected speech allows comparison of processes and features in single words and connected speech. The Diagnostic Evaluation of Articulation and Phonology (DEAP; Dodd, Hua, Crosbie, Holm, & Ozanne, 2002, 2006) contains useful pictures to elicit a short sample efficiently. The DEAP provides norm-referenced scores for an appropriate age range of children and is standardized on a U.K. and an Australian population (Dodd et al., 2002) as well as on a U.S. population (Dodd et al., 2006). Listening to the child talking in a relaxed and confident interaction is essential to estimate intelligibility outside clinical tasks and an important ongoing check on generalization of clinical gains.

Phonological Awareness Assessment

Much of the PA literature on dyslexia describes assessments that require a verbal response from children. However, in the case of children with SSD, their inevitable mismatches in production make it difficult to interpret their performance and to disentangle PA from the effects of output phonology/articulation. Assessing PA and representations of children with SSD requires receptive tasks that need nonverbal or yes/no responses. Subtle variations in task performance can make a considerable difference to the demands on a child and tap different aspects of processing. A detailed consideration of tasks and task demands can be found in Catts, Wilcox, Wood-Jackson, Larrivee, and Scott (1997) and in Stackhouse and Wells (1997).

Several standardized assessments of PA abilities are available. It is important that the standardization sample is relevant to the specific child and context because different ages of school entry and exposure to literacy teaching in different countries can lead to different rates of PA development around 4–6 years. In the United Kingdom the Preschool and Primary Inventory of Phonological Awareness (PIPA; Dodd, Crosbie, McIntosh, Teitzel, & Ozanne, 2000) is particularly useful, being standardized on a U.K. and an Australian sample from 3;0 to 6;11, covering children at the typical age of attendance for therapy. The Phonological Abilities Test (Muter, Hulme, & Snowling, 1997) also has U.K. norms for 5–7 years. They can both be used to give a norm-referenced assessment of a child's general PA abilities. The Comprehensive Test of Phonological Processing (CTOPP; Wagner, Torgesen, & Rashotte, 1999) was normed on a U.S. sample of individuals ages 5–24 years.

Table 10.1. Results of Preschool and Primary Inventory of Phonological Awareness (PIPA) Phoneme Isolation subtest for 42 children ages 4;0–4;6 with speech sound disorders

	Phoneme Isolation raw score (max = 12)	Phoneme Isolation standard score
Mean	1.33	7.69
Range	0–11	6–15
SD	2.88	2.05

Key: SD, standard deviation.

However, tests of PA tend to show floor effects at the younger ages. Table 10.1 shows the PIPA Phoneme Isolation subtest scores for the 42 children who took part in Hesketh, Dima, and Nelson's (2007) study. Note both the wide range and the low expectations in that a raw score of 1 out of 12 achieves a standard score within the normal range. In fact, for children ages 4;0–4;5, a raw score of 0 is recorded as a standard score of 7 (regarded as within normal limits) because so many children in the standardization sample were unable to perform this task. This makes the decision as to whether a child actually has a problem in PA on commencement of therapy far from clear cut.

Assessment of Phonological Representations

Hulme et al. (2002) saw PA tasks as a window onto a child's phonological representations, but there is now interest in assessing representations directly. Anything requiring spoken output will be a clouded window in the case of children with SSD; therefore, receptive judgment activities are necessary, such as the mispronunciation judgment tasks described by Rvachew, Ohberg, Grawburg, and Heyding (2003) and Sutherland and Gillon (2005). PA tasks that require children to make judgments about the sound structure of words not spoken by the tester also demand access to internal representations. An example might be sorting pictures according to their initial sound, when the pictures are not named by either the tester or the child. However, such tasks are very difficult for young children, and an inability to carry them out at a metacognitive level does not necessarily indicate that the representations themselves are immature. Moreover, appropriate norms are not yet available. However, norms on the simpler mispronunciation judgment tasks are beginning to appear (Claessen, Heath, Fletcher, Hogben, & Leitão, 2009; Sutherland & Gillon, 2005).

Assessment Specific to the Individual Child

Detailed assessment and analysis of a child's speech system leads to the identification of one or more candidates for the priority intervention focus. It is then necessary to carry out further assessment directly related to the potential target sounds, investigating auditory discrimination and stimulability, following a psycholinguistic profile (Stackhouse & Wells, 1997; see also Chapter 9), and assessing the child's PA and internal representations for words specifically containing that target.

THEORETICAL BASIS

Dominant Theoretical Rationale for the Intervention Approach

The Typical Development of Phonological Awareness and Phonological Representations

Phonological Awareness

The typical development of PA has been well described. The general pattern is that children move from large-unit (word, syllable, rime) to small-unit (phoneme) awareness, the latter having a reciprocal relationship with early literacy development, particularly letter knowledge. A summary of approximate age levels is discussed in this section; more detail can be found in reviews such as in Gillon (2004). Subtle variations in tasks (e.g., matching versus isolation/identification versus oddity judgments) can make a considerable difference in the level of difficulty at any level of structure, and there is wide variation in children's ability younger than age 5. In addition, different age of school entry and exposure to literacy activities across countries can affect early development, as shown by the different Australian and U.K. PIPA norms established by Dodd and Gillon (2001).

Although very young children can show some implicit knowledge of sounds in words, it is not until the fifth year that a conscious awareness of word structure can reliably be demonstrated. Most children demonstrate very little explicit PA at 4 years but begin to be able to segment words into syllables and to make some rhyme judgments between 4 and 5 years. By age 5, more than half are likely to match rhymes, although it may be after 5 before the majority are successful on rhyme oddity tasks. It was not until 6 years that more than 50% of children studied by Webster and Plante (1995) passed the rhyme detection task. Webster and Plante's results may differ from those in other studies because approximately half the children had SSD. The earliest *phoneme* awareness skill is word-initial phoneme matching or identification, developing from around 4;6 to 5;0, often before children are confident with rhyme judgments. Task nuances are important here, as children may be able to say the sound a word starts with but not be able to identify other words that start with the same sound. Sensitivity to single consonants at the ends of words may follow quite quickly, but awareness of the constituent sounds in consonant clusters is more difficult. Phoneme manipulation skills such as movement, addition, or deletion of phonemes from words are not usually established in children younger than 6 years of age.

Researchers increasingly are suggesting that rime and phoneme skills may be dissociable and reflect separate processes, making a differential contribution to literacy and possibly to speech development and change. The separation of rime and phoneme awareness has been demonstrated in children with typical development (Carroll, Snowling, Hulme, & Stevenson, 2003), Down syndrome (Snowling, Hulme, & Mercer, 2002), and isolated SSD (Hesketh, Adams, & Nightingale, 2000; Hesketh, Dima, & Nelson, 2006;). In this work, small-unit phoneme awareness is generally seen as the more important factor for literacy development (Gillon, 2005; Hulme et al., 2002), and it is thought that mastery of rhyme is not an essential precursor to phoneme level awareness (Anthony & Francis, 2005; Hesketh, Dima, & Nelson, 2006). Conversely, Mann and Foy (2007) found a closer association between rhyme awareness and speech production abilities in U.S. preschool children ages 4–6 years.

Phonological Representations

Another important issue in a child's phonological processing is the status of his or her phonological representations. Development of both PA and phonological representations may reflect vocabulary growth. As a child acquires more lexical items and the differences among those items become more subtle, a finer-grained representation is necessary to be able to distinguish among them in recognition, storage, and retrieval (Metsala, 1999). The detail, accuracy, and readiness of these representations are seen as critical factors in early reading (Snowling & Hayiou-Thomas, 2006), and they are becoming a focus of interest in the areas of both literacy and SSD. Claessen et al. (2008) presented data on typically developing Australian children at 5;5 (end of preprimary year) and 7;9 (end of year 2) using a mispronunciation detection task. Although most participants at both ages were easily able to identify correct pronunciations and reject incorrect ones, there were a significant number of children who found the tasks difficult, especially rejection of incorrect productions. These children (bottom quartile) performed worse at both PA tasks and early literacy achievement, suggesting the assessment of phonological representations in the (Australian) preschool year can be a valuable predictor of outcome.

Phonological Awareness and Phonological Representations in Children with Speech Sound Disorders

Phonological Awareness

A significant body of research has shown that, as a group, children with SSD show PA difficulties; for reviews, see Gillon (2004) and Hesketh et al. (2007). However, it is clear that there is considerable variability of performance and overlap of ability between children with SSD and typically developing children. There are children with good speech and poor PA (at risk for dyslexia) and children with poor speech and good PA. PA ability does *not* show a close association with the severity of the output SSD (Hesketh, 2004; Holm, Farrier, & Dodd, 2008; Sutherland & Gillon, 2005). Raitano, Pennington, Tunick, Boada, and Shriberg (2004) found that children with a history of SSD, even when it had resolved, had lower PA skills than typically developing peers at ages 5–6. However, the delay was greater in children whose SSD persisted or in children who had an accompanying language problem. Holm et al. (2008) described different patterns of PA ability according to speech output pattern; children with consistent but atypical speech features performed worse overall than those with delayed or inconsistent speech.

How specific is the link between speech problems and PA? Webster and Plante (1995) examined this in children with and without speech problems between 3;6 and 6;0, assessing rhyme and alliteration detection in an odd one-out format. When age was accounted for within this mixed group, they found that the lower a child's output score, the lower his or her PA ability. However, other studies specifically of children with SSD (e.g., Hesketh, Adams, & Nightingale, 2000) have shown no significant correlation between speech severity and PA. There is little evidence about specific speech errors being linked to specific difficulties in awareness of those sounds or patterns.

Phonological Representations

Interest has extended to consider the internal phonological representations of children with SSD. Are they, in some children, reduced in their detail or inaccurate in their specification (reflecting the inaccuracies in output)? Rvachew (2006) and Rvachew and Grawburg (2006) found that receptive vocabulary size and speech perception skills before children entered kindergarten were associated with concurrent PA abilities and predicted PA at the end of the kindergarten year. Rvachew's "speech perception" was assessed by a mispronunciation identification task—children were presented with a picture and a spoken word and had to decide whether or not the word was correct (errors differed in the initial consonant). Rather than being a relatively peripheral perception activity, this task required access to stored lexical forms and therefore went to the heart of interest in the accuracy of phonological representations. If speech perception could be shown to be accurate for nonlexical tasks, for example same/different judgments on speech sounds or nonwords (Stackhouse & Wells, 1997), but errors were made on *lexical* accuracy judgments, then the detail or accuracy of lexical representations would be suspect.

As with PA, evidence suggests that children with SSD do on average perform worse than age-matched children on tasks that tap into phonological lexical representations. Sutherland and Gillon (2005) found 4-year-old children with SSD performed worse on two receptive tasks—accuracy judgments about familiar words (the mispronunciation identification task again) and learning and making accuracy judgments about novel words. There was a wide range of abilities within the group, and almost complete overlap with the range of scores from typically developing peers (e.g., on the accuracy judgment task the group range was 10–27 out of 30 items for the children with SSD, whereas the range for typically developing peers was 12–29 items). Sutherland and Gillon concluded that the tasks used were appropriate for the population and age but that changes to the stimulus items may have increased sensitivity in differentiating between the groups. Sutherland and Gillon (2007) showed that these children continued to show poorer performance on phonological representation tasks at age 4;10 and 5;4. Only a moderate correlation between phonological representation tasks and PA skills was shown in this small group of children, and this is an area that requires further investigation.

Literacy and Phonological Awareness

Children may vary in the way and the age at which they learn to read and spell due to individual strengths and weaknesses and the education policy of their home country. Nevertheless, several stages are commonly identified in alphabetic languages (Frith, 1985). An early core vocabulary may be learned on the basis of whole-word recognition, involving visual features (the logographic stage). The next step involves acquiring letter knowledge and learning systematic letter–sound correspondences (the alphabetic stage). Words are read and spelled using analysis of their component phonemes and graphemes, and PA plays an extremely important role at this stage. Finally, children begin to recognize larger word segments such as morphemes and to read and spell by analogy with similar words (the orthographic stage). Now, grapheme–phoneme conversion for each letter is not carried out, and the context of longer linguistic units begins to influence processing. Reading comprehension becomes more salient than decoding, and language begins to play a more important part than PA. Language skills such as vocabulary and grammar are more important in reading comprehension and contribute increasingly as children become fluent decoders and read more complex texts.

In the United Kingdom, there is a great emphasis on phonics in the early stages of teaching literacy, emphasizing the segmentation and synthesis of sounds and letters in order to recognize and spell words. PA is therefore a particularly crucial skill in learning literacy in the U.K. educational system. Development of phonological and phonemic awareness also forms part of literacy policy in the United States (Ehri et al., 2001). Other countries, such as New Zealand, place more emphasis on whole-word recognition and the use of linguistic context as stepping stones to literacy.

Some children do not learn to read and write easily. When the literacy difficulty is out of step with other cognitive abilities, the problem is labeled dyslexia, although debate continues about whether the underlying difficulties are any different than in children without a literacy/cognitive discrepancy. A large amount of literature exists on specific dyslexia, much of which identifies an impairment in phonological processing (see Vellutino et al., 2004, for a detailed review). This would hinder children in establishing firm letter–sound (grapheme–phoneme) links and cause a delay in the early encoding and decoding stages of reading and spelling. It would explain the frequent dyslexic pattern of particular difficulty in reading or spelling *non*words (Snowling & Hayiou-Thomas, 2006), which is in effect what children have to do every time they deal with a word they have never read or written before.

Literacy in Children with Speech Sound Disorders

If PA is an important factor in literacy acquisition and if children with SSD, as a group, have lower-than-average PA skills, then are children with SSD at risk for literacy difficulties? When the SSD is part of a broader picture of language problems, the answer is fairly clearly yes. Widespread evidence suggests that children with language disorders go on to have problems in reading and writing, although these are not entirely due to phonological limitations. Bishop and Snowling (2004) and Snowling and Hayiou-Thomas (2006) argued that phonology and other (semantic/grammatical) language difficulties will interact to cause problems in both early reading *and* in the later stages when broader language skills are drawn on to support comprehension as well as decoding of text. Because of their double impairment in phonological and other language skills, children with specific language impairment are at greater risk for long-term reading and writing difficulties than are children with dyslexia. Rvachew (2007) found language rather than phonological skills to be the main predictor of word reading at the end of first grade.

For children with isolated SSD (i.e., whose language and cognitive abilities are within normal limits), there is conflicting evidence. Bishop and Adams (1990) and Catts (1993) both found that children with pure SSD went on to show literacy skills within the normal range. Nathan, Stackhouse, Goulandris, and Snowling (2004) also found that literacy development in children with SSD was not significantly different from their typically developing peers, whereas children with both speech *and* language difficulties had a higher risk of literacy problems. However, Bird, Bishop, and Freeman (1995) and Webster, Plante, & Couvillion (1997) showed children with speech difficulties to have literacy problems even in the absence of language delay, and Nathan et al. (2004) did find that persisting speech difficulties made children vulnerable to literacy difficulties. Carroll and Snowling (2004) argued that children with speech problems are at a high risk of literacy problems because of limitations in phonological processing and phonological representations.

The answer may lie in the individual variability of children with SSD; those who have consistent speech patterns, which include developmentally atypical errors, are more likely to show PA and literacy problems (Holm et al., 2008; Leitão, Hogben, & Fletcher, 1997). PA may be the important factor. Hesketh (2004) showed that PA ability after a period of intervention predicted whether children with a history of isolated SSD went on to perform within the normal range for single-word reading and spelling. The group average showed PA, single-word reading, and spelling all within the normal range at ages 6;6–7;6, although 4 of 35 individuals had reading and spelling scores more than 1 standard deviation below the norm, defined as a poor literacy outcome. PA scores had been measured at the end of an earlier period of therapy (Hesketh, Adams, Nightingale, & Hall, 2000; age range 3;6–5;0), and children who performed in the bottom quartile range (of a normative sample) at that age were classified as having poor PA skills. PA skills were the strongest predictor of literacy in a multiple regression analysis, and three of the four children with poor literacy outcome fell within the poor PA group at the earlier assessment. Nathan et al. (2004) followed children with SSD only, children with speech and language difficulties, and typically developing controls at nursery (preschool), reception class (kindergarten), and year 1 (first grade). They assessed auditory input tasks, speech output, PA, and literacy. Phoneme awareness showed a moderate-to-strong correlation with literacy skills in children with speech problems, but rime awareness did not, thus confirming the idea that rime awareness is a dissociable and less important factor than phoneme level skill. Rvachew (2007) showed that children with SSD and *poor* PA skills prior to kindergarten entry performed worse at nonword decoding than children with SSD and *good* PA skills at the end of first grade. Both groups, however, were within normal limits on reading assessment. Children with inconsistent speech errors may be vulnerable to difficulties with spelling (Holm et al., 2008).

Bishop and Adams (1990) proposed a critical age hypothesis that predicts that children whose speech difficulties persist when they start to learn to read are at high risk for literacy problems. This is supported to some extent by the research of Nathan et al. (2004), although the latter recognize the contribution of multiple factors to the problem. They propose a modified hypothesis that predicts good literacy outcome for children with SSD if their speech problems have resolved by the time they begin to learn to read *and* their phoneme awareness is adequate.

Summary

PA is an important factor in early literacy development. Although children with SSD are more likely to have poorer PA skills than the population as a whole, many of them go on to have a good literacy outcome. The persistence of SSD to the point of learning literacy, continuing poor PA skills at commencement of literacy activities, and the presence of an additional language delay are negative prognostic factors.

Levels of Consequences Being Addressed

PA work itself targets a functional limitation underlying both speech and literacy but with the clear goal that those speech and literacy skills will improve as a consequence, which will in turn have a beneficial effect on the child's participation in family, school, and social life.

Target Areas of Intervention

Work on PA alone is likely to improve primarily PA alone. However phonological and phonemic awareness is used alongside and integrated with speech production practice and letter knowledge in order to improve the broader domains of speech and literacy.

The first clear example in the United Kingdom of an intervention approach based on the theory of PA was the Metaphon program (Howell, Hill, Dean, & Waters, 1993). Metaphon was developed in response to growing evidence that children with SSD were, as a group, poorer at PA than age- or phonologically matched typically developing children. The authors saw phonological disorder, therefore, as a cognitive-linguistic problem and devised an intervention designed to stimulate cognitive reorganization, which would in turn result in phonological (speech output) change. Since then, PA has become a very common part, sometimes the main focus, of intervention for children with SSD in the United Kingdom, and is also widely used in the United States and other parts of the world. Our knowledge of the development and influence of PA has increased enormously in the last 15 years, as has the evidence on its use in therapy for SSD. This empirical evidence on clinical effectiveness is reviewed in the following section.

EMPIRICAL BASIS

Intervention Research Outcomes

The theoretical review shows us that speech-language pathologists (SLPs) face a clinical puzzle. SLPs frequently work with children with SSD between 4 and 5 years of age, and many SLPs want to include PA in their intervention to raise awareness of speech sounds and how to change them. However, even typically developing children have not developed phoneme awareness at this age, and most children can only acquire the easier stages with direct teaching. Further research is needed on the level of PA that is necessary for speech change and the degree to which it has to be tackled directly and separately. Research suggests that phonological and phoneme awareness can be taught, teaching PA can have a positive effect on literacy and on morphological awareness, and PA work has an effect on speech. Each of these areas will be discussed and evaluated in more detail in the following sections.

Teaching Phonological Awareness

There is a large body of evidence on the teaching of phonological and phoneme awareness in the general or reading-risk populations. A meta-analysis of 52 studies (Ehri et al., 2001) demonstrated a large, significant effect of *phonemic* awareness instruction on phonemic awareness skills themselves. This analysis established the overall efficacy of teaching phonemic awareness and allows further research to ask more specific questions about different populations.

In a U.K. school cohort-based study, Nancollis, Lawrie, and Dodd (2005) investigated children considered to be at risk of education underachievement because of their low socioeconomic status. They gave all children from selected schools nine sessions (7 hours) of PA intervention shortly before school entry (average age 4;6). Controls, who did not receive the PA package, were a different entry cohort; both groups included children with a range of cognitive and speech-language abilities. Intervention focused on syllable and rhyme awareness activities, including some initial phoneme identification. Assessment 2 years after intervention showed the intervention group had better rhyme awareness and nonword spelling performance but performed significantly worse than controls on phoneme segmentation. A *lack of* group difference in the latter skills could potentially be explained by the predominantly large-unit–based teaching or by the time that lapsed post-intervention, but the differentially *better* performance of the control group is puzzling.

A number of studies have investigated PA teaching and development specifically in the population of children with SSD. Research has consistently shown that, as a group, children with SSD perform worse than their typically developing peers on PA tasks (see Gillon, 2005, and Hesketh et al., 2007, for reviews), and PA is frequently included in therapy, sometimes as the main focus of therapy, for these children. However, research also suggests that 1) the phoneme level of awareness is of particular importance for literacy development (and perhaps speech change), and b) children typically attend therapy for their speech problems in the preschool period, before phoneme awareness develops. So, are we restricted in therapy to tasks that are not the most potent contributors to literacy and speech development? Or are preschool children cognitively ready for higher level tasks and simply waiting for a trigger to development that is usually supplied by exposure to literacy tasks on school entry?

In order to tease out this problem, Hesketh et al. (2007) attempted to teach phoneme awareness skills to preliterate children with SSD. Forty-two children ages 4;0–4;6 were randomly allocated to receive either 20 sessions (10–15 hours) of PA work (moving from rhyme awareness to consonant addition and deletion) or a control general language stimulation program. Postintervention, the PA group achieved significantly better scores than the language stimulation group on three of four phoneme awareness measures. The skill showing the most dramatic effect was that of word-initial phoneme identification, which it seemed that children of this age were ready to learn given some facilitation. For the more advanced skills of phoneme segmentation, addition, and deletion, however, only a minority of the children achieved success. These children tended to be older and with good nonverbal achievement. A number of other studies also showed that intervention before 5 years can stimulate the development of some phoneme-level awareness skills to a limited degree or in a minority of children (Laing & Espeland, 2005; Warrick, Rubin, & Rowe-Walsh, 1993). Denne et al. (2005) randomly allocated 20 children with speech problems, ages 5–7 years, to treatment and no-treatment control groups. Treated children were seen in groups of three for 12 hours of intervention, which consisted of phonological and phoneme awareness tasks including attention to specific speech processes. Opportunities for speech production and corrective feedback were provided alongside the awareness work. Children in the treatment group made significantly more progress on a standardized test of PA than did the untreated children. Hesketh et al. (2007) showed that competence in large units is not a necessary precursor to awareness of phonemes; therefore, intervention can progress to phoneme awareness without ensuring success on rhyme tasks.

Whereas Hesketh et al. (2007) investigated the possibility of teaching PA as a research question in its own right, others have taught PA as a means to improvement in the life skills of speech and reading. In these studies PA achievement was measured alongside other outcomes and is reported in this section. Literacy and speech outcomes from those studies are reported separately in the sections that follow.

Gillon (2000) provided three types of intervention: PA, traditional speech-focused, and a minimal contact consultation/advice model. After therapy, children in the PA group had made significantly more improvement in PA than those in other groups and had caught up to the level of a typically developing comparison group. Participants were ages 5;6–7;6 and were already in school so would be expected to be ready to develop phoneme awareness. Gillon's PA therapy program did involve opportunities for speech production practice. The PA intervention group remained on a level with the controls and significantly better at PA than those who had received traditional therapy when followed up approximately 1 year later (Gillon, 2002). Hesketh, Adams, Nightingale, and Hall (2000) similarly compared PA and production-focused interventions and found that children in both groups made progress in PA. After 10 sessions of intervention, both groups had made a similar amount of change on a battery of PA tasks and there was no longer a significant difference in performance between the children with SSD and typically speaking controls. The lack of difference may in part be because it is impossible to carry out therapy for SSD without drawing attention to sounds in words. Even the most articulatory of approaches require children to listen, copy, and adjust their own productions. Sound-facilitation techniques give visual and verbal instructions on how to produce phonemes, and the child's developing articulatory precision feeds back to refine the stored representations.

Gillon (2005) addressed the apparent conflict between the desire to include phoneme awareness in intervention (frequently delivered to preschool or certainly preliterate children) and the age at which phoneme awareness typically emerges (alongside literacy when children are around 6 years of age). Her participants were 12 children with SSD age 3 years on entry to the study (preschoolers in the New Zealand education system). They received on average 25 sessions (19 hours) of therapy between 3 and 5 years, before school entry. Intervention integrated three areas: speech production, phoneme awareness, and letter knowledge. Phoneme awareness concentrated on awareness of word-initial consonants, later introducing segmentation of simple words into phonemes, and did not include more difficult phoneme manipulation tasks. Progress was compared with that of a control group of age-matched typically developing children. Both groups improved at a similar rate for rhyme awareness and letter recognition, but the children with SSD made a significantly greater gain in phoneme matching. The similar improvement in rhyme without PA intervention supports the idea that rhyme tasks are not an essential component of therapy. There was no difference between the children with SSD and their typically developing peers on the PIPA at school entry or 1 year later. Although the PIPA was not administered prior to therapy, mean performance of children with SSD is usually lower than that of typically developing speakers; therefore, a positive result of the intervention is implied, although not explicitly demonstrated. A second control group consisted of age-matched children with SSD who had received therapy not including specific PA work (although some had experienced Metaphon therapy). At the time of comparison, the children were ages 5;6–7;6, and the average amount of therapy received was comparable with the experimental group. Children in the experimental group scored significantly higher on the PIPA than did the control children, supporting the beneficial effect of the integrated therapy on PA development.

There has been little research into therapy directly targeting phonological representations. However, Rvachew, Nowak, and Cloutier (2004) did just this by giving children intervention based on mispronunciation detection versus a control activity of story listening. Both groups also received standard speech and language therapy. Following intervention, children in the experimental group performed better at mispronunciation detection itself but not in rime and onset detection PA tasks.

The Effect of Phonological Awareness Instruction on Literacy and Language Abilities

The Ehri et al. (2001) meta-analysis showed that phonemic awareness instruction had a moderate impact on reading and spelling, which was stronger when PA activities were linked to letters. It was effective for various types of children (typically developing children, at-risk children, and children with reading disabilities), from (U.S.) preschool to first grade and from differing socioeconomic backgrounds. The review gives further indications on provision. Within these studies, phonemic awareness was most effective when accompanied by letter instruction, when taught in small groups, and when just one or two skills were taught at a time. Optimal length of intervention was between 5 and 18 hours. This provides compelling evidence of the value of phonemic awareness activities for reading acquisition in general, although children with SSD were not specifically included.

Gillon has shown in a series of papers that an approach to therapy that integrates PA and speech practice can have a beneficial effect on literacy outcome. Gillon (2000) demonstrated greater progress on a range of real and nonword reading tasks for children receiving PA intervention than for the groups receiving traditional therapy or advice only. At follow-up 1 year later (Gillon, 2002), the children receiving PA intervention continued to make more progress than the children receiving traditional therapy and were reading at least to an age-appropriate level, although there was a great deal of variability and overlap between the two groups. In Gillon's (2005) study of younger children, the experimental PA-plus-speech group performed significantly higher on real and nonword reading and on spelling than did the children whose therapy was production-based only. Although there was (as ever) a wide range of performance in the group who received PA, they were all reading at or above an age-appropriate level, in contrast to the control group of children with SSD.

In contrast, some studies do not show a clear and lasting benefit for reading. Nancollis et al. (2005) found no effect of PA intervention on reading age or nonword reading 2 years after a period of intervention, both groups performing within normal limits. The participants in this study were not selected as having either speech-language or literacy difficulties but were potentially at risk for underachievement in the latter because of their low socioeconomic background. The findings of Nancollis et al. do not concur with the Ehri et al. (2001) conclusion that PA instruction benefits socioeconomically disadvantaged children and those with normal-range reading; the differences in these studies may be due to the syllable and rhyme focus of Nancollis et al., the nature of the reading assessment, or the 2-year gap between intervention and assessment. Denne et al. (2005) did not find an effect on single-word reading and spelling as both their treated and untreated groups improved, although the PA intervention group did show a significant advantage in nonword reading. The gap between pre- and posttesting in this study was only 2 months, with posttesting following closely after the end of intervention. It may be that more time is required for PA developments to show up in literacy improvement.

The Effect of Phonological Awareness Instruction on Speech

In comparison with the effect of PA on literacy, there is less research regarding whether working on PA affects speech. Some studies have concluded a beneficial effect, at least for some children. Rvachew et al. (2004) found that their experimental group who had received phonological representation therapy had a higher percentage of consonants correct (PCC) postintervention than the control group. Howell et al. (1993) measured change in process use in a case series of 13 children receiving the Metaphon program, showing reduction in processes in all children postintervention. However, varying patterns of change in control processes and other linguistic measures made it impossible to be sure that Metaphon was the specific cause of improvement. Moriarty and Gillon (2006) used PA intervention with three children with childhood apraxia of speech (CAS), arguing that previous typical intervention for this population had overemphasized articulatory drill and ignored the PA limitations. The children described in three single case studies were between 6;3 and 7;3 and received just nine sessions of therapy focusing on an individually chosen phonological process. Intervention involved PA work integrated with speech production opportunities. All children improved (to different degrees) in some aspects of phoneme awareness. Two out of the three children also showed significant speech improvement on the target process with less or nonsignificant change on a control process. The speech of the third (and most severe) child did not show significant improvement. Results from these children suggest that lack of stimulability for the speech target and low nonverbal cognitive ability are negative prognostic indicators, although this would need to be confirmed in further studies.

Other studies have shown that the inclusion of PA activities, which we know to be helpful for literacy, does not impede speech progress. Gillon's focus on PA is predominantly to assist children with literacy development, and because she uses PA in an integrated approach alongside speech production work, it is not possible to identify the specific contribution of PA to progress. However, she has consistently demonstrated that the integration of PA and speech work leads to speech outcomes equally as good as for a similar amount of intervention focused on speech only (Gillon 2000, 2002, 2005). This is an important finding with implications for the effective and efficient provision of therapy for children with SSD. Hesketh, Adams, Nightingale, and Hall (2000) compared the effects of a predominantly PA approach with an intervention focusing on production practice. Sixty-one children ages 3;6–5;0 received 10 sessions of therapy and were assessed immediately postintervention and then again 3 months later. Children in both groups improved more in PCC during intervention than they did in a period with no therapy, but there was no significant difference between the groups in PCC change. Production-based therapy had a significantly greater immediate effect on the specific therapy targets, whereas nonsignificant trends in the results suggest PA intervention may have had a broader and longer-lasting effect on speech output. The latter requires confirmation in further research. As with single-word literacy, Denne et al. (2005) did not find a difference between their treated and untreated groups in PCC, both groups showing some improvement.

Summary of Empirical Basis

An overview of the evidence shows that targeting PA in therapy improves PA, and that children as young as 4 years can be taught simple phoneme awareness tasks. Targeting PA alongside letter knowledge leads to improved literacy performance, and integrating PA with speech work leads to speech improvement as great as that seen with a focus on speech alone. All studies mention a variability, both in PA levels and in response to intervention; those children likely to show the most progress are (unsurprisingly) those at a stage of cognitive readiness to learn phoneme awareness. Tables 10.2 and 10.3 summarize the level of evidence for the research reviewed in this chapter.

Table 10.2. Levels of evidence for studies of treatment efficacy for metaphonological intervention

Level	Description	References
Ia	Meta-analysis of > 1 randomized controlled trial	Ehri et al. (2001)
Ib	Randomized controlled study	Hesketh et al. (2007); Rvachew et al. (2004)
IIa	Controlled study without randomization	Denne et al. (2005);* Gillon (2000, 2002, 2005); Nancollis et al. (2005)
IIb	Quasi-experimental study	Hesketh, Adams, Nightingale, & Hall (2000)
III	Nonexperimental studies, i.e., correlational and case studies	Howell et al. (1993; Moriarty & Gillon (2006)
IV	Expert committee report, consensus conference, clinical experience of respected authorities	—

Adapted from the Scottish Intercollegiate Guidelines Network (http://www.sign.ac.uk).

*Denne et al. (2005) was a randomized study, but numbers were small and postintervention assessors were not blinded to group allocation.

Table 10.3. Topic of the main studies reviewed

Topic	Author	Level
The effect of targeting PA on speech	Howell et al. (1993)	III
The effect of targeting PA on PA skills, reading, and speech	Gillon (2000, 2002) Denne et al. (2005)	IIa IIa
The effect of targeting PA on PA skills and speech	Hesketh et al. (2000)	IIb
The effect of targeting PA on PA skills, reading, and spelling	Ehri et al. (2001)	Ia
The effect of targeting PA and phonological representations on PA, representations, and speech	Rvachew et al. (2004)	Ib
The effect of an integrated PA and speech approach on PA, literacy, and speech	Gillon (2005)	IIa
The effect of targeting PA on PA and single-word reading/spelling	Nancollis et al. (2005)	IIa
The effect of an integrated PA and speech approach on PA, literacy-related skills, and speech in children with CAS	Moriarty & Gillon (2006)	III
The effect of targeting PA on PA skills	Hesketh et al. (2007)	Ib

Key: CAS, childhood apraxia of speech; PA, phonological awareness.

Having reviewed both the theoretical and the empirical evidence relevant to PA, the following is known:

- PA, and particularly phoneme awareness, are important factors in early literacy acquisition. Similar evidence is emerging about internally stored phonological lexical representations.

- Children with SSD, as a group, have poorer PA skills than typically developing peers, and similar evidence is emerging about phonological representations.

- Children with SSD are therefore, as a group, at risk for literacy difficulties, and this risk is significantly greater if they also have delayed language.

- Some children with pure SSD have good PA skills, and this subgroup has a good prognosis for literacy.

- Less is known about the role of PA and representations in speech acquisition and speech change.

- Teaching phoneme awareness leads to improvement in phoneme awareness *and* in literacy in many different populations.

- Some aspects of phoneme awareness (awareness and identification, but not manipulation of phonemes) can be taught to preschool children.

- There is no evidence that PA needs to be taught separately or as a precursor to speech development.

- Integrating PA work into therapy for SSD can have beneficial long-term effects on literacy while achieving equally good speech outcomes as production-focused intervention.

PRACTICAL REQUIREMENTS

Nature of Sessions

As an integrated component of intervention, PA can fit into a variety of models of therapy delivery. It has been described in the literature as part of small-group and individual speech and language sessions, and as a program run in conjunction with education staff. Ehri et al. (2001) concluded that school-based PA instruction in support of literacy was most effective given in small groups, but Gillon (2000, 2005) showed that a metaphonological element can be very successfully incorporated into individual SLP sessions.

Personnel

Intervention should be planned by the SLP as the professional with the relevant knowledge of the child's sound system, PA abilities, and psycholinguistic speech processing profile. Parents, teachers, and classroom support workers are vital sources of information; they know about a child's intelligibility, generalization, overall level of educational and literacy progress, and, specifically, the words or letters they are working on in school. Parents, teachers, and classroom support workers are also vital sources of support in practicing tasks and carrying out programs, *but* they will need ample opportunity to observe and to discuss therapy in order to do this reliably and effectively. Tasks are subtle and require detailed understanding of phonemes and their relationship to letters; minor changes in task presentation or response required can lead to totally different demands on the child. Therefore working through other agents requires accurate and detailed descriptions and demonstrations of how to carry out the tasks.

Dosage

PA intervention has been reported as part of weekly or several-times weekly therapy. Gillon (2000) gave twenty 1-hour individual sessions at the rate of two per week. Participants in Gillon's (2005) study received either two or three blocks of therapy of 4–6 weeks, consisting of one 45-minute individual and one group session per week. Both of the above models led to improvement in PA and speech accuracy. Improvement in children's PA skills has been shown after 18 sessions of 30–45 minutes duration, two or three times a week (Hesketh et al., 2000) and from eight weekly ½-hour sessions (Denne et al., 2005). In summary, studies showing significant effects of PA therapy offered between 10 and 27 hours of intervention.

KEY COMPONENTS

Nature of Goals

The broad goal of PA therapy is to increase the child's awareness of word forms and how his or her own differ from the adult target, with the aim of facilitating speech change and literacy acquisition. Metaphonological awareness should be integrated into or alternated with speech production tasks, making the PA activities specifically relevant to the speech target.

Goal Attack Strategies

As the metaphonological awareness activities are linked to the speech targets, they will follow whatever goal strategy is chosen for speech work. The level of metaphonological awareness demanded of the child will gradually increase along developmental lines.

Description of Activities

General Principles

Many factors determine the details of therapy for children with SSD. The auditory perceptual and discriminatory skills, ease of articulation, attention level, motivation, and confidence of a child will all influence the choice of target, the length of session, and the balance of tasks in it. Likewise with metaphonological activities—these will be used more with some children than others and more at some stages of therapy than others. Dodd and Gillon (2001) stressed that because not all children with SSD have poor PA and not all go on to have literacy difficulties, we should not accept nonspecific PA programs as a standard approach. But integration of metaphonological activities into therapy specifically tailored to a child's speech pattern is different and has been shown by Gillon (2000, 2002, 2005) not to hinder speech progress.

The following description should be read in the context of my typical caseload, which includes children ages 4–10 years (mostly 4–7 years) whose SSD is their most salient communication problem. They are almost all within normal limits for overall cognitive development and receptive language, and they do not have structural or neurological diagnoses. This is the population with which I have most experience in applying metaphonological therapy, and the population on which most research for the approach is based.

For children whose peripheral auditory or articulation skills are low, I am less likely to use metaphonological tasks as a central component of therapy. A child who is unable to discriminate between sounds or words on same–different or ABX tasks (Locke, 1980) is not ready to *reflect* on those sounds in words and on the phonological details of their own speech production. If the failure was in a child with good attention, motivation, cognitive, and linguistic skills, then I would devote some time within sessions to working on auditory skills, helping him or her to discriminate among widely differing lexical stimuli, gradually narrowing to widely differing initial phonemes and achieving confidence at that level. Then the child would be ready to identify the more subtle distinctions between his or her errors and target, to begin to isolate phonemes within words, and to reflect on ways in which his or her speech needs to change. Because there is little evidence to suggest that it is necessary to master syllable segmentation or rhyme awareness before moving on to simple phoneme level tasks, I would not include these as a precursor to phoneme awareness. If the problem appeared to be the child's overall cognitive/linguistic maturity, then I would not emphasize metaphonological awareness in therapy until he or she appeared ready to benefit.

Children who cannot easily produce a target sound and need articulation practice at a single-sound or nonsense-syllable level will need to prioritize production attempts during the session. PA activities drawing attention to the new sound can be useful intervening tasks to take the pressure off potentially frustrating practice. Integration of the metaphonological and production elements can take place as soon as the child is attempting the target sound/process at word level. It is vital to bear in mind the child's articulation capacity. Grunwell said of phonological therapy that "the changes in speech production need to take place not so much in the mouth but in the mind of the child" (1987, p. 280).

Change, however, has to happen in the mouth as well, and advances in PA will not be reflected in speech improvement until the child can easily produce the new lexical forms. Because it is not closely correlated with the severity of the SSD, the relative contribution of PA to the problem has to be assessed on an individual basis. This will determine the weighting of metaphonological work and the way in which it is integrated with production practice.

It can be argued that metaphonological work is not essential for those children who have good PA and whose difficulties are primarily on the motor side. However, the addition of minimal pair tasks to emphasize the *need* to change speech alongside increased metalinguistic awareness of *how* to change it can make therapy more efficient. It can also support continued progress during breaks in therapy and aid generalization to processes other than the immediate target. It may be that a child's lexical representations are accurate and PA abilities are within the normal range but stored automatic motor programs remain in immature form. In such a case, therapy needs to provide many opportunities for production practice, but metaphonological work drawing attention to the target can help remind the child of the need to override the automatic production with a new version.

If, as research tells us, PA progresses from large to small units, is it necessary to teach every step in the typical developmental order? Clinical research evidence says no, this is not necessary (Anthony & Francis, 2005; Carroll et al., 2003; Hesketh et al., 2006). It is also acknowledged that rhyme awareness can be stimulated by more general language activities (Gillon, 2005). Awareness of phonemes and their presence in different word positions seems intuitively to be more relevant in changing common speech processes. Within the phoneme level, however, there are a multitude of task variations that make different demands on the child. For example, commonly used tasks requiring awareness of word-initial phonemes include

- Initial phoneme isolation (e.g., "Tell me the first sound in...")

- Phoneme identification from a given target across words (e.g., "Find me all the words beginning with...")

- Phoneme isolation and identification across words (e.g., "This puppet's name is Dan. Find me all the toys that start with the same sound as his name.")

- Odd one-out tasks (e.g., "Which of these words is the odd one out: *cat, car, fan, comb?*")

Within these examples it is hard to predict precisely which will be hardest for an individual child, although isolation and identification is usually harder than identification from a given target, and some suggest that odd-out tasks can be difficult for many children (Hulme et al., 2002).

Phonemes are made more tangible in therapy by linking them to either memorable pictures or to graphemes. I include written letters on materials presented to children, but the extent to which we rely on them depends on the literacy level of the child. For the purposes of speech intervention, the child needs to understand what sound we are discussing and, in working on speech, I will prioritize this understanding over the desire to reinforce letter knowledge. However, graphemes will be used and mentioned more and more as children become more familiar with literacy at school. The introduction of letters can restrict word choice; as well as being pictureable and within a child's vocabulary, it may be necessary to use only words that are regularly spelled, or to avoid digraphs. I may therefore choose to ignore letters for certain tasks in order to include words that are useful for speech practice but that have unhelpful spellings.

The key components of my therapy approach include

- A detailed assessment from which the priority target is identified

- Articulation work if necessary to allow the child to produce the target sounds in isolation and in simple words

- Minimal pair tasks to confront the child with his or her problem and give the child the motivation to change

- Metaphonological work to help the child work out the mismatches in his or her speech and how to move toward the adult pattern

- Production practice to allow new motor patterns to become established and automatic

Although assessment will be the first step, the rest is not a staged program, and elements will overlap and return to prominence as necessary. I encourage phoneme-level awareness of the structure of words to help children understand how their speech differs from the normal template and how to change it in order to become more intelligible. In the longer term, this increased metaphonological awareness will underpin their development of reading and spelling. PA is not seen as a skill in its own right but is linked with speech tasks and with letters in order to support speech change and literacy.

Practical Examples

The following is a possible session plan for Rowan, a girl age 4;9, whose most salient speech features are stopping, deaffrication, backing, voicing, and cluster reduction, leading to a marked overuse of the voiced velar plosive. Rowan is in reception class (kindergarten), but with a July birthday she is one of the youngest in her year and is described by her teacher as slightly immature and not finding phonic and literacy work easy. She recognizes some letters, but picture cards are a better link to phonemes for her at the moment.

In a child with a strong sound preference, my aim would be to break up the resulting oversized phoneme. Rowan collapses /t/, /d/, /s/, /z/, /ʃ/, /tʃ/, /dʒ/, and /k/ to [g]. On imitation she can produce recognizable attempts at all the above except the alveolar plosives. By focusing on the sounds [s] and [tʃ], we can extend the child's range of manner, place, and voicing, and by contrasting them with her current favorite [g], we raise awareness of sounds and how her own production differs from the adult target. You could add other sounds in as well, but because this child is only 4;9, I would want to keep things relatively simple. Rowan can produce both [s] and [tʃ] easily in isolation and with effort word-initially. The tasks below use single-syllable words with the target sounds at the beginning. In addition, the session of course starts and ends with social exchanges, discussion of progress during the week, interpretation of performance within the session, and explanation of tasks for home practice.

Examples of some of the tasks are modeled on the accompanying DVD. Because of time constraints, the DVD clips show only those aspects that are primarily metaphonological. Within a whole session. I include tasks that are more output focused to give children plenty of opportunities to produce the target speech features, plus I frequently ask for spoken attempts at the words within the metaphonological tasks. Table 10.4 describes a whole session that incorporates the core metaphonological therapy aims (i.e., to make Rowan think about the structure of words in ways that are directly relevant to her speech patterns and to integrate this with production practice).

As Rowan begins to have consistent success at the phonemic awareness tasks, the emphasis will shift more to production practice with the awareness activities being used as reminders when necessary. When the target changes, (maybe to introduce new sounds, or to extend use of [s] and [tʃ] to other word positions), phoneme awareness tasks are given more prominence again. As she becomes more confident in literacy, letter names would be given more prominence in feedback and explanations, although it is necessary to check her knowledge with what she has learned at school, especially for the digraph *ch*.

In this particular suggested plan there happen to be no minimal pair tasks, but I use them often in therapy to demonstrate to children the need to change their speech and the improvement in being understood when they do use the expected sound in the expected word position. Understanding both the need for change and how to achieve it are powerful drivers for speech development in children with SSD. Even in a child who has age-appropriate PA skills, metaphonology will form a component of my intervention, and in any case, I do not see how it is possible to engage a child in practicing and changing speech without stimulating or demanding some awareness of sounds in words. On the other hand, I never provide therapy that focuses only on PA. It is always an integrated part of an approach that will involve some speech production practice, too.

Of course the activities described are only a small sample of possible tasks, and there are many subtle variations that can make them more difficult, more literacy based, more physically active, or more fun. Encouraging metaphonological awareness can be integrated into almost any therapy task and adapted to any phonological goal. Several excellent resources are available that provide further therapy suggestions, for example, Schuele and Boudreau's (2008) practical advice based on research evidence and clinical experience. Gillon's materials from her whole series of intervention studies are generously available on the University of Canterbury's College of Education web site (http://www.education.canterbury.ac.nz/people/gillon/resources.shtml).

Materials and Equipment Required

The equipment required is low-tech and standard within SLP clinical and educational settings. The basic need is a way of making abstract phonemes/sounds into concrete entities that a child can think about. When children are moving into literacy, written letters may

Table 10.4. Example session plan for Rowan

Instructions	Materials
Task 1. Reminder of sounds	
Remind Rowan that we are thinking about words that begin with certain sounds. Introduce each sheet in turn, point out the letter, remind her how the picture is linked to the sound, and ask her to imitate each one.	Large sheet of paper for each sound [s], [tʃ], and [g], showing both the letter and a picture cue
Task 2. Sorting words according to their initial consonant	
Spread the sheets of paper out in front of Rowan. Shuffle the pictures so that the order is not predictable and Rowan has to think, not guess. Explain to Rowan that you will say the words and she will work out which sound it begins with and put the picture on the corresponding sheet. Feedback reinforces why she is right or wrong (e.g., "That's right, *soap* has an [s] at the beginning" *or* "You've chosen the [g] picture. If *soap* had a [g] at the beginning, it would sound like this, [gəʊp]. Let's listen again").	Sheets from task 1. Pictures of words beginning with each of the three sounds
Task 3. Production practice	
Praise Rowan for sorting out the pictures and remind her they are now in piles beginning with the same sound. Also remind her that she often uses [g] on too many words and we are practicing saying words with the sounds they need at the beginning. By going through the pictures one pile at a time, we should get a high rate of success and as much error-free production practice as possible because Rowan can concentrate on getting the output right and not have the added load of switching sound all the time. (Alternatively, you could integrate production practice into task 2 and ask Rowan to say each word after she's sorted it.) Praise should reinforce why she was successful (e.g., she used the right sound at the beginning of the words, she had worked out what that sound was).	Sheets with the pictures on them as they ended up at the end of the last task
Task 4. Mispronunciation detection	
Explain to Rowan that she is now the teacher and has to tell you whether you are saying words right or wrong. Shuffle the cards and say the words, getting approximately half right and half wrong but not in a predictable pattern. All mistakes on [s] and [tʃ] words should be to substitute Rowan's typical initial [g]. Feedback reinforces why words were right or wrong. For each item you said incorrectly, ask Rowan to identify which sound you used and which sound it should have been, and then ask her to say each word. This task taps phonological representations by asking Rowan to match her internal template for a word against someone else's production.	Set of 12 pictures of words with word-initial [s], [tʃ], and [g] (four of each). Use different pictures/words from the previous tasks.
Task 5. Categorization by initial sound and production practice	
Mix together all the pictures. Explain to Rowan that you are going to play a game with the words beginning with [s] and [tʃ] and that she will help you sort them out from the words beginning with [g]. As you say each word Rowan indicates whether to keep it or discard it [g] words). This should be very quick as it is a revision of task 3. Then play a game such as lotto with the [s] and [tʃ] initial words offering lots of production opportunities.	All pictures used so far. Lotto game for the 16 [s] and [tʃ] words
Task 6. Categorization from internal representation	
This task is the same as task 2, but this time you don't say the words aloud. Explain to Rowan that once again she is to work out which sound a word begins with but this time you're not going to say it and neither is she. She just needs to think about the word quietly and put it on the right picture. (It's best if children do this silently, otherwise their own incorrect production can mislead them. However, many children do at least a whispered rehearsal, as can be seen in the DVD demonstration). This is a more difficult task tapping internal representations, and it may be that Rowan would not succeed on it at 4;9. If it is too hard it can be turned back into task 2 by the therapist saying the words. Give one final round of production practice as you put each card away.	Set of six pictures of words with word-initial [s], [tʃ], and [g] (two for each sound) selected from those used in the session so far. Sheets from tasks 1–3.
Summary	
Summarize for Rowan what she has achieved (e.g., thinking about the sounds in words, working out which sound should be at the beginning of a word, and using that knowledge to help her say words well).	

be the main support, but for younger children it is often useful to have a picture link, too (e.g., a snake for [s]). Activities can be computer-based, and it is possible to make (selective) use of the extensive literacy support resources. Relevant speech-specific computer resources are available, too, such as the Phoneme Factory Sound Sorter (Wren & Roulstone, 2005) and the Speech Assessment and Interactive Learning System (SAILS; AVAAZ Innovations, 1994). The skilled clinician will use a range of approaches to keep sessions varied and interesting, but specialist equipment is not essential.

ASSESSMENT AND PROGRESS MONITORING TO SUPPORT DECISION MAKING

The research evidence shows that working on PA is both effective and efficient. Therefore, within day-to-day clinical work there is no need to re-demonstrate to experimental levels the specific contribution of metaphonological tasks to a child's progress. However, regular recording of performance on tasks and careful noting of differential performance across tasks allows clinically sensible decisions about the amount and type of meta phonological work that is appropriate for an individual child. These decisions will be informed by consultations with parents and teachers.

PA abilities can be formally assessed using standardized tools as listed earlier. PA in young children is variable, confidence intervals on tests are wide, and PA ability may well be influenced by speech intervention. For these reasons, assessment of PA *following* speech intervention may be a more reliable guide to a child's PA level and prognosis for early literacy (Hesketh, 2004). Children with a relatively pure SSD are at a low risk for literacy acquisition problems (Snowling & Hayiou-Thomas, 2006). However, within this population, PA abilities are an important predictor: Hesketh (2004) showed that PA delay at the end of therapy meant that children were more likely to have reading difficulties at 6;6–7;6, whereas children whose PA skills were within normal limits after therapy almost all went on to perform within the normal range in single-word reading and spelling. This chapter has been concerned with metaphonological components of therapy for speech problems. However, if PA remains low after speech has reached an acceptable level and particularly if language is also delayed, then further PA intervention may be indicated, focusing specifically on literacy. Whether this is seen as the SLP's role varies across services.

CONSIDERATIONS FOR CHILDREN FROM CULTURALLY AND LINGUISTICALLY DIVERSE BACKGROUNDS

PA ability is not language specific. There is evidence of transferability of phonological processing skills across even diverse languages such as English to French, Portuguese, and Chinese, where PA ability tested in a child's first language predicts literacy achievement in both the child's first and second language (see Lafrance & Gottardo, 2005, for a review). The sequence of development of PA from large to smaller unit awareness is also common across languages, although detailed patterns of development may differ depending on the salience of phoneme boundaries, the complexity of syllable structure, stress versus syllable timing, the number of phonemes, and phonotactic constraints (Anthony & Francis, 2005; Lafrance & Gottardo, 2005). Learning to read progresses at different rates and may involve different stages according to the regularity of a language's orthography; reading of transparent languages such as Spanish and Dutch is learned more quickly than reading English and can be more fully mastered by reaching the alphabetic stage (Seymour, Aro, & Erskine, 2003). The downside of this is that impairments in PA can have a greater effect on learning to read a "shallow" orthographic language, more so than in English in which development of visual and orthographic strategies is necessary and potentially compensatory.

The ease of integration of metaphonological work may vary across languages. Linking PA with literacy in languages such as Spanish is made easier by the regular and transparent correspondence between phonemes and letters. Whatever the features, however, because PA is a universal skill, an increased awareness of the individual phonemes of a word should generalize bidirectionally among languages in multilingual children. Although it might be necessary to address separately phonological speech errors specific to the individual languages, work on PA in one language should prepare the child for thinking about word structure in the other.

CASE STUDIES

Joey

Joey, age 4;6, was a very chatty, confident boy who was largely unintelligible to strangers and showed little insight into his speech. At school, although his peers were beginning to recognize some letters and their sounds, he was having difficulty hearing sounds in words and retaining letter knowledge. Joey had good syllable structure but stopped all fricatives and affricates, also fronting velars and postalveolar consonants to the alveolar position. He was an enthusiastic participant in therapy games but had little metaphonological awareness of what or how to change. The introduction of too many sounds, either in PA tasks or in a cycles approach to production, had left Joey confused in the past. It was therefore decided to focus on the labiodental fricatives /f/ and /v/. He could produce [f] word-initially with a gap before the vowel but never used it spontaneously. We did not worry about voicing distinctions, accepting [f] for either fricative.

In the first two sessions of therapy, Joey made excellent progress in producing word-initial labiodental fricatives with increasing accuracy and fluency within therapy tasks. However, as soon as we attempted to put these words into phrases, or to use /f/ and /v/ word-finally, Joey's lack of awareness about word structure became very apparent. He had no idea where the target sounds should go and simply continued to use a labiodental at the beginning of each word or phrase.

Because he was more tuned in to word-initial sounds, we prioritized the production of /f/- or /v/-initial words in phrases for the next two sessions. Using blocks to represent the words, we helped Joey first to identify how many words there were in a spoken phrase (either two or three) and, when he was confident in doing that, to identify which word contained the target sound. He put a sticker on the appropriate block and then attempted to repeat the phrase, with the sticker acting as a location cue for the fricative.

In three further sessions we used smaller blocks to represent the separate phonemes in consonant-vowel-consonant words. Joey was not able to segment words but did learn to identify the word position of the target sounds and was then able to produce a word-final labiodental fricative with some effort. In the last session he was able to identify which word in a short phrase contained a word-final /f/ or /v/ and was able to produce the fricative if it was in the final word of the phrase. Each of the seven sessions began and ended with a reminder of the target sounds linked to their written letters, and there were many more reminders about the target sounds and many production opportunities in each session.

At the end of this period of therapy, Joey was producing a labiodental fricative in word-initial and final positions and was much more aware of what he needed to do, but he still consistently stopped both /f/ and /v/ in conversation. When he was seen after a break of 6 weeks, his progress had generalized to spontaneous speech, and Joey was using labiodental fricatives whenever required. In working on further speech targets, he showed much better awareness of the sounds and their position in words; initial progress was slower because alveolar and postalveolar fricatives were less stimulable, but once articulation was established, their transfer into words was quicker. Joey's teacher reported improving letter-sound knowledge, and by the end of the school year his performance was in line with his peers.

Nick

Nick, age 9;6, has a history of language and reading delay. Following intervention his receptive language scores are now within normal limits but he continues to have difficulty with both reading and spelling. His PA abilities on formal testing are 2 standard deviations below the norm, and his speech is frequently unintelligible. Nick's speech and spelling errors are particularly obvious in word endings, consonant clusters in any position, and polysyllabic words, and he has had little idea how to correct them. He is able to articulate most English consonants but does not have access to a robust underlying phonological representation or output motor program.

Because of his age and continuing literacy difficulties, therapy incorporates written forms in every task. We select words to be as structurally simple (other than the target feature) and as regularly spelled as possible, and we are focusing on initial clusters and word-final single consonants. Words are segmented and the components written onto individual squares of paper that Nick manipulates to produce new written words, which he then says aloud. We might start with asking Nick to form the word *wig*, then to select the appropriate letters to change it to *will*, to *win*, and to *wish*. For clusters, Nick might be asked which letter he needs to add, and where in the word, to change *lock* to *block* or *sick* to *stick*. The latter is much harder for him. Regular meetings with his school support worker allow back up of work between sessions.

Because of his age and profile, PA work with Nick has a heavy involvement of letters, and requires manipulation rather than just identification of sounds. Because of the severity of his problems, he can hardly be described as a success story yet, but PA is an essential skill for Nick to make progress, and he is beginning to be more analytical in both his spelling and in changing his speech when communication breaks down.

STUDY QUESTIONS

1. What is the difference between phonological and phonemic awareness?

2. At what age do typically developing children normally begin to develop phoneme-level awareness?

3. Why is work on phoneme-level awareness likely to be a good preparation for literacy development in children with SSD?

4. How can metaphonological work be integrated with speech and literacy components of intervention?

5. What is the evidence for the beneficial effect of including metaphonological awareness in intervention on 1) speech and 2) literacy?

FUTURE DIRECTIONS

Within the field of SSD, PA-based therapy has a particularly rich theoretical and clinical research base. Within the last 5 years there has been increasing interest in the related topic of phonological representations, the stored knowledge we have about the phonological form of words. Tasks have been developed that attempt to assess the detail and accuracy of children's representations, but we are as yet only in the preliminary stages of understanding this topic. The task most applicable to children around 4 years of age is mispronunciation detection. Studies have used different rules for creating the mispronunciations, and we need to know more about whether vowels or consonants are most appropriately used in assessment/intervention, whether children's own mispronunciations are harder for them to detect, and whether this fairly broad brush task is a sensitive enough tool. That is, if children can successfully detect mispronunciations, does this necessarily mean that their underlying lexical representations are fully specified? Conversely, if a child shows apparent problems on assessment of phonological representations, does this necessarily mean the representations themselves are inadequate, or might it be a metalinguistic difficulty in reflecting on phonological knowledge?

We need to know more about the level of PA that is necessary to change speech and to update phonological representations. The evidence shows that PA is a useful addition to therapy that promotes both speech change and literacy development, but it is also clear that most children develop speech perfectly well without a conscious ability to reflect on word structure at the phoneme level. If a child is struggling with metaphonological aspects of therapy, should we abandon it and take an approach that requires less active learning? This might yield better results for speech in the short term but is likely to leave the child vulnerable to literacy difficulties later. At what age is metaphonological intervention most efficient? Should we ensure that children are stimulable for speech sounds before we spend time on PA tasks involving those sounds? How efficient is the approach for children with additional language or cognitive problems?

In summary, we already know a lot about the mechanisms of PA and the benefits of metaphonological intervention. Efficiency of provision and the relationship between metaphonological awareness and underlying phonological representations are important areas for future research.

SUGGESTED READINGS

Carroll, J.M., Snowling, M.J., Hulme, C., & Stevenson, J. (2003). The development of phonological awareness in preschool children. *Developmental Psychology, 39,* 913–923.

Gillon, G.T. (2004). *Phonological awareness: From research to practice.* New York: Guilford Press.

Hesketh, A., Dima, E., & Nelson, V. (2007). Teaching phoneme awareness to pre-literate children with speech disorder: A randomized controlled trial. *International Journal of Language and Communication Disorders, 42*(3), 251–271.

Sutherland, D., & Gillon, G.T. (2007). Development of phonological representations and phonological awareness in children with speech impairment. *International Journal of Language and Communication Disorders, 42*(2), 229–250.

REFERENCES

Anthony, J.L., & Francis, D.J. (2005). Development of phonological awareness. *Current Directions in Psychological Science, 14*(5), 255–259.

AVAAZ Innovations, Inc. (1994). Speech Assessment and Interactive Learning System (Version 1.2) [Computer software]. London, Ontario, Canada: Author.

Bird, J., Bishop, D.V.M., & Freeman, N.H. (1995). Phonological awareness and literacy development in children with expressive phonological impairment. *Journal of Speech and Hearing Research, 38,* 446–462.

Bishop, D.V.M., & Adams, C. (1990). A prospective study of the relationship between specific language impairment, phonological disorders and reading retardation. *Journal of Child Psychology and Psychiatry, 31*(7), 1027–1050.

Bishop, D.V.M., & Snowling, M.J. (2004). Developmental dyslexia and specific language impairment: Same or different? *Psychological Bulletin, 130*(6), 858–886.

Carroll, J.M., & Snowling, M.J. (2004). Language and phonological skills in children at high risk of reading difficulties. *Journal of Child Psychology and Psychiatry, 45*(3), 631–640.

Carroll, J.M., Snowling, M.J., Hulme, C., & Stevenson, J. (2003). The development of phonological awareness in preschool children. *Developmental Psychology, 39,* 913–923.

Catts, H.W. (1993). The relationship between speech-language impairments and reading disabilities. *Journal of Speech and Hearing Research, 36,* 948–958.

Catts, H.W., Wilcox, K.A., Wood-Jackson, C., Larrivee, L.S., & Scott, V.G. (1997). Towards an understanding of phonological awareness. In C.K. Leong & R.M. Joshi (Eds.), *Cross-language studies of learning to read and spell* (pp. 31–52). Amsterdam: Kluwer Academic Publishers.

Claessen, M., Heath, S., Fletcher, J., Hogben, J., & Leitão, S. (2009). Quality of phonological representations: A window into the lexicon? *International Journal of Language & Communication Disorders, 44*(2), 121–144.

Denne, M., Langdown, N., Pring, T., & Roy, P. (2005). Treating children with expressive phonological disorders: Does phonological awareness therapy work in the clinic? *International Journal of Language and Communication Disorders, 40*(4), 493–504.

Dodd, B., Crosbie, S., McIntosh, B., Teitzel, T., & Ozanne, A. (2000). *Pre-school and Primary Inventory of Phonological Awareness.* London: Pearson PsychCorp.

Dodd, B., & Gillon, G.T. (2001). Exploring the relationship between phonological awareness, speech impairment and literacy. *Advances in Speech-Language Pathology, 3*(2), 139–147.

Dodd, B., Hua, Z., Crosbie, C., Holm, A., & Ozanne, A. (2002). *Diagnostic Evaluation of Articulation and Phonology.* London: Pearson PsychCorp.

Dodd, B., Hua, Z., Crosbie, S., Holm, A., & Ozanne, A. (2006). *Diagnostic Evaluation of Articulation and Phonology (DEAP).* San Antonio, TX: Pearson Assessment.

Ehri, L.C., Nunes, S.R., Willows, D.M., Schuster, B.V., Yaghoub-Zadeh, Z., & Shanahan, T. (2001). Phonemic awareness instruction helps children learn to read: Evidence from the National Reading Panel's meta-analysis. *Reading Research Quarterly, 36*(3), 250–287.

Frith, U. (1985). Beneath the surface of developmental dyslexia. In K.E. Patterson, J.C. Marshall, & M. Coltheart (Eds.), *Surface dyslexia* (pp. 301–330). London: Lawrence Erlbaum Associates.

Gillon, G.T. (2000). The efficacy of phonological awareness intervention for children with spoken language impairment. *Language, Speech, and Hearing Services in Schools, 31,* 126–141.

Gillon, G.T. (2002). Follow-up study investigating the benefits of phonological awareness intervention for children with spoken language impairment. *International Journal of Language and Communication Disorders, 37*(4), 381–400.

Gillon, G.T. (2004). *Phonological awareness: From research to practice.* New York: Guilford Press.

Gillon, G.T. (2005). Facilitating phoneme awareness development in 3- and 4-year-old children with speech impairment. *Language, Speech, and Hearing Services in Schools, 36*(4), 308–324.

Grunwell, P. (1987). *Clinical phonology* (2nd ed.). Kent, England: Croom Helm.

Hesketh, A. (2004). Early literacy achievement of children with a history of speech problems. *International Journal of Language and Communication Disorders, 39*(4), 453–468.

Hesketh, A., Adams, C., & Nightingale, C. (2000). Metaphonological abilities of phonologically disordered children. *Educational Psychology, 20*(4), 484–498.

Hesketh, A., Adams, C., Nightingale, C., & Hall, R. (2000). Phonological awareness therapy and articulatory training approaches for children with phonological disorders: A comparative outcome study. *International Journal of Language and Communication Disorders, 35*(3), 337–354.

Hesketh, A., Dima, E., & Nelson, V. (2006, May). *Should we spend time working on rhyme?* Paper presented at the Royal College of Speech and Language Therapists National Conference, Belfast, Ireland.

Hesketh, A., Dima, E., & Nelson, V. (2007). Teaching phoneme awareness to pre-literate children with speech disorder: A randomized controlled trial. *International Journal of Language and Communication Disorders, 42*(3), 251–271.

Holm, A., Farrier, F., & Dodd, B. (2008). Phonological awareness, reading accuracy and spelling ability of children with inconsistent phonological disorder. *International Journal of Language and Communication Disorders, 43*(3), 300–322.

Howell, J., Hill, A., Dean, E., & Waters, D. (1993). Increasing metalinguistic awareness to assist phonological change. In D. Messer (Ed.), *Critical influences on child language acquisition and development* (pp. 209–228). London: Macmillan.

Hulme, C., Hatcher, P.J., Nation, K., Brown, A., Adams, J., & Stuart, G. (2002). Phoneme awareness is a better predictor of early reading skill than onset-rime awareness. *Journal of Experimental Child Psychology, 82*(1), 2–28.

Lafrance, A., & Gottardo, A. (2005). A longitudinal study of phonological processing skills and reading in bilingual children. *Applied Psycholinguistics, 26*(4), 559–578.

Laing, S.P., & Espeland, W. (2005). Low intensity phonological awareness training in a preschool classroom for children with communication impairments. *Journal of Communication Disorders, 38*(1), 65–82.

Leitão, S., Hogben, J., & Fletcher, J. (1997). Phonological processing skills in speech and language impaired children. *European Journal of Disorders of Communication, 32*(2, Special Issue), 91–111.

Locke, J.L. (1980). The inference of speech perception in the phonologically disordered child. Part II: Some clinically novel procedures, their use, some findings. *Journal of Speech and Hearing Disorders, 45*(4), 445–468.

Mann, V.A., & Foy, J.G. (2007). Speech development patterns and phonological awareness in preschool children. *Annals of Dyslexia, 57*(1), 51–74.

Metsala, J.L. (1999). Young children's phonological awareness and nonword repetition as a function of vocabulary development. *Journal of Educational Psychology, 91*(1), 3–19.

Moriarty, B.C., & Gillon, G.T. (2006). Phonological awareness intervention for children with childhood apraxia of speech. *International Journal of Language and Communication Disorders, 41*(6), 713–734.

Munro, N., Lee, K., & Baker, E. (2008). Building vocabulary knowledge and phonological awareness skills in children with specific language impairment through hybrid language intervention: A feasibility study. *International Journal of Language and Communication Disorders, 43*(6), 662–682.

Muter, V., Hulme, C., & Snowling, M.J. (1997). *Phonological Abilities Test.* Oxford, England: Pearson.

Nancollis, A., Lawrie, B.-A., & Dodd, B. (2005). Phonological awareness intervention and the acquisition of literacy skills in children from deprived social backgrounds. *Language, Speech, and Hearing Services in Schools, 36*(4), 325–335.

Nathan, L., Stackhouse, J., Goulandris, N., & Snowling, M.J. (2004). The development of early literacy skills among children with speech difficulties: A test of the "critical age hypothesis." *Journal of Speech, Language, and Hearing Research, 47*(2), 377–391.

Raitano, N.A., Pennington, B.F., Tunick, R.A., Boada, R., & Shriberg, L.D. (2004). Pre-literacy skills of subgroups of children with speech sound disorders. *Journal of Child Psychology and Psychiatry, 45*(4), 821–835.

Rvachew, S. (2006). Longitudinal predictors of implicit phonological awareness skills. *American Journal of Speech-Language Pathology, 15*(2), 165–176.

Rvachew, S. (2007). Phonological processing and reading in children with speech sound disorders. *American Journal of Speech-Language Pathology, 16*(3), 260–270.

Rvachew, S., & Grawburg, M. (2006). Correlates of phonological awareness in preschoolers with speech sound disorders. *Journal of Speech, Language, and Hearing Research, 49*(1), 74–87.

Rvachew, S., Nowak, M., & Cloutier, G. (2004). Effect of phonemic perception training on the speech production and phonological awareness skills of children with expressive phonological delay. *American Journal of Speech-Language Pathology, 13*(3), 250–263.

Rvachew, S., Ohberg, A., Grawburg, M., & Heyding, J. (2003). Phonological awareness and phonemic perception in 4-year-old children with delayed expressive phonology skills. *American Journal of Speech-Language Pathology, 12*(4), 463–471.

Schuele, C.M., & Boudreau, D. (2008). Phonological awareness intervention: Beyond the basics. *Language, Speech, and Hearing Services in Schools, 39*(1), 3–20.

Seymour, P.H.K., Aro, M., & Erskine, J.M. (2003). Foundation literacy acquisition in European orthographies. *British Journal of Psychology, 94*, 143–174.

Snowling, M.J., & Hayiou-Thomas, M.E. (2006). The dyslexia spectrum: Continuities between reading, speech, and language impairments. *Topics in Language Disorders, 26*(2), 110–126.

Snowling, M.J., Hulme, C., & Mercer, R.C. (2002). A deficit in rime awareness in children with Down syndrome. *Reading and Writing: An Interdisciplinary Journal, 15*, 471–495.

Stackhouse, J., & Wells, B. (1997). *Children's speech and literacy difficulties.* London: Whurr.

Sutherland, D., & Gillon, G.T. (2005). Assessment of phonological representations in children with speech impairment. *Language, Speech, and Hearing Services in Schools, 36*(4), 294–307.

Sutherland, D., & Gillon, G.T. (2007). Development of phonological representations and phonological awareness in children with speech impairment. *International Journal of Language and Communication Disorders, 42*(2), 229–250.

Vellutino, F.R., Fletcher, J.M., Snowling, M.J., & Scanlon, D.M. (2004). Specific reading disability (dyslexia): What have we learned in the past four decades? *Journal of Child Psychology and Psychiatry, 45*(1), 2–40.

Wagner, R., Torgensen, J., & Rashotte, C. (1999). *Comprehensive Test of Phonological Processing.* Austin, TX: PRO-ED.

Warrick, N., Rubin, H., & Rowe-Walsh, S. (1993). Phoneme awareness in language-delayed children: Comparative studies and intervention. *Annals of Dyslexia, 43*, 153–173.

Webster, P.E., & Plante, A.S. (1995). Productive phonology and phonological awareness in preschool children. *Applied Psycholinguistics, 16*(1), 43–57.

Webster, P.E., Plante, A.S., & Couvillion, L.M. (1997). Phonologic impairment and pre-reading: Update on a longitudinal study. *Journal of Learning Disabilities, 30*(4), 365–375.

Wren, Y., & Roulstone, S. (2005). Phoneme Factory Sound Sorter [Computer software]. Malmesbury, England: SEMERC.

Computer-Based Interventions

Yvonne Wren, Sue Roulstone, and A. Lynn Williams

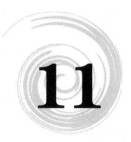

ABSTRACT

Computer-based interventions (CBIs) allow speech-language pathologists (SLPs) access to a variety of phonological and articulatory intervention approaches more efficiently and conveniently than traditional picture stimuli. Two major advantages of CBIs include access and time efficiency, which are important benefits to busy clinicians with large caseloads. Although a number of intervention software programs are available for children with speech sound disorders (SSD), they still lag behind the development and use of CBI for language disorders in children. The majority of CBI programs for children with SSD primarily focus on phonemic speech disorders in young children from the ages of 3 to 11 years.

INTRODUCTION

Computers, as technological tools, provide access to intervention materials and newer models of intervention by practitioners and, thereby, have the potential to decrease the length of intervention for the individuals they serve. Masterson, Wynne, Kuster, and Stierwalt (1999) suggested that continued technological developments in our field would result in improved intervention tools, as well as increased access for practitioners to use these tools. Furthermore, computer technology can optimize practitioners' treatment outcomes with children by reducing the time investment in assessing speech disorders and planning intervention that is tailored to the specific needs of individual children (Masterson & Rvachew, 1999).

It is not the intention to describe or evaluate here every software title that could be used as part of an intervention program for children with SSD. However, mention will be made of some computer programs that the authors have been involved in developing and also of those that have been published and written about in the literature. Readers are encouraged to consider the potential for using a diverse range of software as part of any intervention program with children with SSD. This chapter discusses some of the considerations that clinicians need to make as they select software to support interventions.

Benefits of Computer-Based Interventions

A number of studies have found a positive effect from using computers with children to enhance learning in schools (Lonigan et al., 2003; Nicolson, Fawcett, & Nicolson, 2000; Singleton & Simmons, 2001; van Daal & Reitsma, 2000; Wise, Ring, & Olson, 2000). Benefits have included greater efficiency with regard to the time taken to reach given targets and improved motivation.

These benefits also apply when using computers in speech-language pathology. Jamieson (2004), for example, found that the computer is more engaging than traditional tabletop therapy for children with SSD, suggesting that children are more attentive to therapy which includes use of software. Another advantage is the facility of computers to deliver therapy in a controlled and consistent manner, which is not possible using tabletop techniques. As Veale (1999) pointed out, computers can allow greater accuracy of performance measurement, deliver auditory information more precisely than through the spoken medium, and offer consistent and controlled presentation of stimuli that does not differ in terms of intonation or other suprasegmental features.

Burton, Meeks, and Wright (1991) noted that the relationship between child and clinician was altered by the use of a computer. They consider that in a tabletop activity, the SLP acts as taskmaster, whereas using a computer in therapy facilitates a partnership between the SLP and child. Indeed, Nelson and Masterson (1999) explained that using a computer in therapy enables a child to exert some control in the therapy situation, for example, deciding when and how often instructions are given.

Schery and O'Connor (1997) added the point that computers are nonjudgmental and patient, in a way that even the most understanding of therapists cannot be. Furthermore, computers provide undivided attention and allow training to proceed at the child's pace. Schery and O'Connor commented that computers can also be used to provide immediate reinforcement, whereas the use of animation and graphics can assist in sustaining interest in the task.

TARGET POPULATIONS

Primary Populations

Computers have been successfully used in interventions with children with SSD (Shriberg, Kwiatkowski, & Snyder, 1986, 1989, 1990; Wren & Roulstone, 2008). Generally, CBI would be most appropriate for children who are at least 3 years of age who have SSD that has either a functional or organic basis. Although the few studies reported in the literature have included primarily children with functional speech disorders, children with organically based speech disorders, such as hearing impairment and cleft lip and palate, could also benefit from CBI with appropriate consideration of the physical and sensory factors, which are discussed in the Assessment Methods for Determining Intervention Relevance section later in this chapter.

Secondary Populations

Although CBIs for children with SSD are typically designed for children with articulation and phonological impairments, some programs can also be used with children learning English as a second language (ESL). For example, *SCIP: Sound Contrasts in Phonology* (Williams, 2006) includes vowel contrasts as one of the contrastive intervention options, which can be used to address vowel errors that are common in ESL speakers.

For children with motor-based speech disorders, such as dysarthria or apraxia, phonetic approaches are typically implemented. However, children diagnosed with childhood apraxia of speech (CAS) might benefit from the linguistic-based approaches included in some software programs, such as those described in this chapter, which include contrastive intervention approaches. Studies support the use of linguistic approaches in treating CAS (e.g., Forrest, 2002; Forrest & Morrisette, 1999; Williams, Epperly, Rogers, & Feltes, 1999).

ASSESSMENT METHODS FOR DETERMINING INTERVENTION RELEVANCE

Assessing the suitability of a child to use CBI requires an evaluation of the child's physical and cognitive capabilities. In most cases, this will not result in the decision that computers should not be used, but rather that some adaptation should be made to enable a child to benefit from the particular software program.

When physical dexterity is limited, alternative input devices such as touch screens, switches, joysticks, and trackballs can be used. When a child's vision is affected, adaptations can often be made to the software such as increasing font and picture size and using high-contrast colors. In certain cases, perhaps with older children or children working independently with a computer, the use of screen reader software that converts text to speech may be advised. The use of increased volume or visual feedback in place of auditory feedback may be needed when a child has a hearing impairment. When a child has difficulty in focusing attention, the use of software with reduced screen activity could be helpful.

Beyond that, the assessment of whether or not a child is a suitable candidate for CBI should be identical to whichever intervention approach is embedded in the content of the software used or the way in which it is employed. In this way, the theory and choice of intervention drives the selection of materials and software rather than the computer program dictating what intervention can be offered. As Cochran and Masterson stated, "Selection of goals should precede and drive the choice of any teaching materials, including computer activities" (1995, p. 217).

THEORETICAL BASIS

Dominant Theoretical Rationale for the Intervention Approach

As a clinical tool, CBI does not adhere to a specific theoretical framework. In some cases, software programs are allied to a particular approach to therapy; in others the software could be used in a variety of ways, each of which supposes an alternative rationale to the therapy given. The software is a means of delivering a particular type of therapy, the rationale for which comes from the SLP.

This section presents the theoretical framework of two software programs that have been developed by the authors. Each program is based on a different set of theoretical assumptions regarding SSD and how intervention needs to be structured to address the impairments. It is therefore encumbent upon the SLP to select the software program that is aligned with, or can be used in such a way as to be consistent with, his or her theoretical principles of intervention.

The first of these two software programs is the Phoneme Factory Sound Sorter (PFSS) program (Wren & Roulstone, 2005). This software was designed to be used with a psycholinguistic approach to remediation of SSD (see Chapter 9). This approach is based on a theoretical model of speech processing consisting of three key levels: speech input, stored lexical representations, and speech output. Impairment in a child's speech development arises from a breakdown at one or more points at or between these levels. Intervention from a psycholinguistic perspective uses information gained in assessment and profiling activities to isolate particular areas of breakdown, which can then be targeted specifically through tasks that are designed to incorporate a child's strengths. Often intervention activities may draw on published materials and approaches, such as minimal pairs (see Chapter 2), stimulability (see Chapter 8), Nuffield Dyspraxia Programme (see Chapter 7), perceptual (see Chapter 12), and metaphonological (see Chapter 10).

A second software program, SCIP (Williams, 2006), is based on the linguistic and conceptual theoretical framework of phonemic contrasts and the role of phonemes in a language. As such, SCIP can be used with any of the contrastive phonological approaches, including minimal pairs (see Chapter 2), multiple oppositions (see Chapter 3), the complexity approaches of maximal oppositions and treatment of the empty set (Gierut, 1989, 1990; see also Chapter 4); and vowel contrasts. The theoretical basis of these contrastive approaches is elaborated within the chapters for each approach.

Other software programs, such as the Speech Assessment and Interactive Learning System (SAILS; AVAAZ Innovations, 1994), are based on a different set of assumptions regarding the nature of the underlying impairment of SSD. Specifically, SAILS assumes a perceptual basis as an important foundation for acquiring a phonology. Consequently, this software program is based on a perceptual intervention approach (see Chapter 12).

Beyond the differences in theoretical orientations that are encompassed in different software programs, many of the CBIs integrate evidence-based learning principles into the intervention activities. One principle of learning involves *density of responses*, which is assumed to facilitate learning. CBI incorporates high response rates through the ease and automaticity of stimulus presentation. Another learning principle incorporated into many CBIs involves the structure of activities along a continuum from high to low. Finally, diversity in training with regard to exemplars, context, and partners has been shown to facilitate learning and generalization (e.g., Wilcox, Kouri, & Caswell, 1991). Contextual and partner diversity factors can easily be incorporated with CBI to include additional stimuli, work at different levels (e.g., word, sentence), and use small-group intervention sessions to encourage peer interactions and monitoring.

In summary, theoretical frameworks differ across software programs with each program based on a specific set of assumptions related to intervention of SSD. This section presented software programs with three different theoretical perspectives: psycholinguistic, linguistic, and perceptual. Although the theoretical frameworks might differ, the various CBI programs integrate principles of learning within the structure of the program and the intervention activities.

Levels of Consequences Being Addressed

CBI programs vary in the range of levels of functioning that are addressed in a child with SSD. Specifically, what is addressed will depend partly on the software program used, but also on the way in which it is employed. Generally, however, the levels of consequences that are *directly* addressed within the International Classification of Functioning, Disability and Health for Children and Youth (ICF-CY; World Health Organization [WHO], 2007) framework include the Body Function component, and specifically Articulation functions (b320). With regard to this domain, CBI focuses on *production* to increase sound production accuracy. Some programs, such as the PFSS and SAILS, also focus on the Perception/Discrimination domain (b230) in which intervention is directed at improving the child's discrimination of speech sounds that are produced in error. An *indirect* ICF level that CBI programs incorporate is the Activity and Participation component; specifically the domain of Communication (d3), with the goal of increasing speech intelligibility.

Target Areas of Intervention

As with levels of functioning, the areas of intervention that can be targeted using CBIs are broad. The choice of software will in part determine what is targeted, but the theoretical approach of the clinician will also be crucial.

The PFSS (Wren & Roulstone, 2006), for example, can be used to target a range of speech input, stored lexical representations, and speech output skills. The program contains seven games targeting phoneme detection, phoneme blending, minimal pairs, and rhyme awareness. Each can be customized to select target and contrast consonants and word structure consistent with a child's needs. In this way, an activity could be designed for a child who shows a fronting error pattern in his or her speech, whereby the target consonants are the velars /k/ and /g/ and the contrast consonants are the child's usual substitutes for these phonemes: [t] and [d].

If the psycholinguistic speech processing profile for this child shows that his or her particular area of breakdown is at the lower level of input processing, the SLP might select nonwords within word type. In contrast, if the child's level of breakdown on the profile is within stored lexical representations, real words could be selected within word type and the "sound off" option selected in the software so that the SLP can help the child to make judgments based on his or her own internal phonological representations of the words rather than in response to an auditory presentation. These judgments might relate to determining the onset (initial phoneme) or coda (final phoneme) of a word using only the picture of the word as a stimulus; or they might relate to whether or not two words rhyme, again with only the pictures of these words as stimuli. The specific activity carried out will depend on the options selected within PFSS.

Clinicians can also use PFSS to target output where needed. Nonword and real word repetition can be carried out with the program, with a choice of word position (initial, medial, or final). The Phoneme Blending game, which requires children to listen to individual phonemes in the correct sequence and blend them together to make a word, can also be used to give a child practice at articulating real words from verbally presented segments.

As noted previously, SCIP (Williams, 2006) was designed to implement the contrastive phonological approaches. As such, it targets homonymy, either directly or indirectly, which occurs when children have limited sound inventories and produce one sound for several different adult target sounds. SCIP has a large resource of rhyming contrastive sound pairs that can be used to develop treatment materials for simplification processes (or substitution errors), as well as syllable structure processes (or deletion errors) that occur in word-initial or word-final positions. SLPs can develop individualized treatment materials using any of the contrastive intervention approaches.

The SAILS program (see Chapter 12) focuses on the importance of providing children with precise auditory input. Children are required to listen to and judge correct and incorrect recordings of real speech productions of pictured words containing sounds that are in error in their everyday speech.

Some software titles aimed at intervention for children with SSD have a less clear theoretical framework. Earobics (Cognitive Concepts, 1999), for example, has been criticized by Diehl (1999), who argued that the conceptual base for the program is unclear. She adds that the games within the program are based on two opposing theories—auditory perception and metaphonological awareness. Nevertheless SLPs could select to use those activities that fit with the theoretical framework employed in their work with children with SSD.

Other software programs make use of acoustically modified speech but are essentially targeting language skills and are therefore not addressed in this chapter (e.g., Fast-ForWord (Scientific Learning, 1998); Phonomena (MindWeavers, 2004). Lexion (2006) is a program used by many Swedish schools and contains several activities for use in developing phonological awareness skills among others. However, as this program is essentially aiming to help children with literacy or language difficulties, this title is not covered in detail here.

EMPIRICAL BASIS

Computer-Based Research Outcomes

Despite the growth in software for use in SSD intervention, there is relatively little published research on its effectiveness. A number of reasons explain this. First, as described previously, computer-based approaches to therapy are not an intervention in and of themselves. Rather, the computer is a means by which intervention is delivered and the type of intervention offered will be determined by the theoretical approach held by the clinician. Indeed, one piece of software could be used by two or more clinicians, each using the software in a different way to support alternative theoretical views.

Viewing the computer in this way places it on par with any other tool or resource used to assist in the delivery of therapy. Few investigations have looked into the effectiveness of using ColorCards in intervention for SSD, for example. What is important, then, is that the intervention strategy used by the clinician, and the content of that intervention, is supported by evidence.

Second, to evaluate CBIs as a whole would be to suggest that all CBIs are equal. However, the range of software that is available requires that individual software titles are evaluated with regard to their contribution to change in children's SSD rather than the use of a computer per se.

Nevertheless some investigations have been carried out that look specifically at the contribution of computers in speech-language pathology intervention for children with SSD. A series of early investigations using computers in intervention was carried out by Shriberg and colleagues (Shriberg et al., 1986, 1989, 1990). They compared the use of computers with a tabletop paper presentation of an assessment task and two intervention activities—production of target sounds in words and phrases and sound elicitation tasks. In each case, a clinician facilitated the task. In all three studies they found that computers and tabletop modes of delivering therapy were equally effective, efficient, and engaging for the children in the investigation.

From these exploratory studies, Shriberg and colleagues concluded that computers, "offer attractive alternatives to standard clinical materials" (1990, p. 649). However, since this time, there have been dramatic advances in the way that computers can be used for intervention. In the Shriberg studies the computer presentation was simply a repetition of the tabletop task except for the fact that the material was presented on a computer screen. In this respect, the computer was more of a visual aid. Today, software offers much more flexibility in the way that the child can interact with the computer and in the type of activity that can be carried out. Moreover, animations and enhanced graphics are more available nowadays due to faster loading time.

The Shriberg studies used a traditional articulation approach in their use of a computer in intervention. Other studies have been published that have used computers in intervention following a different theoretical approach. Rvachew, Rafaat, and Martin (1999), for example, used the SAILS computer program to explore the importance of speech perception in intervention for SSD. In this exploratory study, 13 children received speech perception training using the SAILS program and stimulability training prior to receiving the cycles approach to therapy; the speech perception training was delivered by a speech aide trained to use SAILS, and an SLP conducted the stimulability training. Their progress was compared with that of another 10 children who received cycles alone and no computer intervention or stimulability training. They found that the group who received prior training in speech perception and stimulability made greater progress in those sounds that were unstimulable or poorly perceived before treatment than those who did not receive this training. However, the study was not designed to assess the particular contribution of the computer software.

In this way, a computer has been used as a means of delivering an intervention that was under investigation. In another study, the progress of children receiving a computer intervention was specifically compared with children who were receiving the same intervention via tabletop methods (Wren & Roulstone, 2008). The intention in the Wren and Roulstone study was to identify the relative contribution of using a computer as a means to deliver the therapy. As Nelson and Masterson commented,

> If SLPs could show that use of computers in intervention resulted in desirable changes in communicative skills over a shorter time than with traditional modes of treatment, there would be a compelling case for funding computer hardware and software purchases and providing the needed time and training for clinicians. (1999, p. 70)

In this small scale exploratory study, 33 children were randomly assigned to one of three therapy conditions: computer therapy, tabletop therapy, or no therapy. The type of input provided in the two therapy groups consisted of activities consistent with the psycholinguistic approach to intervention (see Chapter 9). Therapy to individual children could be customized according to specific need in either group. In line with local provision, children received one session from an SLP per week for 8 weeks, together with two follow-up sessions each week with a non-SLP who had observed the therapy session. Children from all three groups were assessed pre- and posttherapy on measures of speech output using the Goldman-Fristoe Test of Articulation, Second Edition (GFTA-2; Goldman & Fristoe, 2000), Sounds-in-Words subtest.

The findings showed that children in both therapy groups made significant improvement by the posttherapy assessments. Although the children in the computer group had made greater progress than those in the tabletop group, this difference was not significant. This would suggest then that the computer program used in this study could be used as an additional resource for SLPs as progress made was equivalent to that using a tabletop approach, but that there would be no greater effectiveness in using this method of delivery. However, what was notable was that the children who received no therapy also made significant progress during the time of observation, and, although the two therapy groups made more progress than the no therapy group as a whole, there were no significant differences among all three in the amount of progress made over time.

Closer analysis of the findings showed considerable variation in the performance of individuals within each group. Indeed, those children who were stimulable for their target sounds showed greater progress over time regardless of which group they were in. This finding is consistent with that of Shriberg and colleagues' (1986, 1989, 1990) finding that there are individual differences in the way children respond, and there is a need to identify those children who would benefit most from this mode of therapy.

The outcome of the Wren and Roulstone (2008) study is the understanding that evaluation of software is secondary to an evaluation of the theoretical approach that underpins the intervention given. In a planned replication of the study, participants will be carefully screened to ensure that those who are not stimulable for the target sounds receive pretherapy stimulability and perception training in line with that given in the Rvachew et al. (1999) study. With a more carefully defined and homogeneous group, it should be possible to accurately measure the impact of the intervention, whether delivered by tabletop or computer. With this information, it would then be possible to see whether the computer presentation offers greater efficiency to the clinician.

Following a similar line of inquiry, Overby, Williams, and Bernthal (2008) compared intervention conditions of CBI and traditional tabletop (TAB) with four preschool-age children. Using a multiple baseline across behaviors design, each child received minimal pair therapy on one goal in each intervention condition in a counterbalanced training order. Two nonstimulable, noncognate sounds from two different manner categories were selected for treatment for each child. The treatment materials for both conditions were generated by the SCIP software program to control for the visual representation of contrastive word pairs. Treatment continued in each condition until the child achieved 50% increase in performance above the baseline mean or until a total of 14 treatment sessions were completed. To control for number of responses, treatment in each session stopped once the child completed 40 responses. The children were seen twice weekly for 30-minute individual therapy sessions.

Outcomes compared treatment and generalization performance, as well as measures of social valence and social validity, between the two intervention conditions. Social valence data were gathered on the children's preference of treatment condition. Following completion of treatment of both target sounds, children were given a choice of which treatment condition they preferred for the last five treatment sessions. In addition, clinicians and parents completed a questionnaire regarding which condition was preferred, as well as which condition they felt resulted in the greater improvement for the child.

The results indicated that children achieved moderate-to-high levels of treatment performance on their treated sounds in both conditions, with the noted exception of one child who did not make any improvement on his target in the TAB condition. Slightly higher levels of performance were observed in the CBI condition; some generalization that occurred in the CBI condition did not occur in the TAB condition. In terms of treatment efficiency and treatment effects, the CBI condition was slightly faster (4.5 average sessions compared with 5.5 average TAB sessions) with slightly higher treatment and generalization performance (73% treatment and 5% generalization compared with 48.25% and 0% for TAB condition). Effect size was calculated using percentage of nonoverlapping data (PND). The PND for TAB was .43, which corresponds to "ineffective" treatment outcomes, whereas the PND for CBI was .75, which is interpreted as an "effective" treatment.

With regard to social valence and social validity, the results from the questionnaire data indicated that although the children split 50-50 on preferred treatment condition, three children indicated that the TAB condition was easier and chose that condition to complete the final five treatment sessions. Parents' responses were equivocal with two parents reporting improvement in the TAB condition, one reporting improvement in the CBI condition, and one reporting no difference. Clinicians' ratings of the two conditions were also equivocal. On a 5-point rating scale, clinicians rated the TAB condition an average of 4.5 and the CBI condition an average of 4.4.

The results from this investigation indicate that both treatment conditions were effective. That is, children achieved criteria (50% above the baseline mean) in an average of five treatment sessions in both treatment conditions. Findings from this study indicate that CBI is at least as effective as traditional tabletop intervention.

In a pilot efficacy study, Vicini, Northern, Williams, Lewis, and Caperton (2006) examined the effectiveness of CBI with three kindergarten boys. All three children addressed the error pattern of gliding using the SCIP software program during ten 30-minute small-group therapy sessions. Two of the boys worked on [w] ~ /l, ɹ/ word-initially using the multiple oppositions approach, while the third boy worked on [w] ~ /ɹ/ word-initially using minimal pairs. All children demonstrated improvements in the short intervention period, with the two children who received the multiple oppositions approach evidencing the greatest gains on treatment and generalization performance. These results indicate that CBI was effective in children making improvement during a brief treatment period of only 10 sessions that were 30 minutes in length within a group setting.

The contribution of CBIs is not limited to interactive activities however. Williams (2006) developed SCIP to provide clinicians with a database of picture illustrations for more than 2,000 words and more than 6,000 nonsense words. The program incorporates contrastive word pairs for substitution and omission patterns and enables clinicians to develop individualized treatment sets for individual children. The PFSS software (Wren & Roulstone, 2006) provides a similar facility for producing picture materials for use on screen or on paper. Materials can be selected according to initial or final sound and individual items chosen from a large database of illustrations.

The value of this facility should not be underestimated. McKinley and Williams (2003) completed a feasibility study comparing the time taken for SLPs to develop materials for intervention using a card file method versus a computerized method (SCIP). They found that it took three times as long to produce picture materials using the card index compared with the SCIP software. CBIs then can also be evaluated with regard to the way in which they can improve efficiency of delivering tabletop approaches.

In summary, the empirical basis for CBIs is in its infancy. There is a need for more rigorous evaluations of the use of software in delivering therapy. A first step, however, is to ensure that the approach to therapy that underpins the method of delivery and provides the content of activities is valid. With that information, it is then possible to understand the contribution that individual software titles can offer, keeping in mind that an evaluation of CBI cannot be based on a single program. Olsen and Wise (2006) summarize the situation by explaining that independent research is needed to identify what works in intervention, how, and for whom.

Summary of Levels of Evidence

Table 11.1 summarizes the evidence available in the field of CBI for children with SSD. Each of the studies described in the previous section are included and tabled according to their methodology and resulting level of evidence. Comments are added relating to the quality and limitations of each study which should be considered when interpreting the findings.

PRACTICAL REQUIREMENTS

Nature of Sessions

CBIs will vary in the way sessions are carried out. As with other aspects of CBIs, the way sessions are delivered and the timing of sessions will be determined by the theoretical approach driving the content of the intervention. The computer is a tool rather than a type of intervention.

However, using a computer within a program of intervention may affect the running of sessions in a number of ways. To start with, some software programs enable children to work independently at times without the need for an accompanying adult to facilitate each session. Often, the SLP will set up the activities for a child and see the child at an agreed time to review progress and set new goals, but in between sessions, the child can practice independently. When this is the case, it is possible that sessions can be more frequent as the need for a teacher, parent, or SLP is reduced. It is possible that a child could use the computer with headphones in the corner of a classroom at a regular time each day, for example.

The types of software that are compatible with working in this way tend to be those based on auditory discrimination type activities and linked to the psycholinguistic, metaphonological, and perceptual interventions. In these cases, children are not required to produce a verbal response, but need to interact with the software on screen to an auditory judgment task. As such there is no requirement for either an adult or the computer to judge the child's production of speech targets.

Using a computer to assist in delivering therapy might often be assumed to be an isolated task in which individual therapy is more suited. However, with today's interactive whiteboards, there is no reason why a computer cannot be used within group sessions as well. This would have the added advantage of providing more naturalistic conversational opportunities to encourage carryover of taught targets from the therapy session to everyday speech. Moreover, the availability of computers within classrooms, clinics, and homes means that, in many cases, intervention can be carried out in a range of settings.

Personnel

Using a computer as part of a therapy regime for children with SSD requires a skilled clinician to determine the precise program and settings needed to match the child's specific needs. Schery and O'Connor (1997) argued that because of the systematic structure of software programs, intervention using computers can be used by classroom assistants or others to work effectively with a child. However, the caveat to this is that the program

Table 11.1. Levels of evidence for studies of treatment efficacy for computer-based interventions

Level	Description	References	Quality appraisal/caveats to interpretation
Ia	Meta-analysis of > 1 randomized controlled trial	—	
Ib	Randomized controlled study	Wren & Roulstone (2008)	Study may be underpowered; amount of therapy was relatively small compared with other studies
IIa	Controlled study without randomization	—	
IIb	Quasi-experimental study	Shriberg et al. (1989, 1990)	Children receive both modes of therapy in randomly determined counterbalanced order; sample limited to university clinic attendees; small numbers for exploratory studies
		Rvachew et al. (1999)	No information is given about how the children are recruited and selected. The study was not designed to identify the particular contribution of computer-based intervention and makes no claims about the impact of computer-based intervention. The two studies are carried out sequentially; numbers are not sufficient to carry out formal statistical comparisons and so no adjustment is made for baseline differences between the two groups.
		Overby et al. (2008)	Children received both modes of intervention in randomly assigned counterbalanced order; small sample size.
III	Nonexperimental studies, i.e., correlational and case studies	Vicini et al. (2006)	Children had received traditional therapy with the tabletop mode prior to this study; small sample size; short study period (10 sessions).
IV	Expert committee report, consensus conference, clinical experience of respected authorities	—	

Adapted from the Scottish Intercollegiate Guidelines Network (http://www.sign.ac.uk).

must be carefully matched to the child's developmental needs, and this process will need to be carried out by the clinician.

In support of this is the review of studies using computers in therapy by Cochran and Nelson (1999). They considered comparisons of clinician-guided CBI with clinician-guided activities using traditional materials in language intervention (O'Connor & Schery, 1986; Ott-Rose & Cochran, 1992) and phonological therapy (Shriberg et al., 1989, 1990) and concluded that the clinician is crucial to the success of a therapy program using computers. Indeed, they comment that computers are best viewed as enhancing therapy practices rather than replacing them. As Nelson and Masterson summarized, "Like clinician delivered therapy . . . success is dependent on the clinician" (1999, p.70).

That said, it is those who are in most regular contact with a child who will be able to facilitate their use of the computer for the purposes of intervention. As such, teachers, parents, and any others who see the child frequently could work alongside the clinician in delivering the intervention. In some cases, this may require the non-SLP to observe the intervention session with the clinician to understand what is required and to ensure the child both carries out the activities as often as needed and is able to benefit the most from the computer intervention between SLP visits. When the intervention is entirely delivered using software, it may be sufficient for the nonclinician to talk with the SLP to understand what is required between SLP visits.

Dosage

The correct dosage for CBI to be maximally effective has yet to be established and indeed is likely to vary for different software programs and different underlying approaches to intervention. However, the key feature of CBI, that it can be accessed away from the clinic situation, provides the facility for frequent and intense intervention in a variety of settings, which is difficult to match with other types of intervention.

KEY COMPONENTS

The key components of a CBI will depend on the software used to deliver that intervention. To illustrate the process, the two programs designed by the authors are described here in more detail.

Phoneme Factory Sound Sorter

Nature of Goals

The PFSS (Wren & Roulstone, 2006) provides a range of customizable activities that allow the clinician to target skills that may be shown to be weak following assessment and profiling. The activities predominantly target input skills such as minimal pairs discrimination, phoneme segmentation, rhyme recognition, and phoneme blending. Goals would usually be selected by an SLP, although an accompanying software program, the Phoneme Factory Phonology Screener (Wren, Roulstone, & Hughes, 2006), could also be used to provide broad guidance as to the types of activities that would be suitable for the child on the PFSS.

Goal Attack Strategies

A range of skills and targets can be addressed either simultaneously or sequentially using the PFSS. Targets can be updated as often as needed with the option to archive old activities.

Description of Activities

The PFSS consists of seven games that target five areas: sound/symbol matching, phoneme detection, phoneme blending, minimal pairs discrimination, and rhyme awareness.

Depending on the settings selected, these can be used to address a range of levels on the psycholinguistic framework described by Stackhouse and Pascoe (see Chapter 9).

Following detailed assessment of the child, the clinician uses the data to identify appropriate activities and settings, as well as suitable targets. Options for selection in the phoneme detection and blending games begin with word type. Dependent on the child's profile, it may be more appropriate to work at the level of the nonword or individual sound. Alternatively, the clinician may feel the child needs to hear the target sound within words or even sentences. Following selection of word type, there is the option to select up to four target consonants and four contrast consonants. In this way, a clinician could choose to work on a single pair of consonants that have been reduced by the child to homophones or to work across a range of consonants.

The clinician is then asked to select word position so that targets can be embedded within words in initial, medial, or final word position or within clusters or polysyllables. (This option is dependent on previous selections, thus when single sounds have been selected in word type, the option for word position is unavailable). Sound symbol pictures can be selected whereby letters only are used or letters with accompanying pictures are given. Finally for the phoneme detection game, having the sound on or off is an option. This allows the clinician to work at a higher level of processing whereby the child needs to access the target word in his or her head and then make judgments on this rather than being given the word as an auditory cue. The phoneme blending activity has two different options: selecting length of time between presentation of phonemes and selecting number of stimulus pictures in the game.

Options for selection for the minimal pair discrimination and rhyme awareness activities are slightly different. Word type, target, and contrast consonants are available as in the phoneme detection and blending games. Word structure is also available for the minimal pairs game whereas the rhyme awareness will always place the target in initial position. Instead, the clinician has the option for sounds and pictures to be present or absent. In this way, the game can be targeted to a lower or higher level of processing: When sound and pictures are available, the child is given maximum support to succeed at the task and is able to use internal representations of words as well as the auditory and visual stimulus. With one or more of these taken away, support is reduced and the child is increasingly reliant on his or her own internal representations of a word.

Once selected by the clinician, a range of activities is available for the child and is customized to his or her specific needs based on his or her psycholinguistic profile. The child is easily able to access games through the login screen, and help is provided on screen to learn how to operate the games. Usually a single demonstration of the game by the clinician is sufficient for the child to understand how to proceed.

Often therapy sessions begin with the sound/symbol matching activity, which serves to familiarize the child with the pictures used to represent sounds in other games in the program. Phoneme detection games require the child to listen to a sound, nonword, or word or refer to his or her internal representation of a real word and identify the phoneme either in initial, medial, or final position in the word. In the phoneme blending activity, the child has to listen to the presentation of a number of phonemes in sequence, which make up one of the words pictured on the screen. Minimal pair discrimination requires the child to identify one of a pair of words or nonwords that differ from each other in one phoneme only. And finally, the rhyme awareness games ask children to judge whether or not items rhyme.

With all the activities, children receive rewards for correct responses and feedback for those that are incorrect. Records of each performance are taken and stored.

Materials and Equipment Required

The key equipment needed in addition to the software itself is a computer that can run the program and that is easily accessible to the child in question. This last point is crucial if the child is to have regular access to the software for the purposes of achieving maximum improvement in minimum time.

Sound Contrasts in Phonology

Nature of Goals

As noted previously, SCIP (Williams, 2006) is based on the contrastive approaches to phonological intervention, and therefore can be used to design and implement any of the contrastive approaches. Consequently, the nature of the goals for the contrastive approaches in SCIP is to reduce homonymy by inducing phonemic splits. For each of the contrastive approaches, contrastive word pairs can be created and stored in individual electronic files for each child.

The basis of target selection can be determined by the specific contrastive approach, or according to the target selection approach chosen by the SLP. For example, different contrastive approaches are based on different target selection approaches. Specifically, multiple oppositions uses the metric distance in selecting up to four phonetically diverse targets from one rule set; whereas, maximal oppositions and empty set use nonproportional contrasts in choosing one or two target sounds that represent independent and maximally distinct phonemes in contrastive word pairs. Alternatively, clinicians can choose targets based on other criteria, such as developmental norms, markedness, or phonological complexity, regardless of the contrastive approach.

Goal Attack Strategies

A given child may have a number of goals, each of which can be developed to be addressed by different contrastive approaches. That is, a given child might exhibit a large phoneme collapse that is addressed using multiple oppositions, and a second rule or error pattern that affects only one or two target sounds that can be addressed using a different contrastive approach, such as minimal pairs. In addition, different goal attack strategies can be employed to address multiple goals. The SLP can use SCIP to implement intervention using any of the three goal attack strategies described by Fey (1986): horizontal (or simultaneous), vertical (or sequential), or cyclical. The choice of goal attack strategies will likely be influenced by a number of factors, including severity of the SSD, length and frequency of the sessions, individual or group sessions, and presence of additional goals (e.g., language, fluency, phonological awareness).

Description of Activities

SCIP is primarily a resource tool for SLPs to develop contrastive word pairs for any of the five contrastive phonological intervention approaches. As such, clinicians can use the illustrations in any activities they design. In addition, the illustrations can be printed out and used in intervention activities away from the computer, or the child can work with the contrastive word pairs at the computer.

SCIP generates all the possible rhyming word pairs for the sound contrasts in the specified position. The SLP can choose to include nonsense words, which will significantly increase the number of contrasts that are possible. SLPs can also customize the contrastive stimuli to include specific vowel contexts to address phonological rules that might be conditioned by the vowel context. The option for selecting specific vowel contexts in SCIP (front/back vowels, high/low vowels, and tense/lax vowels) can also be chosen to provide facilitating contexts; for example, choosing back vowels to facilitate learning of velar /k/.

Materials and Equipment Required

For both PFSS and SCIP, the key equipment needed is a computer that is able to run the software and that is easy for the child and clinician to access.

ASSESSMENT AND PROGRESS MONITORING TO SUPPORT DECISION MAKING

As with any approach to the treatment of children with SSD, assessment is carried out through both formal and informal procedures and information is gathered in a variety of ways. CBI can make a contribution to this process through specific screening software such as the Phoneme Factory Screener (Wren et al., 2006) and Computerized Articulation and Phonology Evaluation System (CAPES) (Masterson & Bernhardt, 2002) or through speech analysis software such as the PROPH module in Computerized Profiling (Long, Fey, & Channell, 2007).

During the process of intervention, CBI is unique in its ability to record performance on tasks automatically. Both PFSS and SCIP have built-in data collection features, which record a child's performance on individual tasks and displays that information on graphs to show change over time.

CONSIDERATIONS FOR CHILDREN FROM CULTURALLY AND LINGUISTICALLY DIVERSE BACKGROUNDS

CBIs may permit fewer alterations in how they are used compared with other resources used with children with SSD. An ability to customize to an individual child's needs provides flexibility but in most cases the computer activity will need to be carried out in a prescribed fashion for the game to work. In contrast, a tabletop activity can be altered as the clinician sees fit throughout a session.

This feature is both a strength and a weakness. Its strength is that it enables non-SLPs to use the software in the precise way in which the clinician has set a program for a child. In contrast, with tabletop tasks, confusion in how activities should be carried out and their specific purpose can often lead to unintentional changes in both the execution of the activity and the outcome. This feature can be considered a weakness however, as CBI can be less open to adaptation for users who are not native speakers of the language used in the software or for whom the cultural references are invalid.

This becomes apparent for software produced in the English-speaking countries. Titles produced in the United States with a standard U.S. accent will have some usefulness for a U.K. and Australian audience, but there is likely to be greater emphasis on the word-final [ɪ] sound than would typically be required in a U.K. market. Moreover, some of the pictures and vocabulary will be unfamiliar to many children in U.K. schools. For example, when the U.S. software uses the word *pitcher*, children in the United Kingdom would name the item *jug*. Similarly, U.K.-produced software is less likely to reflect the specific cultural context of U.S. children.

In situations in which children speak different languages to that of the software, it may be necessary to reconfigure the program when possible to set up word lists that are relevant for the particular child. In some programs, it is possible to add material, such as pictures or voice recordings, which may make the program more flexible for an individual child's needs. Think About, for example, a program produced by Granada Assessment in the United Kingdom, allows users to add their own dialogue to given picture stories, whereas Chatback, by Xavier Educational Multimedia, has a facility for recording speech and producing waveforms for any sound, word, or sentence.

CASE STUDY

Jemma was 9;6 and had been working with an SLP since she was a small child. She had some language and learning difficulties but also severe SSD—making her unintelligible to most people who were not familiar with her. On assessment, using the Diagnostic Evaluation of Articulation and Phonology (Dodd, Crosbie, Zhu, Holm, & Ozanne, 2002), she achieved a percent consonants correct score of 26%. She demonstrated stopping of fricatives, weak syllable deletion, fronting of velars, cluster reduction, and gliding. Vowels were generally intact.

A psycholinguistic assessment revealed that Jemma showed difficulties across many areas of the profile with inaccurate motor programs, possibly due to poor input processing and limitations at the level of single-sound imitation. An intervention program was planned around developing Jemma's low-level input and output skills for the fronting error pattern. The PFSS program was used to provide nonword discrimination and repetition tasks using velar consonants as targets and their alveolar equivalents as contrasts. From this, she moved on to real-word tasks in initial and final word position in rhyme detection, phoneme detection, and sound blending tasks.

Jemma's activities using the computer program were carried out at school on a regular basis, working with a teaching assistant. The SLP saw Jemma when she needed to update the settings on the program. She also provided additional ideas to supplement the work of the computer program in other settings during the school day, such as ideas for rhyming songs to sing and worksheets using *g* words to try at home.

Initially, Jemma was unable to produce /g/ in isolation, and, although she was stimulable for /k/, she did not use it in connected speech. Following her work using PFSS, she was reliably able to produce /g/ in isolation and was starting to produce it in consonant vowel combinations during intervention activities. Her use of /k/ improved to the point in which she was able to use the sound spontaneously in everyday speech.

Given the severity of Jemma's speech, language, and learning difficulties, she continued to have problems with her intelligibility and needed ongoing speech-language pathology after her progress with velars. However, PFSS helped her to make progress with two sounds that had previously been the target of many periods of intervention where no perceptible progress had been made.

A second case study of CBI is provided for a brief, small-group intervention for two children using SCIP. Both children exhibited severe SSD characterized by extensive phoneme collapses, resulting from phonotactic inventory, positional, and sequence constraints. Nate was 5;9 and produced 46 errors out of the 77 sounds assessed on the GFTA-2 (Goldman & Fristoe, 2000). He also exhibited frequent vowel errors. Nate's predominant error patterns included stopping/devoicing of word-final obstruents, and idiosyncratic gliding of fricatives and fricative clusters word-initially. Suzanne, 5;11, produced 67 errors out of the 77 sounds assessed on the GFTA-2. She exhibited two complementary word-initial error patterns that resulted in backing of obstruents to [g] or backing of sonorants to [h].

Each child received intervention using multiple oppositions, which were developed for two of their primary error patterns. Treatment profiles were developed for each child using SCIP, which included five contrastive word pairs for each of the goals. Nate met treatment criterion on all six target sounds and achieved generalization criteria on all word-initial targets. For Suzanne, training criteria was met for five of her eight target sounds, of which three targets also achieved the generalization criterion. Nate and Suzanne continued to receive intervention using SCIP at the completion of this brief intervention study. Nate met all therapy objectives following 25 additional sessions over a 7-month period and was discharged from therapy. His final GFTA-2 results indicated that he correctly produced 76 of 77 sounds tested, and all vowel errors were resolved. Suzanne completed all of her therapy objectives following an extra 45 sessions during an 11-month period. Her final GFTA-2 results demonstrated that she only produced 5 errors of the 77 sounds assessed.

STUDY QUESTIONS

1. In what ways do computer software programs supplement traditional tabletop intervention approaches?

2. What assessment considerations should be made by the SLP in implementing a CBI program?

3. What intervention approaches can be implemented with computer software programs?

FUTURE DIRECTIONS

CBIs for children with SSD are still in their infancy. Some specific software programs have been designed to complement particular intervention approaches. Other published software titles can be used in a way that makes them compatible with particular intervention approaches.

Given that using computers in speech-language pathology has been shown to increase engagement in some students (Jamieson, 2004; Shriberg et al., 1990) and there is evidence to support their use in education (Becta, 2002a, 2002b), we should be looking to how such technology can become an everyday part of our therapy repertoire as clinicians. The need to retain a theoretical basis for our work remains, however. The software should never drive the intervention—it should be viewed as a means of delivering a therapy regime that has credibility in terms of its explanation for the impairment and an evidence base for intervention. We should encourage and promote the development of new software and technologies that can support existing evidence-based interventions. Further research is needed to establish the precise contribution of varied technologies to the intervention process, and in particular whether or not their use provides a more efficient means of delivering therapy.

SUGGESTED READINGS

Rvachew, S., Rafaat, S., & Martin, M. (1999). Stimulability, speech perception skills and the treatment of phonological disorders, *American Journal of Speech-Language Pathology, 8,* 33–43.

Shriberg, L., Kwiatkowski, J., & Snyder, T. (1986). Articulation testing by microcomputer. *Journal of Speech and Hearing Disorders, 51,* 309–324.

Shriberg, L., Kwiatkowski, J., & Snyder, T. (1980). Tabletop versus microcomputer-assisted speech management: Stabilisation phase. *Journal of Speech and Hearing Disorders, 54,* 233–248.

Shriberg, L., Kwiatkowski, J., & Snyder, T. (1990). Tabletop versus microcomputer-assisted speech management: Response evocation phase. *Journal of Speech and Hearing Disorders, 55,* 635–655.

Wren, Y., & Roulstone, S. (2008). A comparison between computer and tabletop delivery of phonology therapy. *International Journal of Speech-Language Pathology, 10,* 346–363.

REFERENCES

AVAAZ Innovations. (1994). Speech Assessment and Interactive Learning System (Version 1.2) [Computer software]. London, Ontario, Canada: Author.

Becta. (2002a). *ImpaCT2: The impact of information and communication technologies on pupil learning and attainment.* Nottingham, England: DfES Publications.

Becta. (2002b). *ImpaCT2: Learning at home and school—Case studies.* Nottingham, England: DfES Publications.

Burton, E., Meeks, N., & Wright, K. (1991). Opportunities for using computer in speech and language therapy: A study of one language unit. *British Journal of Disorders of Communication, 26,* 207–217.

Cochran, P.S., & Masterson, J.J. (1995). NOT using a computer in language assessment/intervention: In defence of the reluctant clinician. *Language, Speech, and Hearing Services in Schools, 26,* 213–222.

Cochran, P.S. & Nelson, L.K. (1999). Technology applications in intervention for pre-school age children with language disorders. *Seminars in Speech and Language, 20,* 203–217.

Cognitive Concepts. (1999). Earobics [Computer software]. Evanston, IL: Author.

Diehl, S.F. (1999). Listen and learn? A software review of Earobics. *Language, Speech, and Hearing Services in Schools, 30,* 108–116.

Dodd, B., Crosbie, S., Zhu, H., Holm, A., & Ozanne, A. (2002). *The Diagnostic Evaluation of Articulation and Phonology.* London: Pearson PsychCorp.

Fey, M.E. (1986). *Language intervention with young children.* Boston: Allyn & Bacon.

Forrest, K. (2002). Are oral-motor exercises useful in the treatment of phonological/articulation disorders? *Seminars in Speech and Language, 23,* 15–25.

Forrest, K., & Morrisette, M. (1999). Feature analysis of segmental errors in children with phonological disorders. *Journal of Speech and Hearing Research, 42,* 187–194.

Gierut, J.A. (1989). Maximal opposition approach to phonological treatment. *Journal of Speech and Hearing Disorders, 54,* 9–19.

Gierut, J.A. (1990). Differential learning of phonological oppositions. *Journal of Speech and Hearing Research, 33,* 540–549.

Goldman, R.M., & Fristoe, M. (2000). *Goldman-Fristoe Test of Articulation* (2nd ed.). Circle Pines, MN: American Guidance Service.

Jamieson, G. (2004). *Children's attention on tabletop versus computer administered phonology therapy.* Unpublished bachelor's dissertation, College of St Mark and St John, Plymouth, England.

Lexion. (2006). Lexion [Computer software]. Sweden: Frölunda Data.

Long, S., Fey, M., & Channell, R.W. (2007). Computerized Profiling (Version 9.70) [Computer software]. Cleveland, OH: Case Western Reserve University.

Lonigan, C.J., Driscoll, K., Phillips, B.M., Cantor, B.G., Anthony, J.L., & Goldstein, H. (2003). A computer assisted instruction phonological sensitivity program for pre-school children at risk for reading problems. *Journal of Early Intervention, 25,* 248–262.

Masterson, J.J., & Bernhardt, B. (2002). CAPES: Computerized Articulation and Phonology Evaluation System [Computer software]. San Antonio, TX: Pearson Assessment.

Masterson, J.J., & Rvachew, S. (1999). Use of technology in phonological intervention. *Seminars in Speech and Language, 20*(3), 233–249.

Masterson, J.J., Wynne, M.K., Kuster, J.M., & Stierwalt, J.A.G. (1999). New and emerging technologies: Going where we've never gone before. *ASHA/Leader, 41,* 16–20.

McKinley, N., & Williams, A.L. (2003). *Sound Contrasts in Phonology (SCIP) Phase II.* NIH NIDCD Progress Report.

MindWeavers. (2004). Phonomena [Computer software]. Oxford, England: Author.

Nelson, L.K., & Masterson, J.J. (1999). Computer technology: Creative interfaces in service delivery. *Topics in Language Disorders, 19,* 68–86.

Nicolson, R.T., Fawcett, A.J., & Nicolson, M.K. (2000). Evaluation of a computer based reading intervention in infant and junior schools. *Journal of Research in Reading, 23,* 194–209.

O'Connor, L., & Schery, T. (1986). A comparison of microcomputer-aided and traditional language therapy for developing communication skills in non-oral toddlers. *Journal of Speech and Hearing Disorders, 51,* 356–361.

Olsen, R., & Wise, B. (2006). Computer-based remediation for reading and related phonological disabilities. In M. McKenna, L. Labbo, R. Kieffer, & D. Reinking (Eds.), *International handbook of literacy and technology* (Vol. 2, pp. 57–74). Mahwah, NJ: Lawrence Erlbaum Associates.

Ott-Rose, M., & Cochran, P.S. (1992). Teaching action verbs with computer-controlled videodisk vs. traditional picture stimuli. *Journal for Computer Users in Speech and Hearing, 8,* 15–32.

Overby, M., Williams, A.L., & Bernthal, J. (2008, November). *Comparison of two treatment conditions for young children with speech sound disorders.* Technical session at the annual convention of the American Speech-Language-Hearing Association, Chicago.

Rvachew, S., Rafaat, S., & Martin, M. (1999). Stimulability, speech perception skills and the treatment of phonological disorders. *American Journal of Speech-Language Pathology, 8,* 33–43.

Schery, T., & O'Connor, L. (1997). Language intervention: Computer training for children with special needs. *British Journal of Educational Technology, 28,* 271–279.

Scientific Learning. (1998). Fast ForWord [Computer software]. Oakland, CA: Author.

Shriberg, L., Kwiatkowski, J., & Snyder, T. (1986). Articulation testing by microcomputer. *Journal of Speech and Hearing Disorders, 51,* 309–324.

Shriberg, L., Kwiatkowski, J., & Snyder, T. (1989). Table-top versus microcomputer-assisted speech management: Stabilisation phase. *Journal of Speech and Hearing Disorders, 54,* 233–248.

Shriberg, L., Kwiatkowski, J., & Snyder, T. (1990). Table-top versus microcomputer-assisted speech management: Response evocation phase. *Journal of Speech and Hearing Disorders, 55,* 635–655.

Singleton, C., & Simmons, F. (2001). An evaluation of 'Workshark' in the classroom. *British Journal of Educational Technology, 32,* 317–330.

van Daal, V.H.P., & Reitsma, P. (2000). Computer-assisted learning to read and spell: Results from two pilot studies. *Journal of Research in Reading, 23,* 181–193.

Veale, T. (1999). Targeting temporal processing deficits through Fast ForWord: Language therapy with a new twist. *Language, Speech, and Hearing Services in Schools, 30,* 353–362.

Vicini, C., Northern, J., Williams, A.L., Lewis, K., & Caperton, K. (2006, October). *Computer-based intervention in phonology: It's about time.* Poster presentation at the annual convention of the Tennessee Association of Audiologists and Speech-Language Pathologists, Franklin, TN.

Wilcox, M.J., Kouri, T.A., & Caswell, S.B. (1991). Early language intervention: A comparison of classroom and individual treatment. *American Journal of Speech-Language Pathology, 1,* 49–62.

Williams, A.L. (2006). SCIP: Sound Contrasts in Phonology (Version 1.0) [Computer software]. Greenville, SC. Thinking Publications.

Williams, A.L., Epperly, R., Rodgers, J.R., & Feltes, L. (1999, November). *Treatment efficacy in phonological intervention: Clinical case studies.* Paper presented at the annual convention of the American Speech-Language-Hearing Association, San Francisco.

Wise, B.W., Ring, J., & Olson, R.K. (2000). Individual differences in gains from computer assisted remedial reading. *Journal of Experimental Child Psychology, 77,* 197–235.

World Health Organization. (2007). *International classification of functioning, disability and health for children and youth (ICF-CY).* Geneva: Author.

Wren, Y., & Roulstone, S. (2005). Phoneme Factory Sound Sorter [Computer software]. London: GL Assessment.

Wren, Y., & Roulstone, S. (2008). A comparison between computer and tabletop delivery of phonology therapy. *International Journal of Speech-Language Pathology, 10,* 346–363.

Wren, Y., Roulstone, S., & Hughes, A. (2006). Phoneme Factory Phonology Screener [Computer software]. London: GL Assessment.

Speech Perception Intervention

Susan Rvachew and Françoise Brosseau-Lapré

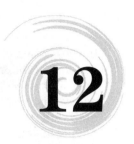

12

ABSTRACT

Difficulties with phonological processing are central to speech sound disorders (SSD). The goal of speech perception interventions is to help the child develop a detailed internal model of the acoustic-phonetic characteristics of the phonemes that the child misarticulates. The Speech Assessment and Interactive Learning System (SAILS; AVAAZ Innovations, 1994) is a computer-based speech perception intervention during which the child listens to natural recordings of the target word produced by adult and child talkers with and without SSD. On each trial, the child indicates whether or not the stimulus was an exemplar of the target word. Studies have shown that the use of SAILS significantly enhances children's response to standard speech therapy.

INTRODUCTION

The inclusion of speech perception training in speech therapy has a long history in speech-language pathology, dating back at least to the 'ear training' procedures recommended by Van Riper (1963). The motivation for including such procedures as part of interventions for children with SSD has not changed: The goal is to ensure that the child has a detailed internal representation of the acoustic-phonetic characteristics of the target phoneme that serves as a model against which the child can compare his or her own productions. A stable acoustic-phonetic representation allows the child to discover the articulatory gestures that result in the desired speech output and achieve consistent productions of the target phoneme across a variety of phonetic contexts and communication goals.

Research conducted during the past few decades has validated the importance of ensuring stable acoustic-phonetic representations to the achievement of good speech outcomes (for review, see Rvachew, 2007a). At the same time, this research has improved our knowledge of optimal practices for perceptual training and has explained why the original live-voice ear training procedures were not always effective (Shelton, Johnson, Ruscello, & Arndt, 1978). Computer technologies offer an opportunity to improve the efficiency and effectiveness of perceptual approaches to intervention.

This chapter focuses specifically on the computer-based speech perception intervention known as SAILS. The child's task is to indicate whether or not the stimulus presented on each trial constitutes the target word. The program was designed to be consistent with the best research on effective practices for improving speech perception skills. The key features of the intervention include 1) the nature of the stimuli, 2) the type of training task, 3) the feedback provided by the software, and 4) the role of the speech-language pathologist (SLP) or assistant when conducting the intervention. Each of these aspects of the intervention will be discussed in turn.

Research with second-language learners suggests that exposure to highly variable natural stimuli provides the best foundation for perception learning (Kingston, 2003; Lambacher, Martens, Kakehi, & Marasinghe, 2005; Lively, Logan, & Pisoni, 1993; Nishi & Kewley-Port, 2007). In keeping with this principle, the treatment levels of each SAILS model consist of natural recordings of the target word, half articulated correctly by various child or adult talkers with typical speech development and half misarticulated by various child talkers with SSD. Correct exemplars vary from highly prototypical versions of the target phoneme to versions that are less distinct members of the target phoneme class. The incorrect exemplars cover the full range of commonly occurring misarticulations of the target phoneme. Although it is possible for the SLP to conduct a similar intervention using his or her own voice (Locke, 1980b), it would not be possible for the SLP to replicate this degree of variability in stimulus presentation. Furthermore, SLPs find it difficult to imitate misarticulations that are phonetically similar to authentic child productions (Gardner, 1997). Rvachew (1994) showed that exposure to the full range of exemplars provided more effective support for the child's acquisition of correct /ʃ/ articulation than did a restricted set involving a single talker and a prototypical exemplar of the target word.

The SAILS task is a two-alternative, forced-choice identification procedure involving real words. Basic research has established clearly that an identification task is superior to a discrimination task for inducing categorical perception (Guenther, Husain, Cohen, & Shinn-Cunningham, 1999). Another alternative to the identification task is auditory bombardment, a procedure in which the child listens passively to the presentation of words or sentences containing the target phoneme (Hodson & Paden, 1983; Van Riper, 1963). No experimental studies have directly investigated the relative effectiveness of asking the child to make explicit responses to the stimuli when compared with a passive listening procedure. However, the results of Rvachew, Rafaat, and Martin (1999), as described later in this chapter, suggested that an explicit identification task is more effective than auditory bombardment.

Related to the issue of passive listening versus explicit responses is the provision of feedback about the accuracy of the child's responses. McClelland, Fiez, and McCandliss (2002) demonstrated that Japanese-speaking adults learned to perceive the /ɹ/–/l/ contrast when the intervention involved identification of fixed blocks of training stimuli presented with feedback. This training condition was completely ineffective without feedback, thus validating the use of explicit feedback for correct and incorrect responses by the SAILS program.

SAILS provides visual feedback for correct responses—specifically, a new item is added to a scene shown on the left side of the screen. Providing reinforcement without information can be counterproductive because in some circumstances, external reinforcers undermine the child's intrinsic interest in an activity (Cameron, Pierce, Basko, & Gear, 2005). For this reason, the visual feedback is intended to act more as a counting device that helps the child judge the passage of time. It is expected that informative feedback will be provided by the adult who is mediating the child's interaction with the program. Although the software is designed to allow independent play by the child, this feature has not been used in any of the intervention studies conducted to date. Rather, an adult provided informative feedback if the child pointed to the wrong response alternative and did not allow the child to advance to the next trial until the missed trial was re-presented and the child selected the correct response alternative.

TARGET POPULATIONS

Primary Populations

SAILS was developed for use with children with SSD and has been tested in studies targeting 4- and 5-year-old children with moderate or severe primary SSD. All children with SSD that was secondary to some other condition (e.g., craniofacial anomalies, hearing impairment, frank motor impairments) were specifically excluded from these studies. Speech perception training was expected to be an effective intervention for these children because a large body of research indicated that phonological processing difficulties are central to most cases of primary SSD. Shriberg and colleagues have proposed that the most common subtypes of children with primary SSD are Speech Delay–Genetic and Speech Delay–Otitis Media with Effusion (estimated to comprise approximately 60% and 30% of the total population of children with primary SSD, respectively). Both etiologies are presumed to result in difficulties with processing speech input that lead in turn to inaccurate speech output (Shriberg, 1994; Shriberg, Austin, Lewis, McSweeny, & Wilson, 1997).

Evidence for the genetic basis of SSD is growing along with increasing evidence for a genetic link between SSD and dyslexia, another developmental disorder associated with a core impairment in phonological processing (Lewis et al., 2006; McGrath et al., 2007; Pennington, 2006; Shriberg et al., 2005; Smith, Pennington, Boada, & Shriberg, 2005; Stein et al., 2004; Tunick & Pennington, 2002). A large body of empirical evidence confirms that, as a group, children with SSD demonstrate significant difficulties with a variety of tasks involving phonological processing, including measures of speech perception (Broen, Strange, Doyle, & Heller, 1983; Cohen & Diehl, 1963; Hoffman, Daniloff, Bengoa, & Schuckers, 1985; Hoffman, Stager, & Daniloff, 1983; Rvachew & Jamieson, 1989; Sherman & Geith, 1967), phonological awareness (Bird, Bishop, & Freeman, 1995; Larrivee & Catts, 1999; Nathan, Stackhouse, Goulandris, & Snowling, 2004; Raitano, Pennington, Tunick, Boada, & Shriberg, 2004; Rvachew, 2007b; Webster, Plante, & Couvillion, 1997), long-term repetition priming (Munson, Baylis, Krause, & Yim, 2006), and nonword repetition (Munson, Edwards, & Beckman, 2005b). This body of research provides a strong rationale for targeting these children's phonological processing abilities as a means to correcting their overt articulation errors.

The proposed link between SSD and otitis media with effusion (OME) is controversial due to mixed research findings, with prospective large sample studies confirming a link in some cases (Klausen, Moller, Holmefjord, Reisaeter, & Asbjornsen, 2007) but not others (Campbell et al., 2003). These mixed findings reflect the complex relationships among OME, speech and language outcomes, and a variety of moderating and mediating variables that include age of onset of the OME (Rvachew, Slawinski, Williams, & Green, 1999), family socioeconomic status (SES; Johnson et al., 2000), caregiving environment (Roberts et al., 1998), and genetic factors (McGrath et al., 2007). Children with a history of chronic OME have been observed to have difficulties with speech perception and phonological awareness (Clarkson, Eimas, & Marean, 1989; Nittrouer, 1996; Teele, Klein, Chase, Menyuk, & Rosner, 1990). Therefore, in those cases in which the child with SSD has a positive OME history, attention to the child's speech perception skills is warranted.

In conclusion, it is reasonable to expect that most children with SSD will benefit from a speech perception intervention. SLPs are charged with determining whether an intervention is likely to be of benefit to a particular child, however. No studies to date have involved large enough samples to identify interactions between child characteristics and response to the intervention, and thus it is not clear which specific children are the most appropriate candidates for this intervention.

It is clear that children with primary SSD are a heterogeneous group, even with respect to phonological processing abilities, and thus it is reasonable to ask whether all children with primary SSD will benefit equally from a speech perception intervention. Rvachew and Grawburg (2006) described speech perception and phonological awareness performance for 95 preschoolers with SSD. Speech perception was assessed using SAILS, targeting the phonemes [k, l, ɹ, s]. Scores were averaged across these four phonemes and compared with performance on the same assessment by age- and SES-matched children with typically developing speech. When examining total test scores, only 38% scored below normal limits. Closer examination of the data revealed that 74% of the children failed the speech perception test for at least one of the four phonemes targeted, however, reflecting the fact that children's speech perception impairments are not global in nature, but rather are tied to the specific phonemes that they misarticulate (for further discussion of this point, see Locke, 1980a, 1980b; Rvachew & Jamieson, 1995). For example, all nine children who misarticulated /s/ and/or /θ/ in Rvachew and Jamieson's (1989) study failed to perceive the contrast between /s/ and /θ/ when asked to identify a synthetic continuum of words that differed in the spectral characteristics of the fricative onset. Overall, it appears that most if not all children with primary SSD will have difficulty perceiving at least some of the phonemes that they misarticulate and are thus candidates for speech perception intervention.

Secondary Populations

Older children with residual errors have not been included in any studies designed to assess the efficacy of SAILS; but, given findings of speech perception and phonological awareness difficulties among this population, it is possible that a perceptually based approach to intervention may benefit these children (Preston & Edwards, 2007; Shuster, 1998). Children with secondary SSD associated with speech perception difficulties might also benefit from the intervention, although these other populations have not been involved in clinical trials of SAILS to date. Children whose speech delay is secondary to cleft palate (Whitehill, Francis, & Ching, 2003) or Down syndrome (Keller-Bell & Fox, 2007) have been found to have difficulty with speech perception tasks. Second language learners may also benefit from the intervention because their speech differences reflect an inability to perceive nonnative phoneme contrasts (Rvachew & Jamieson, 1995). Beyond considering the child's speech perception abilities, cognitive and motivational factors must be taken into account. We have found that children younger than 4 years of age have difficulty understanding the SAILS task. Children who are much older may consider the graphics to be unappealing.

Table 12.1. Expected performance on certain Speech Assessment and Interactive Learning System (SAILS) modules

Module	Prekindergarten (mean age = 59 months)		Kindergarten (mean age = 71 months)		First grade (mean age = 89 months)	
	M	*SD*	*M*	*SD*	*M*	*SD*
/l/: lake	87.00	8.06	91.92	10.96	92.29	10.31
/k/: cat	78.60	7.17	77.31	10.79	81.43	12.87
/ɹ/: rat	79.46	10.92	82.31	8.51	85.70	12.61
/s/: Sue	71.52	8.64	80.26	8.38	81.24	7.59
All four	77.70	6.60	82.09	6.10	84.12	6.68

Note: These scores, expressed as percent correct responses per module, were obtained from 35 children recruited from child care and preschools. The children were normally developing and spoke English as their first language according to their parents and teachers. On entry to the study, socioeconomic status was rated for each child's family by combining the parents' occupation and level of education to yield a Blishen score. The resulting Blishen scores ranged from 31 (high school not completed) to 101 (professional credentials), with a mean of 58 (some postsecondary education). Thirteen of the children attended French immersion schools although English was their home language. Goldman-Fristoe Test of Articulation percentiles were within normal limits (mean [*M*] = 45.03; standard deviation [*SD*] = 18.53), as were Peabody Picture Vocabulary Test standard scores (*M* = 112.43; SD = 11.02). The children's speech perception abilities were assessed during the spring of the prekindergarten, kindergarten, and first-grade years when their average ages were 59, 71, and 89 months of age.

ASSESSMENT METHODS FOR DETERMINING INTERVENTION RELEVANCE

Determining appropriateness of the intervention should involve assessing the child's ability to perceive the phoneme contrasts that will be targeted in speech therapy. SAILS is configured to provide information about the child's perception of the phonemes /k, f, l, s, θ, ʃ, ʧ, ɹ/ in the word-initial position. Additional modules, targeting /st/ in word-initial position and /k, f, l, s, ɹ, st, nd/ in word-final position are under development. Normative data have been collected for four of the SAILS modules targeting /l, k, ɹ, s/ in word-initial position, as shown in Table 12.1. As a general rule, approximately 70% correct performance is the lower limit of normal performance at age 4 years for any phoneme. Split-half reliability for these modules was determined to be .82 (Rvachew & Grawburg, 2006).

THEORETICAL BASIS

Dominant Theoretical Rationale for the Intervention Approach

From the perspective of the representation approach (Munson, Edwards, & Beckman, 2005a), phonological development is driven by the gradual accretion of knowledge in multiple representational domains, especially acoustic-phonetic, articulatory-phonetic, and lexical. Typical and atypical development in each of these domains will be discussed in turn. The achievement of acoustic-phonetic knowledge of the sound system of one's native language is a gradual process, beginning before birth and continuing through late childhood. Access to speech input, coupled with statistical learning processes, leads the infant to discover the sound categories that are specific to the language being learned as well as the language-specific acoustic properties of those sound categories (Maye, Werker, & Gerken, 2002). Well before the emergence of receptive or expressive knowledge of word meanings, the infant has learned to attend differentially to phonetic contrasts that are represented in the speech input, with language-specific perception of vowels developing during the first 6 months and language specific processing of consonants observed before the end of the first year of life (Werker & Curtin, 2005). Ongoing refinements in the stability of the child's acoustic-phonetic knowledge of the sound properties of words continue through late childhood (Edwards, Fox, & Rogers, 2002; Hazan & Barrett, 2000). Stable acoustic-phonetic representations allow the child to perceive speech contrasts and recognize words despite the large range of acoustic variability that is associated with differences among talkers, phonetic contexts, communicative goals, and environmental conditions. Any disruption in the child's access to speech input will interfere with speech perception development, including both severe and mild hearing impairment (Houston, Pisoni, Kirk, Ying, & Miyamoto, 2003; Polka & Rvachew, 2005). However, more central impairments in phonological processing can interfere with the abstraction of stable acoustic-phonetic representations from speech input. For example, infants with a family history of dyslexia show differences in speech processing that are reflected in electrophysiological and behavioral measures of phonological processing from birth through school age (Leppanen, Pihko, Eklund, & Lyytinen, 1999; Lyytinen et al., 2004; Lyytinen, Eklund, & Lyytinen, 2005; Pihko et al., 1999). Phonological processing impairments in individuals with dyslexia are associated with structural and physiological differences in the left perisylvian cortex (McCandliss & Noble, 2003; Ramus, 2004). Given documented genetic, cognitive, and symptom overlap between dyslexia and SSD (Lewis et al., 2006; Pennington, 2006), it is reasonable to assume that a neurological impairment in phonological processing underlies delayed phonological development in at least some children with SSD.

The development of flexible articulatory-phonetic representations allows the child to produce accurate speech sounds within a variety of phonetic contexts, despite developmental change in the structure of the vocal tract. The process begins with the emergence of speechlike babble, typically between 7 and 10 months of age (Oller, 2000), and continues with gradual improvements in speech accuracy and precision through late childhood (Smit, Hand, Freilinger, Bernthal, & Bird, 1990; Smith & Kenney, 1998). During babbling, the infant is learning the mapping between acoustic-phonetic targets and the articulator configurations required to achieve those targets. Structural and functional motor impairments will have an impact on the development of appropriate articulatory-phonetic representations from an early age (Chapman, Hardin-Jopnes, Schulte, & Halter, 2001; Levin, 1999; Rvachew, Creighton, Feldman, & Sauve, 2005). By definition, children with primary SSD do not have overt difficulties with motor function; they may, however, demonstrate more subtle deficiencies in speech motor control (Gibbon, 1999; Gibbon, Hardcastle, & Dent, 1995). Impoverished access to self-produced auditory feedback impairs the development of appropriate articulatory-phonetic representations even when the integrity of the articulatory system is intact. The importance of auditory feedback is evidenced by delayed development of speechlike babble in infants with hearing impairment (Eilers & Oller, 1994; Koopmans-van Beinum, Clement, & van den Dikkenberg-Pot, 2001; Rvachew et al., 1996; Rvachew, Slawinski, et al., 1999). Such feedback is critical to the infant's developing knowledge of the relationship between acoustic-phonetic targets and the vocal tract configurations that result in the production of those targets. The specificity of acoustic-phonetic representations themselves play an important role in the development of speech motor control (Perkell et al., 2000), and thus the poor speech accuracy observed in children with phonological processing impairments is to be expected.

Lexical processes have an impact on both phonetic and phonological knowledge. In particular, speech perception and vocabulary development are tightly linked (Rvachew, 2006). Children who have more advanced speech perception skills as infants produce larger vocabularies as toddlers (Tsao, Huei-Mei, & Kuhl, 2004). Vocabulary size predicts speech perception performance among older children (Edwards et al., 2002). Lexicality of stimulus items has an impact on speech perception performance (Chiappe, Chiappe, & Siegel, 2001; Walley & Flege, 1999). Nonword repetition is enhanced when the consonant sequences that make up the nonword stimulus are commonly occurring with the child's lexicon (Munson et al., 2005b; Munson, Kurtz, & Windsor, 2005; Munson, Swenson, & Manthel, 2005). Neighborhood density and word frequency have an impact on phonological awareness because a rapidly growing lexicon demands greater specificity of phonetic representations for words in order to facilitate lexical access when lexical items have many similar-sounding neighbors (Bruno et al., 2007; Garlock, Walley, & Metsala, 2001; Metsala, 1997). The pressure to reorganize the lexicon gives rise to abstract phonological categories at the prosodic, segmental, and featural levels.

Given that phonological knowledge is derived from interactions among these three knowledge domains (acoustic-phonetic, articulatory-phonetic, and lexical), why develop an intervention that focuses preferentially on the specificity of the child's acoustic-phonetic representations? First, speech perception plays a key role in the acquisition of speech production accuracy from an early age. For example, differences in language input lead to cross-linguistic differences in speech perception in the first year of life and in production in the second year of life (de Boysson-Bardies, Halle, Sagart, & Durand, 1989; Polka, Rvachew, & Mattock, 2007; Rvachew, Alhaidary, Mattock, & Polka, 2008; Rvachew, Mattock, Polka, & Menard, 2006). Furthermore, speech perception skills predict growth in articulation abilities over time in older children (Rvachew, 2006). Second, as reviewed earlier, it is well established that children with SSD as a group have significantly poorer speech perception and phonological processing skills than do children with typically developing speech. In fact, these difficulties with acoustic-phonetic knowledge are more salient among this population than difficulties with phonological knowledge (Munson et al., 2006; Munson et al., 2005b). Overall, these studies indicated that children with SSD have nonadult-like acoustic-phonetic representations—their perceptual categories are too broad, encompassing both correct and incorrect productions of a given phoneme. Finally, it appears that speech therapy programs rarely address this speech perception impairment directly, leading to disappointing results. The findings reported by Shuster (1998) are both striking and distressing in this regard—a group of children who were discharged from therapy after failing to progress had no ability to identify incorrect and correct versions of /ɹ/ despite 2 years of therapy targeting this phoneme. SAILS was designed to ensure that children know what the target phoneme is supposed to sound like as they embark on the task of learning to produce it accurately.

Levels of Consequences Being Addressed

SAILS targets speech perception difficulties directly and speech accuracy indirectly and is thus primarily concerned with functional limitations. It has been demonstrated that the intervention leads to improved speech intelligibility, which should impact social participation. Resolution of the child's phonological impairment should contribute to the prevention of reading disability, thus diminishing the likelihood of school failure and underemployment.

Target Areas of Intervention

SAILS addresses the child's speech perception abilities with a two-alternative, forced-choice task, the goal of which is to identify words that are good exemplars of the target against a background of varied authentic misarticulations of the target phoneme. The task helps the child to develop more specific acoustic-phonetic representations for the phonemes that the child misarticulates, with the goal of enhancing the child's response to speech therapy that targets the child's articulatory-phonetic and phonological knowledge of the misarticulated phonemes.

EMPIRICAL BASIS

Research Outcomes

The first study involving SAILS (Rvachew, 1994) was designed to determine if speech perception training would facilitate children's response to a behaviorist intervention for remediation of /ʃ/ misarticulations. Twenty-seven children ages 42–66 months with moderately delayed articulation skills but typical language development participated. All of the children were unstimulable for the target phoneme (/ʃ/) during pretesting. The children were randomly assigned to three different intervention conditions. All of the children received six once-weekly intervention sessions. A research assistant administered 60 SAILS training trials at the beginning of each session. Subsequently, 20 minutes of articulation therapy, targeting the /ʃ/ phoneme, were provided by the first author who was blind to the child's speech perception training condition. The difference between intervention conditions lay solely with the nature of the recorded stimuli presented during the speech perception training trials. Children in Group 1 listened to a variety of naturally produced exemplars of the word *shoe*, half produced correctly and half produced incorrectly. Children in Group 2 listened to a single well-produced token of the word *shoe* and a single well-produced token of the word *moo*, each token being presented 30 times. Group 3 children listened to the words *cat* and *Pete*. Outcomes were assessed by an SLP who was blind to the child's condition assignment.

Group 1 demonstrated the greatest improvement in speech perception performance, but Group 2 also showed significant gains in speech perception ability. Group 3 did not show any improvement in speech perception scores between the pre- and postintervention assessments. With respect to improvements in speech production ability, all outcome measures indicated that Group 1 children made significantly more progress than Group 2 children who made significantly more progress than Group 3 children. In fact, only one child in Group 3 achieved stimulability for the target phoneme in isolation. On the other hand, six children in each of Groups 1 and 2 achieved stimulability in isolation, and some children in Group 1 achieved mastery at the spontaneous sentence level. One explanation for the impact of the SAILS intervention in this study is that the children developed a strong internal representation for the /ʃ/ phoneme, which allowed them to monitor the accuracy of their own productions and self-correct their errors. Parents of children in Group 1 reported that their children engaged in self-practice when alone.

The next study involving SAILS was a nonexperimental comparison of the cycles approach, with and without the inclusion of SAILS (Rvachew, Rafaat, et al., 1999). In the first year of this study, children received 12 weeks of small-group therapy modeled after the cycles approach (Hodson & Paden, 1983). Prior to the onset of the intervention, the children's stimulability and perceptual knowledge of the target phonemes was assessed. Measurable improvements in production accuracy probes for these targets were observed if the child was stimulable for the sound and/or had good perceptual knowledge of the targeted phoneme category prior to intervention. When the child's speech perception performance for the target phoneme was poor or the child was unstimulable for the target, gains were unlikely to occur. Overall, measurable gains in production accuracy were observed for only 40% of the phonemes that were targeted during the 12-week intervention. In the second year of this study, children received the same small-group intervention except that the first three group sessions were replaced with individual therapy during which phonetic placement was used to ensure stimulability of intervention targets, and SAILS was used to ensure good perceptual knowledge of the target phonemes. Postintervention, improved performance was observed for 80% of all intervention targets, regardless of preintervention level of speech perception skills and stimulability.

Wolfe, Presley, and Mesaris (2003) randomly assigned nine children, ages 41–50 months, to receive either production training alone (Production condition) or production training combined with SAILS (Perception condition). Each child received between 9 and 17 intervention sessions targeting three phonemes with a horizontal goal attack strategy. Mean perception test scores improved from 6.58 to 9.03 for the Perception group and from 7.33 to 7.67 for the Production group. On average, target-specific production probe scores improved from 0.83 to 5.42 for the Perception group and from 0.40 to 3.80 for the Production group. Nonparametric statistical analyses revealed a significant advantage to the Perception condition when the child demonstrated poor perception of the target phoneme prior to intervention.

The most recent study of the SAILS approach also involved preschool-age children with moderate or severe SSD (Rvachew, Nowak, & Cloutier, 2004). This study was designed to examine the effect of SAILS on more global aspects of speech performance as well as on the development of phonological awareness skills. Thirty-four children with multiple speech errors received 16 once-weekly intervention sessions. These sessions were conducted by SLPs who were free to use any approach to speech therapy that they felt was appropriate. After each speech therapy session, an undergraduate student research assistant helped the child's parent administer a 10- to 15-minute computer-based intervention. The experimental group received SAILS, targeting a different phoneme in word-initial or -final position each week. The control group listened to computerized books and answered questions about the pictures. The questions were provided to the parent in the form of a script based on standard dialogic reading techniques. The SLPs who were responsible for the children's speech therapy programs were blind to the specific intervention that was provided during these sessions. Speech samples were recorded pre- and postintervention by an SLP who was not involved in the child's speech therapy program and who was not aware of whether the child was in the experimental or control group. Improvements in production accuracy during picture naming and conversation were significantly greater for the children who received SAILS in comparison with children who received the dialogic reading intervention (see Figure 12.1). Follow-up testing 1 year later revealed that 50% of the experimental group achieved normalized speech prior to first-grade entry in comparison with 19% of the control group. Improvements in phonological awareness skills were equivalent in the two groups, however.

Summary of Levels of Evidence

Each of the four studies just described represents a high level of evidence for the effectiveness of SAILS as a means to improve children's acoustic-phonetic knowledge of

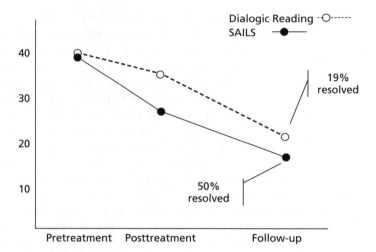

Figure 12.1. Changes in number of errors on the GFTA-2 for children who were randomly assigned to receive either SAILS or a dialogic reading intervention in Rvachew et al. (2004). Percentage of children whose speech delay has resolved as indicated by GFTA-2 percentiles within normal limits (i.e., above 16th) is also indicated for each group.

phonemes that they misarticulated and to facilitate their learning of the articulatory gestures required for the accurate production of these sounds, as summarized in Table 12.2. In three of the studies, the children were randomly assigned to an experimental condition that included SAILS or a control condition that did not involve SAILS. One study was a controlled experiment that compared equivalent groups without randomization. Improvements were observed on study-specific probes that corresponded to the children's speech therapy targets as well as on more global measures of speech production accuracy in picture naming and conversational contexts.

PRACTICAL REQUIREMENTS

Nature of Sessions

The intervention is provided individually, either concurrently with regular speech therapy or in sessions that precede the regular speech therapy program. In Rvachew, Rafaat, and Martin (1999), all SAILS sessions occurred concurrently with stimulability training but prior to the onset of group phonological therapy. In the other studies, SAILS was provided concurrently with speech therapy that was based on either a traditional approach targeting specific phonemes or the cycles approach targeting phonological processes.

Personnel

SAILS can be provided by a communication disorders assistant, a research assistant, or the child's parent supported by a research assistant. The assistants should be trained to set up the software and provide appropriate feedback to the child when he or she points to the wrong response alternative. The SLP should determine in advance the phonemes

Table 12.2.   Levels of evidence for studies of intervention efficacy for Speech Assessment and Interactive Learning System (SAILS)

Level	Description	References
Ia	Meta-analysis of > 1 randomized controlled trial	—
Ib	Randomized controlled study	Rvachew (1994); Wolfe et al. (2003); Rvachew et al. (2004)
IIa	Controlled study without randomization	Rvachew, Rafaat, & Martin (1999)
IIb	Quasi-experimental study	—
III	Nonexperimental studies, i.e., correlational and case studies	—
IV	Expert committee report, consensus conference, clinical experience of respected authorities	—

Adapted from the Scottish Intercollegiate Guidelines Network (http://www.sign.ac.uk).

that would be targeted and the order in which the phonemes would be targeted for each child.

Dosage

In the four studies that have examined the effectiveness of SAILS, the use of SAILS significantly boosted children's response to standard speech therapy approaches with the time devoted to SAILS being 20–60 minutes per target phoneme. In every case, all speech perception training was conducted individually, and the child's exposure to SAILS lasted no longer than 15 minutes in any given session. The number of sessions varied from 3 to 16. No studies have been conducted to determine the optimal timing, frequency, or intensity of speech perception training.

KEY COMPONENTS

Nature of Goals

It is expected that SLPs will select the SAILS modules that correspond to their specific goals—in other words, perception training should target the phonemes that the child misarticulates. This practice proved successful in Rvachew (1994) and Rvachew, Rafaat et al. (1999). In Rvachew et al. (2004), all children experienced the same SAILS training modules in the same order regardless of their error patterns and regardless of the phonemes that were being targeted during their regular speech therapy sessions. It is likely that most, if not all, of these children misarticulated many of the phonemes that were targeted in the standard program because their speech delay was severe enough to encompass a large number of phonemes. It seems possible that SAILS may have general as well as phoneme-specific effects on children's perceptual abilities, perhaps by heightening children's awareness of certain aspects of speech (e.g., the spectral characteristics of the noise portion of words involving fricatives) and by indirectly encouraging them to monitor their own speech accuracy. Nonetheless, the ideal strategy is to link SAILS intervention goals to the goals targeted during speech therapy.

Goal Attack Strategies

No studies have investigated the most efficient goal attack strategy for integrating SAILS into a speech therapy program. On the basis of prior experience with the intervention, however, it is recommended that SAILS be integrated with procedures for teaching correct articulatory placement and promoting frequent speech production practice.

Description of Activities

The SAILS activity is completely controlled by the computer, as shown in the accompanying video demonstration. It is a very simple activity in which the child hears the recording of a word and then points to a picture of the target word or to a picture of a large X in order to indicate whether or not the word sounded like an exemplar of the target. The advantages of the commercial software are that the program provides interesting visual feedback as well as a record of the child's performance on each trial. In the absence of the SAILS software, a similar procedure could be developed by recording a sentence such as "Is this a rat?" from all of the individuals on your caseload using a computer-based recording device. Each resulting wave file could be inserted into a PowerPoint slide along with a picture of a rat. Children who are receiving therapy for /ɹ/ would listen to the sentence presented with each slide and answer the question based on the accuracy of the recorded production of the word *rat*.

Materials and Equipment Required

The original version of SAILS that was used in all of the studies described herein is no longer commercially available. A new version of SAILS is currently under development for use with any computer that has a sound card. Information about access to the new version can be obtained from the first author. The stimuli should always be presented to the child through good quality headphones with a flat frequency response through 20 kHz.

ASSESSMENT AND PROGRESS MONITORING TO SUPPORT DECISION MAKING

A standard articulation/phonology assessment tool should be used to identify the phonemes that the child misarticulates. Typically, the child's speech perception difficulties will be restricted to those phonemes that he or she misarticulates (Locke, 1980a; Rvachew & Jamieson, 1995). Two SAILS modules are provided for each target phoneme so that one module can be used for intervention, whereas the other can be used during the preintervention assessment, for target selection, and/or for monitoring the child's progress.

CONSIDERATIONS FOR CHILDREN FROM CULTURALLY AND LINGUISTICALLY DIVERSE BACKGROUNDS

The SAILS stimuli were recorded from native English speakers who grew up in western or central Canada. Locally recorded stimuli should be recorded for use with speakers of other dialects of English (e.g., Australian English) or speakers of other languages. A French version is under development and an American Spanish version is planned.

CASE STUDIES

Case examples of two children with SSD who participated in the Rvachew et al. (2004) study are described to provide insight into the benefits of including a perceptual intervention in the speech therapy program. The two children were selected for these case studies because they achieved outcomes that were representative of their groups.

SAILS group participant 7 was 4;5 at the time of the preintervention assessment, when he presented with a moderate SSD, his score on the Goldman-Fristoe Test of Articulation–Second Edition (GFTA-2; Goldman & Fristoe, 2000) being at the 4th percentile rank and percent consonants correct (PCC) being 66 in conversation. His receptive vocabulary skills were in the average range (percentile rank of 48) as assessed on the Peabody Picture Vocabulary Test–Third Edition (PPVT-III; Dunn & Dunn, 1997). On measures of speech perception and phonological awareness ability, he achieved 74% and 13% correct responses, respectively. He received sixteen 45-minute speech therapy sessions on a weekly basis. The clinician, who was instructed to treat the child as she felt appropriate, reported that she selected a traditional approach and horizontal target selection strategy to target word-initial /l/ clusters in word-initial position, /k/, /g/, and /ʃ/ in word-initial and -final position, and auxiliary verbs. After each regular speech therapy session, his mother administered SAILS to him with guidance from a research assistant.

Six months after the onset of the intervention, his score on the GFTA-2 improved to the 17th percentile rank, and his PCC was 80. He had also made progress with regard to speech perception and phonological awareness (90% and 74% correct responses, respectively). One year after the onset of the study, he achieved a percentile rank of 44 on the GFTA-2 and a PCC of 94. He obtained a perfect score on the test of phonological awareness. His receptive vocabulary skills were at the 68th percentile rank as measured on the PPVT-III. As shown in a partial transcript of his pre- and postintervention spontaneous speech (see Figure 12.2), it is clear that he made great progress during the study, enabling him to begin school with intelligible speech and a firm foundation for the acquisition of reading.

Control group participant 8 was 4;8 at the time of the preintervention assessment. He obtained similar scores to participant 7 at the onset of the study (percentile rank of 3 on the GFTA-2; PCC of 51; speech perception: 77% correct; phonological awareness test 15%; and percentile rank of 40 on the PPVT-III). During regular therapy sessions, his SLP employed a traditional approach and a horizontal goal attack strategy to target /s/ clusters, /k/ and /g/ in word-initial position, and unspecified expressive language goals. Following these sessions, he participated in a dialogic reading activity targeting vocabulary knowledge and verbal reasoning conducted by his mother who was given a script consisting of increasingly complex and abstract questions about the story and illustrations presented in computerized books.

Participant 7 Before SAILS Intervention

SLP: What's happening here?
Child: [his hɝʔɪn aʊʔ ə də wɪndo]

SLP: OK, he's looking out of the window. And then what happens?
Child: [də bebi dɛd aʊʔ ɛn do an də dad]

SLP: The baby gets out and goes on the dog. And then what?
Child: [ɛn hi waʔ hɪm tu də bɛd]

SLP: Can you tell me more?
Child: [dɛn hi jɝpʰ aʊtʰ]

SLP: Then he what?
Child: [dɛn hi jɝps aʊtʰ]

SLP: Are you allowed to jump on the beds at your house? No? How come?
Child: [bitʌz aɪ tɛn ʤʌ mam bɪtni bɛd]

SLP: You're allowed to jump on Brittany's bed? Do you think it might get broken? No? What would happen if you fell off?
Child: [aɪ wʊ bʌmp maɪ hɛd]
SLP: Yeah, you'd better be careful. . .

Participant 7 After SAILS Intervention

SLP: What's happening here?
Child: [də bebi gaɾʌp]

SLP: Uh-huh.
Child: [hi klaɪmd aʊtʰ an də dag]

SLP: He climbed right out of his crib and onto the dog.
Child: [sʌmtaɪm aɪ do an də da ɛn aɪ seɪ gɪdi ʌp bʌt hi don laɪk ɪt i wʌn aʊʔ də weɪ]

SLP: You do that to your dog?
Child: [jɛ wɛn hi sɪɾɪn daʊn]

SLP: How about over here?
Child: [dɛɝ an də bɛd]

SLP: What do you think they're doing?
Child: [stændɪn an də bɛd]

SLP: I was thinking that maybe they were jumping on the bed. Do you jump on the beds at your house?
Child: [jɛə sʌmtaɪm bə mʌm seɪ no]

SLP: How come your mom says no?
Child: [bikʌz mami hæv tʰu waʃ ɪt]

SLP: Oh.
Child: [bikʌz wɛn aɪ ʤʌmp an də bɛd i seɪ do? du ɪt wɪ maɪ koz an ju maɪ fa daʊn]

SLP: I think that she's worried you might fall and hurt yourself.
Child: [aɪ wont fal ɛn hɝt mʌsɛf ɪt kʌmfi ɛn ɪf aɪ fal ɛn bʌmp mʌsɛf də bɛd wɛl laɪk ɪt al ʃaft]

SLP: Yeah, but what if you fell off the bed onto the floor?
Child: [aɪ wʊd nɛvɚ du dæt dæt wʊd nɛvɚ hæpɛn tu mi]

Figure 12.2. Partial transcripts of pre- and postintervention speech samples recorded from a child who participated in the SAILS condition in Rvachew et al. (2004).

At the postintervention assessment, he obtained a percentile rank of 1 on the GFTA-2, and a PCC of 62. His speech perception and phonological awareness test scores also indicated no improvement. One year after the onset of the study, he continued to present with a moderate SSD (percentile 4 on the GFTA-2, PCC of 86). He had made similar gains to participant 7 on the phonological awareness test, obtaining a perfect score. His vocabulary was now in the higher average range, at the 87th percentile. As shown in a partial transcript of participant 8's pre- and postintervention spontaneous speech (see Figure 12.3), this child did not achieve intelligible speech during the intervention period.

Participant 8 Before Control Intervention

SLP: What d'ya think?
Child: [wʌ daɪ owi twa pʰipo tʰɔɪn nɑp hɪm bebisɪts]
SLP: Pardon me?
Mother: Only real people babysit him.
SLP: That's right. I sure would not leave a dog to look after a baby.
Child: [maɪ dɑd bebisɪt miːnː]
SLP: Pardon me?
Child: [maɪ dʌ bebisɪt miːnː]
SLP: Your dog babysits you?
Child: [maɪ dæij]
SLP: Your dad. I'll bet your dad does a much better job than a dog would do.
Mother: Where did the dog take her?
Child: [bɛɪdʂ]
Mother: And what are they doing there?
Child: [ævɪn næpʰ]
SLP: What is it?
Mother: Having a nap.
SLP: I don't think they're napping. Better look again. What do you see?
Child: [beɪn]
SLP: Playin. Oh!
Child: [bebi jeɪn daʊn ɪn gaʂ tʰæni ʌpʰ]
SLP: OK. I was thinking that maybe they're jumping on the bed. Do you think they are?
Child: [nou] [wai bɛbi]
SLP: What about the baby?
Child: [bebi weɪ daʊ̆]
SLP: Baby's laying down. OK.
Child: [wɛɪʂ] [bebi tʰa dʌo hɪm do no haʊ]
SLP: The baby can't jump. He doesn't know how. OK.

Participant 8 After Control Intervention

SLP: If you had a dog would you let a baby look after him?
Child: [m m] [maɪ gaʃowi be ʌwaʊ̆ds]
SLP: This dog plays around too. Let's check it out.
Child: [ɪm jʊkɪn aʊ də wɪndo]
SLP: He is looking out the window. Yeah, and then what happens?
Child: [ʌ bebi gʌm aŋ ə gaːg]
SLP: Yeah. He sure does. . . .It's mom's room. What do they do there?
Child: [ə bebi jeɪ̆ daʊn ɛ̃ gaː tʌnɪn ʌp]
SLP: The baby's lying down and the dog's standing up. I was thinking that maybe they were jumping on the bed. Do you think?
Child: [nowaɪ hɪm an hɪm tʰɪptʰoʂ ɛ̃ hɪm an bi]
SLP: Pardon me? I didn't understand that part.
Child: [mebi wəs dʌmpan hɪm wəʂ dʌmpɪn mebi hɪm dʌmpɪn an hɪs bʌm]
SLP: Oh. He was jumping on his bum. Do you jump on the beds at your house?
Child: [maɪ mʌm aɪ kæ̃ dʐʌmp a maɪ weŋ maɪŋ ɪs ʌ bʌʔbɛds]
SLP: Pardon me?
Child: [aɪ ɛvə bʌŋkbɛds]
SLP: You have a bunk bed. So if you jumped on your bed you'd hit your head, right?
Child: [aɪ dʌmp an ɪ tapʊ ɪs waɪ du ə wuf]
SLP: That's right, you'd go right through the roof.

Figure 12.3. Partial transcripts of pre- and postintervention speech samples recorded from a child who participated in the control condition in Rvachew et al. (2004).

The final outcomes were very different for these two children. Participant 7 achieved intelligible speech after 6 months, whereas participant 8 presented with moderate SSD throughout the intervention and follow-up phases of the study. Participant 8 did show significant progress in vocabulary development, however. Interestingly, both children made equivalent gains on the test of phonological awareness, highlighting the important roles of both speech perception and vocabulary development to the emergence of phonological awareness skills in preschool children, as described in Rvachew and Grawburg (2006).

STUDY QUESTIONS

1. Describe the key features of SAILS with respect to the stimuli, the task, the feedback provided, and the role of the clinician.

2. What are the goals of SAILS?

3. What is the level of evidence that supports the efficacy of SAILS?

FUTURE DIRECTIONS

Research is focused on extending the SAILS approach to other languages and confirming the efficacy of SAILS in randomized control trials with children speaking Canadian French. Furthermore, we seek to identify the optimal combination of interventions for ensuring that children with SSD begin school with good enough phonological awareness abilities to benefit from formal reading instruction. We are also conducting research with adult learners of a second language to identify the optimal stimulus characteristics for perceptual learning. Studies that compare computer-based perceptual training with live-voice procedures such as receptive minimal activities would be valuable. Direct comparisons of SAILS with auditory bombardment are also required. Finally, large sample studies that investigate interactions between child characteristics and response to different types of phonology interventions are clearly required.

SUGGESTED READINGS

Munson, B., Edwards, J., & Beckman, M.E. (2005). Phonological knowledge in typical and atypical speech-sound development. *Topics in Language Disorders, 25*(3), 190–206.

Rvachew, S. (2007). Perceptual foundations of speech acquisition. In S. McLeod (Ed.), *International guide to speech acquisition* (pp. 26–30). Clifton Park, NY: Thomson Delmar Learning.

REFERENCES

AVAAZ Innovations, Inc. (1994). Speech Assessment and Interactive Learning System (Version 1.2) [Computer software]. London, Ontario, Canada: Author.

Bird, J., Bishop, D.V.M., & Freeman, N.H. (1995). Phonological awareness and literacy development in chil-

dren with expressive phonological impairments. *Journal of Speech and Hearing Research, 38*, 446–462.

Broen, P.A., Strange, W., Doyle, S.S., & Heller, J.H. (1983). Perception and production of approximant consonants by normal and articulation-delayed preschool children. *Journal of Speech and Hearing Research, 26*, 601–608.

Bruno, J.L., Manis, F.R., Keating, P., Sperling, A.J., Nakamoto, J., & Seidenberg, M.S. (2007). Auditory word identification in dyslexic and normally achieving readers. *Journal of Experimental Child Psychology, 97*, 183–204.

Cameron, J., Pierce, W.D., Basko, K.M., & Gear, A. (2005). Achievement-based rewards and intrinsic motivation: A test of cognitive mediators. *Journal of Educational Psychology, 97*, 641–655.

Campbell, T.F., Dollaghan, C.A., Rockette, H.E., Paradise, J.L., Feldman, H.M., Shriberg, L.D., et al. (2003). Risk factors for speech delay of unknown origin in 3-year-old children. *Child Development, 74*, 346–357.

Chapman, K.L., Hardin-Jopnes, M., Schulte, J., & Halter, K.A. (2001). Vocal development of 9-month-old babies with cleft palate. *Journal of Speech, Language, and Hearing Research, 44*, 1268–1283.

Chiappe, P., Chiappe, D.L., & Siegel, L.S. (2001). Speech perception, lexicality, and reading skill. *Journal of Experimental Child Psychology, 80*, 58–74.

Clarkson, R.L., Eimas, P.D., & Marean, G.C. (1989). Speech perception in children with histories of recurrent otitis media. *Journal of the Acoustical Society of America, 85*, 926–933.

Cohen, J.H., & Diehl, C.F. (1963). Relation of speech sound discrimination ability to articulation-type speech defects. *Journal of Speech and Hearing Disorders, 28*, 187–190.

de Boysson-Bardies, B., Halle, P., Sagart, L., & Durand, C. (1989). A cross-linguistic investigation of vowel formants in babbling. *Journal of Child Language, 16*, 1–17.

Dunn, L.M., & Dunn, L.M. (1997). *Peabody Picture Vocabulary Test–Third Edition (PPVT-III)*. Circle Pines, MN: American Guidance Service.

Edwards, J., Fox, R.A., & Rogers, C.L. (2002). Final consonant discrimination in children: Effects of phonological disorder, vocabulary size, and articulatory accuracy. *Journal of Speech, Language, and Hearing Research, 45*, 231–242.

Eilers, R., & Oller, D. (1994). Infant vocalizations and the early diagnosis of severe hearing impairment. *Journal of Pediatrics, 124*, 199–203.

Gardner, H. (1997). Are your minimal pairs too neat? The dangers of phonemicisation in phonology therapy. *European Journal of Disorders of Communication, 32*, 167–175.

Garlock, V.M., Walley, A.C., & Metsala, J.L. (2001). Age-of-acquisition, word frequency, and neighborhood density effects on spoken word recognition by children and adults. *Journal of Memory and Language, 45*, 468–492.

Gibbon, F.E. (1999). Undifferentiated lingual gestures in children with articulation/phonological disorders. *Journal of Speech, Language, and Hearing Research, 42*, 382–397.

Gibbon, F.E., Hardcastle, W.J., & Dent, H. (1995). A study of obstruent sounds in school age children with speech disorders using electropalatography. *European Journal of Disorders of Communication, 30*, 213–225.

Goldman, R.M., & Fristoe, M. (2000). *Goldman-Fristoe Test of Articulation* (2nd ed.). Circle Pines, MN: American Guidance Service.

Guenther, F.H., Husain, F.T., Cohen, M.A., & Shinn-Cunningham, B.G. (1999). Effects of categorization and discrimination training on auditory perceptual space. *Journal of the Acoustical Society of America, 106*, 2900–2912.

Hazan, V., & Barrett, S. (2000). The development of phonemic categorization in children aged 6-12. *Journal of Phonetics, 28*, 377–396.

Hodson, B.W., & Paden, E.P. (1983). *Targeting intelligible speech: A phonological approach to remediation*. Boston: College-Hill Press.

Hoffman, P.R., Daniloff, R.G., Bengoa, D., & Schuckers, G. (1985). Misarticulating and normally articulating children's identification and discrimination of synthetic [r] and [w]. *Journal of Speech and Hearing Disorders, 50*, 46–53.

Hoffman, P.R., Stager, S., & Daniloff, R.G. (1983). Perception and production of misarticulated /r/. *Journal of Speech and Hearing Disorders, 48*, 210–215.

Houston, D.M., Pisoni, D., Kirk, K.I., Ying, A., & Miyamoto, R.T. (2003). Speech perception skills of deaf infants following cochlear implantation: A first report. *International Journal of Pediatric Otorhinolaryngology, 67*, 479–495.

Johnson, D.L., Swank, P.R., Owen, M.J., Baldwin, C.D., Howie, V.M., & McCormick, D.P. (2000). Effects of early middle ear effusion on child intelligence at three, five, and seven years of age. *Journal of Pediatric Psychology, 25*, 5–13.

Keller-Bell, Y., & Fox, R.A. (2007). A preliminary study of speech discrimination in youth with Down syndrome. *Clinical Linguistics and Phonetics, 21*, 305–317.

Kingston, J. (2003). Learning foreign vowels. *Language and Speech, 46*, 295–349.

Klausen, O., Moller, P., Holmefjord, A., Reisaeter, S., & Asbjornsen, A. (2007). Lasting effects of otitis media with effusion on language skills and listening performance. *Acta Otolaryngology, 543*, 73–76.

Koopmans-van Beinum, F.J., Clement, C.J., & van den Dikkenberg-Pot, I. (2001). Babbling and the lack of auditory speech perception: A matter of coordination? *Developmental Science, 4*, 61–70.

Lambacher, S.G., Martens, W.L., Kakehi, K., & Marasinghe, C.A. (2005). The effects of identification training on the identification and production of American English vowels by native speakers of Japanese. *Applied Psycholinguistics, 26*, 227–247.

Larrivee, L.S., & Catts, H.W. (1999). Early reading achievement in children with expressive phonological disorders. *American Journal of Speech-Language Pathology, 8*, 118–128.

Leppanen, P.H.T., Pihko, E., Eklund, K.M., & Lyytinen, H. (1999). Cortical responses of infants with and without a genetic risk for dyslexia: II. Group effects. *Neuroreport, 10,* 969–973.

Levin, K. (1999). Babbling in infants with cerebral palsy. *Clinical Linguistics and Phonetics, 13,* 249–267.

Lewis, B.A., Shriberg, L.D., Freebairn, L.A., Hansen, A.J., Stein, C.M., Taylor, H.G., et al. (2006). The genetic bases of speech sound disorders: Evidence from spoken and written language. *Journal of Speech, Language, and Hearing Research, 49,* 1294–1312.

Lively, S.E., Logan, J.S., & Pisoni, D. (1993). Training Japanese listeners to identify English /r/ and /l/. II: The role of phonetic environment and talker variability in learning new perceptual categories. *Journal of the Acoustical Society of America, 94,* 1242–1255.

Locke, J.L. (1980a). The inference of speech perception in the phonologically disordered child. Part I: A rationale, some criteria, the conventional tests. *Journal of Speech and Hearing Disorders, 45,* 431–444.

Locke, J.L. (1980b). The inference of speech perception in the phonologically disordered child. Part II: Some clinically novel procedures, their use, some findings. *Journal of Speech and Hearing Disorders, 45,* 445–468.

Lyytinen, H., Aro, M., Eklund, K., Erskine, J., Guttorm, T., Laakso, M., et al. (2004). The development of children at familial risk for dyslexia: Birth to early school age. *Annals of Dyslexia, 54,* 184–220.

Lyytinen, P., Eklund, K., & Lyytinen, H. (2005). Language development and literacy skills in late-talking toddlers with and without familial risk for dyslexia. *Annals of Dyslexia, 55,* 166–192.

Maye, J., Werker, J.F., & Gerken, L. (2002). Infant sensitivity to distributional information can affect phonetic discrimination. *Cognition, 82,* B101–B111.

McCandliss, B., & Noble, K.G. (2003). The development of reading impairment: A cognitive neuroscience model. *Mental Retardation and Developmental Disabilities Research Reviews, 9,* 196–205.

McClelland, J.L., Fiez, J.A., & McCandliss, B.D. (2002). Teaching the /r/-/l/ discrimination to Japanese adults: Behavioral and neural aspects. *Physiology and Behavior, 77,* 657–662.

McGrath, L.M., Pennington, B.F., Willcutt, E.G., Boada, R., Shriberg, L.D., & Smith, S.D. (2007). Gene x environment interactions in speech sound disorder predict language and preliteracy outcomes. *Development and Psychopathology, 19,* 1047–1072.

Metsala, J.L. (1997). An examination of word frequency and neighborhood density in the development of spoken-word recognition. *Memory and Cognition, 25,* 47–56.

Munson, B., Baylis, A., Krause, M., & Yim, D.-S. (2006, June 30–July 2). *Representation and access in phonological impairment.* Paper presented at the 10th Conference on Laboratory Phonology, Paris, France.

Munson, B., Edwards, J., & Beckman, M.E. (2005a). Phonological knowledge in typical and atypical speech sound development. *Topics in Language Disorders, 25*(3), 190–206.

Munson, B., Edwards, J., & Beckman, M.E. (2005b). Relationships between nonword repetition accuracy and other measures of linguistic development in children with phonological disorders. *Journal of Speech, Language, and Hearing Research, 48,* 61–78.

Munson, B., Kurtz, B.A., & Windsor, J. (2005). The influence of vocabulary size, phonotactic probability, and wordlikeness on nonword repetitions of children with and without specific language impairment. *Journal of Speech, Language, and Hearing Research, 48,* 1033–1047.

Munson, B., Swenson, C. L., & Manthel, S.C. (2005). Lexical and phonological organization in children: Evidence from repetition tasks. *Journal of Speech, Language, and Hearing Research, 48,* 108–124.

Nathan, L., Stackhouse, J., Goulandris, N., & Snowling, M.J. (2004). The development of early literacy skills among children with speech difficulties: A test of the "critical age hypothesis." *Journal of Speech, Language, and Hearing Research, 47,* 377–391.

Nishi, K., & Kewley-Port, D. (2007). Training Japanese listeners to perceive American English vowels: Influence of training sets. *Journal of Speech, Language, and Hearing Research, 50,* 1496–1509.

Nittrouer, S. (1996). The relation between speech perception and phonemic awareness: Evidence from low-SES children and children with chronic otitis media. *Journal of Speech and Hearing Research, 39,* 1059–1070.

Oller, D.K. (2000). *The emergence of the speech capacity.* Mahwah, NJ: Lawrence Erlbaum Associates.

Pennington, B.F. (2006). From single to multiple deficit models of developmental disorders. *Cognition, 101,* 385–413.

Perkell, J., Guenther, F.H., Lane, H., Matthies, M.L., Perrier, P., Vick, J., et al. (2000). A theory of speech motor control and supporting data from speakers with normal hearing and with profound hearing loss. *Journal of Phonetics, 28,* 233–272.

Pihko, E., Leppanen, P.H.T., Eklund, K.M., Cheour, M., Guttorm, T.K., & Lyytinen, H. (1999). Cortical responses of infants with and without a genetic risk for dyslexia: I. Age effects. *Neuroreport, 10,* 901–905.

Polka, L., & Rvachew, S. (2005). The impact of otitis media with effusion on infant phonetic perception. *Infancy, 8*(2), 101–117.

Polka, L., Rvachew, S., & Mattock, K. (2007). Experiential influences on speech perception and speech production in infancy. In E. Hoff & M. Shatz (Eds.), *Blackwell handbook of language development* (pp. 153–172). Oxford, England: Blackwell Publishing.

Preston, J.L., & Edwards, M.L. (2007). Phonological processing skills of adolescents with residual speech sound errors. *Language, Speech, and Hearing Services in Schools, 38,* 297–308.

Raitano, N.A., Pennington, B.F., Tunick, B.F., Boada, R.,

& Shriberg, L.D. (2004). Pre-literacy skills of sub-groups of children with speech sound disorders. *Journal of Child Psychology and Psychiatry, 45*, 821–835.

Ramus, F. (2004). Neurobiology of dyslexia: A reinterpretation of the data. *TRENDS in Neurosciences, 27*, 720–726.

Roberts, J.E., Burchinal, M.R., Zeisel, S.A., Neebe, E.C., Hooper, S.R., Roush, J., et al. (1998). Otitis media, the caregiving environment, and language and cognitive outcomes at 2 years. *Pediatrics, 102*, 346–354.

Rvachew, S. (1994). Speech perception training can facilitate sound production learning. *Journal of Speech and Hearing Research, 37*, 347–357.

Rvachew, S. (2006). Longitudinal prediction of implicit phonological awareness skills. *American Journal of Speech-Language Pathology, 15*, 165–176.

Rvachew, S. (2007a). Perceptual foundations of speech acquisition. In S. McLeod (Ed.), *The international guide to speech acquisition* (pp. 26–30). Clifton Park, NY: Thomson Delmar Learning.

Rvachew, S. (2007b). Phonological processing and reading in children with speech sound disorders. *American Journal of Speech-Language Pathology, 16*, 260–270.

Rvachew, S., Alhaidary, A., Mattock, K., & Polka, L. (2008). Emergence of the corner vowels in the babble produced by infants exposed to Canadian English or Canadian French. *Journal of Phonetics, 36*, 564–577.

Rvachew, S., Creighton, D., Feldman, N., & Sauve, R. (2005). Vocal development of infants with very low birth weight. *Clinical Linguistics and Phonetics, 19*(4), 275–294.

Rvachew, S., & Grawburg, M. (2006). Correlates of phonological awareness in preschoolers with speech sound disorders. *Journal of Speech, Language, and Hearing Research, 49*, 74–87.

Rvachew, S., & Jamieson, D.G. (1989). Perception of voiceless fricatives by children with a functional articulation disorder. *Journal of Speech and Hearing Disorders, 54*, 193–208.

Rvachew, S., & Jamieson, D.G. (1995). Learning new speech contrasts: Evidence from learning a second language and children with speech disorders. In W. Strange (Ed.), *Speech perception and linguistic experience* (pp. 411–432). Timonium, MD: York Press.

Rvachew, S., Mattock, K., Polka, L., & Menard, L. (2006). Developmental and cross-linguistic variation in the infant vowel space: The case of Canadian English and Canadian French. *Journal of the Acoustical Society of America, 120*(4), 2250–2259.

Rvachew, S., Nowak, M., & Cloutier, G. (2004). Effect of phonemic perception training on the speech production and phonological awareness skills of children with expressive phonological delay. *American Journal of Speech-Language Pathology, 13*, 250–263.

Rvachew, S., Rafaat, S., & Martin, M. (1999). Stimulability, speech perception and the treatment of phonological disorders. *American Journal of Speech-Language Pathology, 8*, 33–34.

Rvachew, S., Slawinski, E.B., Williams, M., & Green, C.L. (1996). Formant frequencies of vowels produced by infants with and without early onset otitis media. *Canadian Acoustics, 24*, 19–28.

Rvachew, S., Slawinski, E.B., Williams, M., & Green, C.L. (1999). The impact of early onset otitis media on babbling and early language development. *Journal of the Acoustical Society of America, 105*, 467–475.

Shelton, C.M., Johnson, A.F., Ruscello, D.M., & Arndt, W.B. (1978). Assessment of parent-administered listening training for preschool children with articulation deficits. *Journal of Speech and Hearing Disorders, 43*, 242–254.

Sherman, D., & Geith, A. (1967). Speech sound discrimination and articulation skill. *Journal of Speech and Hearing Research, 10*, 277–280.

Shriberg, L.D. (1994). Five subtypes of developmental phonological disorders. *Clinics in Communication Disorders, 4*, 38–53.

Shriberg, L.D., Austin, D., Lewis, B.A., McSweeny, J.L., & Wilson, D.L. (1997). The Speech Disorders Classification System (SDCS): Extensions and lifespan reference data. *Journal of Speech, Language, and Hearing Research, 40*, 723–740.

Shriberg, L.D., Lewis, B.A., Tomblin, J.B., McSweeny, J.L., Karlsson, H.B., & Scheer, A.R. (2005). Toward diagnostic and phenotypic markers for genetically transmitted speech delay. *Journal of Speech, Language, and Hearing Research, 48*, 834–852.

Shuster, L.I. (1998). The perception of correctly and incorrectly produced /r/. *Journal of Speech, Language, and Hearing Research, 41*, 941–950.

Smit, A.B., Hand, L., Freilinger, J.J., Bernthal, J.E., & Bird, A. (1990). The Iowa articulation norms project and its Nebraska replication. *Journal of Speech and Hearing Disorders, 55*, 779–798.

Smith, B.L., & Kenney, M.K. (1998). An assessment of several acoustic parameters in children's speech production development: Longitudinal data. *Journal of Phonetics, 26*, 95–108.

Smith, S.D., Pennington, B.F., Boada, R., & Shriberg, L.D. (2005). Linkage of speech sound disorder to reading disability loci. *Journal of Child Psychology and Psychiatry, 46*, 1057–1066.

Stein, C.M., Schick, J.H., Taylor, G., Shriberg, L.D., Millard, C., Kundtz-Kluge, A., et al. (2004). Pleiotropic effects of a chromosome 3 locus on speech-sound disorder and reading. *American Journal of Human Genetics, 74*, 283–297.

Teele, D.W., Klein, J.O., Chase, C., Menyuk, P., & Rosner, B.A. (1990). Otitis media in infancy and intellectual ability, school achievement, speech, and language at age 7 years. *Journal of Infectious Diseases, 162*, 685–694.

Tsao, F., Huei-Mei, L., & Kuhl, P.K. (2004). Speech perception in infancy predicts language development in the second year of life: A longitudinal study. *Child Development, 75*, 1067–1084.

Tunick, R.A., & Pennington, B.F. (2002). The etiological relationship between reading disability and phonological disorder. *Annals of Dyslexia, 52,* 75–97.

Van Riper, C. (1963). *Speech correction: Principles and methods.* Upper Saddle River, NJ: Prentice Hall.

Walley, A.C., & Flege, J. (1999). Effect of lexical status on children's and adults' perception of native and nonnative vowels. *Journal of Phonetics, 27,* 307–332.

Webster, P.E., Plante, A.S., & Couvillion, M. (1997). Phonologic impairment and prereading: Update on a longitudinal study. *Journal of Learning Disabilities, 30,* 365–376.

Werker, J.F., & Curtin, S. (2005). PRIMIR: A developmental framework of infant speech processing. *Language Learning and Development, 1,* 197–234.

Whitehill, T.L., Francis, A.L., & Ching, C.K.-Y. (2003). Perception of place of articulation by children with cleft palate and posterior placement. *Journal of Speech, 46,* 451–461.

Wolfe, V., Presley, C., & Mesaris, J. (2003). The importance of sound identification training in phonological intervention. *American Journal of Speech-Language Pathology, 12,* 282–288.

Nonlinear Phonological Intervention

B. May Bernhardt, Karen D. Bopp,
Bonnie Daudlin, Susan M. Edwards, and Susan E. Wastie

13

ABSTRACT

Nonlinear phonology refers to phonological theories that describe the hierarchical representation of phonological form from the prosodic phrase to the individual feature. The theories provide a comprehensive framework for analyzing phonological systems and apply to all speakers, with the perspective that even a "simple lisp" occurs in context. The theories have motivated analyses, goal-setting methodology, treatment strategies, and activities for clinical practice. This chapter provides an overview of the theories, intervention studies, and treatment ideas, capturing the spirit of "fun-ology."

INTRODUCTION

Nonlinear phonology encompasses phonological theories of the past 3 decades that describe the hierarchical representation of phonological form from the prosodic phrase to the individual feature. Phonologists assume nonlinear representation, thus the term *nonlinear* is seldom stated. In order to distinguish nonlinear phonology from other perspectives in this book, however, the adjective *nonlinear* is retained. This chapter presents an overview of theories, clinical research applications, and studies, including treatment ideas (e.g., Bernhardt, 1992, 1994a, 1994b, 2005; Bernhardt & Stemberger, 1998, 2000; Bernhardt, Stemberger, & Major, 2006; Bernhardt & Stoel-Gammon, 1994).

TARGET POPULATIONS

Nonlinear phonology refers to the entire phonological system; thus, general principles concerning nonlinear phonological assessment and treatment pertain across ages and etiologies. A comprehensive set of analyses may be particularly useful for someone with a

The authors would like to acknowledge and thank the families and colleagues who have contributed to the enterprise of clinical application of nonlinear phonology since 1988. Thank you also to our Guest Speech Fairy, Carmine Bernhardt; to Travis Bernhardt for the footage; and to Flicker Filmworks and Daniel Santiago for editing. Funding for the projects has come from the BC Medical Services Foundation, the BC Health Research Foundation, the Canadian Language and Literacy Network, and various grants at the University of British Columbia.

moderate to severe impairment in speech production. However, all phonemes occur in context and thus, the phonological hierarchy is relevant also for clients with only single-phoneme mismatches. Although assessment may indicate no apparent effects of structural or segmental context, intervention may need to take context (the phonological hierarchy) into account in order to facilitate initial production of a phone or to promote generalization of the target into running speech.

Nonlinear frameworks have been used for the following groups: 1) typically developing children (Ayyad & Bernhardt, 2007, Kuwaiti Arabic; Bernhardt & Stemberger, 1998; Ullrich, 2004, German); 2) children with primary speech production impairments (Bernhardt, 1990, 1992; Bernhardt, Brooke, & Major, 2003; Bernhardt & Gilbert, 1992; Edwards, 1995; Von Bremen, 1990); 3) children with speech and morphosyntactic production impairments (Bernhardt, 1990; Bernhardt, Brooke, et al., 2003; Bopp, Bernhardt, & Johnson, 1995); 4) children and adolescents with hearing and speech impairments (Ayyad & Bernhardt, 2007; Bernhardt, Gick, Bacsfalvi, & Ashdown, 2003); 5) children with autism (McGee, 2006); 6) children and adults with cleft palate (Bernhardt, Bacsfalvi, Gick, Radanov, & Williams, 2005; Bernhardt, Doan, & Stoel-Gammon, 1995); 7) children, adolescents, and adults learning English /ɹ/ (Adler-Bock, Bernhardt, Gick, & Bacsfalvi, 2007; Gick, Bernhardt, Bacsfalvi, & Wilson, 2008; Modha, Bernhardt, Church, & Bacsfalvi, 2008); and 8) adults with Down syndrome (Fawcett, Bacsfalvi, & Bernhardt, 2008). The treatment activities described later in this chapter are suitable for young children. Other supports such as electropalatography and ultrasound have been used for older individuals (Adler-Bock et al., 2007; Bernhardt, Gick et al., 2003, 2005; Gick et al., 2008; Modha et al., 2008).

ASSESSMENT METHODS FOR DETERMINING INTERVENTION RELEVANCE

Nonlinear phonological assessments have the same general objectives as other communication assessments: 1) to identify whether the client is communicating as effectively as he or she, the family, or others would like in terms of Body Structure/Function, Activities, and Participation (World Health Organization [WHO], 2001); 2) to provide baseline information; 3) to assess whether there are other factors associated with the domain of inquiry; and 4) to determine a management plan.

Many assessment methods are similar to those based on other frameworks: case history-taking and baseline testing, including both a speech sample and evaluations of other domains (e.g., oral mechanism, hearing, language and voice, motor abilities, cognitive, social or academic function). For speech samples, the objective is to obtain sufficient words for nonlinear analysis using audio and, when possible, video recording and online transcription notes. Narrow transcription of the recordings is recommended using an auditory anchor (e.g., Ladefoged, 2004) and/or acoustic analysis to help classify unfamiliar productions. For a basic clinical nonlinear analysis, about 75–80 different words can be sufficient, if these words contain all the phonemes of the language and a wide variety of word structures. Additional words may be needed to answer specific questions. However, if a client produces few words during assessment, even those few words can provide information for short-term goal setting. The sample will optimally include both single words and connected speech; single-word elicitations can ensure content coverage of the language, and connected speech samples can provide information about targets in context and prosody (Bernhardt & Holdgrafer, 2001a, 2001b; Masterson, Bernhardt, & Hofheinz, 2005). Nonlinear phonological analysis provides an overview of all phonological domains, and can be quantitative and/or qualitative. Computer programs increase efficiency of quantitative analysis (Masterson & Bernhardt, 2001; Rose & Hedlund, 2008). However, qualitative scanning analyses (e.g., Bernhardt & Stemberger, 2000) can also provide comprehensive information for management planning. If management is to include treatment, targets and treatment strategies are then determined as the final step of assessment (see Nature of Goals section later in this chapter).

THEORETICAL BASIS

Dominant Theoretical Rationale for the Intervention Approach

By the 1970s, linear organization of phonological form was considered insufficient to account for phonological phenomena. By positing autonomous (autosegmental) hierarchically organized, representational levels (tiers) for tones and vowels, Goldsmith (1979) was able to account for previously inexplicable tonal phenomena, for example, patterns in which a tone could become associated with more than one vowel, or vice versa. The concept of autonomous hierarchically organized, representational tiers was then adopted to explain other phenomena. For example, it is assumed that phonological alternations or patterns reflect the immediate environment; that is, nasals in English taking the place of articulation of the following surface-adjacent stop (*monkey* versus *paint*). However, assimilation can also occur between surface-distant elements (*dub* /dʌb/ > [bʌb]). If consonants and vowels are viewed to be on different tiers, the /d/ and /b/ of *dub* can be viewed as underlyingly adjacent as consonants, and thus able to affect each other.

Figures 13.1 and 13.2 outline the various tiers of the phonological hierarchy. Segments are viewed as intermediary levels of representation, dominating hierarchically organized features and being dominated by larger prosodic units (e.g., syllables, feet).

Considering structure above the segment, research by Kahn (1980) and others supported the inclusion of syllable structure in phonological representations. Syllables can be divided into onsets and rimes (Bernhardt & Stemberger, 1998; Kenstowicz, 1994). The onset encompasses all consonants preceding the most sonorous element of the syllable (generally a vowel); the rime encompasses the most sonorous element of the syllable (nucleus or peak) and any postnuclear consonants (the coda). For example, in the word *flute*, /fl/ is the onset and /ut/ is the rime with /u/ being the nucleus and /t/ the coda.

Theories also posit a timing tier between the segmental and syllable tiers. The timing tier accounts for phenomena such as compensatory lengthening, in which vowel lengthening maintains syllable timing after coda deletion (e.g., *bit* /bɪt/ > [biː]). Timing units in the rime of the syllable (weight units, moras) also relate to stress assignment in some languages (Hayes, 1989, 1995). Short (usually lax) vowels are considered to have one mora, and long vowels or diphthongs, two moras. In some quantity-sensitive languages (e.g., English), codas following lax vowels also appear to be moraic (Hayes, 1995), for example, *bun* having two moras (one for the vowel and one for /n/). Syllable-onset consonants are considered nonmoraic because they are not relevant for stress assignment. In modern English, intervocalic consonants following lax vowels (as in *bunny*) have shortened to singletons, leaving one mora for the lax vowel, one for the unstressed

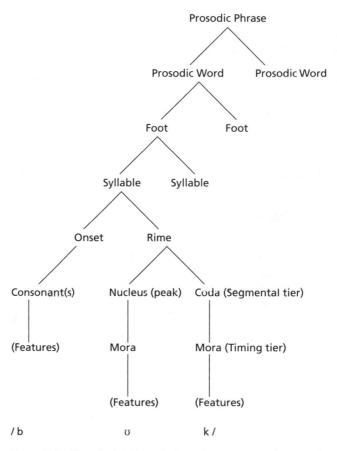

Figure 13.1. Phonological hierarchy from the segment to the prosodic phrase.

vowel /i/, and none for the medial consonant. In terms of moras, then, *bunny* is equivalent to *bun*, the latter having one mora for /ʌ/ and one for /n/. (This concept can be used in intervention, as described later).

Above the syllable tier, the stressed syllables are grouped with unstressed syllables into feet. Feet are described in terms of direction of prominence, that is, which part of the foot is stressed. A word with a right-prominent, weak-Strong (wS) or iambic foot is *gui-TAR*. In contrast, *TAR-get* is left-prominent, Strong-weak (Sw), or trochaic. English has a predominance of trochaic patterns. Feet are grouped further into prosodic words, which have at most one primary stress. Finally, words are grouped into prosodic phrases, which may have additional or alternative positions of prominence. During development, children may show restrictions on any aspects of prosodic structure (e.g., on the number of timing units per syllable, on the complexity of onsets or rimes, on the number of syllables per word or foot; Bernhardt & Stemberger, 1998).

Below the segment, nonlinear theories posit hierarchical organization of features (e.g., Bernhardt & Stemberger, 1998; McCarthy, 1988; Sagey, 1991). Features are considered autonomous, hierarchically organized elements that can combine and recombine into segments. Major organizing features (or nodes), such as Place, Laryngeal, and Root

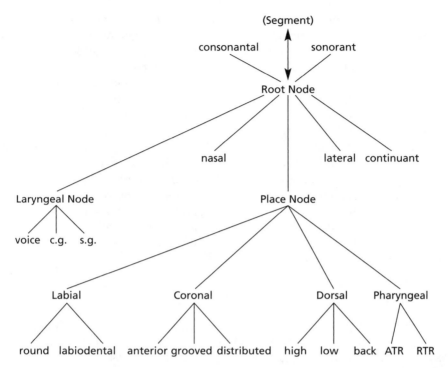

Figure 13.2. Feature hierarchy below the segment. ATR, advanced tongue root; RTR, retracted tongue root; c.g., constricted glottis; s.g., spread glottis.

(manner; see Figure 13.2) are defined as dominating more specific types of features. Most accounts show manner features attached to or near the Root node, the link to the segmental tier (i.e., manner features are thus higher than place and laryngeal features in the hierarchy). Definition of place features shows differences from previous accounts (Chomsky & Halle, 1968). For example, [Labial] is viewed as distinct from the feature [anterior] (now designated solely as a feature of [Coronal], or tongue tip and blade articulations); subsidiary features of [Coronal] have been designated for tongue shape, for example [+grooved] or [−grooved], or airflow pattern [+distributed] or [−distributed]; vowels, /k/ and /g/ are designated as [Dorsal] rather than velar, because [Dorsal] refers to the tongue body, the primary active articulator. Laryngeal features now describe both the state of the glottis as [+constricted] (glottal stops; creaky voice) or [+spread] (/h/, aspirated stops, voiceless fricatives for English) and as vibrating/nonvibrating (voicing; Bernhardt & Stemberger, 1998, 2000; Kenstowicz, 1994). Accounts vary in the description of exact features and their locations and in assumptions of assigned feature values (0, +, −; see Bernhardt & Stemberger, 1998, 2000).

Across the phonological hierarchy, there remains a general distinction between what is considered frequent/less complex (unmarked) and infrequent/complex in phonological systems. The term *default* is now often used to designate unmarked elements. For prosodic structures, noncomplex onsets, nuclei, rimes, and feet are generally considered defaults, although for some children bimoraic syllables/feet/words may be a default (Bernhardt & Stemberger, 1998). The features of /t/ are considered to be default consonant features for many languages: [−continuant] (stop), [−voiced] and [Coronal, +anterior] (alveolar) (although children may have defaults that differ from those of the target language, Bernhardt & Stemberger, 1998). Generally, segments are represented underlyingly by their nondefault features. For example, /m/ is [+nasal] and [Labial], but /n/ is [+nasal] because it has default [Coronal] place. Predictable features of /m/ ([+consonantal], [+sonorant] and [+voiced], given [+nasal]) are not included in characterization of /m/ (Bernhardt & Stemberger, 1998). Phonological development involves the gradual mastery of the nondefaults of the target language and alignment of the defaults with the adult system.

If development does not occur naturally at a rate acceptable to stakeholders, intervention may be warranted. The perspective taken here does not assume a clear dividing line between articulation and phonology; thus, nonlinear phonological intervention has a dual focus: development of more well-defined underlying representations (awareness building) and actual speech production (e.g., imitation, phonetic facilitation, rate control). The best outcome is intelligible, age-appropriate speech production in conversation. However, a profound hearing impairment or aberrant oral mechanism potentially could limit expectations for "perfect" speech.

Levels of Consequences Being Addressed

Nonlinear phonological intervention primarily addresses Body Function impairments in speech perception and production (WHO, 2001). Activity level skills are sometimes addressed in addition in terms of phonological awareness skills, which refer to various levels of the phonological hierarchy and promote literacy acquisition. The treatment strategies and activities described in this chapter are designed to engage the client's interest in speech communication and to enhance communicative effectiveness, that is, Participation-level skills (WHO, 2001).

Target Areas of Intervention

The major focus of intervention is awareness and production of phonological form. Communicative effectiveness and client comfort in communication are also objectives of treatment. Related areas can include phonological awareness, morphosyntax, and the lexicon. Phonological awareness activities typically include awareness of various levels of the phonological hierarchy: the prosodic phrase, word, syllable, onset, rime, and segment. Morphosyntax requires production of prosodic phrases (with a variety of stressed and unstressed elements) and often production of complex word shapes (through addition of morphemes to a base form: *bat–bats*). The lexicon can be enhanced through introduction of new words and enhanced access to the form of established words.

EMPIRICAL BASIS

Nonlinear Phonological Intervention Research Outcomes

This section focuses on treatment studies relating to preschoolers with primary speech production impairments. All studies had individual, clinic-based treatment, with parents participating actively in the 45-minute sessions and conducting home activities. For the smaller-scale studies, the first author conducted the entire investigation. The two larger group studies involved community speech-language pathologists (SLPs), who collected data and conducted the intervention after participating in a 2-day workshop given by the university research team at the outset of the study (see further details later); research assistants not blind to the sample or child completed the phonetic transcriptions of four major speech samples per study. For all but the last study, speech samples were elicited using objects and pictures with a 164-word list (Bernhardt, 1990). For the final study (Bernhardt, Brooke et al., 2003), the *Photo Articulation Test–Third Edition* (PAT-3; Lippke, Dickey, Selmar, & Soder, 1997) was used to increase efficiency. Connected speech samples confirmed target selection and speech production outcomes. For the two larger group studies, nonstandardized assessments of phonological awareness were also conducted. (All studies also included other language, hearing, and oral mechanism evaluations.)

All studies were quasi-experimental in nature (see Table 13.2) and are classified here as exploratory, efficacy, or effectiveness studies (Olswang, 1998). Studies had single-subject designs involving alternating treatment in a multiple baseline, ABCBC format.

1. *Exploratory single-subject design studies:* Bernhardt (1990), with six preschoolers, had two 6-week treatment blocks, each containing two sub-blocks for word structure development and two for feature/segment development; program sequence was counterbalanced across participants. Von Bremen (1990), a study of 5-year-old identical twins, had the same timing, but for the first two blocks, one twin was assigned to structural goals and the other twin to segmental goals. Both studies had a final 6-week treatment block designed to meet the child's needs. Edwards (1995) studied two 3-year-old boys, following the general principles and methods of the first two studies, but allowing flexibility in timing and goal sequence in order to follow the children's developmental paths more closely; this study had twice-weekly therapy for 16 weeks and was a pilot for a 1997 study discussed later.

2. *A quasi-experimental efficacy study* (described in detail in Major & Bernhardt, 1998): A 1994 study had 19 participants ages 3–5 years, and was conducted three times a week in various agencies by local SLPs over 16 weeks. The first author provided phonological analyses and determined goal sequence and treatment conditions, counterbalancing these across children. Phonological awareness was tested before and after the first two 6-week treatment blocks. Both phonological production and awareness were targeted in a third 4-week child-centered treatment block.

3. *A quasi-experimental effectiveness study:* A 1997 study (reported by Bernhardt, Brooke, et al., 2003) had 15 participants (ages 3–6) and a small reference control group (eight children). It also involved local SLPs, who conducted their own analyses (based on phonetic transcripts received from the university research assistant) and planned the individualized intervention program with confirmation by the first author. The study included two 8-week treatment blocks of two sessions per week each. Phonological awareness was targeted in the second block only. Both word structure and feature/segment targets were balanced in the treatment programs, but with greater flexibility than the earlier studies by the author and colleagues, in order and time spent on each target and with no counterbalancing across participants.

Key questions and results for the studies are presented below and in Table 13.1.

1. *Higher level, faster gain?* Treatment was designed to effect change at various levels of the phonological hierarchy. Top-down hierarchical effects were expected (i.e., a

Table 13.1. Does higher-level form develop at a faster rate in intervention?

Study	Results
Bernhardt (1990), 6 children ages 3-6	1. Significantly faster gain for higher level word structures than segments (Block 1, 6/6 participants; Block 2, 5/6 participants) 2. Faster rate of change for higher-level features: 4/6 participants
Von Bremen (1990), 5-year-old twin boys with identical phonology, one assigned to structure and one to segments	1. The "structural" twin mastered his targets and those of his brother in two treatment blocks (when his twin's targets were not known). 2. The "segmental" twin took three blocks to achieve his own and his brother's targets (when they were directly targeted). 3. Higher-level features showed a faster rate of change.
1994 study: 19 preschoolers	Significantly greater gain for word structure versus consonant match pre-post: a 22% gain in word shape match, compared with a 13% gain in consonant match ($t = 2.11038$, $p = .042$).
1997 study: 15 children ages 3–6	1. The fastest-developing target was CVCV. 2. A nonsignificant advantage for word structure targets (21.4% gain compared with 18.9% for consonants).

faster rate of change for higher-level elements after treatment). Results converge across the studies: higher-level elements generally showed greater and faster change.

2. *Onset-rime focus versus mora focus in word structure development?* The question was whether treatment highlighting onset-rime divisions or alternatively, moraic constituents, might be more facilitative of word structure development (Bernhardt, 1990). No significant differences were noted in a Kolmogorov-Smirnov cumulative frequency evaluation for the six children. However, it was considered that using both approaches may have facilitated the accelerated gains in word structure development.

3. *Phonological intervention and development of phonological awareness?* Research hypotheses were that there would be treatment effects of both nonlinear phonological intervention and direct phonological awareness (metaphonology) intervention. In the 1994 study, phonological awareness skills were not targeted directly in the first 12 weeks of intervention, but there was a significant group improvement in phonological awareness skills ($Z = -2.08$, T1 to T2, $p < .05$). Four weeks later, after which phonological awareness skills were directly targeted, there was a slightly larger positive group effect ($Z = -2.15$, T2 to T3, $p < .05$). A follow-up study 3 years later (Bernhardt & Major, 2005) found that most children were performing in the average range on a number of speech, language, and literacy tasks. These longer-term results may have reflected the earlier nonlinear phonological intervention that had a focus on word structure. The two children who showed no significant gains in phonological awareness skills by the end of the 1994 study had below-average literacy skills in early elementary school, suggesting it is important to follow individuals at risk.

4. *Efficacy-style versus effectiveness-style studies?* The question was whether a study more in keeping with clinical practice would have equivalent results to a more rigidly investigator-controlled study. The 1997 study (32 instead of 48 sessions) gave greater control to the SLPs, although they followed the general principles and methods introduced at the outset of the study. There was no significant difference in average gain in percent consonant match (PCM, including deletions) for the 1994 and 1997 studies (16.4% average gain for 1994, 18.96% for 1997, each with a standard deviation of 12.1%) or percent vowel match (PVM, 15% gain in both).

In summary, quasi-experimental data support the application of intervention based on nonlinear phonological analysis and treatment strategies. The 1997 study suggests that SLPs, with training, can facilitate significant change in child speech production through this approach. The data also suggest that there are benefits to focusing systematically on word structures in treatment. The phonological awareness results imply that it is important to monitor those skills at the beginning of phonological intervention and intermittently throughout the intervention program. If a child does not benefit indirectly in terms of phonological awareness from the intervention for speech production, direct phonological awareness training is warranted.

Summary of Levels of Evidence

Nonlinear phonological intervention studies range from case studies (e.g., Bernhardt, MacNeill, & Bohlen 1994; Noble-Wiebe, MacFarlane, & Bernhardt, 1994) to quasi-experimental studies (Bernhardt, 1990, 1992; Bernhardt et al., 2003; Bernhardt & Gilbert, 1992; Edwards, 1995; Major & Bernhardt, 1998) to studies with nonrandomized controls (Bernhardt, 2007). Randomized control trials remain to be done (see Table 13.2).

PRACTICAL REQUIREMENTS

Nature of Sessions

The format of nonlinear phonological intervention (i.e., the number, frequency, and length of sessions or service delivery model) is independent of the theories. The nonlinear analyses and the development of treatment strategies require the direct involvement of an SLP, but the highly active participation of the client and caregivers is paramount. Ideally, the service delivery model will reflect the needs of the client. In reality, service delivery limitations may affect selection and order of goals and treatment strategies (see Nature of Goals section later in this chapter).

Table 13.2. Levels of evidence for studies of treatment efficacy for nonlinear phonological intervention

Level	Description	References
Ia	Meta-analysis of > 1 randomized controlled trial	—
Ib	Randomized controlled study	—
IIa	Controlled study without randomization	—
IIb	Quasi-experimental study	Adler-Bock et al. (2007); Bernhardt (1990, 1992); Bernhardt et al. (2005); Bernhardt, Brooke, et al. (2003); Bernhardt, Gick et al. (2003); Bernhardt & Gilbert (1992); Edwards (1995); Fawcett et al. (2008); Gick et al. (2008); Major & Bernhardt (1998); Modha et al. (2008). Von Bremen (1990).
III	Nonexperimental studies, i.e., correlational and case studies	Additional studies not reported here
IV	Expert committee report, consensus conference, clinical experience of respected authorities	—

Adapted from the Scottish Intercollegiate Guidelines Network (http://www.sign.ac.uk).

Personnel

Although the SLP is involved in terms of analysis, program planning, and intervention, parents/caregivers/family members are integral throughout the process from the assessment onwards. In addition, other personnel (e.g., teachers, speech assistants) may help with treatment and generalization activities in addition to documentation of progress.

Dosage

The amount of time needed per client is very individualized, reflecting the client needs and availability and the service delivery constraints of the interventionists.

KEY COMPONENTS

Nature of Goals

For speech production, Bernhardt and Stemberger (2000) describe four basic types of nonlinear intervention goals. Other goals of treatment may include general communicative effectiveness and phonological awareness, such as the skills in identifying rhymes, onsets, segments, or syllable and rhythm patterns.

For intervention targets, there are two major divisions, leading to four types of goals (see Table 13.3): 1) a division between prosodic (syllable and word) structure targets and targets for features and segments, and 2) a division between new individual elements (either prosodic or feature) and new locations for or combinations of at least partially established elements (as in the later empirical studies). *New individual elements* are those that are assessed to be absent or marginal (emerging) in the client's phonological system. For example, if /k/, /g/, and /ŋ/ are missing or marginal, a *new individual feature* could be [Dorsal]. *New individual prosodic structures* could entail new word lengths in syllables, new word and/or phrasal stress patterns, and/or new word shapes in terms of consonant (C)/vowel (V) sequences (e.g., CVC, CCVC). *New combinations of features* could entail combination of an existing [Labial] feature from /p/ with an existing [+continuant] for /s/ to make a new fricative, /f/. *New locations for old elements* could entail moving a segment or feature from one word position where that segment exists to an already established structural position where it does not exist (e.g., targeting fricatives word-

Table 13.3. Nonlinear phonological intervention goal types

Domain	New form	Existing forms targeted in new structures or combinations
Prosodic structure	New word lengths New stress patterns New word shapes (CV sequences)	New word position for existing features and word position; e.g., [+continuant] fricatives copied from coda to onset New sequences for existing form; e.g., Coronal-Labial (*top*), when Labial-Coronal (*pot*) exists
Segments and features	New individual features; e.g., [+lateral], [−voiced], and so forth	New simultaneous feature combinations

initially if there are other word-initial consonants and word-final fricatives, thereby strengthening a particular word position). A new location might additionally involve setting up new sequences of features across partially established word positions.

The first step in target selection is to determine if the four types of targets demonstrate needs for intervention. If this is the case, one or two needs per category type are identified as potential candidates for the first period of intervention. Decisions are made about the assumed relative ease of the various targets, with the perspective that it may be prudent to choose some that are already partially established (or stimulable) and some that are less so. It is assumed that nondefault features and structures are more important for development of the phonological system (more contrasts and intelligibility) than the more readily available (easier, more frequent) default features and structures (Bernhardt, 1990, 1992). The client's views and other needs and strengths are also taken into account (Bernhardt et al., 2006). Once a set of targets has been identified, the sequence of targets can be determined. If a cycles approach to targeting is selected, the sequence of targets may not be as critical.

Service delivery considerations also play a role in target selection. If a client can attend therapy frequently, and home practice is feasible, a full set of targets or the most complex nondefault targets may be chosen at the outset. Compromises may be necessary if service delivery is to be limited for any reason.

Goal Attack Strategies

The nonlinear phonological framework described in Bernhardt and Stemberger (2000) (and utilized in the intervention studies) works well with a cycles approach to goal attack. However, there have been no empirical studies contrasting the cycles approach to a sequential or simultaneous approach with the particular nonlinear framework.

Table 13.4. Treatment activities*

Target	Focus	Activity description
Word structure: CVC V: primarily lax C2: stop or nasal	Mora focus	Example: *The Red Riding Hood Rag/Rap.* Each of the words at the end of the lines has an audible, and often visible, "moraic beat" both on the vowel and the coda.
Word structure: CCVV /s/ clusters with divisible onsets	/s/: treated as add-on to existing onset	Example: *s - - no, s-no > snow.* The snake *s* hisses at the others, who say *no* (*s-no,* and so on). They do this gradually faster. The /s/ finally joins up to [no] and, magically, *snow* falls.
Word structure: CCVV Clusters with sonorant in C2 position	/sC/ treated as indivisible unit	Example: *sn-ow* (*sn-oh!*). Two linked-up characters move together, each pronouncing their part of the cluster: [s][n]. They meet a third party, "O." Once all together, *snow* falls.
Positional target: Coronal-Labial place sequences (targeting assimilation or metathesis)	CVV CVV > CVVCVV > CVVC	Examples: *Day Bee, Dayby, Dayby, Dabe* (and so forth) Place sequences are introduced in open-syllable words such as *day, bee,* then in CVV.CVV words (e.g., *Dayby*), and finally in CVVC words (e.g., *Dabe*)
Positional target: C from coda to onset	Alternations	Example: Word-final /p/ *up > pup.* Marchers say *up up upupup* until *pup* results.

*Supplemental DVDs with additional activities in both English and Spanish are available on request from the authors.

Description of Activities

Presented on the companion DVD to this book and described in Table 13.4 are illustrative activities for promotion of new word structures (using onset-rime and mora constituents). The activities as demonstrated are for awareness development but can be adapted for direct production practice with various levels of cuing (auditory, visual, tactile-kinesthetic). For new feature/segmental targets, similar assumptions are made as in generative phonological approaches, that is, that a feature is being targeted, not a specific segment (except in the case of the feature [+lateral] for /l/, which applies to one phoneme) and that perceptual contrasts, awareness, and imitation techniques with cuing are facilitative. (Two supplemental DVDs with additional activities [one for English, one for Spanish] are available from the first author; these include more word structure activities, including stress patterns, and feature combination activities.)

Materials and Equipment Required

At the outset, a word list is needed for data collection that encompasses the structures and segments across word positions of the language in question. Audio- and, if possible, video-recording equipment is needed. A set of forms can be helpful for the nonlinear analysis, such as those in the Bernhardt and Stemberger (2000) workbook. Computer support for analysis (Masterson & Bernhardt, 2001; Rose & Hedlund, 2008) can increase accuracy and efficiency if quantification is desired. For treatment activities, there are many options that will suit clients and clinicians. Our approach has been to use some older well-known activities, and for children, to supplement these with creative activities that fit the child and target, using props, costumes, wands, and a warped sense of fun-ology.

ASSESSMENT AND PROGRESS MONITORING TO SUPPORT DECISION MAKING

For monitoring progress, short probes with trained and untrained words can be given to the child at the end of one cycle or the beginning of the next. It is probably unnecessary to probe in every session unless there is some particular reason for doing so (e.g., to monitor small changes in articulation or conversational use). Families and clients can also document progress informally or formally. The SLP can visit the classroom or schoolyard to listen in for conversational use of targets. If there is no progress after two treatment cycles, then reevaluation of the targets, goal attack, and treatment strategies is warranted. In an ideal world, treatment would be terminated when the client has age-appropriate speech production in conversation most of the time. In reality, agencies or families may have time limits for service, and some clients may not be ready for significant change at that point in their life. Ultimately, the decision about termination depends on the client and service provider.

CONSIDERATIONS FOR CHILDREN FROM CULTURALLY AND LINGUISTICALLY DIVERSE BACKGROUNDS

If there are no materials available for assessment in a given language, it is first necessary to determine the phonological aspects of the language through literature searches and work with native speakers. Comprehensive nonlinear analyses require the following facts about a language: the phonetic inventory by word position, the feature system by word position and sequence (including information about defaults and nondefaults), the number and type of possible onsets, intervocalic consonants and codas, the syllable types, the foot structures, and the types of prosodic words and phrases; in addition, information is needed about the allophonic, morphological, and morphophonemic alternations of the language.

Elicitation of data samples can be through connected speech or carefully constructed single-word lists, developed with native speakers. A cross-linguistic study is under way, following the Bernhardt and Stemberger (2000) approach; there are now word lists for German (Ullrich, 2008); Mandarin (Bernhardt, Ayyad, Stemberger, Ullrich, & Zhao, in press); Kuwaiti Arabic (Ayyad & Bernhardt, 2007); Icelandic, Slovene, and Spanish; word lists for additional languages are under development. (Word lists are available from the first author.) Ideally, a phonetically trained native speaker will transcribe the speech samples, but a person trained well in transcription of nonEnglish can (and may be obliged to) do the transcription in clinical contexts if the target word is known and there is a recording of a native speaker for comparison purposes.

For analysis, the CAPES (Masterson & Bernhardt, 2001) computer program can analyze data in any language through its Connected Speech (open entry) module (which can have single words or connected speech), as can PHON, a CHILDES program (Rose & Hedlund, 2008). For qualitative analyses, there are scan analysis forms for German (Ullrich, 2008) and Mandarin (Zhao, Bernhardt, & Stemberger, 2008), with a Spanish form under development and others planned for each of the languages of the project.

Finally, it is important to work in a way that matches the personal, cultural, demographic, and linguistic characteristics of each client. The knowledge required in order to match cultural expectations requires partnerships with the relevant cultural communities and ongoing study.

CASE STUDY

The following case study is a fictionalized account of a 4-year-old child. Pretreatment, this child demonstrated strong needs for word structure development and lesser needs for segmental/feature development. Word shape match (accuracy) was about 15% overall (with 8% match for CVC and 50% match for CVCV). The child's PCM was 25%; PVM was 65%. Nasals, stops, and glides were at mastery level (see Table 13.5).

Emergent (occasional) word-initial consonants included the labiodental and voiceless coronal fricatives and affricate and /l/. Word-medially, intervocalic /m/, and glides were established; /n/ and stops were emergent. Word-finally, only /m/ was established. Substitution patterns and individual or combination feature needs in word-initial position were as follows (underlined feature is the key target; parentheses indicate a lesser need).

Table 13.5. Consonant inventory for a child pretreatment (age 4;0).

Feature	Word-initial	Medial onset	Word-final
[+consonantal]	m n pʰ **tʰ** kʰ b **d g** (f v s̪ ts s ʃ̪ tʃ l)	**m** (n p b̲w̲ t k g)	m
[−consonantal]	**w j** h (ʔ)*	ʔ **w** (h̲)	((ʔ))

Note: There were no medial coda consonants. Regular font, match with adult target; **bold,** match plus substitution; underlined, substitution only. Parentheses indicate marginal use.
*Glottal stop as onset to vowel-initial words in isolation.

1. /ɹ/, (/f/, /v/) > [w]. *read* [wi] (feather [wɛwə], van [wæ̃])

    Needs: (1) Feature combination [Labial] & [<u>Coronal</u>] & [Dorsal]: /ɹ/
    (2) Feature combination [Labial] & [+continuant] & [−<u>sonorant</u>]: /f/, /v/)

2. /l/ > [j]. *leaf* [ji]

    Need: [+lateral] (1/7 match pretreatment)

3. Coronal fricatives/affricates: *thumb* [sˡʌ̃m], *see* [sˡi], *shoe* [tʰʌː], *zipper* [tʰĩweɪ], *chicken* [tʰeĩ], *judge* [dʌ]

    Needs: (1) [+grooved] for sibilants, [−grooved] for interdentals
    (2) Feature combination for voiced fricatives and affricate: [<u>+continu-</u> <u>ant</u>] and [−sonorant] and [<u>+voiced</u>] (1/11 match pretreatment)

The intervention program for the first two 6-week treatment blocks is shown in Table 13.6.

New individual word structures included bimoraic syllables targeted with both diphthongs and CVC (lax vowel plus coda). Moras were emphasized rhythmically, highlighting the two parts of the diphthong (C)VV and the lax vowel and coda (CVC). The C2 of C1VC2V was considered a positional goal for structure because the shape CVCV was relatively well-established in terms of timing unit slots. The C1 and C2 onsets were highlighted in activities such as "Day-Bee" (see Table 13.4); the two CVV syllables were first produced separately, and then incorporated into CVV.CVV words. The new feature was [+lateral] for /l/ and the new feature combination, voiced fricatives. In the third treatment block, CVC, CVCV, CCVC, and /l/ were targeted.

Posttreatment, considerable gains were evident:

1. Word shapes: 100% match for CVCV, 72.7% for CVC, and 47.5% overall

2. PCM 50%, PVM 83.5%

3. Voiced fricatives: Word-initially (targeted), a gain from 1/11 to 3/6 and generalizations to untargeted word positions; word-medially, 5/10 match posttreatment and word-finally, /v/ and /z/ were emergent (4/17 matches)

4. /l/: No gain as singleton; /pl/ emergent

5. Word-initial /ɹ/: Emergent

Table 13.6. One child's nonlinear phonological intervention targets

Domain	New elements	New locations or combinations of elements
Word structure	Bimoraic syllables CVC: C2 /s/ or /k/ CVV: Caɪ, Caʊ (C1 = stops, nasals, glides)	CVCV C1: stops, nasals, glides C2: coronal flap, /p/, /f/
Features and segments	+lateral: In CVV (long vowel, not diphthong) or CV/m/	[+continuant] and [−sonorant] and [+voiced]: /v/, /z/, /dʒ/ In CVV (not diphthong) or CV/m/

Note: The above targets were for two treatment blocks of 6 weeks each. In the third 4-week treatment block, CVC, CVCV, CCVC, and /l/ were targeted.

Segmentally, the child's speech was within age limits posttreatment. Structurally, there were still needs for clusters and coda use in longer words. In terms of phonological awareness and morphosyntax, the child's skills improved during the study. In a follow-up test at the end of kindergarten, the child scored within normal limits on a standard articulation test, and in the low–average range for reading and phonological awareness (although still showed minimal spelling skills).

STUDY QUESTIONS

1. What constituted the four types of treatment goals for the child and why?

2. Why were the CVC and CVV treated together for the child and how?

3. Why would the child's academic progress need to be monitored?

FUTURE DIRECTIONS

The ideas presented in this chapter are just a sample of possible assessment and intervention applications of nonlinear phonology. The first author and colleagues are creating clinical applications of nonlinear phonology for languages other than English: German, Mandarin, Arabic, Spanish, Slovene, Bulgarian, and Icelandic, to start. Randomized control trials with large groups of participants are also planned. Regarding everyday clinical application, it has been found that SLPs, with training, can implement effective nonlinear phonological intervention. As current theories find their way into training programs, it is expected that more clinicians will implement intervention that focuses on the various levels of the phonological hierarchy.

SUGGESTED READINGS

Bernhardt, B.H., & Stemberger, J.P. (1998). *Handbook of phonological development: From a nonlinear constraints-based perspective.* San Diego: Academic Press.

Bernhardt, B.H., & Stemberger, J.P. (2000). *Workbook in nonlinear phonology for clinical application.* Austin, TX: PRO-ED.

Bernhardt, B., & Stoel-Gammon, C. (1994). Nonlinear phonology: Clinical application. *Journal of Speech and Hearing Research, 37,* 123–143.

REFERENCES

Adler-Bock, M., Bernhardt, B.M.H., Gick, B., & Bacsfalvi, P. (2007). The use of ultrasound in remediation of /r/ in adolescents. *American Journal of Speech-Language Pathology, 16*(2), 128–139.

Ayyad, H., & Bernhardt, B.M.H. (2007, June 22–23). *Phonological patterns in the speech of an Arabic-speaking Kuwaiti child with hearing impairment compared with a bilingual Arabic-English 2-year-old.* Paper presented at the Child Phonology Conference, Seattle.

Bernhardt, B.M.H. (1990). *Application of nonlinear phonological theory to intervention with six phonologically disordered children.* Unpublished doctoral dissertation, University of British Columbia, Vancouver, British Columbia, Canada.

Bernhardt, B.M.H. (1992). The application of nonlinear

phonological theory to intervention. *Clinical Linguistics and Phonetics, 6,* 283–316.

Bernhardt, B.M.H. (1994a). The prosodic tier and phonological disorders. In M. Yavaş (Ed.), *First and second language acquisition* (pp. 149–172). San Diego: Singular Press.

Bernhardt, B.M.H. (1994b). Phonological intervention techniques for syllable and word structure development. *Clinics in Communication Disorders, 4*(1), 54–65.

Bernhardt, B.M.H. (2005). Selection of phonological goals and targets: Not just an exercise in phonological analysis. In S.F. Warren & M.E. Fey (Series Eds.) & A.G. Kamhi & K.E. Pollock (Eds.), *Communication and language intervention series: Phonological disorders in children—Clinical decision making in assessment and intervention* (pp. 109–120). Baltimore: Paul H. Brookes Publishing Co.

Bernhardt, B.M.H., Ayyad, H., Stemberger, J.P., Ullrich, A., & Zhao, J. (in press). Nonlinear phonology: Clinical application adaptations for Arabic, German and Mandarin. In J. Guendouzi, P. Loncke, & M.J. Williams (Eds.), *The handbook of psycholinguistic and cognitive processes: Perspectives in communication disorders.* London: Taylor & Francis.

Bernhardt, B.M.H., Bacsfalvi, P., Gick, B., Radanov, B., & Williams, R. (2005). Exploring electropalatography and ultrasound in speech habilitation. *Journal of Speech-Language Pathology and Audiology, 29,* 169–182.

Bernhardt, B.M.H., Brooke, M., & Major, E. (2003, July). *Acquisition of structure versus features in nonlinear phonological intervention.* Poster presented at the Child Phonology Conference, University of British Columbia, Vancouver, British Columbia, Canada.

Bernhardt, B.M.H., Doan, A., & Stoel-Gammon, C. (1995). Phonological and phonetic analysis of cleft palate speech. In K. Elenius & P. Branderud (Eds.), *Proceedings of the XIIIth International Congress of Phonetic Sciences, 4* (pp. 108–115). Stockholm: KTH and Stockholm University.

Bernhardt, B., Gick, B., Bacsfalvi, P., & Adler-Bock, M. (2005). Ultrasound in speech therapy with adolescents and adults. *Clinical Linguistics and Phonetics. 19*(6/7), 605–617.

Bernhardt, B.M.H., Gick, B., Bacsfalvi, P., & Ashdown, J. (2003). Speech habilitation of hard of hearing adolescents using electropalatography and ultrasound as evaluated by trained listeners. *Clinical Linguistics and Phonetics, 17*(3), 199–216.

Bernhardt, B.M.H., & Gilbert, J. (1992). Applying linguistic theory to speech-language pathology: The case for nonlinear phonology. *Clinical Linguistics and Phonetics, 6,* 123–145.

Bernhardt, B.M.H., & Holdgrafer, G. (2001a). Beyond the basics I: The need for strategic sampling for in-depth phonological analysis. *Language, Speech, and Hearing Services in Schools, 32,* 18–27.

Bernhardt, B.M.H., & Holdgrafer, G. (2001b). Beyond the basics II: Supplemental sampling for in-depth phonological analysis. *Language, Speech, and Hearing Services in Schools, 32,* 28–37.

Bernhardt, B.M.H., & Major, E. (2005). Speech, language and literacy skills three years later: Long-term outcomes of nonlinear phonological intervention. *International Journal of Language and Communication Disorders, 40,* 1–27.

Bernhardt, B.M.H., & Stemberger, J.P. (1998). *Handbook of phonological development: From a nonlinear constraints-based perspective.* San Diego: Academic Press.

Bernhardt, B.M.H., & Stemberger, J.P. (2000). *Workbook in nonlinear phonology for clinical application.* Austin, TX: PRO-ED.

Bernhardt, B.M.H., Stemberger, J., & Major, E. (2006). General and nonlinear phonological intervention perspectives for a child with a resistant phonological impairment. *Advances in Speech-Language Pathology, 8,* 190–206.

Bernhardt, B.M.H., & Stoel-Gammon, C. (1994). Nonlinear phonology: Clinical application. *Journal of Speech and Hearing Research, 37,* 123–143.

Bopp, K., Bernhardt, B.M.H., & Johnson, C. (1995, June). *The effects of phonological intervention on the development of grammatical production in children with severe impairments in both phonological and grammatical production.* Poster presented at the annual SRCLD conference, Madison, WI.

Chomsky, N., & Halle, M. (1968). *The sound pattern of English.* Cambridge, MA: The MIT Press.

Edwards, S.M. (1995). *Optimal outcomes of nonlinear phonological intervention.* Unpublished master's thesis, University of British Columbia, Vancouver, British Columbia, Canada.

Fawcett, S., Bacsfalvi, P., & Bernhardt, B.M.H. (2008). Ultrasound as visual feedback in speech therapy for /r/ with adults with Down syndrome. *Down Syndrome Quarterly, 10*(1), 4–12.

Gick, B., Bernhardt, B.M.H., Bacsfalvi, P., & Wilson, I. (2008). Ultrasound imaging applications in second language acquisition. In J. Hanson Edwards & M. Zampini (Eds.), *Phonology and second language acquisition* (pp. 309–322). Amsterdam: John Benjamins.

Goldsmith, J. (1979). *Autosegmental phonology* (Doctoral dissertation, MIT, 1976). New York: Garland Press.

Hayes, B. (1989). Compensatory lengthening in moraic phonology. *Linguistic Inquiry, 20,* 253–306.

Hayes, B. (1995). *Metrical stress theory: Principles and case studies.* Chicago: The University of Chicago Press.

Kahn, D. (1980). Syllable-based generalizations in English phonology (Doctoral dissertation, MIT, 1976). *Outstanding dissertations in linguistics series.* New York: Garland Press.

Kenstowicz, M. (1994). *Phonology in generative grammar.* Cambridge, MA: Blackwell.

Ladefoged, P. (2004). *Vowels and consonants* (2nd ed.). Oxford, England: Blackwell.

Lippke, B.A., Dickey, S.E., Selmar, J.W., & Soder, A.L. (1997). *Photo Articulation Test–Third Edition.* Austin, TX: PRO-ED.

Major, E., & Bernhardt, B.M.H. (1998). Metaphonological skills of children with phonological disorders before and after phonological and metaphonological intervention. *International Journal of Language and Communication Disorders, 33,* 413–444.

Masterson, J., & Bernhardt, B.M.H. (2001). *Computerized articulation and phonology evaluation system (CAPES).* San Antonio, TX: Pearson Assessment.

Masterson, J., Bernhardt, B.M.H., & Hofheinz, M. (2005). A comparison of single words and conversational speech in phonological evaluation. *American Journal of Speech-Language Pathology, 14,* 229–241.

McCarthy, J.J. (1988). Feature geometry and dependency: A review. *Phonetica, 43,* 84–108.

McGee, C. (2006). *Phonological awareness skills of children with autism spectrum disorder.* Unpublished master's thesis, University of British Columbia, Vancouver, British Columbia, Canada.

Modha, G., Bernhardt, B.M.H., Church, R., & Bacsfalvi, P. (2008). Case study using ultrasound to treat /ɹ/. *International Journal of Language and Communication Disorders, 43*(3), 323–329.

Olswang, L. (1998). Treatment efficacy research. In C. Frattali (Ed.), *Measuring outcomes in speech-language pathology* (pp. 134–150). New York: Thieme.

Rose, Y., & Hedlund, G. (2008). PHON. Retrieved November 7, 2008, from http://childes.psy.cmu.edu/phon/

Sagey, E.C. (1991). *The representation of features and relations in non-linear phonology: The articulator node hierarchy* (Doctoral dissertation, MIT, 1986). New York: Garland Press.

Ullrich, A. (2004). *Nichtlineare Analyse des phonologischen Systems deutschsprachiger Kinder —Theoretische Eröterung und Konsequenen für die sprachtherapeutische Praxis* [Nonlinear analysis of the phonological systems of German-speaking children—Theoretical discussion and consequences for speech therapy practice]. Unpublished Master's thesis, University of Würzburg, Germany.

Ullrich, A. (2008). *Nichtlineare Phonologische Diagnostik (NILPOD)* [Nonlinear phonological assessment]. Unpublished manuscript.

Von Bremen, V. (1990). *A nonlinear phonological approach to intervention with severely phonologically disordered twins.* Unpublished master's thesis, University of British Columbia, Vancouver, British Columbia, Canada.

World Health Organization. (2001). *ICF: International classification of functioning, disability and health.* Geneva, Switzerland: Author.

Zhao, J., Bernhardt, B.M.H., & Stemberger, J.P. (2008). *Nonlinear scan analysis for Mandarin.* Unpublished manuscript.

Dynamic Systems and Whole Language Intervention

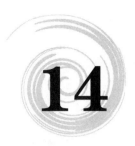

Paul R. Hoffman and Janet A. Norris

ABSTRACT

Principles of whole language and dynamic systems learning are used to structure intervention for preschool children's phonological development within the context of interactive storybook reading. Phonological development is targeted simultaneously with development of discourse structure, semantic, syntactic, morphological, and letter-sound knowledge. The interventionist uses conversational strategies including models, expansions, and extensions along with visual representations of letter–sound relationships and word meaning to enhance children's development of phonological units and patterns. The intervention can be implemented through collaboration with parents and teachers. Data currently support its use with preschool children of varying abilities.

INTRODUCTION

Whole language and dynamic systems accounts of oral and written language development propose that phonological development interacts with development of larger language patterns including discourse structures, sentences, words, and grammatical morphemes. Children develop oral and written phonological abilities as a natural consequence of their communicative interactions with adults, including interactive storybook reading. Thus, intervention should seek to develop phonological aspects of language as parts of larger language patterns while enhancing the transition to learning written language patterns. The intervention described in this chapter uses oral language facilitation techniques and visual tools representing letter–sound and printed word-meaning relationships to enhance phonological development within storybook reading.

Three visual tools, exemplified in Figure 14.1, are described here: Phonic Faces, MorphoPhonic Faces, and Phonic Faces storybooks (Norris, 2003). Phonic Faces are drawings that incorporate letters within the faces of characters who are producing speech sounds. Placement of the letters provides a cue to the production of the speech sound most often associated with the letter. The upper right-hand corner of the figure shows the faces representing the *Ll*-[l] and *Kk*-[k] letter–sound relationships. *L* is incorporated into the character's raised tongue tip as a cue to [l] production. *K* is incorporated into the raised back of the tongue as a cue to [k] production. The lower right-hand corner of the

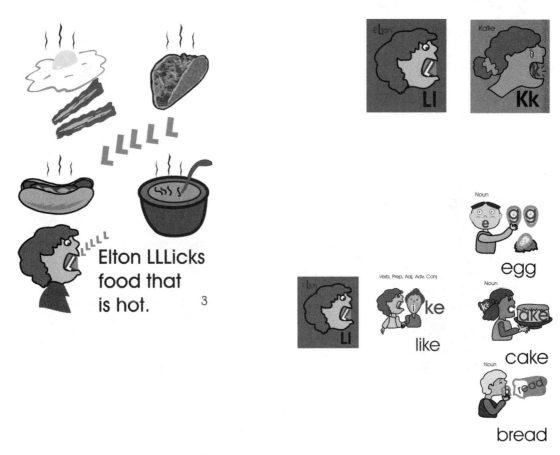

Figure 14.1. Visual tools in which letter–sound and word–meaning relationships are visually represented using Phonic Faces and MorphoPhonic Faces. (From Norris, J.A. [2003]. *Phonic Faces: Manual and picture cards* [2nd ed.]. Baton Rouge, LA: Ele-Mentory; reprinted by permission.)

figure contains examples of MorphoPhonic Faces, which use a Phonic Face to represent the first letter-sound of the most frequently occurring words in children's storybooks. The remainder of the word is overlaid with a drawing that represents a meaning of the word. The upper left-hand corner of the figure shows a page from a Phonic Face storybook. Each book targets a single letter–sound relationship by using a Phonic Face as a character in a narrative, including numerous words containing the letter, and using the letter to signal the production of the isolated sound. These oral language techniques and visual tools can be applied in a variety of settings and can be used by teachers and parents as well as speech-language pathologists (SLPs).

TARGET POPULATIONS AND ASSESSMENT
METHODS FOR DETERMINING TREATMENT RELEVANCE

This intervention is potentially applicable to all children demonstrating phonological delay but is particularly important for preschool children with concomitant delays in acquisition of vocabulary, grammar, and discourse aspects of language who are also at risk for failure to develop written language abilities in school. When an SLP diagnoses a pre-school child as demonstrating primarily a phonological delay, there is approximately a 60% probability that the child will also exhibit delayed language development (Shriberg & Austin, 1998). The diagnosis of phonological delay leads some SLPs to delay intervention for other aspects of language while they target speech sound development despite correlational studies demonstrating that phonological development is strongly related to development of other aspects of oral and written language (Larrivee & Catts, 1999; Paul & Jennings, 1992; Paul & Smith, 1993). This strategy contributes to delayed acquisition of expressive morphemic and syntactic knowledge, which will become measurable and is eventually associated with problems in written language (Fey, Catts, Proctor-Williams, Tomblin, & Zhang, 2004). In contrast, our approach seeks to improve speech sound production simultaneously with other aspects of language organization using oral language scaffolding techniques such as modeling and expansion that have been shown to be effective in increasing the complexity of children's language at a variety of language levels.

Our assessment methods describe the child's organization of language across a broad range of language structures from the phonological through the narrative (Hoffman & Norris, 2002). A parent interview is expected to reveal delayed acquisition of early language milestones including onset of babbling, use of first words, extent of vocabulary development, and use of two-word and larger syntactic constructions. The child's speech would be described as unintelligible, and the child might be showing signs of withdrawal or frustration when communicative attempts fail. We would supply the child with developmentally appropriate toys that could be used to represent commonly occurring childhood events such as mealtime, shopping, or going to the park. At first we would observe the child's solo play to determine the level of independent organization of pretend actions and potential talking about character actions, motives, plans, and emotional reactions. Judgments would be made regarding the complexity of the discourse structure the child uses to organize events into socially appropriate sequences of actions, cause–effect relationships, and intentionality of characters.

Next, we would join the child's play, using scaffolding techniques to see what the child adds to this organization when adult assistance is provided. We would engage the child in interactive storybook reading and would probe the use of visual strategies to prompt improved performance (Hoffman & Norris, 2006). Video recordings of these interactions would be analyzed and transcript data compared with normative data for the child's ability to organize the discourse structure of events, the semantic complexity of the child's utterances, the child's overall syntactic stage, number of different words used, syllable structures produced, phonetic inventory, and percentage of consonants correct (PCC). Table 14.1 displays some of the expectations for 3- and 4-year-old children that we use as a guide to describing a child's development and for setting long-term goals. The Processor column of this table refers to the language processors described in Figure 14.2. Detailed descriptions of these expectations are available in Norris and Hoffman (2001), with extensive data regarding phonetic and phonological characteristics of development found in McLeod (2009).

THEORETICAL BASIS

Our theory of language development is based on principles of connectionism and dynamic systems as represented in Figure 14.2 (Norris & Hoffman, 2001). This model's connectionistic traits include its simultaneous activity of the full range of language proces-

Table 14.1. Examples of language performance expectations for 3- and 4-year-olds

Processor	3-year-old	4-year-old
Prior Knowledge (Metalinguistic knowledge of written language)	Locates words of text versus pictures Knows words are read from left to right Names rhyming words Attempts writing using scribbles	Names letters on page Names sound at beginning of word Creates rhyme by altering first sound Says sound associated with letter Recognizes some sight words Writing attempts include some letters
Macrostructure (Narrative structure of routine events and stories)	Extended topic maintenance for contextualized topics Recounts past personal experiences and can predict future events in real or imaginary situation based on present evidence Narratives are organized by time and physical causality	Recounts observed past events with errors of cohesion Narratives include sequences of plans and attempts that are reactions to the preceding actions outcomes rather than the course of an overall plan Learns from verbal explanations
Connotative Meaning (Inferences and Interpretations)	Complex sentences express Mental states "I know . . . I wish . . . " Causality "but, so, or, if" Time "before, after" Produces dialogue for familiar and less familiar social roles (e.g., parent, police officer)	Uses complex sentences expressing facts, rules, beliefs, attitudes Facial expression and body language convey humor, tease, protest, show off
Denotative Meaning (Description of attributes of people and objects and their actions)	MLU 2.50–3.99 Elaborated noun phrases include size, color, texture, shape, and so forth Verb phrases are elaborated to express past events; modal verbs are used for future possible events and intentionality	MLU 4.00–4.99 All basic sentence types organized
Referential Meaning Words representing people, objects, actions, and so forth	Vocabulary of 1,000 words organized as slot-filler categories in denotative sequences Abstract words for color, texture, size, shape, location Words expressing desires, feelings, thoughts Developing grammatical morphemes	Vocabulary of 1,500 words Slot-filler categories transforming into hierarchies
Canonical/Categorical (Syllable structures and phonemes)	PCC 82% Clusters /tw, kw/ /p, b, t, d, k, g, m, n, ŋ, f, v, s, z, h, w, l, j/	PCC 90% Clusters /tw, kw, sp, st, sk, sm, sn, sl, pl, bl, kl, gl, pr, br, tr, dr, kr/ /p, b, t, d, k, g, m, n, ŋ, f, v, s, z, ʒ, h, w, l, j, ʤ, ʧ/

Key: MLU, mean length of utterance; PCC, percentage of consonants correct.

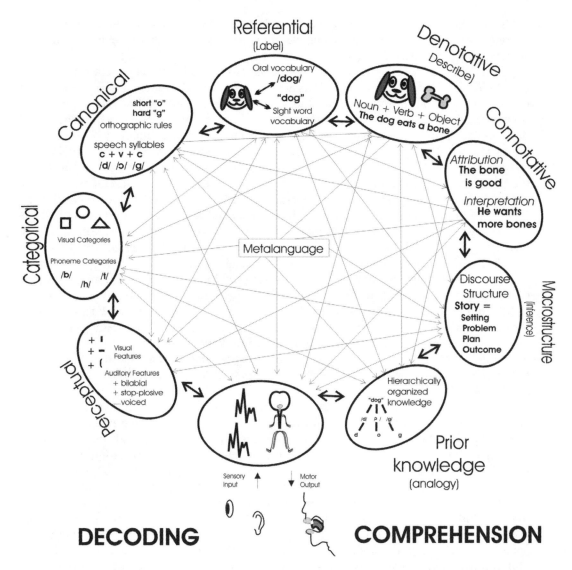

Figure 14.2. Model of language processes. (From Norris, J.A. [2003]. *Phonic Faces: Manual and picture cards* [2nd ed.]. Baton Rouge, LA: EleMentory; reprinted by permission.)

sors, the multidirectional interaction of processors, and self-organizing learning that is driven by the input of models of language during active language processing. These traits lead to intervention in which multiple language units are targeted for simultaneous improvement, development in each processor enhances development in the other processors, and organization within processors is affected by provision of models of language prior to and following the child's conversational turns. The model's dynamic properties include the context-sensitive nature of the units being developed in each processor and the temporal nature of the patterns developing within each processor (Elman, 1995). Context sensitivity is embodied in the intervention's targeting of phonemic or syllabic development through the development of words used in a variety of sentence and topic contexts. The units that are targeted for development include narratives and a variety of sentence types, each of which structures temporal plans for words, syllables, speech sounds, and gestures.

The *Sensory-Motor Processor* at the bottom of the model represents the child's coding of sensory inputs resulting from interaction with the environment. Of particular interest to phonological intervention are the auditory, visual, and tactile-kinesthetic sensations related to speech sound production and print recognition. SLPs manipulate input patterns to improve phonological organization by modeling the production of sounds, syllables, and words prior to a child's speech attempts. These models result in the child's language system making small adjustments within and between all of the processors so that the patterns within the child's system become more adult-like in an incremental fashion. Adult models that follow a child's speech sound errors by expanding or recasting the child's utterance also result in better phonological production on the part of the child as they engage in play with toys (Camarata, 1993) and storytelling (Hoffman, Norris, & Monjure, 1990, 1996). Following a child's error production with a binary choice that contrasts the child and adult productions of a pattern (e.g., "did you say [dɔ] or [dɔg]?") provides both an expansion of the phonological form of the child's utterance and a model for part of the child's next utterance (Bellon-Harn, Hoffman, & Harn, 2004; Weiner & Ostrowski, 1979). Adult–child interactions using Phonic Faces and MorphoPhonic Faces increase the speech attempts of nonverbal children (Banajee, 2007), the speech sound accuracy of preschool children with severe (Hoffman & Norris, 2004; Kaufman & Norris, 2007) and moderate (Nettleton & Hoffman, 2005) phonological delays, and the development of letter-sound awareness among typically developing 2-year-olds (McInnis, 2008; Terrell, 2007) (see Table 14.2).

The *Perceptual Processor* organizes patterns of sensory-motor features such as vowel length, voice onset time, and formant frequencies. These phonetic features relate the tactile-kinesthetic feelings of speech movement patterns, such as lifting the tongue tip, with the auditory effects of the movement, such as a change in formant frequency trajectories. These features include the visible movements of articulators of other people, such as lip rounding. Incomplete development of features in the Perceptual Processor results in the appearance of substitution processes such as stopping of fricatives and gliding of liquids that affect classes of phonemes in the Categorical Processor (discussed next). Interventions that focus on these individual movements by isolating them from speech production do not appear to facilitate speech sound production accuracy among children with phonological disorders (Ruscello, 2008). Phonological interventions target the development of these features through the production of words that differ either minimally or maximally in terms of feature contrasts (Williams, 2005). Children exposed to print also develop patterns for visual features of text (e.g., the lines, circles, and curves of letter symbols). Our use of Phonic Faces and MorphoPhonic Faces is intended to provide the child with visual cues to phonetic features that should be incorporated into phoneme production and word production as well as letter features to be used in reading and writing.

The *Categorical Processor* develops phonemes and letter symbols. Each phoneme organizes sequences of gestural and auditory features. The phoneme /b/ organizes a sequence of gestures such as velum raising, lip closing, and lip opening, which are related to a sequence of auditory features such as a silent period, a sudden burst of energy, and a short voice onset time. The letter *B* develops to include links to a vertical line and one or two (*B*) loops extending to the right of the line. The Phonic Face representation for *Bb*

Table 14.2. Levels of evidence for studies of treatment efficacy for dynamic systems and whole language intervention

Level	Description	References
Ia	Meta-analysis of > 1 randomized controlled trial	—
Ib	Randomized controlled study	McInnis (2008); Terrell (2007)
IIa	Controlled study without randomization	—
IIb	Quasi-experimental study	Nettleton & Hoffman (2005)
III	Nonexperimental studies, i.e., correlational and case studies	Hoffman & Norris (2004); Kaufman & Norris (2007)
IV	Expert committee report, consensus conference, clinical experience of respected authorities	—

Adapted from the Scottish Intercollegiate Guideline Network (www.sign.ac.uk).

blends these representations by overlapping the loops of the letter on the lips of the speaker. Development of phonemes involves relating a large number of context-sensitive allophones with slightly different combinations of features to one another as the child learns to produce the phoneme in many different syllables and words.

The *Canonical Processor* develops sequences of phonemes or letters. Oral language units include syllables and subsyllabic units such as onsets and rimes. Graphemic units include digraphs such as *ph* and *gh* that are associated with a single phoneme and letter sequences associated with syllabic onsets (e.g., *tr*) and rimes (e.g., *ough*). Canonical phonological development typically begins in babbling with CV and reduplicated CVCV syllable shapes, with a smaller percentage of VC syllables. These babbled syllables are incorporated into the first words produced by the child. Over the course of development more complex syllable shapes emerge including consonant clusters as parts of onsets and final consonants and clusters as parts of rimes. The original tendency toward production of CV syllables results in the appearance of phonological processes such as final consonant deletion and consonant cluster reduction. Children's spelling errors also include these tendencies (Hoffman & Norris, 1989) as the child mentally rehearses a word while seeking to create a spelling pattern to represent it. Traditional interventions provide practice in syllabic production as a separate phase of intervention (Van Riper, 1978). Phonological interventions target canonical sequences, such as CVC syllables, through practice in perception and production of groups of words that include the pattern (Hodson & Paden, 1991) or groups of words that contrast depending upon their syllable structure (Williams, 2005).

The *Referential Processor* develops units representing words and morphemes. Connections of a word unit to the processors on the left side of the model establish its phonological characteristics including sequences of syllables and phonemes. These perceptible connections also represent more concrete word meanings—labels for visually observable and otherwise perceptible objects and people. Connections to the units on the right side of the model establish the word's syntactic properties and more abstract meanings. Increasing the number of words and morphemes in the Referential Processor provides the need to refine the units and connections among the phonologically related processors on the left side of the model so that the words and morphemes can be understood and expressed clearly. Toddlers with slow expressive language development (SELD) develop words more slowly while also producing less complex syllable shapes, fewer different consonants, and a lower percentage of correctly produced consonants (Paul & Jennings,

1992). Intervention for 2-year-olds with SELD that targeted development of specific vocabulary items and two-word combinations expressing actions through parent–child interaction has been shown to result in increased phonological development including expanded use of complex syllables and the use of a wider variety of speech sounds (Girolametto, Pearce, & Weitzman, 1997).

The *Denotative Processor* develops knowledge of the primary or explicit meanings of actions making up daily routines and the language patterns used to talk about actions. Some of the earlier developed multiword language patterns are verb-related sequences in which a particular verb is associated with patterns of other words. For example, a 2-year-old child was observed to use the verb *cut* only in the construction *cut* _____ (e.g., *cut paper*) while using the word *draw* in a wider variety of constructions, such as *draw* _____ (e.g., *draw doggie*), *draw* _____ *on* _____ (e.g., *draw doggie on paper*) and _____ *draw on* _____ (e.g., *I draw on paper*) (Tomasello, 2003). The slots in these sequences represent groups of words that appear in these particular sequential patterns. These early word constructions are combined to form more complex structures such as the subject-verb-object structure in which a variety of people, objects, and actions can occur in the slots formed to represent events, for example, *Mommy drinks coffee. Baby drinks milk. Baby eats cookies.* The child also learns to refer to attributes of objects, *big cookie*, and to incorporate these elaborations into his or her descriptions of actions, such as *Baby eats the big cookie.*

Development of the ability to express denotative meaning interacts with phonological development as seen in the findings that toddlers' speech sound accuracy is better for object labels than action words (Camarata & Schwartz, 1985). In addition, teaching the use of bound morphemes in sessions that involved thematically related storybook reading, art projects, and singing songs resulted in improved phonological performance by preschoolers with SELD (Tyler, Lewis, Haskill, & Tolbert, 2002). The targeted morphemes—third person regular, past tense, possessive, and plural—all require the development of syllable final consonants and consonant clusters in the Canonical Processor and an /s/ phoneme in the Categorical Processor. The children's learning of these morphological structures appears to have induced learning of the syllabic shape and phonemic parts of the morphological structures.

The *Connotative Processor* develops secondary meanings that must be interpreted or inferred. These include physical cause–effect relationships; predictions of future events; figurative meanings; and mental states of others including emotions, motivations, goals, and thoughts. These secondary meanings are often expressed within complex syntactic structures that are more likely to include speech sound production errors. Prediction of possible future events utilizes modal verb structures (e.g., *John will go to the store*). Cause–effect relationships are expressed in complex sentence constructions such as, *The bottle broke because the baby pushed it.* Mental states are expressed in structures such as *I know that* + Sentence or *He thinks that* + Sentence and *He wants to* + Verb Phrase. An intervention targeting increased production of interpretations within a storytelling task also resulted in increased appropriate production of consonants (Hoffman et al., 1990, 1996).

The *Macrostructure Processor* develops knowledge of the patterns of social events and narrative discourse. Typical narratives sequence elements including setting, problem, internal reaction, plan, attempt, and outcome to highlight the solving of a socially important problem. Problem solving in the lives of children is a common theme in children's storybooks that must be mastered as part of early literacy development. Children with SELD who showed delayed phonological development at 2–3 years also showed delayed narrative development at 4 years, with their stories including fewer propositions that were not as well coordinated as stories of typically developing children (Paul & Smith, 1993). Children with phonological disorders produce more speech errors when they tell or retell narratives (Dubois & Bernthal, 1978), play with an adult (Andrews & Fey, 1986), or talk about decontextualized topics (Morrison & Shriberg, 1992) than when they name pictures. Intervention in which an adult scaffolds the repeated telling of a small number of stories by preschool children with SELD has been shown to increase the children's use of syntactic complexity and phonological form (Hoffman et al., 1990, 1996).

The *Prior Knowledge Processor* structures information about the physical and social worlds into hierarchies that may be organized in multiple schemes. Included here is the knowledge the child has gained from engagement in the macrostructure events of early childhood and from formal learning that occurs in school. School topics structure knowledge into topically organized areas of social studies, sciences, arts, and print conventions. Development of these knowledge structures includes development of literacy-related abilities, such as phonemic awareness, knowledge of print conventions, reading, writing, and the ability to interpret analogies. Children with histories of expressive phonological disorders appear to be at risk for failure to develop printed word recognition skills in first grade (Larrivee & Catts, 1999). Teaching children with delayed speech sound development to segment words into sounds, to blend sounds into words, and to read and spell words that included the child's error sounds resulted in increases in speech sound production that were comparable with a traditional articulation intervention and provided increased phonemic awareness and printed word reading ability (Gillon, 2002). Teaching phonemic awareness is better accomplished when the visual-auditory associations are embodied in letter–sound relationships than when letters are not used (Ehri et al., 2001).

EMPIRICAL BASIS

Our evidence for the use of narrative-based interventions augmented by visual tools includes case studies for a child with SELD (Hoffman & Norris, 2004) and a 4-year-old with severe impairment in development of speech sound production (Kaufman & Norris, 2007). It also includes a single-subject design study of 4-year-olds with SELD (Nettleton & Hoffman, 2005). Finally, it includes randomized control studies and experimental/control group comparisons of 2-year-olds with typical language development (McInnis, 2008; Terrell, 2007). Child participants included in these various studies show the value of this intervention throughout development across an oral to literate language continuum.

LONG-TERM CASE STUDY FOR A CHILD WITH SLOW EXPRESSIVE LANGUAGE DEVELOPMENT

Hoffman and Norris (2004) followed the case of a boy, ND, with SELD between the ages of 20 and 60 months. He was identified as exhibiting SELD at 20 months because he began babbling at 14 months, his first word was produced at 18 months, and he had yet to combine two words when first seen at 20 months. He actively participated in routine events with appropriate action sequences suggesting some knowledge of these routines. He used utterances such a "bye bye" and "night night" only to label whole events, but failed to use true words to label objects and people, or to describe actions. His play was limited to object manipulation with rapidly shifting focus from one toy to another. He did not talk while playing. Attempts to scaffold functional play related to routine events or to elicit verbal participation were resisted by breaking off social contact and whining.

From 2 to 3 years, ND participated in a narrative-based preschool program in which small groups of children were engaged in storybook reading and more contextualized explorations of storybook-related concepts in art, symbolic/pretend play, snack time, and outside play. Goals included 1) acting out three- to four-step sequences of actions in functional play; 2) using words and word combinations to request, protest, and comment; 3) labeling storybook characters/objects; and 4) describing actions of characters and characteristics of objects in storybooks. ND demonstrated improvements toward all of these goals. His performance on a standardized measure of receptive language rose from below the 3rd percentile to above the 10th percentile. Standardized measures of expressive language and phonology did not improve. However, he was improving his organization of phonological aspects of language as seen in his increasing PCC, production of appropriate syllable shapes, and an increasing phonetic inventory. Increased production of final consonants and consonant clusters can be seen as Canonical Processor improvements. Increases in his phonetic inventory from [b, d, t, g, n, w, j, h] to [b, p, t, d, k, g, m, n, f, s, z, θ, tʃ, w, j, h] suggest an expansion of his control of phonetic features to include more voiceless sounds, fricatives, and affricates—which can be seen as Perceptual Processor improvements

Between ages 3 and 5 years, ND's preschool program incorporated the use of the visual tools described here in storybook reading and writing activities. Goals between ages 3 and 5 years were expanded to include 1) interpreting character emotion and cause–effect relationships; 2) making inferences based on knowledge of story structure and routine events; 3) increasing complexity of story retelling; 4) using more specific, complex language to request, protest, comment, and command; and 5) improving literacy development, including letter name recognition and letter–sound relationships. This period was marked by a rapid increase in receptive language development (from the 12th to the 50th percentile), which was followed by developments in expressive language (from the 4th to 30th percentile) and phonological development (from below the 1st to the 27th percentile). He continued to develop his production of syllable structures so that all final consonants were represented by 4 years and all consonants in clusters were represented by 5 years. He continued to refine his production of phonemically appropriate consonants so that his PCC for the production of single words reached 100% at 5 years. In addition, ND's score on an early reading test was in the high-normal range (85th percentile) as he entered kindergarten.

ND's improved organization of phonological characteristics of language occurred without a clinical focus targeting particular syllable shapes, phonemes, or features and without specific periods of practice in syllable or single word production. The speech sound production practice that occurred was always in a context of communicating about topics related to narrative themes established by storybooks and a focus on letter–sound relationships as part of storybook reading and writing. The interventionists supplied models and expansions targeting phonological levels of organization while at the same time targeting use of appropriate discourse structures, syntax, morphology, and word choice. Phonological development appears to have occurred following the development of receptive and expressive vocabulary, morphology, and syntactic organization.

SHORTER-TERM CASE STUDY OF A CHILD
WITH SUSPECTED CHILDHOOD APRAXIA OF SPEECH

Kaufman and Norris (2007) described a case study of a 4-year-old boy who was expressing himself using hummed intonation contours without discernable consonant productions following 18 months of traditional articulation intervention. His receptive language skills were in the average range, but his expressive language skills were measured to be at an 8-month level. Intervention was provided in 18 hour-long sessions that included talking about the pictures and then reading the text in storybooks, supported by Morpho-Phonic Face cards for characters, objects, and actions. The adult modeled utterances that could be used to talk about the actions depicted in the pictures and text while pointing out the articulatory cue on the morphophonic card for words in the utterance. For example, in talking about a storybook picture in which a boy is pulling his sister in a wagon, MorphoPhonic Face cards for *boy*, *girl*, *wagon*, *pull*, and *ride* were used to cue talking about the characters and their actions. The adult pointed to the Phonic Face sound at the beginning of each word, modeled the sound at the beginning of the word, and modeled the whole word. The child's speech attempts were followed by recasts that included appropriate phonological characteristics of the words.

During the nine sessions of the fall semester, the number of imitated and spontaneously produced words including distinguishable consonants increased from 2 in the first session to more than 50 in the ninth session. Following the semester break, the child's production of spontaneous words increased to more than 100, averaging about 200 per session in the spring semester. The number of imitated words declined to an average of about 10 per session. From preintervention to postintervention, this child demonstrated a variety of improvements in his expressive phonological abilities. His standard score on the Goldman-Fristoe Test of Articulation-2 (Goldman & Fristoe, 2000) increased from unscorable to 57. At pretest he produced no consonants correctly; at posttest he correctly produced /p, b, k, g, m, w, h, s, z, ʃ/ in at least one word context.

Single-Subject Design Studies of Preschoolers
with Slow Expressive Language Development

Nettleton and Hoffman (2005) used a multiple baseline across speech sounds design to study development of [f] and [ʃ] production in words and knowledge of the F-[f] and SH-[ʃ] letter–sound relationships by four 4-year-olds with SELD. In 15-minute sessions the adult and child interactively read a Phonic Face book using individual Phonic Faces to point out letter–sound relationships. In each session, the interventionist introduced the Phonic Face card by pointing out the relationship between the letter and its placement in the character's mouth and the speech gesture related to the sound's production. This introduction was followed by reading the text of the storybook one page at a time, first word by word and then as a sentence. After reading the single words, the adult read the whole sentence, followed by the child's reading of the whole sentence. The child's productions of the targeted sound were followed by expansions in which the adult repeated the word with a lengthened sound while pointing to the Phonic Face card. On each page the child was asked to find each targeted letter, to name the letter, to say the sound cued by the letter, and to read the word. On a number of the pages in the book targeting [f], there are numerous *f*s in the picture indicating the sound being made by either the character blowing a candle or the fan blowing air. These *f*s were pointed to and read as a sequence of [f] sounds.

Following a baseline measurement period during which a book focusing on the letter *G* was read, the book highlighting the relationship between *F*-[f] was introduced. All four children increased their production of [f] in words, as part of the name of the letter *F* (i.e., the syllable [εf]), and as an isolated [f] representing the sound "said by" the letter *F*. None of these measures for *SH*-[ʃ] improved during this period, indicating that it was the storybook reading that affected [f] production. All of the children were readily stimulable for production of [f] in isolation prior to the introduction of the *F* storybook. In the next two sessions the *SH* book was read. Three of the four children improved their production of [ʃ] in words. The child who did not improve his production of [ʃ] in words was not readily stimulable for production of an isolated [ʃ] prior to the intervention. All of the children improved their production of isolated [ʃ] as the sound produced by the letters *SH*. In sum, these results suggest that this form of storybook reading may improve fricative production for children who are stimulable for the sounds being targeted in a short period of time. Further research is needed to determine if this technique is successful in improving production of a sound that is not stimulable.

Two Studies of Typically Developing 2-Year-Olds

Terrell (2007) repeatedly read an alphabet book with typically developing 2-year-olds, talking about letter–sound associations and the occurrence of sounds in pictured words. Each page of the book included a Phonic Face representation of a letter–sound relationship and three words starting with that letter represented both in pictures and text. The adult helped the child control turning the pages of the book and pointed to and talked about the targeted letter on each page, the sound it produced, and the words that it occurred in. For example, on the *K* page the adult said something such as "Here's Katie. She likes the letter *K*. *K* says [kə, kə, kə]. Here's a *kite*, a *kitten*, and a *key*. Those all start with the [kə] sound. Do you hear it? [kə] *kite*, [kə] *kitten*, [kə] *key*." If the child spontaneously pointed to a letter or picture on the page, it was labeled and then given a print or phoneme reference. For example, if a child pointed to a pig, then the experimenter might say, "Yes, that's a pig. Look. It starts with the [pə] sound, 'pig.' I see the letter *P* at the beginning of the word *pig*." After 18 book readings, each lasting about 10 minutes, the children in the randomly selected experimental group outperformed the children in a control group in letter name knowledge, letter–sound association, and production of speech sounds in words.

McInnis (2008) taught 16 typically developing 2-year-olds to read eight printed words using MorphoPhonic Face cards compared with eight words taught with plain text cards within a game format over a period of eighteen 20-minute sessions. The posttest results showed a significant effect in which children were able to recognize more plain text versions of words taught using the MorphoPhonic Face cards than those taught with the plain text cards. They were also better able to read words represented with either a MorphoPhonic Face or with a combination of plain text plus a Phonic Face card representing the first sound compared with plain text representations. On average, the children made significant gains in measures of phonological awareness and early literacy development.

These studies provide preliminary evidence that productive phonology and knowledge of letter–sound relationships can be improved through interactive storybook reading in which the adult uses visually enhanced text to talk about letter–sound relationships. The weaknesses in these data involve the varying levels of experimental control presented by the types of study conducted and the trade-off between experimental control and treatment fidelity. Our case studies of younger children with more severe speech production impairments (Hoffman & Norris, 2005; Kaufman & Norris, 2007) provide measures of improvements in speech and language production for interventions that most resemble the overall strategy described in this chapter. However, these studies lack the control of extraneous variables provided by either a control group or single-subject design. The study that included single-subject design controls (Nettleton & Hoffman, 2005) is less like the procedures described here, as they become more focused on particular speech sound targets and more constrained in intervention time. The studies that showed the efficacy of use of visual strategies using relatively large numbers of children in either a control group or a within-subjects control-sound design (McInnis, 2008; Terrell, 2007) included participants who were typically developing rather than identified as phonologically delayed.

PRACTICAL REQUIREMENTS

The underlying premise of this intervention, that phonological aspects of word productions should be coordinated with language structures up to the level of discourse structures, demands that intervention sessions be relatively long so that narrative topics can be organized and explored. Our long-term case intervention was provided within a 2-hour-long preschool program for small groups of children. The short-term case study intervention used 1-hour-long, individual sessions. The much shorter (20-minute) individual sessions employed in the single-subject design studies were able to show a treatment effect only because intervention was focused on one sound at a time.

This intervention strategy can be applied in a variety of settings including individual or small-group sessions and can be provided by SLPs, teachers, or parents in clinic-, school-, or home-based settings. The oral language-enhancing techniques that we employ such as models, expansions, and binary choices were all discovered as parts of naturally occurring parent–child interactions in literate home environments and are taught for use by SLPs and early education teachers. Phonic Face cards, Phonic Face books, and MorphoPhonic Face cards have been successfully used by parents (Norris & Hoffman, 2003, 2004) and Head Start teachers (Brazier-Carter, Norris, & Hoffman, 2004) after minimal training. In these studies, the teachers and parents were briefly introduced to how Phonic Faces represent letter–sound relationships or how the MorphoPhonic Faces represent the first letter-sound and meaning of the words. The interventionist modeled an interactive book-reading style using the books and cards followed by sessions conducted by the parent and teacher demonstrating increased use of appropriate strategies.

KEY COMPONENTS

The important components of this intervention include the provision of meaningfully structured information to talk about oral language facilitation techniques and the use of visual tools to support the process of categorizing and interrelating inputs across the multiple language processors. The interventionist organizes contexts in which adult and child explore a narrative topic, which can include play, snack, art, daily routines, or book reading. The complexity of the context and the complexity of the parts that the child is asked to supply within the interaction depend upon the child's developmental level. Some children may only be able to play at the level of a series of single actions, whereas others can engage in highly symbolic, narrative play in which they talk about characters' emotional reactions, plans, and reactions to outcomes of attempts to solve a problem. (For a detailed discussion of developmental levels, see Norris and Hoffman, 2001.)

The apparent purpose of the adult–child interaction to the child is to collaborate in topic development as a part of their ongoing conversation. The primary conversational focus is on topic development rather than on the child's speech and language goals and performance. In this manner the adult's questions, models, expansions, and comments regarding underdeveloped aspects of the child's language and speech may be perceived by the child as help in topic construction rather than criticisms of child performance.

The interaction between adult and child is dynamic, with changes in the input provided by the adult in each conversational turn based on the level of the child's preceding turn. As the child participates in topic elaboration, his or her responses should reflect better organization of the information, as seen in a change from the child's initial attempt. For example, the following topic extensions to a child's utterance "The dog" provide the child with models of connotative to hierarchical organizations of the child's topic: "The dog is wagging his tail," "The dog is happy," "The dog will lick the boy's hand," "Dog begins with Dedra's [d] sound." If the child uses some of this input to produce a more complex utterance by producing a description of the action "The dog licks hand" and/or improves the phonological characteristics of the words "the dog," the adult judges that the language input was effective. When the child fails to participate with increased language complexity, the inputs must be adjusted to include a reduced level of complexity.

Nature of Goals

The overall goal of intervention is to increase refinement throughout the constellation processors, which will result in better child performance in all areas of speech and language. Table 14.1 includes expectations for typically developing children's performance that we use to develop long-term goals for a 2-semester period of time. For example

Macrostructure: Child will talk about an observed event or tell a story that includes character mental states, intentions, and goals

Connotative: expressed in complex sentence structures

Denotative: with coherent references across sentences, elaborated noun phrases, verb phrases with appropriate auxiliary verbs, and grammatical morphemes

Referential: using specific vocabulary and appropriate pronoun reference

Canonical: containing appropriately produced syllable structures

Categorical: and phonemes

Perceptual: including fricative, affricate, and liquid features.

These long-term objectives may also be expressed as expected improvements in standard scores on norm referenced measures of phonology, receptive and expressive vocabulary, syntactic development, and story structure.

Shorter-term objectives would be written to sample behaviors representative of development across the areas of knowledge within specific contexts. Objectives would first be supported with visual scaffolds, then with the scaffolds removed. For example, while reading a storybook, the child will

Prior knowledge: Match a Phonic Face card with a word-initial letter in a storybook and state that the word begins with the target letter and sound produced in isolation. For example "The word *fan* begins with the letter *F;* it starts with the sound [f]."

Macrostructure: Retell a portion of a story from a book that includes a sequence of plan + attempt + outcome.

Denotative: Use complex sentence structure to explain the plan + attempt sequence.

Connotative: Use appropriate sentence structures and pronouns to describe action sequences.

Referential: Use specific nouns, verbs, and appropriate grammatical morphemes.

Canonical: Produce appropriate final consonants and consonant clusters.

Categorical: Produce all contrasting phonemes

Multiple Goals Across Time

The goal of dynamic intervention is to facilitate children's development so that they will have the integrated communication skills needed to succeed in their current and future environments. Thus, intervention must be preventive as well as remedial. For example, 1- and 2-year-old children need to acquire the speech and language skills to communicate, play, and talk about picture books to prepare them for the decontextualized talk demanded of preschoolers. Children 3–4 years old should be acquiring the speech, language, phonological awareness, and literacy skills needed to support early reading development in kindergarten to prevent literacy failure. School-age children should be acquiring the phonological, language, and phonics skills needed for spelling, written language decoding, and reading comprehension at a grade-appropriate level. Intervention must facilitate development synergistically across the entire constellation. Putting one area on hold such as vocabulary or language while articulation skills are developed creates a system that is not synergistic and cannot function in a manner that will adequately support the learning demands in the child's current or future environment.

Materials and Equipment Required

Repeated book reading is an excellent context for intervention because the visual illustrations and text provide highly stable and replicable input. Within and across sessions, the same pictures or text can be talked about repeatedly. Each repetition may enhance language variability as more complex ideas and wording are introduced when the child expresses more basic ideas independently. The information that has become more familiar through this redundancy will have more established dynamic patterns, making it easier to talk about the story with each exposure. More attention and processing can be devoted to small changes that add refinement to the story, such as a shift in articulation or the letter–sound relationships in the text.

For younger children, illustrated books with a good story line and interesting events make excellent contexts for facilitating change. Storybooks typically elicit talk about people and events with little regard to sound or print. Alphabet books, such as the book used by Terrell (2007) with 2-year-olds, elicit talk about letters, sounds, and sounds in word positions, but at the expense of talk about meaning. Phonic Faces books seek to span these two genres.

Using Phonic Faces books, children are cued to attend to and produce sounds in isolation and within words throughout the book reading. The adult augments this attention to other letter-sounds using Phonic Face cards such as Elton and Katie shown in the upper right-hand corner of Figure 14.1. For example, if a child's reading of the word *likes* does not include final consonants, the interventionist could add the Phonic Face sequence of Elton and Katie and explain that the word starts with the letter *L* and the [l] sound and that means lifting the front of the tongue like Elton does. And the word *like* ends with the [k] sound.

During intervention, other words containing a range of sounds can be phonemically cued before and after the child attempts the words using sequences of Phonic Face cards. In addition, MorphoPhonic Face cards such as those shown in the lower left-hand corner of Figure 14.1 are used to easily manipulate slot filler categories that extend the story topic and provide redundant practice of sentence structures, such as "Elton likes eggs" and "Elton likes bread." MorphoPhonic cards representing the grammatical morphemes such as the plural "s" can be added to cue further refinements within these sentence structures.

Visual cues such as these provide the network with stable inputs that can be examined before, during, and following a production attempt. Auditory models disappear rapidly, whereas visuals provide more time for the information to be processed and the multiple cues integrated. The print in the text of the book can provide cues to sentence length, even for nonreaders (one word must be said for each printed word), and letter cues can be used to prompt sound-in-word position. Visuals can be used to provide feedback, such as, "Here is the sound you wanted (pointing to target mouth on card), but here is the sound your mouth made (placing the card for the child's production next to the intended sound)." Features in the visual cue can be pointed out and modeled for the child to imitate, and later attempted more independently when shown the card without a direct model. As an added benefit, phonemic awareness and alphabet skills are learned simultaneously.

Patterns of Interaction

Although materials provide the tools for dynamic intervention, interactions guide the creation of new space states and trajectories. In these interactions, scaffolding strategies (Norris & Hoffman, 1993) are used to engage the child in storytelling, with each turn eliciting a change in at least one region of the network. The focus may shift from picture interpretation to vocabulary word to phoneme to sound production from turn to turn as the child is helped to tell the story with greater complexity and increasing independence.

In our video example (see the accompanying DVD), the child, diagnosed with apraxia, is first introduced to the Elton story. As the character's picture on the book cover is introduced, attention is drawn to Elton's sound through the adult's explanations of the letter–sound relationship and phonetic features of [l] production, models of [l] production, and opportunities to produce [l] in isolation and as part of words.

Clinician: "This is the story about Elton (pointing to the character) and he makes the [l] sound (pointing to the raised tongue). He gets his tongue up tall to make the [l] sound. Elton (produced with an exaggerated [l]). Can you do that?

Child: (nonresponsive)

The adult then models the prolonged [l] and the child imitates the prolonged [l].

The adult points to the book title and starts to read the title. She stops to focus on the *L*-[l] letter–sound relationship. However, this child's development of phonemic categories and canonical structures requires the addition of many sounds, particularly those at the end of syllables, so the interventionist targets other sounds to improve the production of the words used in the story.

Clinician: "Okay, and it says 'Elton likes' (pointing to print) . . . can you say that?"

Child: "[laɪ]"

Clinician: "Ok, and there's another sound I hear (add Katie Phonic Face) at the end of the word . . . *like*"

Child: "[laɪk]"

Clinician: "*Like.* You got it! You can feel that little explosion at the end of the word (models with emphasis on final [k]), *like.*"

Child: "[laɪk]"

The attention returns to the title and its meaning.

Clinician: "And I wonder what Elton likes to do (holds the morphophonic vocabulary card for *lick* below the written word). Let's figure it out, it has the [l] sound at the beginning, and the [k] at the end . . . .*lick.*"

Child: "[lɪk]"

Clinician: "That's right, let's make that [l] sound, *lick* (produced with a lengthened [l])."

Child: "[lɪk]"

The clinician then reads the title and the child shadows each word, producing phonemes correctly. The picture is examined and a meaning-focused question asked:

Clinician: "Let's see what food he likes. What do you see?"

Child: "I don't know."

The interaction then goes on to talk about foods, with an alternating focus on meaning and articulation. Many phonemes are addressed during this talk (e.g., [g] in *egg;* final consonants for *hot, dog,* and *soup;* and words with more complex syllable structures such as *bacon* and *pepper*). The words are always generated within meaningful sentences, with cloze used to provide the child an opportunity to co-construct sentences with increasing length and complexity. Many word approximations the child produces are followed by recasts.

Clinician: "He tried to lick the food, but it was too _____."

Child: "Too [ha]."

Clinician: "Hot."

Child: "[hat]"

Clinician: "Hot, you're right. He burned his _____."

Child: no response.

Clinician: "[tə]_____."

Child: (no response)

Clinician: "Tongue."

Child: "[təŋ]"

Clinician: "He burned his *tongue*."

These interactions serve to develop all aspects of the child's language knowledge synergistically. Changes in speech productions are motivated by meaningful communication that takes place within extended discourse, expresses complex ideas, and is produced within longer syntactic utterances than the child produces spontaneously. The addition of new words, morphemes, and syntactic forms each requires changes from the current phonology across levels from features to phonemes to canonical structures. Phonology is refined when a new discrimination or distinction is needed to differentiate one meaningful word from a similar word. The more words a child develops, the more the self-organizing network forms and refines the underlying phonological categories within the system. The words include those that refer to concepts, such as nouns and verbs, but also morphemes that mark elements of time and status, and cohesive ties that refer to old, new, and given information throughout discourse. Thus, any development in language knowledge, including lexical, morphosyntactic, discourse, pragmatic, and metalinguistic elements, will both refine and be refined by phonology, leading to more accurate speech production.

ASSESSMENT AND PROGRESS
MONITORING TO SUPPORT DECISION MAKING

Progress is monitored by sampling products of the child's emerging speech and language system. Long-term progress can be determined through changes in standardized language and phonological tests, as well as through speech and language samples derived from clinical sampling or the child's classroom work. The most comprehensive view would be gained by assessing a complex language structure such as an oral report or retelling a story that has been read within the classroom.

Short-term progress can be monitored using probes. Depending on the child's developmental level, she or he could be asked to construct a story using a wordless picture book, to read and retell an episode of a story, or relate a recently experienced event from the classroom. Probes may be taken at the end of a session or on a weekly schedule. The clinician should be careful to keep the familiarity of the probes at an even level during a range of assessments. For example, the picture used to elicit a story might be one that was previously explored in intervention, a novel picture accompanied by an adult-modeled story, or a novel picture with no support provided for the story. The ideas that comprise the main points of the story as well as several details can be typed on a scoring form. As the child tells the story, the adult checks off the ideas from the story told by the child and indicates each sentence that is longer than the child's current mean length of utterance (MLU). These behaviors can usually be recorded as the child is telling the story. Key words in the story could be chosen for transcription and analysis for the occurrence of syllable structure or phonemic errors. Thus, in a few minutes a fairly representative sample of the child's language and phonology can be obtained that can be compared with a baseline, as well as with the previous probe, to ascertain whether progress is being made.

When intervention is failing, it means that the inputs to the system cannot be assimilated. New information must be familiar enough to be assimilated into existing structures but have sufficient novel or contrasting elements to create the discontinuity needed to effect change. For some children the zone or range of input between the known and the incomprehensible is very limited. For example, some children can learn when a picture is located immediately in front of them (i.e., the child is seated at a table with the clinician immediately next him or her, pointing to salient information) but not when the same picture is at a distance (i.e., the child is seated in a chair with the adult holding the picture in front of him or her, as in group storybook reading). The picture viewed by itself can be too difficult for the child to comprehend when there is not sufficient information in the illustration for the words and the visual images to overlap within the network (e.g., the story is about a girl who lost her dog, but the picture only shows her talking to her friend). In this case the picture and text maintain a distanced relationship and the words alone may be insufficient for the child to derive meaning. Likewise, the picture may be comprehensible, but the adult may be using an MLU or vocabulary choices that are too complex for the child to internalize. Conversely, the child may not be able to see changes in states or action from pictures and may need input in which props show the actions represented in the picture.

CONSIDERATIONS FOR CHILDREN FROM CULTURALLY AND LINGUISTICALLY DIVERSE BACKGROUNDS

The processors in the model of language use and development that underlie this intervention are meant to represent general processes that would be active in the language learning of all children. The details of the patterns developed within and across processors would depend on the structure of the language inputs that the child's system receives. As long as the adult providing the intervention is speaking the language to be learned, it is expected that the child will develop phonemes, syllable structures, and other patterns appropriate to the target language. However, available data for these techniques are derived from a small number of English-speaking countries. Components of this intervention, including the use of story construction (Hoffman et al., 1990, 1996), are reportedly used by 25% of the SLPs who responded to a questionnaire in Australia (McLeod, 2007). A focus on building phonological awareness and letter-sound knowledge has been used in New Zealand (Maclagan & Gillon, 2007).

The adult–child interaction patterns used in this intervention are largely based on studies of parent–child interaction among middle class families in the United States. Adults in social groups that do not afford as much attention to giving children conversational turns and using their own conversational turns to elaborate on children's utterances may find the use of these strategies more difficult to manage than techniques that more closely match their typical interactions with children. Although there are data suggesting that families in lower socioeconomic environments use fewer of these techniques (Hart & Risley, 1995), we have gathered a small amount of data suggesting that teachers in a Head Start program were able to swiftly make significant changes in their use of these storybook reading techniques with minimal training; for example, by increasing their letter-sound referencing (Brazier-Carter et al., 2004). As expected, the models of language they provided for the children in their storybook reading included appropriate models of their own dialect.

Our use of storybooks with Western, linear problem-solving narrative structures may be challenging for African American students who may be more familiar with a cyclical story structure (Bidell, Hubbard, & Weaver, 1997). However, other books with differing story structures could be chosen as materials. The letter–sound relationships in whatever books are used would be similar and could be portrayed with the Phonic Face representations. The interventionist could choose to discuss two ways of reading words— one as the way the children speak the words and the other as the way the author would read the words.

STUDY QUESTIONS

1. How would learning to describe the characters and actions in a story such as "Goldilocks and the Three Bears" lead to improved production of the allophones of /ɪ/, final consonants, and consonant clusters in words?

2. How would labeling letters on a storybook page and talking about the sounds produced by the letters provide a child with practice in production of isolated sounds and syllables?

3. How does repetition of a child's production of a word (e.g., child says "da," followed by the adult saying "dog") provide an expansion of the word's phonological form that may improve the child's phonological organization?

FUTURE DIRECTIONS

The intervention strategy outlined in this chapter has the theoretical potential to affect development of the array of processors in the child's system, and thus a wide variety of potential outcomes would be expected to improve simultaneously. The studies cited typically measured a relatively small number of these potential dependent variables at any one time. Future research is needed to determine what combinations of outcomes are most likely. The available data are based on small numbers of children. Further single-subject design studies are needed to specify in greater detail the children who are most likely to benefit, followed by randomized control group studies to provide the highest level of experimental control. Finally, the available studies have all been conducted within our research group, so the generalizability of these results to other clinician-researchers needs to be determined.

SUGGESTED READINGS

Hoffman, P.R., & Norris, J.A. (2002). Phonological assessment as an integral part of language assessment. *American Journal of Speech-Language Pathology, 11*, 230–235.

Hoffman, P.R., & Norris, J.A. (2006). Visual strategies to facilitate written language development. In S.F. Warren & M.E. Fey (Series Eds.) & R.J. McCauley & M.E. Fey (Vol. Eds.), *Communication and language intervention series: Treatment of language disorders in children* (pp. 347–382). Baltimore: Paul H. Brookes Publishing Co.

Hoffman, P.R., Norris, J.A., & Monjure, J. (1990). Comparison of process targeting and whole language treatments for phonologically delayed preschool children. *Language, Speech, and Hearing Services in Schools, 3*, 102–109.

Norris, J.A., & Hoffman, P.R. (2001). Language development and late talkers: A connectionist perspective. In R.G. Daniloff (Ed.), *Connectionist approaches to clinical language problems* (pp. 1–109). Fairfax, VA: TechBooks.

REFERENCES

Andrews, N., & Fey, M.E. (1986). Analysis of the speech of phonologically impaired children in two sampling conditions. *Language, Speech, and Hearing Services in Schools, 17*, 187–198.

Banajee, M.H. (2007). *Effect of adapted Phonic Faces story books on phonological skills with severe expressive language disorders.* Unpublished doctoral dissertation, Louisiana State University, Baton Rouge, LA.

Bellon-Harn, M.L., Hoffman, P.R., & Harn, W.E. (2004). Use of cloze and contrast word procedures in repeated storybook reading: Targeting multiple domains. *Journal of Communication Disorders, 37*, 53–75.

Bidell, T.R., Hubbard, L.J., & Weaver, M. (1997, April). *Story structure in a sample of African-American Children: Evidence for a cyclical story schema.* Paper presented at the Biennial meeting of the Society for Research in Child Development, Washington, DC.

Brazier-Carter, P., Norris, J.A., & Hoffman, P.R. (2004, November). *Print and meaning referencing in Head Start reading of alphabet-storybooks.* Poster session presented at the American Speech-Language-Hearing Association national convention, Philadelphia, PA.

Camarata, S.M. (1993). The application of naturalistic conversation training to speech production in children with speech disabilities. *Journal of Applied Behavior Analysis, 26*, 173–182.

Camarata, S.M., & Schwartz, R.G. (1985). Production of object words and action words: Evidence for a relationship between phonology and semantics. *Journal of Speech and Hearing Research, 26*, 50–53.

Dubois, E.M., & Bernthal, J.E. (1978). A comparison of three methods for obtaining articulatory responses. *Journal of Speech and Hearing Disorders, 43*, 295–305.

Ehri, L.C., Nunes, S.R., Willows, D.M., Schuster, B.V., Yaghoub-Zadeh, Z., & Shanahan, T. (2001). Phonemic awareness instruction helps children learn to read: Evidence from the national reading panel's meta-analysis. *Reading Research Quarterly 36*(3), 250–287.

Elman, J. (1995). Language as a dynamical system. In R.F. Port & T. van Gelder (Eds.), *Mind as motion: Explorations in the dynamics of cognition* (pp 195–223). Cambridge, MA: The MIT Press.

Fey, M.E., Catts, H.W., Proctor-Williams, K., Tomblin, J.B., & Zhang, X. (2004). Oral and written story composition skills of children with language impairment. *Journal of Speech, Language, and Hearing Research, 47*, 1301–1318.

Gillon, G.T. (2002). The efficacy of phonological awareness intervention for children with spoken language impairment. *Language, Speech, and Hearing Services in Schools, 31*, 126–141.

Girolametto, L., Pearce, P.S., & Weitzman, E. (1997). Effects of lexical intervention on the phonology of late talkers. *Journal of Speech, Language, and Hearing Research, 40*, 338–348.

Goldman, R., & Fristoe, M. (2000). *Goldman-Fristoe Test of Articulation-2.* Circle Pines, MN: American Guidance Service.

Hart, B., & Risley, T.R. (1995). *Meaningful differences in the everyday experiences of young American children.* Baltimore: Paul H. Brookes Publishing Co.

Hodson, B., & Paden, E. (1991). *Targeting intelligible speech: A phonological approach to remediation* (2nd ed.). San Diego: College-Hill Press.

Hoffman, P.R., & Norris, J.A. (1989). On the nature of phonological development: Evidence from normal children's spelling errors. *Journal of Speech and Hearing Research, 32*, 787–794.

Hoffman, P.R., & Norris, J.A. (2002). Phonological assessment as an integral part of language assessment. *American Journal of Speech-Language Pathology, 11*, 230–235.

Hoffman, P.R., & Norris, J.A. (2004, November). *Phonological changes resulting from language therapy: A self-organizing system.* Seminar presented at the

American Speech-Language-Hearing Association national convention, Philadelphia, PA.

Hoffman, P.R., & Norris, J.A. (2005). Intervention: Maipulating complex input to support self-organization of a neuro-network. In S.F. Warren & M.E. Fey (Series Eds.), & A.G. Kamhi & K.E. Pollock (Vol. Eds.), *Communication and language intervention series: Phonological disorders in children—Clinical decision making in assessment and intervention* (pp. 139–155). Baltimore: Paul H. Brookes Publishing Co.

Hoffman, P.R., & Norris, J.A. (2006). Visual strategies to facilitate written language development. In S.F. Warren & M.E. Fey (Series Eds.) & R.J. McCauley & M.E. Fey (Vol. Eds.), *Communication and language intervention series: Treatment of language disorders in children* (pp. 347–382). Baltimore: Paul H. Brookes Publishing Co.

Hoffman, P.R., Norris, J.A., & Monjure, J. (1990). Comparison of process targeting and whole language treatments for phonologically delayed preschool children. *Language, Speech, and Hearing Services in Schools, 3,* 102–109.

Hoffman, P.R., Norris, J.A., & Monjure, J. (1996). Effects of narrative intervention on a preschooler's syntactic and phonological development. *National Student Speech Language Hearing Association Journal, 23,* 5–13.

Kaufman, E., & Norris, J.A. (2007, November). *Eliciting speech using pictured sounds from a nonverbal preschooler.* Poster session presented at the American Speech-Language-Hearing Association national convention, San Diego, CA.

Larrivee, L.S., & Catts, H.W. (1999). Early reading achievement in children with expressive phonological disorders. *American Journal of Speech-Language-Pathology, 8,* 118–128.

Maclagan, M., & Gillon, G.T. (2007). New Zealand English speech acquisition. In S. McLeod (Ed.), *The international guide to speech acquisition* (pp. 257–268). Clifton Park, NY: Thomson Delmar Learning.

McInnis, A.T. (2008). *Phonemic awareness and sight word reading in toddlers.* Unpublished doctoral dissertation, Louisiana State University, Baton Rouge, LA.

McLeod, S.J. (2007). Australian English speech acquisition. In S. McLeod (Ed.), *The international guide to speech acquisition* (pp. 241–256). Clifton Park, NY: Thomson Delmar Learning.

McLeod, S.J. (2009). Children's speech acquisition. In J.E. Bernthal, N.W. Bankson, & P. Flipsen (Eds.), *Articulation and phonological disorders: Speech sound disorders in children* (pp. 385–405). Boston: Pearson.

Morrison, J.A., & Shriberg, L.D. (1992). Articulation testing versus conversational speech sampling. *Journal of Speech and Hearing Research, 35,* 259–273.

Nettleton, S., & Hoffman, P.R. (2005, November). *Phonic Faces v animated literacy alphabets in preschool phonological intervention.* Poster session presented at the American Speech-Language-Hearing Association national convention, San Diego, CA.

Norris, J.A. (2003). *Phonic Faces.* Baton Rouge, LA: Ele-Mentory.

Norris, J.A., & Hoffman, P.R. (1993). *Whole language intervention for school-age children.* San Diego: Singular Publishing. Norris, J.A., & Hoffman, P.R. (2001). Language development and late talkers: A connectionist perspective. In R.G. Daniloff (Ed.), *Connectionist approaches to clinical language problems* (pp. 1–109). Fairfax, VA: TechBooks.

Norris, J.A., & Hoffman, P.R. (2003, November 14). *Use of alphabet storybooks to increase print referencing in parent–child reading.* Poster session presented at the American Speech-Language-Hearing Association national convention, Chicago, IL.

Norris, J.A., & Hoffman, P.R. (2004, November 19). *Print and meaning referencing in parent-child reading of alphabet-storybooks.* Poster session presented at the American Speech-Language-Hearing Association national convention, Philadelphia, PA.

Paul, R., & Jennings, P. (1992). Phonological behavior in toddlers with slow expressive language development. *Journal of Speech and Hearing Research, 35,* 99–107.

Paul, R., & Smith, R.L. (1993). Narrative skills in 4-year-olds with normal, impaired, and late-developing language. *Journal of Speech and Hearing Research, 36,* 592–598.

Ruscello, D.M. (2008). Nonspeech oral motor treatment issues related to children with developmental speech sound disorders. *Language, Speech, and Hearing Services in Schools, 39,* 380–391.

Shriberg, L.D., & Austin, D. (1998). Comorbidity of speech-language disorder: Implications for a phenotype marker for speech delay. In S.F. Warren & J. Reichle (Series Eds.) & R. Paul (Vol. Ed.), *Communication and language intervention series: Vol. 8. Exploring the speech-language connection* (pp. 73–117). Baltimore: Paul H. Brookes Publishing Co.

Terrell, P.A. (2007). *Alphabetic and phonemic awareness in toddlers.* Unpublished doctoral dissertation, Louisiana State University, Baton Rouge, LA.

Tomasello, M. (2003). *Constructing a language: A usage-based theory of language acquisition.* Cambridge, MA: Harvard University Press.

Tyler, A.A., Lewis, K.E., Haskill, A., & Tolbert, L.C. (2002). Efficacy and cross-domain effects of a morphosyntax and a phonology intervention. *Language, Speech and Hearing Services in Schools, 33,* 52–66.

Van Riper, C. (1978). *Speech correction: Principles and methods* (6th ed.). Upper Saddle River, NJ: Prentice Hall.

Weiner, F., & Ostrowski, A. (1979). Effects of listener uncertainty on articulatory inconsistency. *Journal of Speech and Hearing Disorders, 44,* 487–493.

Williams, A.L. (2005). A model and structure for phonological intervention. In S.F. Warren & M.E. Fey (Series Eds.) & A.G. Kamhi & K.E. Pollock (Vol. Eds.), *Communication and language intervention series: Phonological disorders in children—Clinical decision making in assessment and intervention* (pp. 189–200). Baltimore: Baltimore: Paul H. Brookes Publishing Co.

Morphosyntax Intervention

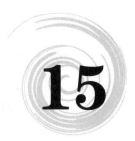

Ann A. Tyler and Allison M. Haskill

ABSTRACT

The morphosyntax intervention focuses on speech indirectly through targeting language structures that mark tense and agreement, and, therefore, involves final clusters. It is an integrative approach that is ideal for preschool children who have a comorbid speech sound disorder (SSD) and expressive language impairment characterized by morphosyntactic difficulties. The intervention can be delivered in weekly individual and group sessions in clinical, preschool, and early childhood classroom settings. As many as four grammatical morphemes are targeted, each for 1 week, in a cycle that can be repeated or in one that can involve alternating the intervention with speech intervention every other week. Teaching methods involve stories from children's literature, focused stimulation activities, and elicited production activities, all of which can be varied in level of difficulty.

INTRODUCTION

The morphosyntactic intervention, *Months of Morphemes* (Haskill, Tyler, & Tolbert, 2001), was originally developed as one of the interventions for a research project funded by the National Institutes of Health (DC03358). The project was designed to examine the efficacy of different goal attack configurations targeting *both* speech and language in children with speech and language disorders. Because these children typically experience expressive language disorders characterized by grammatical difficulties, the morphosyntax intervention was developed to focus on structures that interface with phonology and are, at the same time, significant for language development. The intervention is theme-based and uses scripts for implementing hybrid teaching procedures that include features of both clinician-directed and child-centered techniques. The intervention uses a cycles approach involving 1-month cycles in which a different target is the focus each week. Because of its design and use of children's literature, other language skills are inherently practiced and modeled in the activities designed for each target.

TARGET POPULATIONS

Primary Populations

The primary population the intervention was designed for is preschoolers, ages 3;0 through 6;0, who exhibit morphosyntactically based language disorders and comorbid

SSD. In this group, children whose mean length of utterance (MLU) is at least 2.0 are prime candidates for this intervention.

Secondary Populations

Because this intervention focuses on tense and agreement markers (i.e., finite morphemes) and was designed for children with morphosyntactically based language disorder, that impairment is the primary prerequisite for use of the approach. As such, other populations with morphosyntactic impairments may be candidates for this intervention. Children exhibiting an expressive language impairment characterized by morphosyntactic difficulties that is secondary to a primary etiology such as hearing impairment, as well as those with primary SSD, may be candidates. Estimates of the co-occurrence of language impairment and SSD range from 35%–60% in clinical samples of preschoolers with either of these impairments (Botting & Conti-Ramsden, 2004; Conti-Ramsden & Botting, 1999; Rapin & Allen, 1983; van Daal, Verhoeven, & van Balkom, 2004). Shriberg (2004) also estimated from a large data set that the probability of expressive language disorder is 40%–60% in his speech delay-genetic subgroup, the proposed largest, etiologically determined subgroup of children presenting with childhood SSD. This group manifests co-occurring speech, language, and/or reading impairments affected by cognitive-linguistic processes. These preschoolers with comorbid speech and language impairments are prime candidates for the morphosyntactic intervention because of the surface interactions affecting morphophonemic forms that result, for example, when a child omits final consonants/clusters, thereby prohibiting use of certain grammatical morphemes (e.g., if bat→/bæ/ then plural ba*ts* or third-person singular regular ba*ts* also become /bæ/).

Evidence suggests that even when a child does not display final consonant deletion/ cluster reduction, finite morpheme production is more compromised for children with co-occurring language and speech disorder than language disorder alone (Rvachew, Gaines, Cloutier, & Blanchet, 2005). Haskill and Tyler (2007) examined morpheme use in subgroups of children with language impairment, separating those with language impairment only from those with both speech and language impairments; within this latter group, a group with final consonant deletion/cluster reduction was separated from those without this error pattern. The children with final consonant deletion/cluster reduction had the lowest accuracy, as expected, on a finite morpheme composite (FMC) percentage from spontaneous conversation. Children with both speech and language impairment (but no final consonant deletion/cluster reduction) displayed significantly lower finite morpheme accuracies, by approximately 20%, than children with language-only impairment, indicating relatively greater severity of involvement. Compared with children with language impairment only, those with concomitant speech disorder are more vulnerable for difficulty with tense and agreement markers and, thus, especially appropriate candidates for an intervention focused on these morphemes. In contrast, nonfinite (i.e., noun related) morpheme accuracies were similar across the subgroups, other than the one displaying final consonant deletion/cluster reduction.

Although the preschool age range is the ideal window for this intervention due to the typical acquisition course of grammatical morphemes and phonology, older children with developmental delay or English language learners may also benefit from this intervention. The prerequisite expressive language level of Brown's (1973) Stage II (minimum MLU = 2.0) is required for children optimally to benefit from focused stimulation and production tasks aimed at stimulating the primary morpheme targets of the intervention.

Those targets, which focus on tense and agreement, are regular past tense *–ed*, uncontractible and contractible copula *BE* verbs, regular third-person singular, and irregular past tense. Although developmentally, some of these morpheme targets are mastered in stages beyond that encompassing the predicted age for an MLU = 2.0 (22–37 months; Miller & Chapman, 1981), their age ranges of mastery overlap the age range of MLU Stage II (Brown, 1973; Miller & Chapman, 1981). Not only must children be linguistically ready, they must be cognitively ready to combine words and modify them with markers.

ASSESSMENT METHODS FOR DETERMINING INTERVENTION RELEVANCE

To determine the appropriateness of using the morphosyntactic intervention with a particular child, assessment should include at a minimum standardized tests and/or nonstandardized tasks that allow determination of level of morphosyntactic functioning. Ideally, language sample analysis provides the most naturalistic reflection of a child's morphological usage, and computerized analysis procedures (e.g., Systematic Analysis of Language Transcripts [SALT], Miller & Chapman, 2000) allow calculation of morpheme percent accuracy in obligatory contexts. Language sampling contexts can be designed to provide multiple opportunities for production of specific morphemes. In the interest of time, however, language assessment tools that have proven particularly well suited for assessing morphological performance are the Structured Photographic Expressive Language Test–Preschool 2 (SPELT-P2; Dawson et al., 2005), the Rice/Wexler Test of Early Grammatical Impairment (RWTEGI; Rice & Wexler, 2001), and subtests of the Clinical Evaluation of Language Fundamentals–Preschool 2 (CELF-P2; Wiig, Secord, & Semel, 2004)—Word Structure and Recalling Sentences in Context. In addition, for children with SSD, identification of such a disorder through standardized testing is necessary.

Children for whom this intervention was designed all performed below 1 standard deviation (*SD*) less than the mean on a standardized expressive language measure. Language sample analyses were also completed using language samples that were collected in the children's preschool setting and involved spontaneous conversation during play with a replica house and accessories, as well as with a wordless picture book. The language samples contained at least 200 utterances and multiple opportunities for each of the finite morphemes across narrative and play-based conversational contexts. An FMC was calculated (Bedore & Leonard, 1998; Rice, Wexler, & Cleave, 1995). This reflected the combined percent correct usage of the following finite morphemes: regular past tense *–ed*, third-person singular regular *–s*, contractible and uncontractible copula *BE* verbs, and uncontractible and contractible auxiliary *BE* forms. Finite morpheme usage for children in the study sample averaged 42% in obligatory contexts.

THEORETICAL BASIS

Dominant Theoretical Rationale for the Intervention Approach

The theoretical rationale for the morphosyntactic intervention is twofold: 1) targeting finite morphemes is of prime importance due to the disproportionate impact they have on early linguistic development, which has a potential cascading effect on later language developments; and 2) cross-domain generalizations achieved by triggering interactions between domains of the linguistic system, in this case morphosyntax and phonology, have potential for increased efficiency when children display difficulties in these two domains.

Finite Morphemes Are of Prime Importance

Finite morphemes were selected as the primary targets of this intervention because numerous studies at the time it was developed indicated these morphemes are particularly vulnerable in children with specific language impairment (SLI; Bedore & Leonard, 1998; Leonard, Eyer, Bedore, & Grela, 1997; Marchman, Wulfeck, & Ellis Weismer, 1999; Rice, 1999). Finite morphemes such as the third-person singular regular (e.g., *–s* in *she runs*) reflect tense (present) and agreement (third person: she), as do both copula and auxiliary *BE* forms *is, are, am, was,* and *were.*

Although subgroups of children with language disorders display difficulties across different clusters of linguistic domains, a core feature of most clusters is difficulty in syntax and morphology. It has long been documented that development of grammatical morphology in children experiencing language disorders is protracted (deVilliers & deVilliers, 1973). In addition, finite morphology has been shown to be disproportionately problematic and hypothesized to interact with syntactic development as well (Leonard, 1998; Rice & Wexler, 1996, 2001; Rice et al., 1995). Not only do results of numerous studies indicate that preschoolers with SLI perform more poorly on these morphemes in comparison to nonfinite ones, they suggest that these impairments have a protracted course, whereas other impairments such as lexical diversity, show relatively greater improvement with age (Goffman & Leonard, 2000). Children with SLI show reduced accuracy in obligatory contexts well into early elementary school in comparison with their typically developing peers (Norbury, Bishop, & Briscoe, 2001; Rice, Wexler, & Hershberger, 1998).

Results of other studies have shown that the slow growth in tense morpheme productivity may be one of the earliest signs of a long-standing language disorder (Hadley & Holt, 2006). In addition, there is independent treatment evidence that shows treating selected tense and agreement morphemes leads to gains, although modest, for the targets (Camarata, Nelson, & Camarata, 1994; Leonard, Camarata, Brown, & Camarata, 2004). Generalization to untreated tense and agreement morphemes occurs to a lesser extent (Leonard, Camarata, Brown, & Camarata, 2004; Leonard, Camarata, Pawlowska, Brown, & Camarata, 2006). A further reason for selecting finite morphemes is that there is some indication nonfinite morphemes will also improve without direct treatment, as the finite morphemes are being targeted (Willet, 2001).

Finite morphology is also significant for children with SLI because it may have an impact on syntactic development. In the "morphosyntactic perspective," finite morphology holds a pivotal place in the development of sentence type elaborations (Rice & Wexler, 1996, 2001). As in a yes/no question that requires inversion of the copula, sentence structure rules and finite morphology are interconnected. An additional case for economy can be made in targeting finite morphemes because of the interconnectedness of finite verbs and sentence structure.

There is not agreement about the underlying cause of grammatical impairments in SLI, as evidenced by the array of theories proposed. Two broad categories, however, can be identified, one focusing on linguistic impairments involving faulty rules or misapplication of linguistic paradigms, and the other focusing on a broader cognitive-linguistic processing impairment. Within the former category, a more circumscribed grammatical impairment is proposed, whereas theories in the latter category suggest a generalized slower processing system (Dollaghan, 2004; Hayiou-Thomas, Bishop, & Plunkett, 2004;

Leonard, 1998) or phonological working memory limitations (Conti-Ramsden, Botting, & Faragher, 2001).

The morphosyntactic intervention with its focus on a linguistic form, by default, would appear to support the assumption of a linguistic impairment; however, such a focus does not eliminate consideration of a cognitive processing component, nor the incorporation of techniques designed to enhance cognitive-linguistic processing. The intervention does focus more squarely on impairment of Body Function, in language, with respect to the World Health Organization's (WHO's) *International Classification of Functioning, Disability and Health* (ICF; 2001). The morphosyntactic intervention indirectly addresses activity limitations and participation restrictions that result from a speech and language impairment. For example, scripted conversational activities included in the intervention to provide production practice for specific finite morphemes are designed to be implemented in group settings, where communication for forming relationships and educational purposes may be enhanced.

Cross-Domain Generalizations May Be Triggered by Linguistic Interactions

The second rationale for the morphosyntactic intervention rests on the assumption that there are multiple interactions among developing linguistic domains and that these may be harnessed or maximized during intervention, thus achieving gains that extend beyond the domain that is immediately being targeted. In the case of children with SSD and expressive language impairments, particularly morphosyntactic, several researchers have addressed potential interactions among linguistic domains. Marshall and van der Lely (2003) in their "computational grammatical complexity hypothesis" suggested that not only may there be a core grammatical impairment (i.e., faulty rules), but this might affect other rule systems such as phonology (van der Lely, 2004, 2005). Akin to the cognitive-linguistic processing accounts of SLI that focus on grammatical limitations, Chiat (2001) proposed a phonological theory of SLI with core phonological processing impairments that result in influences on lexical and syntactic development. Disruptions in mapping arise because phonological characteristics influence morpheme productions in various populations. Similarly, Stemberger (2003) has shown that phonological characteristics may influence the processing of English inflections. Phonological characteristics of past tense verbs and their errors with respect to cluster phonotactics, rime characteristics, and frequency were examined (Stemberger, 2002, 2003). Results verified that the regular *–ed* affix is phonologically restricted; thus, phonological factors can prevent morphemes from appearing.

It has also been argued that connectionist models, as well as optimality theory, both of which suggest that phonological and morphological processing occur in parallel, best explain child error data and impairments in speech and language disorders (Bernhardt & Stemberger, 1998; Stemberger, 2002). What appear to be specific morphological impairments that have been accounted for by proposing separate "rule" and "associative" memory systems can be more parsimoniously explained with connectionist models. These contrast even with accounts discussed previously that suggest there are autonomous impairments in phonology and morphology (Marshall & van der Lely, 2003). If the interactions suggested in these connectionist theories occur, we should be able to maximize efficiency by designing interventions that capitalize on cross-domain generalizations, that is, indirect gains in untreated structures. In the case of a morphosyntactic intervention, a number of mechanisms might be responsible for change in phonology, depending to a large extent on what the intervention focuses on. For example, an intervention that focuses on bound morphemes such as the plural, past tense *–ed*, or third-person singular *–s*, whose allomorphs create morphophonemically complex forms, might cause specific improvements in final consonant clusters.

Thus, it can be hypothesized that an intervention that focuses on finite morphemes, and indirectly on clusters, might facilitate improvement in both morphosyntax and phonology. Final clusters used as morphological markers are clearly problematic for children with speech and language impairment. Haskill and Tyler (2007) found that even when children with both speech and language disorders did *not* display final deletions patterns, their consonantal accuracy for final cluster morphemes was only 54%. In addition, treatment-induced improvement in final cluster accuracy might, in turn, facilitate learning of less complex aspects of the ambient phonology such as singletons (Gierut & Champion, 2001). In the Gierut and Champion study, children who were taught initial three-element consonant clusters increased the size of their singleton inventories by the addition, on average, of five untreated sounds.

Alternatively, a broad-based narrative intervention, such as that described by Norris and Hoffman (1990), might induce phonological changes because speech sounds are repeatedly practiced as part of a larger narrative script. Thus, organizational changes in higher linguistic levels simultaneously cause changes in lower linguistic levels (Hoffman, 1992). Similarly, an intervention following the "concentrated normative model," a naturalistic model that recognizes the need for concentrated and/or focused input, should facilitate growth in all linguistic domains. Just as lexical and morphosyntactic growth could occur, so could phonological growth take place within a classroom intervention that stresses the functional and social value of interaction and provides opportunity for both active and passive learning.

Levels of Consequences Being Addressed

With respect to the WHO framework (ICF [2001]) for the functional impact of a speech and language disorder, the morphosyntax intervention targets Activity limitations and Participation restrictions that result from the disorder. Specific Activity and Participation restrictions are encompassed in the broad areas of communication, interpersonal interactions and relationships, and education. The intervention focuses on speaking and conversational skills, within individual as well as group sessions, where social interactions are practiced; these skills all potentially influence educational success.

Target Areas of Intervention

The intervention focuses primarily on grammatical morphemes that mark tense and agreement and secondarily on complex morphophonemic forms such as final consonant clusters. It also indirectly focuses on other areas of language such as vocabulary, direction-following, story-retelling, and social pragmatic skills.

EMPIRICAL BASIS

The evidence base for the morphosyntax intervention consists of five studies at various levels of evidence designed to examine the efficacy of the approach first and then the implementation of the approach under controlled experimental conditions in a public school and university clinic. These studies and the levels of evidence represented are displayed in Table 15.1.

Table 15.1. Levels of evidence for studies of treatment efficacy for morphosyntax intervention

Level	Description	References
Ia	Meta-analysis of > 1 randomized controlled trial	—
Ib	Randomized controlled study	Tyler et al. (2003)
IIa	Controlled study without randomization	Sweat (2003); Tyler et al. (2002)
IIb	Quasi-experimental study	Hide (2007); Tyler & Sandoval (1994)
III	Nonexperimental studies, i.e., correlational and case studies	—
IV	Expert committee report, consensus conference, clinical experience of respected authorities	—

Adapted from the Scottish Intercollegiate Guidelines Network (http://www.sign.ac.uk).

Preliminary Exploration of Generalization

The morphosyntactic intervention is included in this book within a group of integrative approaches for treating SSD. It may also be considered a language-based approach (Tyler, 2002), but can be distinguished from approaches that are conversation-based (Camarata, 1995; Norris & Hoffman, 2005). It is not a conversational approach, but rather an integrative one, precisely because of the nature of the morphophonemic structures it targets. Finite morphemes necessarily require phonotactic forms with singleton or cluster codas (e.g., past tense: *sipped*, third-person singular regular: *puts*, copula: *is*). A focus on these forms in treatment presents an opportunity for generalization to untreated phonotactic structures, final consonants, and clusters, as well as the possibility for the addition or increase in accuracy of constituent phonemes in the child's system. For example, targeting third-person singular through elicited production of the word *kicks* facilitates increased accuracy in production of final singletons /k/ or /s/. Such cross-domain generalization or indirect gains in another linguistic system that does not receive direct intervention should increase efficiency. This extension of learning can also be used to demonstrate that change is the direct result of intervention. Thus, efficacy research for an integrative approach such as the morphosyntax intervention must evaluate potential interactions between phonological reorganization and morphosyntax.

Summary of Levels of Evidence

This section describes in depth the five studies included in Table 15.1. Together they represent a research agenda that began with an exploratory, quasi-experimental investigation of interactive effects of focus on either phonology or language and progressed to a larger study involving efficacy and effectiveness questions. This two-part study had features of Levels Ib and IIa characterized by a control group design, with randomization of the experimental groups, and a wait-list control group. An independent quasi-experimental investigation of cross-domain effects of morphosyntax intervention is also included.

Exploratory Study

In an exploratory study, Tyler and Sandoval (1994) examined cross-domain effects of interventions differentially focused on morphosyntax, phonology, or both domains for six preschoolers with moderate-to-severe disorders in both domains. All children displayed final consonant deletion/cluster reduction, thus providing the opportunity to evaluate the hypothesis that elimination of error patterns affecting final segments/clusters should lead to improvement in grammatical morphemes. Two children were semi-randomly assigned to each of the three types of intervention. An abbreviated multiple baseline across subject pairs and extensive phonological and morphological generalization probes were used, making the study quasi-experimental.

Children who received direct phonological intervention focusing on final consonant deletion/cluster reduction showed a moderate improvement in both phonology and language. Specifically, with regard to morphosyntactic improvement, both children progressed from Brown's Stage II to Late Stage III–Early Stage IV. They both also showed an increase in production of phonetically complex morphophonemic forms evident in a final language sample as well as in generalization probes. One child who received treatment on final /ps, ts/ improved from 0% to 80%–100% accuracy on the plural /z/ and regular past tense forms in probes. The other child was treated on final /n, t/; for this child, plural and possessive /z/ and third-person singular increased in accuracy in generalization probes. In contrast, the two children in this study who received the indirect narrative intervention made no such improvements in phonetically complex morphophonemic forms, although MLU did increase. These results suggest that a phonological focus on final consonants/clusters led to improvement in grammatical morphemes subject to surface-level interactions with phonological forms. When children display final consonant deletion/cluster reduction error patterns, these should take precedence in a treatment program, not only for their potential morphophonemic status but also because they alter basic syllable structure.

Efficacy and Effectiveness Studies

Efficacy of the morphosyntax intervention was tested against an untreated control and the intervention was also compared with a speech intervention and mixed intervention strategies for children with both speech and language disorders.

Evidence supporting the morphosyntax intervention comes from a study that investigated both the efficacy of the intervention in comparison to a no-treatment control and the indirect effects of the intervention on phonological performance (Tyler, Lewis, Haskill, & Tolbert, 2002). This study was part of a larger study (Tyler, Lewis, Haskill, & Tolbert, 2003) involving 47 participants, in which different strategies of scheduling speech and language goals were investigated. The larger design involved four different intervention strategies to which preschool children were randomly assigned, 10 for each group, and a control group of seven formed from a waiting list. The children, ages 3;0–5;11, had *both* speech and language disorders identified through performance on standardized measures that were less than 1 *SD* below the mean for their age group. Intervention strategies were provided twice weekly in one 45-minute group session and one 30-minute individual session in the children's early childhood programs housed in public elementary schools. Outcomes were compared at 12 and 24 weeks postintervention. Due to the nature of this design, with its control group and randomized assignment to different intervention strategies, a high level of evidence was achieved, falling between Levels Ib and IIa (ASHA, 2004). This signifies a well-designed controlled study with and without, in the case of the control group, randomization; that is, 40 participants were randomly assigned to interventions, but the control group was not because it was a group of convenience. Nonetheless, the study achieved a high degree of credibility.

The smaller efficacy study examined the effects of two of the four intervention strategies, both block interventions in which speech or morphosyntax goals received concentrated focus for 12-week blocks, but in different orders (Tyler et al., 2002). The sequence effects of the block interventions, when they occurred in different orders, were also evaluated. The morphosyntax intervention, published as *Months of Morphemes* (Haskill et al., 2001), was applied in one strategy during the first block. It focused on four finite morphemes in cyclical fashion, with repetition of the cycle twice (4 weeks × 3 cycles = 12 weeks). For this "morphosyntax first" strategy, the second block involved 12 weeks of hybrid phonological intervention. This phonological intervention was applied during the first block of the other "speech first" strategy and focused on four phoneme/cluster targets in a similar cyclical fashion. Data were collected at pretreatment and after the first 12-week intervention block. For the control group, data were collected at the beginning and end of a 12-week period, equivalent to one intervention block. Thus, three groups were compared, the controls, the group receiving speech first, and the group receiving morphosyntax first.

Research Outcomes

Change in an FMC and target/generalization phoneme composite was assessed. FMC percentages were calculated from language samples that were collected in the children's preschool setting and involved spontaneous conversational contexts, as described previously in the Assessment Methods for Determining Intervention Relevance section. The target generalization composite (TGC) was a percentage reflecting the accuracy of target and generalization sounds selected for each child from the total number of opportunities for these sounds in the *Bankson-Bernthal Test of Phonology* (BBTOP; Bankson & Bernthal, 1990) words and supplementary words. There were at least three opportunities for each phoneme in word-initial and word-final positions from these words. Children typically had four target phonemes, including several clusters, identified by word position. These targets, as well as their cognates, were identified for generalization in untreated word positions, depending on their accuracy. For example, if a child had initial /k/, final /f/, and initial /s/ as targets, these sounds along with initial /g/, final /v/, and initial /z/, as well as final /k, g/, initial /f, v/, and final /s, z/ were identified for the TGC. There were on average 32 opportunities for assessment of sound productions in single words that were not included as treatment stimuli.

In comparison to the control group, the morphosyntax and hybrid phonological interventions were effective at a statistically significant level in facilitating improvement for their respective targets after 12 weeks. This time period corresponded to the first block during which each group received one of the two different interventions. The average change in finite morphemes for the morphosyntax intervention first group was 14.4% compared with −0.7% for the control group. The average change in speech sound targets and generalization targets for the speech intervention group was 18.7% compared with 3.3% for the control group. Results also revealed a cross-domain effect for the morphosyntax intervention, but no cross-domain effect for the speech intervention. The morphosyntax intervention led to change in speech for the group receiving it, which was significantly greater than the speech change of the control group, with means of 19.3 and 3.3, respectively (Tyler et al., 2002). Furthermore, the effect of morphosyntax intervention on speech for this group was similar to that observed in the group that received the speech intervention; target and generalization sound growth was 19.3% for the morphosyntax first group and 18.7% for the speech first group. Tyler et al. (2002) suggested that targeting finite morphemes involving the production of final clusters, a more difficult aspect of phonology, may have led to improvements in other less complex aspects of the phonology.

Analysis of phonological and morphosyntactic change in the different intervention sequences across 24 weeks (morphosyntax first or speech first) revealed similar changes in both speech and morphosyntax, regardless of the sequence in which children received the interventions. The morphosyntactic first sequence, however, led to slightly better overall morphosyntactic performance; it also led to significant phonological change and continued improvement in phonology when it was the second intervention in the sequence. Tyler et al. (2002) noted that continued investigation of these variables and relationships is warranted.

Researchers have further explored the hypothesis that increased production of final clusters is a byproduct of targeting finite morphemes (Hide, 2007; Sweat, 2003). Hide found that final cluster production increased in accuracy for two of three children who participated in morphosyntax intervention alternated with speech intervention. Sweat examined widespread phonological changes involving the constituent segments of the cluster forms. Final consonant inventories and accuracies of final clusters for the morphosyntax first and speech first groups ($N = 10$ each) from the Tyler et al. (2002) study were examined. The accuracies of final clusters used for marking regular past tense –*ed* and contractible copula *'s* in spontaneous conversation were significantly greater for the group receiving the morphosyntax intervention after 12 weeks. There was also a trend for the group that had received the morphosyntax intervention to have added more age-appropriate and later-developing sounds to their phonetic inventories, although there was no significant group difference for the sheer number of sounds added to the final inventory. It can thus be hypothesized that repeated practice of finite morpheme targets, and therefore certain final clusters, appears to result in increased accuracy in spontaneous language. Cluster types that were produced less accurately by the 47 participants of the large study included /-ts, -ks, gz, -nz, -mz, -nts, -mpt/ used for third-person singular and contractible copula and auxiliary markers. Five of these seven clusters are specifically targeted in the finite morpheme intervention (Haskill et al., 2001) used in the Tyler et al. (2002) cross-domain study.

Although the results of the smaller efficacy study (Tyler et al., 2002) suggested that the morphosyntax intervention facilitated significant gains in both speech and morphosyntax for the participants with comorbid speech and language impairment, results from the larger study complicate the picture (Tyler et al., 2003). In this study, the two-block intervention strategies previously described were compared along with a strategy that involved alternating focus on speech and morphosyntactic goals and a simultaneous strategy. The alternating strategy involved the speech and morphosyntax interventions, each a focus every other week for 8 weeks total. Results from this study indicated that the alternating strategy produced greater morphosyntactic change compared with all other strategies after 24 weeks of intervention. There was no difference among the four strategies, however, for speech gains; they all produced similarly significant gains. This suggests, then, that if a child has comorbid speech and language difficulties, and the goal is to produce gains in both domains, alternating goals among them may be the best strategy in the long run.

PRACTICAL REQUIREMENTS

The morphosyntax approach initially was designed to be implemented in early childhood, elementary school, or clinical settings within a September–May school year calendar (Southern hemisphere: March–November). The cyclical organization of the approach lends itself to meeting other schedules and intervention configurations as well (e.g., semesters in a college clinic).

Nature of Sessions

The morphosyntax approach is structured to include one individual and one small-group session per week. The length of sessions may vary based on the needs of individual settings, but generally 30 minutes for individual and 45 minutes for group sessions is sufficient to complete activities. Groups may consist of two to four children with similar ages and communication goals. The same teaching strategies and activities are used in both individual and group sessions.

Personnel

This scripted approach may be implemented by individuals with training and experience in grammar and child language development and disorders. Complete scripts are found in Haskill et al. (2001). The approach has been implemented successfully by licensed, certified speech-language pathologists (SLPs), graduate and undergraduate speech-language pathology student clinicians, and early childhood special educators. Activities are intended to be functional and felicitous for preschool-age children, and generally involve fine motor, gross motor, and literacy materials that are readily available in typical households or early childhood settings.

To encourage participation of families during intervention, clinicians may distribute a weekly family letter that is provided for each target. These letters list the weekly theme, target structures with examples, children's books, activities from the sessions, and suggested follow-up activities for home. If clinicians have the opportunity to meet with parents, they may also elect to involve families by demonstrating basic facilitating strategies, such as forced choice or focused stimulation. A suggestion for home practice may be as simple as encouraging caregivers to read to their children books containing multiple exemplars of each week's targeted morphosyntactic forms. Clinicians also may provide a specific example of a daily home routine in which targeted forms could be modeled naturalistically. For example, past tense morphemes could be targeted during a cooking routine in which the child recalls the steps taken to bake cookies.

KEY COMPONENTS

Nature of Goals

As indicated previously, the aim of this approach is for children with both SSD and morphosyntactically based language impairment to achieve cross-domain improvement in both phonology and morphosyntax. This is accomplished through the use of thoughtfully selected morpheme goals using a hybrid combination of naturalistic and clinician-directed elicited production techniques in developmentally appropriate, interactive activities.

In the study for which this approach was designed (Tyler et al., 2003), each participant focused on four speech sounds and four grammatical morphemes that were targeted cyclically over the course of one academic year, the equivalent of 24 weeks. Morpheme targets were selected based on several factors: 1) low percent correct usage in preintervention language samples (forms used with 0%–40% accuracy received priority), 2) finiteness (finite morphemes were prioritized over nonfinite forms), and 3) the target morpheme's relation to the child's speech errors.

Goal Attack Strategies

Once individual children's targets are identified, the clinician must decide how to coordinate speech and morphosyntax targets. Though a cycles approach to goal organization (Hodson & Paden, 1991) may be most typically associated with phonological intervention, it also may be useful in intervention targeting morphemes (Fey, Cleave, Long, & Hughes, 1993) and is the method used in the morphosyntax approach described in this chapter. As previously discussed, maximum cross-domain benefits may be achieved by opting for an alternating speech-morphosyntax format. In this strategy, speech sound goals would be targeted one week, followed by a week of morphosyntax focus. A block strategy in which speech or morphosyntax is targeted for three 1-month cycles also may result in both speech and morphosyntactic improvement (Tyler et al., 2002). A third option may be for clinicians to focus on both speech and morphosyntax targets simultaneously in each session. Findings from Tyler et al. (2003), however, suggest that simultaneously targeting morphosyntax and speech goals in the same session is minimally effective. Table 15.2 displays an example schedule for alternating and block strategies.

Description of Activities

Activities are theme-based to enable pragmatically appropriate repetition and introduction of new vocabulary in common experiences. In the original program in which the morphosyntax approach was used, each cycle included activities that conformed to the broad themes of water, animals, and food, respectively. Clinicians may adapt similar activities to meet a variety of other themes using a session planning sheet such as the one provided in Appendix A for this chapter. Session activities are also easily adapted to meet early childhood education standards and interface well with commonly used curricula in the areas of oral language, literacy, socialization, early academic skills, and gross and fine motor development. For each activity, skills used, such as direction following, sequencing, or fine motor, are explicitly listed. Though morphosyntax clearly is the primary emphasis, other language domains such as semantics and pragmatics also are targeted indirectly through the activities. Literacy is incorporated into each session in the form of book sharing or narrative-type tasks. For example, a children's book whose text provides multiple examples of the morpheme target is suggested for each lesson. In addition, supplemental books related to the theme of the session are suggested.

The morphosyntax approach involves both naturalistic and child production and practice opportunities. As such, children have in each session the opportunity to both hear and produce multiple tokens of target morphemes. In each of the two weekly ses-

Table 15.2.   Example schedules for alternating and block strategies for organizing speech and morpheme goals

Alternating	Block
Week 1: morpheme target #1	Week 1: speech OR morpheme target #1
Week 2: speech target #1	Week 2: speech OR morpheme target #2
Week 3: morpheme target #2	Week 3: speech OR morpheme target #3
Week 4: speech target #2	Week 4: speech OR morpheme target #4
Week 5: morpheme target #3	(Repeat for 2 additional cycles per domain, for a total of 24 weeks)
Week 6: speech target #3	
Week 7: morpheme target #4	
Week 8: speech target #4	
(Repeat for 2 additional cycles, for a total of 24 weeks)	

sions, activities include two focused stimulation activities to promote awareness of the target forms as well as one elicited production activity.

Focused Stimulation

Focused stimulation is a frequently used facilitation technique in which the facilitator, generally a clinician or parent, provides numerous contextually relevant examples of a specific linguistic form, which is most typically a semantic or grammatical target (Ellis Weismer & Robertson, 2006; Fey, 1986; Leonard 1981). Researchers have interpreted differently the child's role in focused stimulation activities on a continuum ranging from primarily input-focused with the child having a relatively passive role (e.g., Leonard et al., 1982) to interactive, with the child having a more active role in producing the targeted form (Girolametto, Pearce, & Weitzman 1996).

In the morphosyntax approach, clinicians aim to provide, at minimum, 40 correct (not contrasting or erroneous) examples of the target form, primarily in literacy, narrative, or singing activities. Haskill et al. (2001) included a list of theme-based children's books that contain numerous exemplars of various morpheme targets (e.g., the popular children's book, *Have You Seen My Cat?* [Carle, 1991] contains numerous exemplars of copula *BE* morphemes). Alternatively, "syntax stories," described by Fey and Cleave (1997), may be adapted for use in focused stimulation activities for selected morphemes. For books that are relevant to the selected theme, but do not contain multiple examples of the target form, clinicians may choose to retell or comment on stories, focusing on particular forms. For example, a story originally written in present tense could be adapted for the third-person singular morpheme in a story retelling focused stimulation activity with the clinician narrating in third person (e.g., "The mouse EATS the cookie then CLEANS the floor").

Alliterated or rhyming verses also are used in focused stimulation activities in the morphosyntax approach in the form of traditional or customized songs saturated with target morphemes. Some popular children's songs, such as The Itsy Bitsy Spider, naturally contain target morphemes (regular past tense *–ed: climbed, washed, dried*), whereas others may be adapted (e.g., to focus stimulation on copula *BE:* "Here *IS* a little seed, little seed, little seed. Here *IS* a little seed. Soon it will grow . . ."; Haskill et al., 2001).

Elicited Production

Focused stimulation activities provide numerous, contextually viable opportunities for exposure to target morphemes; however, children may or may not have an opportunity to produce target forms during such activities. Because children receiving the morphosyntax intervention have both morphosyntax and speech sound impairments, and many of the morpheme targets may include weakly stressed, phonetically complex forms (e.g., clusters), production practice was viewed as a logically necessary component to include to complement focused stimulation and recasting efforts. As children progress through the three cycles, the structure and content of focused stimulation activities remains consistent; however, the level of complexity for elicited production activities increases from cycle 1 to 3 (i.e., clinician support decreases gradually from cycle 1 to 3). In the original study on which the morphosyntax approach was based, 20–30 opportunities were created for participants to produce target morphemes in each session.

In cycle 1 of the morphosyntax approach, the maximum amount of clinician support is provided in the form of forced choice questions (Fey & Cleave, 1997). This elicitation technique results in the child's imitation of one of two possible choices, both of which contain the target morpheme. In a third-person singular elicited production activity in which a child is commenting on pictures in a book, the clinician may present a forced choice prompt such as, "Tell me what Jenny does with the flower seeds. She *plants* them or she *waters* them?" It is critically important for both choices to contain the target morpheme, even if the clusters are not the same. Clinicians using forced choice are encouraged to emphasize and respond to the child's use of morphemes, even when the child's response may not be correct in terms of semantics or pragmatics. To avoid potential confusion, it is therefore ideal for the clinician to structure the two choices such that either is viable in terms of morphosyntax, semantics, and pragmatics. For example, in the *plants* versus *waters* example just mentioned, both choices contained the target third-person singular morpheme and both also made sense semantically and pragmatically.

In cycle 2 elicited production activities, the child's task becomes more complex as he or she completes a clinician's utterance using a cloze task, which is in the form of a grammatical closure, or fill-in-the-blank format. The clinician creates an opportunity for the child to use the target morpheme by providing the syntactic organization for an obligatory context, pausing, and looking expectantly when the child is expected to supply the target morpheme to complete the sentence. For example, in a cycle 2 craft activity in which the regular past tense morpheme is being targeted, the clinician may refer to the craft project and say to the child, "Look what Jeff did to the frog's eye, he _____." The child's expected response may be, "glued it." If the child does not respond in this format, the examiner may reelicit the form, recast, or provide a direct model.

The task demand of elicited production activities becomes even more complex in cycle 3, in which preparatory sets are used. In a preparatory set, the clinician uses the target morpheme in a sentence that provides a template for the child. The child is then prompted to use the target morpheme in his or her own new utterance within the same context. An example preparatory set prompt follows in the context of a puppet show.

Clinician: The king eats the grapes. The queen eats the watermelon. Now you tell me about the prince.

Child: He eats the apple.

Preparatory sets are more challenging than direct imitation, forced choice, or cloze tasks because they require the child to use a similar grammatical form in a slightly different context that may involve subjects or root words that differ from the clinician's example utterance.

In each of the three cycles, clinicians are encouraged to respond positively to children's correct responses, emphasizing the morpheme target (e.g., "That's right, she *waters* the seeds"). If the child omits or otherwise incorrectly uses a target morpheme, the clinician is encouraged to respond with a simple expansion recast (repetition of the child's utterance but using the correct grammatical form) or with a "growth recast" (Camarata, Nelson, & Camarata, 1994; Nelson, Camarata, Welsh, Butkovsky, & Camarata, 1996), emphasizing the correct adult form in a new complete sentence that expands on the child's original utterance. For example, the clinician may use an expansion recast, "She *waters* them," or a growth recast, "Oh, she *waters* all of the seeds," in response to the child's utterance with an omitted third-person singular form, "She water them."

In some individual cases, it may be necessary to elicit imitations of a target morpheme, although this elicited production format is not provided in the scripts. As suggested by Fey, Long, and Finestack (2003), imitation may be a useful part of an intervention program, particularly in imitation opportunities that involve the use of contrasting grammatical forms. Furthermore, Fey and colleagues suggested that imitation activities may be beneficial for providing practice with segmental aspects of grammatical production that may be particularly challenging for children who have impairments in both morphosyntax and phonology: the population that is the focus of this chapter. Some children may not be responsive to other production requests and may also readily imitate clinician productions and benefit from such practice.

Materials and Equipment Required

Months of Morphemes (Haskill et al., 2001) contains detailed scripts for use during different elicitation activities. These scripts provide examples of the dialogues between clinicians and children and can be used as a framework for implementing activities or structuring additional activities. Book activities for auditory awareness of session targets are included; full references for these weekly children's literature selections are provided. Supplemental theme-related books are also listed with references in the Bibliography. Materials required for all the activities of a session are listed in a box on the first page devoted to that session. These materials are selected from typical school and household items, such as glue, scissors, crayons, and craft sticks. Some activities require that paper or felt art items be assembled prior to or during the session. For these art projects, patterns and stencils are provided in an appendix along with materials needed and directions for assembly. Weekly family letters that are meant to be photocopied and sent home are also provided for each target. These letters clearly list the theme, book, and activities, as well as provide simple examples of the target and a script to model target morphemes. A template is also provided in an appendix for clinicians to use in creating their own letters. Sample planning and data collection forms are provided as well.

ASSESSMENT AND PROGRESS MONITORING TO SUPPORT DECISION MAKING

Perhaps the most informative, time efficient, and functional means for tracking children's progress under this approach involves language sample analysis pre- and postintervention, and/or, following cycles 1, 2, and 3. It may not be necessary to elicit a lengthy language sample; however, clinicians should deliberately plan to create multiple opportunities for the child to produce each of the four target morphemes within the sample context. An example script for target morpheme elicitation is found in Appendix B for this chapter. Following language sample elicitation, percent correct usage of each individual morpheme target may be calculated by dividing the total number of correct productions of each morpheme by the total number of obligatory contexts. Consistent with Brown (1973), mastery is achieved when the child's percent correct usage exceeds 90% in obligatory contexts. An alternative to calculating percent correct usage of individual morphemes is deriving a composite score reflecting overall percent correct usage of the four morpheme targets. Similar to the previously referenced FMC and to the elicited grammar composite from the RWTEGI (Rice & Wexler, 2001), a composite score may be calculated to reflect the child's combined mean accuracy of the four morpheme targets.

For clinicians who choose to document children's progress on a more regular basis, monitoring may be achieved through examination of each session's data. Percent correct use of morpheme targets in elicited production activities may be achieved through a relatively simple process of dividing correct productions by total opportunities for production. The cycles approach used in this intervention operates on a time-based system as opposed to an accuracy-based system.

In addition to considering pre- and posttreatment language sample analysis or individual session data logs, several standardized and criterion-referenced tests, some of which were referenced in the Target Populations section of this chapter, are available to measure morphosyntactic performance (see Table 15.3). Raw score data on such measures may be beneficial to examine individual children's progress, whereas standard or criterion scores may be helpful in gauging relative standing among peers in morphological performance.

A final option for assessing or monitoring children's morpheme progress involves using an informal probe. The clinician may develop a short (i.e., 4 or 5 items) task in which the child independently has opportunities to use the forms. This could be accomplished with the use of a variety of clinician-generated stimuli. For example, the clinician

Table 15.3. Commercially available measures of expressive morphosyntax

Test	Morphosyntax subtests	Age range (years;months)
Bankson Language Test, 2nd Ed. (Bankson, 1990)	Morphological/Syntactic Rules	3;0–6;11
Clinical Evaluation of Language Fundamentals, 4th Ed. (Semel, Wiig, & Secord, 2003)	Recalling Sentences (RS) & Word Structure (WS)	RS: 6+ WS: 6;0–8;0
Clinical Evaluation of Language Fundamentals, Preschool, 2nd Ed. (Wiig, Secord, & Semel, 2004)	RS & WS	3;0–6;11
Comprehensive Assessment of Spoken Language (Carrow-Woolfolk, 1999)	Syntax Construction	3;0–6;0
Rice/Wexler Test of Early Grammatical Impairment (Rice & Wexler, 2001)	Third Person Singular, Past Tense, *BE*, *DO* probes, Elicited Grammar Composite	3;0–6;11
Structured Photographic Expressive Language Test–Preschool, 2nd Ed. (Dawson et al., 2005)	—	3;0–5;11
Test of Language Development–Primary, 4th Ed. (Newcomer & Hammill, 2008)	Sentence Imitation & Morphological Completion	4;0–8;0

could probe regular past tense forms by asking the child to discuss several actions in a book following a prompt such as, "Tell me what happened here." The RWTEGI (Rice & Wexler, 2001) also contains picture stimuli that may be adapted to probe regular and irregular past tense, third-person singular, auxiliary *BE* and *DO*, and copula *BE*.

Progress monitoring procedures may be valuable for determining if the level of clinician support is sufficient to ensure children's success in the approach. Clinicians are encouraged to be flexible in their use of facilitating strategies in assisting children who do not show improvement in one or more morphemes. If focused stimulation, recasting child productions, and the facilitating strategies used for elicited production activities in a particular cycle do not seem to be meeting the child's needs, the clinician is encouraged to increase support as needed. For example, if a child in cycle 3 does not respond to preparatory sets, the clinician may need to revert to a cloze task or forced choice structures to accommodate the child's needs.

CONSIDERATIONS FOR CHILDREN FROM CULTURALLY AND LINGUISTICALLY DIVERSE BACKGROUNDS

A primary consideration when working with children from culturally and linguistically diverse populations within a morphosyntax approach has to do with target morpheme selection. Morphosyntax-specific impairments may be typical in children with language impairments who speak English and other languages such as Swedish (Hakansson & Nettelbladt, 1993) and French (Paradis & Crago, 2000). However, the interaction between speech and morphosyntax varies cross-linguistically, making goal selection a challenging endeavor for clinicians working with English language learners who have speech and language impairments in both their primary and second languages.

The majority of morphosyntax-based studies referenced in the empirical and theoretical basis sections of this chapter included Standard American English speakers. Several of the morphemic forms that may be targeted in the morphosyntax approach may be inappropriate targets for speakers of non–Standard English languages or dialects. For example, in African American English (AAE), several finite morphemes that are common targets for Standard English speakers with language impairment, such as regular past tense, and contractible *BE* forms are nonobligatory, and therefore, may not be appropriate targets (Paul, 2007; Roseberry-McKibbin, 2008). In Spanish-Influenced English, regular past tense and third-person singular markers are not obligatory (Paul, 2007; Roseberry-McKibbin, 2008). In selected Native American dialects, alternatives to Standard English contractions of *TO BE* forms may be permissible. In Asian English dialects, omissions of auxiliary *BE* forms, past tense verbs, and other inflections may occur (Paul, 2007; Roseberry-McKibbin, 2008). Selection of target morphemes may be further complicated by phonotactic rules of various languages and dialects. For example, in AAE, final consonant deletion and final cluster reduction may be dialectically appropriate (though this is true to a lesser extent for bimorphemic grammatical morpheme contexts, such as *kissed* /kɪst/, than it is for monomorphemic forms, such as *mist* /mɪst/) (Stockman, 1996, 2006). Furthermore, finite morphophonemic forms may not always result in clusters, such as in British or Australian English (e.g., /ɪz/ in *pours*). Clearly, if instruction is taking place in Standard English, both morphosyntactic and phonological factors of the child's language or dialect must be considered when selecting specific targets, or when determining if morphosyntactic-based intervention is appropriate for the child.

The types of language activities and facilitating techniques used in the morphosyntax approach may be effective in meeting needs of culturally and linguistically diverse children and are rooted in selected principles of multicultural teaching (Goldstein, 2000). Materials used mirror what typically would be found in an early childhood classroom, making them functional for young English language learners. Numerous visual aides are incorporated throughout the activities and multiple types of interactions in the forms of role playing and narratives are used, as well as the frequent use of scripts. Importantly, literacy is incorporated into each session. Emerging research suggests that focused stimulation, a primary facilitating technique used in the morphosyntax approach, may be effective for selected groups of English language learners (Thordardottir, Ellis Weismer, & Smith, 1997). Because focused stimulation techniques do not require strict child and adult conversational roles, they may be appropriate for use with individuals with diverse conversational styles (Ellis Weismer & Robertson, 2006). Additional research is needed to support the efficacy of various elicited production techniques that may violate cultural models for interaction. For example, using cloze tasks that may involve the child responding to a clinician's expectant look (which may necessitate close proximity and eye contact), may be problematic when interacting with a child from a cultural background in which direct eye contact is not used.

CASE STUDY

The case provided here to demonstrate the benefits of the morphosyntax intervention for both speech and language is a child who participated in the Tyler et al. (2002, 2003) goal attack studies. Renee was referred by her public school SLP for participation in the Tyler et al. (2003) study that compared different configurations of scheduling both speech and language goals. She qualified for the intervention study by meeting the selection criteria of exhibiting both speech and language performance that was less than 1 *SD* below the mean for her age on standardized tests. At the initial assessment she was 57 months of age and received an Auditory Comprehension standard score of 79 on the Preschool Language Scale–3 (Zimmerman, Steiner, & Pond, 2002) and an Expressive Communication standard score of 75. Her MLU was 3.54 from a spontaneous language sample, 2.4 *SD* below the expected mean for her age, and her nonverbal IQ from the Columbia Mental Maturity Scale (Burgemeister, Blum, & Lorge, 1972) was 107. On the BBTOP, her standard scores for the Word Inventory, Consonant Inventory, and Process Inventory were 65, 66, and 66, respectively. Her percent consonants correct (PCC) calculated from the BBTOP and supplementary words was 57. Renee was randomly assigned to receive the block sequence of morphosyntax intervention first, followed by the hybrid speech intervention. Her four language targets were third-person singular, past tense *–ed*, past tense irregular, and copula *is*. Although speech was not targeted in the first block, goals were identified for measurement through the TGC. Speech targets were initial /l/, initial /s, ʃ/, /s/-clusters, final /tʃ/; generalization targets were final /l/, final /s, z/, final /ʃ/, and initial /z/.

Renee participated in the morphosyntax intervention during an individual 30-minute and a group 45-minute session each week for 12 weeks. After the three 4-week cycles of morphosyntax treatment, her MLU had increased from 3.54 to

Table 15.4. Treatment accuracies for speech and language targets, generalization forms, and summary measures

	Pretreatment	Post 12-week morphosyntax intervention	Post 12-week speech intervention
Speech			
Targets (initial /l, s, ʃ/ /s/-clusters, final /tʃ/)	7%	29%	57%
Generalization	7%	62%	100%
PCC	57%	65%	71%
Language			
Third-person singular regular	7%	28%	44%
Past tense –ed	0%	40%	68%
Past tense irregular	44%	74%	78%
Copula to be	24%	52%	47%
Uncontractible auxiliary to be	50%	86%	15%
Contractible auxiliary to be	17%	27%	80%
MLU	3.54	4.29	4.56

Key: MLU, mean length of utterance; PCC, percentage of consonants correct.

4.29, FMC increased from 19% to 44%, PCC increased from 57% to 65%, and TGC increased from 7% to 44%. Specific results for speech targets, language targets, and their generalization targets are displayed in Table 15.4, along with results after the block of speech intervention, at 24 weeks posttreatment. Results show that language targets displayed greater increases in accuracy when they were the focus during the morphosyntax block; however, third-person singular and past tense –ed continued to show improvement during the speech intervention block. There also appeared to be generalization to the auxiliary form. Renee's speech targets also increased in accuracy during the morphosyntax block, when they were not a focus of intervention, particularly those identified for generalization. Speech targets continued to increase in accuracy when they were directly targeted in the speech block. At the posttreatment assessment, PCC had improved to 71% and the TGC to 78%. In language, MLU showed improvement from 4.29 to 4.56 after the speech block, although FMC increased minimally from 44% to 49%. These data reflect rather dramatic qualitative observations of improvement in Renee's speech and language. Her posttreatment language sample was characterized by the ability to produce a narrative for a wordless picture book using considerably longer utterances and speech that was marked more by sound distortions than omissions and substitutions. Gains in both language and phonology were substantial during the morphosyntax block and, even though both areas improved during the following speech intervention block, gains were more circumscribed to speech.

STUDY QUESTIONS

1. How do we plan for and monitor within- and across-domain generalization in different language domains?

2. How does language-based intervention for phonological disorders lead to cross-domain gains in phonology for some children, though it may not directly target phonology?

3. How can a "hybrid" combination of naturalistic and direct elicitation techniques be implemented to target speech and language goals, and how can these be scheduled in a cycle?

4. What supporting rationale can be provided for interactive effects of morphosyntactic intervention on speech?

FUTURE DIRECTIONS

Findings from preliminary investigations of the morphosyntax intervention indicate that speech and morphosyntactic improvement was observed in varying degrees in children with impairments in both domains, particularly when alternating and block sequenced interventions were used. The morphosyntax intervention was observed to facilitate significant gains in both speech and language in a 12-week block, but it is not known what long-term gains would result from a focus on language only. For example, would a 24-week focus on finite morphemes result in greater change for both speech and language than the alternating focus? The answer to this question is related to another area for additional research, that is, to investigate the impact of targeting certain cluster forms on other cluster forms, as well as on change in constituent singletons following morphosyntax intervention. Gierut and Champion (2001) found that children with SSD who were taught three-element clusters increased the size of their singleton inventories by the addition, on average, of five untreated sounds. It is of note that the singletons that were acquired were not necessarily elements of the clusters that were targeted in treatment.

Future investigations of the morphosyntax approach should also include participants from culturally and linguistically diverse backgrounds because there is extremely limited information available about how to best serve English language learners and speakers of nonstandard dialects who have speech and language impairments.

SUGGESTED READINGS

Haskill, A.M., Tyler, A.A., & Tolbert, L. (2001). *Months of morphemes: A theme-based cycles approach.* Eau Claire, WI: Thinking Publications.

Tyler, A.A., Lewis, K.E., Haskill, A.M., & Tolbert, L.C. (2002). Efficacy and cross-domain effects of a morphosyntax and a phonology intervention. *Language, Speech, and Hearing Services in Schools, 33,* 52–66.

Tyler, A.A., Lewis, K.E., Haskill, A.M., & Tolbert, L.C. (2003). Outcomes of different speech and language goal attack strategies. *Journal of Speech, Language, and Hearing Research, 46,* 1077–1095.

REFERENCES

American Speech-Language-Hearing Association. (2004). *Evidence-based practice in communication disorders: An introduction* [Technical Report]. Retrieved August 2, 2009, from http://www.asha.org/docs/html/TR2004-00001.html#sec2.2

Bankson, N.B. (1990). *Bankson Language Test–Second Edition (BLT-2).* Austin, TX: PRO-ED.

Bankson, N.B., & Bernthal, J.E. (1990). *Bankson-Bernthal Test of Phonology (BBTOP).* Chicago: Riverside.

Bedore, L.M., & Leonard, L.B. (1998). Specific language

impairment and grammatical morphology: A discriminant function analysis. *Journal of Speech, Language, and Hearing Research, 41*, 1185–1192.

Bernhardt, B.H., & Stemberger, J.P. (1998). *Handbook of phonological development*. San Diego, CA: Academic Press.

Botting, N., & Conti-Ramsden, G. (2004). Characteristics of children with specific language impairment. In L. Verhoeven & H. van Balkom (Eds.), *Classification of developmental language disorders: Theoretical issues and clinical implications* (pp. 23–38). London: Lawrence Erlbaum Associates.

Brown, R. (1973). *A first language*. Cambridge, MA: Harvard University Press.

Burgemeister, B., Blum, L., & Lorge, I. (1972). *Columbia Mental Maturity Scale*. San Antonio, TX: Pearson PsychCorp.

Camarata, S.M. (1995). A rationale for naturalistic speech intelligibility intervention. In S.F. Warren & J. Reichle (Series Eds.) & M.E. Fey, J. Windsor, & S.F. Warren (Vol. Eds.), *Communication and language intervention series: Vol. 5. Language intervention: Preschool through the elementary years* (pp. 63–84). Baltimore: Paul H. Brookes Publishing Co.

Camarata, S.M., Nelson, K.E., & Camarata, M.N. (1994). Comparison of conversational-recasting and imitative procedures for training grammatical structures in children with specific language impairment. *Journal of Speech and Hearing Research, 37*, 1414–1423.

Carle, E. (1991). *Have you seen my cat?* New York: Simon & Shuster Children's Publishing.

Carrow-Woolfolk, E. (1999). *Comprehensive Assessment of Spoken Language*. Minneapolis, MN: Pearson Assessment.

Chiat, S. (2001). Mapping theories of developmental language impairment: Premises, predictions and evidence. *Language and Cognitive Processes, 16*, 113–142.

Conti-Ramsden, G., & Botting, N. (1999). Classification of children with specific language impairment: Longitudinal considerations. *Journal of Speech, Language, and Hearing Research, 42*, 1195–1204.

Conti-Ramsden, G., Botting, N., & Faragher, B. (2001). Psycholinguistic markers for specific language impairment (SLI). *Journal of Child Psychology and Psychiatry, 42*, 741–748.

Dawson, J., Stout, C., Eyer, J., Tattersall, P., Foukalsrud, J., & Croley, K. (2005). *Structured Photographic Expressive Language Test–Preschool 2*. Dekalb, IL: Janelle.

deVilliers, J., & deVilliers, P. (1973). A cross-sectional study of the development of grammatical morphemes in child speech. *Journal of Psycholinguistic Research, 2*, 267–268.

Dollaghan, C.A. (2004). Taxometric analyses of specific language impairment in 3- and 4-year-old children. *Journal of Speech, Language, and Hearing Research, 47*, 464–475.

Ellis Weismer, S.E., & Robertson, S. (2006). Focused stimulation approach to language intervention. In S.F. Warren & M.E. Fey (Series Eds.) & R.J. McCauley & M.E. Fey (Vol. Eds.), *Communication and language intervention series: Treatment of language disorders in children* (pp. 175–202). Baltimore: Paul H. Brookes Publishing Co.

Fey, M. (1986). *Language intervention with young children*. San Diego: College-Hill Press.

Fey, M.E., & Cleave, P.L. (1997). Two models of grammar facilitation in children with language impairments: Phase 2. *Journal of Speech, Language, and Hearing Research, 40*, 5–19.

Fey, M.E., Cleave, P., Long, S., & Hughes, D. (1993). Two approaches to the facilitation of grammar in children with language impairment: An experimental evaluation. *Journal of Speech and Hearing Research, 36*, 141–157.

Fey, M.E., Long, S.H., & Finestack, L.H. (2003). Ten principles of grammar facilitation for children with specific language impairments. *American Journal of Speech-Language Pathology, 12*, 3–15.

Gierut, J.A., & Champion, A.H. (2001). Syllable onsets II: Three-element clusters in phonological treatment. *Journal of Speech, Language, and Hearing Research, 44*, 886–904.

Girolametto, L., Pearce, P., & Weitzman, E. (1996). Interactive focused stimulation for toddlers with expressive vocabulary delays. *Journal of Speech and Hearing Research, 39*, 1274–1283.

Goffman, R., & Leonard, R. (2000). Growth of language skills in preschool children with specific language impairment: Implications for assessment and intervention. *American Journal of Speech-Language Pathology, 9*, 151–161.

Goldstein, B. (2000). *Cultural and linguistic diversity resource guide for speech-language pathology*. San Diego: Singular Publishing.

Hadley, P.A., & Holt, J.K. (2006). Individual differences in the onset of tense marking: A growth-curve analysis. *Journal of Speech, Language, and Hearing Research, 49*, 984–1000.

Hakansson, G., & Nettelbladt, U. (1993). Developmental sequences in L1 (normal and impaired) and L2 acquisition of Swedish syntax. *International Journal of Applied Linguistics, 3*, 3–29.

Haskill, A.M., & Tyler, A.A. (2007). A comparison of linguistic profiles in subgroups of children with specific language impairment. *American Journal of Speech-Language Pathology, 16*, 209–221.

Haskill, A.M., Tyler, A.A., & Tolbert, L.C. (2001). *Months of morphemes: A theme-based cycles approach*. Eau Claire, WI: Thinking Publications.

Hayiou-Thomas, M.E., Bishop, D.V.M., & Plunkett, K. (2004). Simulating SLI: General cognitive processing stressors can produce a specific linguistic profile. *Journal of Speech, Language, and Hearing Research, 47*, 1347–1362.

Hide, M. (2007). *Treatment effects on cluster development in the speech of 4-year-old children with speech disorder*. Unpublished master's thesis, University of Canterbury, Christchurch, New Zealand.

Hodson, B.W., & Paden, E.P. (1991). *Targeting intelligible speech* (2nd ed.). Austin, TX: PRO-ED.

Hoffman, P.R. (1992). Synergistic development of phonetic skill. *Language, Speech, and Hearing Services in Schools, 23*, 254–260.

Leonard, L.B. (1981). Facilitating linguistic skills in children with specific language impairment. *Applied Psycholinguistics, 2*, 89–118.

Leonard, L.B. (1998). *Children with specific language impairment*. Cambridge, MA: The MIT Press.

Leonard, L.B., Camarata, S.M., Brown, B., & Camarata, M.N. (2004). Tense and agreement in the speech of children with specific language impairment: Patterns of generalization through intervention. *Journal of Speech, Language, and Hearing Research, 47*, 1363–1379.

Leonard, L.B., Camarata, S.M., Pawlowska, M., Brown, B., & Camarata, M.N. (2006). Tense and agreement morphemes in the speech of children with specific language impairment during intervention: Phase 2. *Journal of Speech, Language, and Hearing Research, 49*, 749–770.

Leonard, L.B., Eyer, J.A., Bedore, L.M., & Grela, B.G. (1997). Three accounts of the grammatical morpheme difficulties of English-speaking children with specific language impairment. *Journal of Speech, Language, and Hearing Research, 40*, 741–753.

Leonard, L.B., Schwartz, R.G., Chapman, K., Rowan, L.E., Prelock, P.A., & Terrell, B. (1982). Early lexical acquisition in children with specific language impairment. *Journal of Speech and Hearing Research, 25*, 554–564.

Marchman, V.A., Wulfeck, B., & Ellis Weismer, S.E. (1999). Morphological productivity in children with normal language and SLI: A study of the English past tense. *Journal of Speech, Language, and Hearing Research, 42*, 206–219.

Marshall, C., & van der Lely, H. (2003, July). *Interactions between morphology and phonology in children with Grammatical SLI*. Presentation at the annual Child Phonology Conference, Vancouver, British Columbia, Canada.

Miller, J.F., & Chapman, R.S. (1981). The relation between age and mean length of utterance in morphemes. *Journal of Speech and Hearing Research, 24*, 154–161.

Miller, J., & Chapman, R. (2000). Systematic Analysis of Language Transcripts (Version 6.1) [Computer software]. Madison, WI: Waisman Center.

Nelson, K.E., Camarata, S.M., Welsh, J., Butkovsky, L., & Camarata, M. (1996). Effects of imitative and conversational recasting treatment on the acquisition of grammar in children with specific language impairment and younger language-normal children. *Journal of Speech and Hearing Research, 39*, 850–859.

Newcomer, P., & Hammill, D. (2008). *Test of Language Development–Primary* (4th ed.). Austin, TX: PRO-ED.

Norbury, C.F., Bishop, D.V.M., & Briscoe, J. (2001). Production of English finite verb morphology: A comparison of SLI and mild-moderate hearing impairment. *Journal of Speech, Language, and Hearing Research, 44*, 165–178.

Norris, J.A., & Hoffman, P.R. (1990). Language intervention within naturalistic environments. *Language, Speech, and Hearing Services in Schools, 21*, 72–84.

Norris, J.A., & Hoffman, P.R. (2005). Goals and targets: Facilitating the self-organizing nature of a neuronetwork. In S.F. Warren & M.E. Fey (Series Eds.) & A.G. Kamhi & K.E. Pollock (Vol. Eds.), *Communication and language intervention series: Phonological disorders in children—Clinical decision making in assessment and intervention* (pp. 77–87). Baltimore: Paul H. Brookes Publishing Co.

Paradis, J., & Crago, M. (2000). Tense and temporality: Similarities and differences between language-impaired and second-language children. *Journal of Speech, Language, and Hearing Research, 43*, 834–848.

Paul, R. (2007). *Language disorders from infancy through adolescence: Assessment and intervention* (3rd ed.). St. Louis: Mosby.

Rapin, I., & Allen, D.A. (1983). Developmental language disorders: Nosologic considerations. In U. Kirk (Ed.), *Neuropsychology of language, reading and spelling* (pp. 155–184). New York: Academic Press.

Rice, M.L. (1999). Specific grammatical limitations in children with specific language impairment. In H. Tager-Flusberg (Ed.), *Neurodevelopmental disorders* (pp. 331–359). Cambridge, MA: The MIT Press.

Rice, M.L., & Wexler, K. (1996). Toward tense as a clinical marker of specific language impairment in English-speaking children. *Journal of Speech and Hearing Research, 39*, 1239–1257.

Rice, M.L., & Wexler, K. (2001). *Rice/Wexler Test of Early Grammatical Impairment* (examiner's manual). San Antonio, TX: Pearson Assessment.

Rice, M.L., Wexler, K., & Cleave, P. (1995). Specific language impairment as a period of extended optional infinitive. *Journal of Speech and Hearing Research, 38*, 850–864.

Rice, M., Wexler, K., & Hershberger, S. (1998). Tense over time: The longitudinal course of tense acquisition in children with specific language impairment. *Journal of Speech, Language, and Hearing Research, 41*, 1412–1431.

Roseberry-McKibbin, C. (2008). *Multicultural students with special language needs: Practical strategies for assessment and intervention* (3rd ed.). Oceanside, CA: Academic Communication Associates.

Rvachew, S., Gaines, B.R., Cloutier, G., & Blanchet, N. (2005). Productive morphology skills of children with speech delay. *Journal of Speech-Language Pathology and Audiology, 29*, 83–89.

Semel, E., Wiig, E.H., & Secord, W. (2003). *Comprehensive Evaluation of Language Fundamentals–Fourth Edition (CELF-4)*. San Antonio, TX: Pearson Assessment.

Shriberg, L.D. (2004). *Diagnostic classification of five subtypes of childhood speech sound disorders (SSD) of currently unknown origin*. Paper presented at the

International Association of Logopedics and Phoniatrics, Brisbane, Queensland, Australia.

Stemberger, J.P. (2002). Overtensing and the effect of regularity. *Cognitive Science, 26*(6), 737–756.

Stemberger, J.P. (2003). *Phonology and morphology occur in parallel in child language production.* Paper presented at the 43rd annual meeting of the Psychonomic Society, Kansas City, MO.

Stockman, I. (1996). Phonological development and disorders in African American children. In A. Kamhi, K. Pollock, & J. Harris (Eds.), *Communication development and disorders in African American children: Research, assessment, and intervention* (pp. 117–153). Baltimore: Paul H. Brookes Publishing Co.

Stockman, I.J. (2006). Alveolar bias in the final consonant deletion patterns of African American children. *Language, Speech, and Hearing Services in Schools, 37*, 85–95.

Sweat, L. (2003). *Comparing the effects of morphosyntax and phonology intervention on final consonant clusters in finite morphemes and final consonant inventories.* Unpublished master's thesis, University of Nevada, Reno.

Thordardottir, E.T., Weismer, S.E., & Smith, M.E. (1997). Vocabulary learning in bilingual and monolingual clinical intervention. *Child Language Teaching and Therapy, 13*, 215–227.

Tyler, A.A. (2002). Language-based intervention for phonological disorders. *Seminars in Speech and Language, 23*, 69–81.

Tyler, A.A., Lewis, K.E., Haskill, A.M., & Tolbert, L.C. (2002). Efficacy and cross-domain effects of a morphosyntax and a phonology intervention. *Language, Speech, and Hearing Services in Schools, 33*, 52–66.

Tyler, A.A., Lewis, K.E., Haskill, A.M., & Tolbert, L.C. (2003). Outcomes of different speech and language goal attack strategies. *Journal of Speech, Language, and Hearing Research, 46*, 1077–1095.

Tyler, A.A., & Sandoval, K.T. (1994). Preschoolers with phonological and language disorders: Treating different linguistic domains. *Language, Speech, and Hearing Services in Schools, 25*, 215–234.

van Daal, J., Verhoeven, L., & van Balkom, H. (2004). Subtypes of severe speech and language impairments: Psychometric evidence from 4-year-old children in the Netherlands. *Journal of Speech, Language, and Hearing Research, 47*, 1411–1423.

van der Lely, H. (2004). Evidence for and implications of a domain-specific grammatical deficit. In L. Jenkins (Ed.), *Variation and universals in biolinguistics* (pp. 117–144). Oxford, England: Elsevier.

van der Lely, H. (2005). Domain-specific cognitive systems: Insight from grammatical specific language impairment. *Trends in Cognitive Sciences, 9*, 53–59.

Wiig, E.H., Secord, W., & Semel, E. (2004). *Clinical Evaluation of Language Fundamentals–Preschool 2.* San Antonio, TX: Pearson Assessment.

Willet, H. (2001). *Effects of treatment on finite morphemes in children with specific language impairment.* Unpublished master's thesis, University of Nevada, Reno.

World Health Organization. (2001). *ICF: International classification of function, disability and health.* Geneva: Author.

Zimmerman, I., Steiner, V., & Pond, R. (2002). *Preschool Language Scale–Fourth Edition (PLS-4).* San Antonio, TX: Pearson Assessment.

Appendix 15A Morphosyntax Session Planning Worksheet

Clinician _____

Child(ren) _____

Theme for cycle _____

Level of support for elicited production activities for this cycle:

____ Forced choice   ____ Cloze task   ____ Preparatory set

	Target form	Focused stimulation activities		Elicited production activities		Home practice	Other
		Session 1	Session 2	Session 1	Session 2		
Week 1							
Week 2							
Week 3							
Week 4							

Materials I already have: Materials I need to obtain:

_____   _____

_____   _____

_____   _____

Example language sample context. Playing with a toy house that has moveable windows and doors and accompanying accessories, including pets, family members, furniture, a boat, and a car.

Morpheme	Example Elicitations	
Present progressive *-ing*	Educator:	Look what this dog is doing!
	Child:	<u>Barking</u>!
Preposition *in*	Educator:	I wonder where I should put this cable.
	Child:	<u>In</u> the house.
Preposition *on*	Educator:	I'm going to put the lamp under the table.
	Child:	No! Put it <u>on</u> the table!
Regular plural *-s*	Educator:	Look, this boy has a cat. I wonder if he has any other <u>pets</u>. *[There are two dogs]*
	Child:	He has two <u>dogs</u>.
Irregular past tense	Educator:	*[Unsnap a piece from the house]* Oh no! Look what happened!
	Child:	It <u>broke</u>!
Possessive *'s*	Educator:	I think this s the <u>mommy's</u> bed. *[Present crib/cradle]*
	Child:	No, it's the <u>baby's</u>!
Uncontractable copula *is, am, are, was, were* (main verb)	Educator:	Have the daddy ask the girl if she<u>'s</u> hungry.
	Child:	<u>Are</u> you hungry?
Articles *a, an, the*	Educator:	I want a bed for my room. I wonder what you would like
	Child:	<u>A</u> chair.
Regular past *-ed*	Educator:	*[Make a figurine jump on the bed]* The sister got in trouble. Daddy wants to know what she did.
	Child:	She <u>jumped</u> on her bed!
Regular third person *-s*	Educator:	This boy <u>runs</u> down the stairs. Look whathis sister does!
	Child:	She <u>eats</u> her dinner
Irregular third person *has, says, does*	Educator:	This dog <u>has</u> a pretty yellow house. Tell me about the kitty.
	Child:	She <u>has</u> a blue pillow.
Uncontractable auxiliary *is, am, are, was, were*	Educator:	Have mommy ask daddy what <u>he's</u> doing.
	Child:	What <u>are</u> you doing?
Contractable copula *is, am, are, was, were* (main verb)	Educator:	Look, he<u>'s</u> the daddy. Tell me about this guy.
	Child:	He<u>'s</u> the baby.
Contractable auxiliary *is, am, are, was, were* (helping verb)	Educator:	I think she<u>'s</u> running really fast!
	Child:	No, she<u>'s</u> going slow!

Naturalistic Intervention for Speech Intelligibility and Speech Accuracy

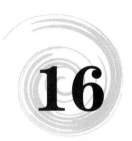

16

Stephen M. Camarata

ABSTRACT

Although speech intervention has long been focused on remediating individual speech sounds (phonemes), children with severe speech sound disorders (SSD) may have low levels of overall intelligibility. Such cases may require intervention that focuses at least initially on increasing overall intelligibility rather than improving individual phoneme production. This chapter presents an overview of naturalistic intervention for speech intelligibility in children with severe SSD. In addition, it presents the application of these techniques to improving speech accuracy for individual phonemes. A theoretical overview, key elements, and empirical support for the model are included. This chapter also discusses adaptations of the techniques for preschool children with severe SSD, children with Down syndrome (DS), and children with autism or autism spectrum disorder.

INTRODUCTION

The primary focus of intervention for children with SSD has long been on production of individual phonemes (e.g., Swift, 1918). A goal of this training is to improve articulation for specific phonemes that are produced inaccurately in the hopes that this will lead to improved overall intelligibility. This approach to treating SSD on a sound-by-sound basis is a fundamental foundation for intervention. Although there are a number of different approaches to the task of teaching phoneme production, most rely on imitation and drill as a primary intervention method (Bernthal, Bankson, & Flipsen, 2009). There can be no doubt that this approach is useful in many cases. However, with the expansion of services to preschoolers and toddlers and the ongoing need of populations with severe SSD, such as individuals with cerebral palsy and DS, it is important to consider overall speech intelligibility as well as speech accuracy for individual phonemes. The purpose of this chapter is to provide a rationale and preliminary evidence for a naturalistic, whole-word approach to intervention for these populations. It is important to bear in mind from the outset that speech accuracy, that is, production of individual phonemes, is not the same construct as intelligibility. And, although intuition would suggest that drilling individual speech sounds will ultimately generalize to words and thus incidentally improve intelligibility, there are currently no data to support this hypothesis in children with severe SSD.

In addition, Shriberg and Kwiatkowski (1982) reported only a modest correlation between percentage of consonants correct (PCC) and intelligibility in children with severe SSD, suggesting that intelligibility and accuracy are not identical constructs in these children. Therefore, it will be worthwhile to consider speech intelligibility and speech accuracy as related but individual constructs.

The Separate but Related Concepts of Speech Intelligibility and Speech Accuracy

From the outset, it is important to differentiate among sound-by-sound production, phoneme-by-phoneme production, and overall intelligibility. Many clinicians may use these terms interchangeably, but speech intelligibility and speech accuracy are actually two separate but empirically related constructs. In this chapter, *intelligibility* is defined as the degree to which the listener understands what the speaker says when the target is uncertain. This definition is a different construct than traditional psychoacoustic studies of intelligibility that are focused on the acoustic parameters that contribute incrementally to the identification of a known target (e.g., Weismer, Kent, Hodge, & Martin, 1988) or that are focused on the incremental contribution of percentage of consonants correct (PCC, a measure of speech accuracy) and prosody to an overall intelligibility index (Shriberg, Austin, Lewis, McSweeny, & Wilson, 1997). Without minimizing the importance of these perspectives on intelligibility, the view of speech intelligibility herein is motivated by an interest in the notion that if adults or peers do not understand the intended message, then the children with severe SSD will receive less frequent speech- and language-facilitating input. Therefore, this chapter is focused on intelligibility within every day conversational contexts.

In contrast, *speech accuracy* refers to the accuracy with which individual speech sounds (phonemes) are produced. Several empirical studies have shown that naturalistic speech intervention has an effect on conversational intelligibility in preschool children with speech and language impairment (Yoder et al., 2005), children with autism (e.g., Koegel, Camarata, Koegel, Ben-Tal, & Smith, 1998), and children with DS (Camarata, Yoder, & Camarata, 2006).

Moreover, a two-tiered approach to intervention in SSD is proposed herein. The first tier includes increasing overall intelligibility so that the number of intended messages are comprehensible to listeners even if the accuracy of individual phonemes remains less than perfect. After the child has reached the point in development in which the majority of messages are understood, the second tier of intervention would focus on improving the accuracy of individual phonemes. Therefore, this chapter includes a rationale and description of naturalistic intervention for improving overall speech intelligibility, which is the proposed first-tier goal. In addition, naturalistic intervention can also be utilized to improve the second tier: speech accuracy.

TARGET POPULATIONS

The target population for naturalistic speech intelligibility and naturalistic speech accuracy intervention is broadly defined as any individual with severe SSD. That is, this approach can be applied to any individual in order to improve overall intelligibility and for increasing the accuracy of individual speech sounds. One could argue that the approach is particularly well-suited to populations that do not readily respond to imitation and drill techniques for improving speech accuracy and most specifically for those with low levels of intelligibility. For example, many children with autism will not imitate speech sounds on demand. Similarly, articulation training techniques that require a preschooler to sit and imitate individual speech sounds may be quite challenging for any child at that age level because didactic instruction often requires that a child sit still and listen for extended time periods in addition to imitating on demand. These skills are not often acquired until school age in many typically developing children. And, children with disabilities are often even less cooperative than typically developing toddlers and preschoolers so that didactic methods may be impractical.

Similarly, if the primary focus of the intervention is to improve intelligibility, then an approach specifically designed to improve the overall ability to generate intelligible messages may be preferable to a sound-by-sound approach for these children. Therefore, in cases in which low intelligibility is a primary characteristic, a speech intelligibility approach that targets improved approximations of the words may be more useful than adopting a speech accuracy approach. Thus, populations such as toddlers and preschoolers with severe SSD resulting in low intelligibility and children with DS who often have low intelligibility would be logical candidates for naturalistic speech intelligibility training.

Primary Populations

Early intervention for SSD is being extended to very young children, so a question arises as to whether preschool children and toddlers will benefit from the kinds of direct instruction that can be useful in older children. For example, Bleile (2003) has described traditional articulation training that has long been used with school-age children. Specifically, this approach includes teaching a child tongue placement for individual phonemes and systematically practicing correct production for each misarticulated sound in isolation. After proficiency is achieved, production moves to the syllable level for additional practice and then to the word level and finally in phrases and sentences.

Interestingly, direct drill techniques evidently are now being applied to toddlers younger than the age of 2 and to preschoolers. But, these latter groups may not have sufficient comprehension or metalinguistic competence to benefit from this imitation and drill approach for individual phonemes. Indeed, most toddlers and preschoolers, including those who are typically developing, do not ordinarily spend time seated at a table engaged in direct instruction. Rather, learning for these populations is often within the context of play. Although some children, even very young children, will sit and imitate, many do not. As Haley, Camarata, and Nelson (1994) reported, for children who do not readily sit at a table and imitate, much of the therapy time may be spent on simply getting compliance. Perhaps worse, for these children, the therapy may become aversive. Therefore, one could argue that a naturalistic, responsive intervention that includes play activities is more likely to match the developmental skills of most toddlers and preschoolers.

Secondary Populations

Children with Down Syndrome

Children with DS (Trisomy 21) often display a number of developmental delays in physical, social, and mental development (Miller, Leddy, & Leavitt, 1999). One major developmental challenge in DS is generating comprehensible and accurate speech within the context of a dynamic, maturing system, which is mediated by input from immature, dynamic speech processing ability. It is perhaps not surprising that the development of speech often goes awry in children with DS, with SSD being a relatively high-incidence condition (Stoel-Gammon, 2001) in these children, typically persisting through adolescence into adulthood, and is often a life-long disabling characteristic of DS. Indeed, virtually all individuals with DS have reduced speech accuracy, and various samples of speech intelligibility indicate that few reach typical levels of speech intelligibility (see Buckley, 1993; Chapman, 1997; Leddy, 1999). In particular, children with DS tend to have impairments that ultimately impact speech intelligibility, which is often below that expected for mental age, language comprehension level, and even vocabulary level (Miller, 1999; Miller, Leddy, & Leavitt, 1999).

During uncontrolled naturalistic conversation, the most frequent language-use context of children with DS, the intended message is often at least partly unknown. Therefore, the extent to which an unfamiliar listener can understand what the child says (i.e., speech intelligibility) is a socially important outcome and should be examined using a socially valid measurement context. Many believe that the speech-intelligibility problems of children with DS are due largely to motor constraints (Miller et al., 1999) and unique vocal tract structures (Leddy, 1999). Not surprisingly, children with DS are routinely enrolled in speech-language pathology therapy with the goal of improving speech accuracy, and ultimately, speech intelligibility. It should be noted that an implicit assumption is that treating speech accuracy will automatically generalize to speech intelligibility, but this doesn't necessarily occur in severe SSD (see Hanson, Yorkston, & Beukelman, 2004). Therefore, one important goal of treatment should be to examine speech intelligibility *and* speech accuracy to ensure that the child's message is identifiable to the listener.

Speech accuracy is the extent to which the child accurately produces the speech sounds in the words he or she uses as compared with the adult version of the words. For example, a child with DS saying [ba wo] for *ball roll* may be *intelligible* because the adult understood the meaning of the child's production, but the *speech accuracy* of the production, if measured in PCC, would be 25% ([b] is correct whereas the final [l] in *ball* and *roll* are incorrect and initial [ɹ] is incorrect in *roll*, so the PCC would be $1 / 4 \times 100 = 25\%$). This example illustrates that assessments of speech accuracy will not necessarily tell us about a child's speech intelligibility. Thus, it is not surprising that studies of children with speech problems indicate that the measures of speech accuracy (e.g., PCC) explain only an average of 16% of the percentage word attempts for which words are transcribed, even though both measures are derived from the same speech samples (Shriberg & Kwiatkowski, 1982; Shriberg, Kwiatkowski, Best, Hengst, & Terselic-Weber, 1986). It is reasonable to consider speech intelligibility as a socially important outcome because this ultimately measures the extent to which listeners can understand what the child says. The distinction between speech accuracy and speech intelligibility is used in the adult disability literature (e.g., dysarthria secondary to stroke; Hanson et al., 2004) and appears to be a useful distinction in children with DS and other children with severe SSD as well.

Children with Autism

Although most children with autism do not display significant SSD, many do. In autism, it has long been known that reinforcing communicative attempts using natural rewards is a very effective method for teaching language (Koegel, O'Dell, & Koegel, 1987). From a social developmental perspective, SSD is unfortunate in this population because children with autism have a reduced or even absent motivation for social communication so that the overall level of communicative attempts is severely restricted. In those children with a speech disorder, when a communicative attempt does occur, reduced speech accuracy and reduced intelligibility make it less likely that the adult will be able to respond to the child's message. In addition, because social interactions in autism are often fragile from the standpoint of maintaining social engagement, it is important for clinician responses to be immediately contingent and as consistent as possible. Therefore, SSD can be particularly devastating in autism because limited opportunities for interaction are available and these become even further disrupted when the child's intended message is unintelligible.

Coupled with this is the pressing need to provide interactions that are rewarding or reinforcing for the child with autism. As with preschoolers and toddlers, many children with autism indirectly or directly resist imitation and drill. This is particularly problematic with traditional articulation training because the meaning of the individual speech sounds is divorced from functional communication. In addition, children with autism are often literal and may lack the fluid reasoning needed to generalize from production of individual speech sounds to words and conversational use. Taken together, this suggests that children with autism are candidates for naturalistic speech intervention for speech intelligibility and for speech accuracy.

Tertiary Population

Children who Stutter

Children who stutter may also be good candidates for naturalistic intervention on speech accuracy. Unlike children with DS or children with autism, the problem is not a lack of intelligibility or a lack of motivation. Rather, Louko, Edwards, and Conture (1990) have suggested that imitation and drill on speech sounds or phonemes increases stuttering. That is, asking a child who stutters to repeatedly imitate individual speech sounds evidently may exacerbate the stuttering rather than improve articulation. Therefore, a more indirect intervention approach must be employed. So, in cases of remediating SSD in children who stutter, naturalistic intervention should be the first option in order to ensure that the intervention for speech disorder does not make the stuttering worse. However, there does not appear to be substantial empirical support for this position other than the case reports by Rather et al.

ASSESSMENT METHODS FOR DETERMINING INTERVENTION RELEVANCE

Traditional methods of assessment for SSD can be utilized in naturalistic intervention. The procedures for selection of targets for speech accuracy are identical to those used in other intervention approaches. Individual phonemes can be selected from articulation testing on standardized instruments such as the Goldman-Fristoe Test of Articulation (Goldman & Fristoe, 2000) or the Arizona Articulation Proficiency Scale (Fudala, 2001). As always, the speech evaluation should include measures of spontaneous production.

With regard to speech accuracy training using naturalistic speech intervention, the choice of targets to evaluate is at the discretion of the clinician. For example, if one wishes to employ the multiple contrast intervention sequence described by Williams (2005), these targets can be trained using naturalistic speech intervention procedures. That is, a naturalistic approach for improving speech accuracy can be applied to *any* goal within *any* theoretical framework for target selection. In this regard, naturalistic speech intervention is an alternative to imitation and drill methods for teaching individual phonemes. And like imitation and drill methods, it can be applied to a wide variety of individual goals. Stated simply, there is no a priori limitation on the targets that can be planned for and emphasized within naturalistic speech accuracy training.

For intelligibility training using naturalistic speech intervention, the assessment should focus on the overall intelligibility of the child's lexical productions. As described previously, overall intelligibility can be a goal that is not necessarily an automatic outcome for speech accuracy training. Because of this, if the focus of training is improving intelligibility, the assessment also must include systematic evaluation of what percentage of the child's productions are readily understood. In practice, the parent can often be used as a "gold standard" because they often can interpret a higher proportion of their child's utterances than outside listeners. Therefore, it may be useful to generate estimates of overall intelligibility for a parent and for an unfamiliar listener. At this time there is no universally accepted method for calculating intelligibility. Many children appear to be attempting words and use predictable suprasegmental envelopes so that the reliability of identifying word attempts or utterance attempts can be reasonably high. In some populations with severe disabilities, however, it can be difficult to distinguish nonmeaningful from meaningful speech. In such cases, using a parent report form such as MacArthur-Bates Communicative Development Inventories (CDIs; Fenson et al., 1994) may be helpful.

It should be noted that the intelligibility score derived from the Arizona Articulation Proficiency Scale (Fudala, 2001) is computed from speech accuracy on the test and thus is an indirect, and perhaps inaccurate, measure of functional intelligibility. It cannot be overemphasized that speech accuracy and speech intelligibility are not interchangeable parameters. It is possible to be highly intelligible while also having poor speech accuracy. Conversely, improving speech accuracy on individual phonemes will not automatically generalize to functional conversational contexts nor to functional intelligibility. Because of this, both aspects of speech production should be assessed. It is also worth noting that vowel errors are particularly disruptive to intelligibility as are phonological processes that affect word-initial consonants such as 1) assimilations that impact the initial consonant and 2) the phonological process of initial consonant deletion. For example, assume four children attempt the word *big* /bɪg/. Furthermore, assume child A produces this word as [bɪ], child B says [bog], child C says [ɪg], and child D says [gɪg]. With the exception of child B, whose production included correct articulation for both consonants (/b/ and /g/, PCC = 100%), all productions have the same PCC of 50%. But the probability that child A's production [bɪ] will be understood as *big* is much higher than child B's production [bog], child C's production [ɪg], or child D's production [gɪg]. In the case of A and B, a lower PCC has a higher probability of being intelligible. Indeed, even 100% PCC doesn't guarantee intelligibility. These examples illustrate why it is important to consider accuracy and intelligibility as separate measures of SSD during assessment and to evaluate each parameter in children with severe SSD.

THEORETICAL BASIS

Dominant Theoretical Rationale for the Intervention Approach

For speech intervention to affect intelligibility in a conversational context, the treatment will probably need to address more than just speech accuracy. Although is it clear that speech accuracy is an important contributor, Weston and Shriberg (1992) also found that syllable structure and grammatical role contributed to conversational speech production accuracy. For preschool children with both SSD and expressive language impairment, it may be particularly important that the speech intervention method address speech within the everyday conversational contexts, which model what the child ultimately will need for intelligible communicative attempts. In addition, phonological recast is hypothesized to provide phonological information at moments when the child is most likely to process the information (Camarata, 1993, 1995, 2003). The temporal proximity and semantic overlap of phonological knowledge recasts may make it easier for the child with unintelligible speech to unconsciously compare their utterance to the adult's recast, thus noticing the phoneme, pitch, stress, rate, and intonation differences between the two. Similarly, unlike phoneme-by-phoneme presentation, the words are produced with natural coarticulation. Many instances of the heightened awareness of these differences increase the probability that the child will develop more accurate representations of the way words are intelligibly produced. The result can be a closer approximation to the adult model even if the child is not yet capable of producing the individual speech sounds with complete accuracy. It should be emphasized that this new information is not just in the form of accurate phonemic categories and thus speech sounds. Proper coarticulation, pitch, stress, rate, and intonation are also modeled in a lexical context. The fact that phonological recasts retain the child's meaning is thought to increase the probability that the new information will be integrated into the child's existing semantic knowledge base (Nelson, 1989). Integration of the new information with existing semantic knowledge may increase the probability that newly learned information will become accessible during naturally occurring conversations (Camarata, 1993).

Given that children with severe SSD can be difficult to understand, one could question whether clinicians will be able to understand the children's utterances frequently enough to deliver accurate phonological recasts. Several factors within the controlled treatment setting facilitate interpretation of the child's speech, thereby enabling appropriate phonological recasts. First, the materials are selected to elicit the word productions in known contexts. This provides a more limited set of items than would be encountered in more open-ended contexts and increases the opportunities for words to be recast. In addition, the actual items are designed to reduce the probability of eliciting homophonous (and thus ambiguous) forms. Finally, the clinicians can be trained to both interpret speech of children with SSD and become increasingly familiar with an individual child's typical topics and phonological substitutions.

Importance of Speech Intelligibility in Development

Children who frequently and clearly communicate are likely to elicit adult input that, in turn, facilitates speech and language development (Camarata & Yoder, 2002; Yoder & Warren, 1993). As children develop linguistic communication, clear communication is usually in the form of comprehensible speech. In contrast, children with poor speech intelligibility will not recruit facilitating input as often as their peers. But developing comprehensible speech is a difficult task. The child must coordinate perceptual input from adults and older peers and generate output using an immature and changing articulatory system (Kent, 1993; Ruark & Moore, 1997). Rather than being an isolated construct, speech intelligibility may be an integral part of a child's ability to access key developmental responses from the environment via transactions (Camarata, 1995; see Figure 16.1). To

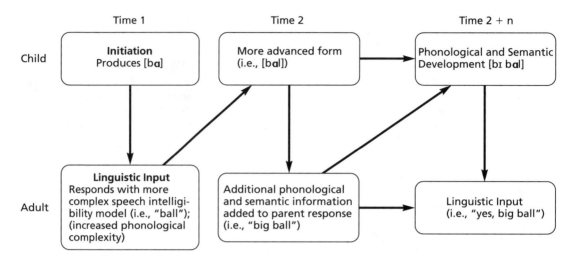

Figure 16.1. Transactional learning of speech.

trigger this transaction, the child's attempt to produce the word *ball* must be comprehensible to the adult so that a teaching model can be elicited.

In this example, the child's immature production of *ball* is responded to immediately with a correct whole-word phonological recast. The response does not include elicitation (e.g., "say ball"), nor does it include a request to imitate the individual phoneme that was incorrect (e.g., "say [l]"). Also, the adult recast does not shift to additional semantic, syntactic, or morphological forms unless the child's production is phonologically accurate and fully intelligible. It is clear that natural language acquisition does not include systematic imitation or drill on individual phonemes or phoneme clusters outside of the word context presented in the form of adult recast. The underlying theory for using naturalistic intervention is that paralleling typical developmental learning processes can be an efficient method for teaching preschoolers speech and language skills when the frequency at saliency of such models is increased over what is occurring in the ambient environment.

Theoretical Considerations for Children with Down Syndrome

The theoretical basis for applying this technique to children with DS includes the rationale presented for preschool children broadly with some important additional considerations. Children with DS often have oral architecture and oral motor skills that differ from their typically developing peers (Kumin, 2001). The overwhelming majority of these individuals continue to have unintelligible or partially intelligible speech even as adults. Because of this, one could argue that it is vitally important to *first* target overall intelligibility as the *primary* goal of speech intervention. Moreover, it is an open question as to whether extensive imitation and drill on production of phonemes in isolation will ultimately improve overall intelligibility in this population. Because of this, the focus of intervention should shift to compensatory productions that allow higher intelligibility when speech accuracy cannot be attained within the constraints of the speech production mechanisms. Thus, there appears to be a strong theoretical rationale for applying naturalistic speech intelligibility training to individuals with DS.

Theoretical Considerations for Children with Autism

Traditional imitation and drill-based articulation training for SSD may not be effective for children with autism due to the nature of this disability (see Koegel et al., 1998). Communication training for children with autism can include discrete trials for word production, but this training is directly contingent on teaching the meaning of the productions to the child with autism by using external rewards. If the words are dissected into phonemic parts, this focus on meaning is no longer a part of the paradigm and may inadvertently result in decontextualized "savant" phoneme production skills that do not readily generalize to word production. For example, if a child with autism is taught to request *cookie* by a clinician holding up a cookie and giving a cookie to the child when they imitate the word *cookie*, the success of this paradigm relies in part on the child's ability to generate a recognizable proximity to the target word. The ecological validity of the paradigm would shift when a cookie is presented while the clinician presents the phoneme /k/ rather than a word model. The child may know the text version of /k/ and associate phoneme production in isolation with this letter rather than a food item symbolically labeled *cookie*. In addition, repeated versions of *cookie* may be confusing when the various individual phonemes are presented; that is, when the object is referenced for /k/ and then /ʊ/ then /k/ for the medial consonant and finally /i/ for the final vowel. In keeping with functional communication (Koegel & Koegel, 2006), the interactions during intervention should have direct application to the naturalistic environments wherein the target behaviors are used. It is difficult to imagine that teaching a child with autism to identify objects based on individual phonemes will readily generalize to functional communication contexts.

Nonspeech Oral Motor Exercises

Many speech-language pathologists (SLPs) recommend and implement nonspeech oral motor exercises in children with severe SSD. Because speech includes motor coordination of the articulators, this approach has a logical appeal, and there are a number of programs that directly or indirectly focus on oral motor exercises in the hopes that these will improve speech articulation. However, despite this intuitive appeal and evidently widespread application, several reviews have indicated that these techniques do not meet minimal standards for evidence-based practice nor do they conform to discoveries in speech motor theory (Powell, 2008; Ruscello, 2008). This point is raised because an explicit argument for applying naturalistic speech intelligibility intervention is the direct functional utility of the approach: The child is taught using words and communicative context, which is the desired outcome. If one's a priori perspective is that oral motor competence must be attained as a prerequisite to improving speech accuracy or speech intelligibility, however, this could be used as a theoretical argument against a naturalistic approach. Yet, there is no evidence that systematically teaching children to move their tongues, pucker their lips, blow bubbles, increase oral awareness, or any other nonspeech oral motor exercise is a necessary requisite skill for speech production or that these exercises contribute to improved speech accuracy or speech intelligibility.

Stated simply, if oral motor competence is viewed as a necessary prerequisite skill for improving speech, a clinician would be skeptical that a naturalistic approach could be successfully applied to children with severe SSD. Therefore, it is important from the outset to objectively point out that it is clear that oral motor exercises are not necessarily prerequisite skills for improving speech accuracy or for improving speech intelligibility (see Ruscello, 2007). From a developmental perspective it is clear that even typically developing toddlers and preschoolers display immature and in some cases poorly developed oral motor coordination, yet they make systematic progress toward improved speech intelligibility and speech accuracy without the benefit of systematic oral motor training. In addition, there is a lack of evidence that such approaches actually result in improved speech accuracy or speech intelligibility above and beyond what one would simply expect due to maturation or to intervention that focuses directly on speech accuracy or speech intelligibility. Thus, the belief that oral motor exercises are an essential prerequisite to improving speech intelligibility or speech accuracy may not be valid counterargument to naturalistic, word-level intervention for severe speech disorder.

Levels of Consequences Being Addressed

The World Health Organization (WHO, 2007) uses the International Classification of Functioning, Disability and Health for Children and Youth (ICF-CY) to quantify levels of the consequences of disruptions in an individual's ability to function in society. In terms of speech errors, the oral facial differences in DS would fall under the definition of impairment both in terms of Body Structure and in terms of Body Function. The functional consequence of these impairments is a disruption in speech development so that both speech accuracy and speech intelligibility are classified under Body Function. Finally, the social consequence of the speech accuracy and speech intelligibility disabilities is limitation in the ability to effectively communicate with others in social situations (Activities and Participation). For other children with speech disorder, the consequences of impairment may be more limited in scope. For example, producing a distorted /ɹ/ (Shriberg, 1980) can be an error in speech accuracy that persists into adulthood. This can be viewed as an impairment in function within the WHO classification system. However, aside from perhaps some limited functional consequences (e.g., listeners mistakenly viewing the speaker as having a foreign accent), this impairment may not have an impact on Activities and Participation.

Employing naturalistic intervention for speech intelligibility or for speech accuracy will directly address the consequences of SSD as they appear in the WHO classification system. Speech intelligibility disorders will inevitably fall into impairment of Body Functions, Activities, and Participation under this system because reductions in intelligibility arising from SSD will have both functional and social consequences. From a broad perspective, SSD would appear to be relatively secondary or even tertiary in development. And, in the case of relatively minor impairments that do not adversely affect function, this perspective is valid. Severe disruptions in speech intelligibility, however, can in fact be a significant condition. For example, individuals with cancer who undergo partial removal of the glossus can experience severe disruptions in both Activities and Participation when this results in impaired speech intelligibility and associated limitations in their functional ability and social and vocational situations. Clearly, disruptions in speech accuracy and more broadly in speech intelligibility could have adverse consequences for a child attempting to successfully communicate in the community, and applying naturalistic speech intelligibility and speech accuracy intervention is consistent with the WHO framework and guidelines.

Target Areas of Intervention

The intervention targets speech production and morphophonology. It can also be adapted to morphosyntax, syntax, and semantic targets and can be used to model social interaction. The approach does not directly target perception, literacy, or cognition.

EMPIRICAL BASIS

It is important to bear in mind that applying naturalistic intervention to the problem of speech intelligibility disorders is a relatively recent (e.g., Camarata, Yoder, & Camarata, 2006) theoretical framework and thus has relatively limited direct experimental tests of the model. With regard to naturalistic intervention for speech accuracy, there is more evidence available. This section describes the empirical basis for naturalistic intervention and includes summaries of studies supporting the application of naturalistic intervention for speech accuracy and studies examining naturalistic intervention for speech intelligibility, including studies of DS and autism. Taken together, although the need for additional randomized clinical trials remains, there is a solid basis of empirical support for the approach.

Summary of Levels of Evidence

The first level of support for this model is found in the studies of naturalistic language intervention, particularly studies focusing on acquisition of morphological or, more precisely, morphophonological targets (see Table 16.1). For example, Camarata, Nelson, and Camarata (1994) presented evidence using a quasi-experiment indicating that generalized use of morphophonological targets was associated with naturalistic intervention that primarily included recasts of the targets. For example, if a child said "three book," the clinician model included the plural form that had been deleted: "three books." Notice that this is incidentally modeling the final phonological cluster needed to indicate plural in English (/ks/). All bound morphemes in English take the form of final affixes, and derivational morphemes also appear as phonological alterations to the root word (e.g., *un*real). Because of this, studies such as that conducted by Camarata, Nelson, and Camarata can be viewed as being akin to phase 1 clinical trials for naturalistic speech intervention. Similarly, a series of studies by Leonard and his colleagues (2004, 2006, 2008) focused on teaching third person singular and regular past tense to children with specific language impairment (SLI). The regular past tense is produced with a phonological form of word-final /t/, /d/, and /əd/ (as in *milked, banned, and hunted*). Regular third person singular is expressed phonologically as word final /s/, /z/, and /əz/ (as in *walks, runs, and seizes*). Leonard et al. (2004, 2006, 2008) reported that both of these forms were acquired at significantly higher rates than control (untreated) forms in a randomized clinical trial. The intervention in the Leonard et al. studies included recast procedures; however, other intervention techniques such as modeling within short stories were also delivered to the children so that this is not a specific experimental test of naturalistic recast intervention. It can be viewed as providing partial indirect evidence in support of naturalistic speech intervention. Additional studies of naturalistic intervention targeting morphological structures are reviewed in Camarata and Nelson (2006) and broadly suggest that morphological recasts can be associated with growth in application of the phonological manifes-

Table 16.1. Levels of evidence for studies of treatment efficacy for naturalistic intervention for speech intelligibility and speech accuracy

Level	Description	References
Ia	Meta-analysis of > 1 randomized controlled trial	—
Ib	Randomized controlled study	Camarata et al. (1994); Leonard et al. (2004, 2006, 2008); Yoder et al. (2005)
IIa	Controlled study without randomization	Crosbie et al., 2005; Tyler et al. 2003
IIb	Quasi-experimental study	—
III	Nonexperimental studies, i.e., correlational and case studies	Camarata (1993); Camarata et al. (2006); Crosbie et al. (2006); Koegel et al. (1998); Smith & Camarata (1999); Weiner (1981)
IV	Expert committee report, consensus conference, clinical experience of respected authorities	—

Adapted from the Scottish Intercollegiate Guidelines Network (http://www.sign.ac.uk).

tations of these forms. Tyler, Lewis, Haskill, and Tolbert (2003) provided support for the notion that studies of morphological acquisition can also be viewed through the lens of phonological goals. In a randomized trial, they reported cross modality effects of phonological training on morphology and of morphological training on phonology. The study included 20 preschool children randomly assigned to phonological, morphological, and control conditions. The implication here is that morphological intervention focusing on bound morphemes can indirectly also have an impact on phonology.

The second source of evidence for applying naturalistic speech intervention can be seen in studies that directly evaluate the effectiveness of this approach for improving speech accuracy. For example, Camarata (1993) provided single-subject data indicating that naturalistic intervention that included phonological recasts was effective for increasing accurate production of misarticulated phonemes. Similarly, Camarata (2002) reported on a randomized clinical trial including 48 preschool children with SSD that included random assignment to control, phonological recast, or imitation and drill conditions. The results indicated that both imitation and drill and naturalistic speech intervention focusing on speech accuracy were effective in increasing generalized spontaneous use of phonemic targets as compared with production for a wait-list control condition. These results are depicted in Figure 16.2.

An additional source of indirect evidence to support recast comes from using lexical or whole-word approaches to phonological intervention. For example, Ingram and Ingram (2001) described a whole-word approach to phonological analysis and intervention and presented details for applying this framework in a case study involving a preschool child (age 4;2) with SSD. Bellon-Harn, Hoffman, and Harn (2004) reported that storybook reading that included cloze and whole-word contrast procedures was associated with improvements in SSD in three kindergarten children. Similarly, Crosbie, Holm, and Dodd (2005) compared "phonological contrast therapy" to "core vocabulary therapy" in 18 children with SSD who were from 4 to 6 years of age. The core vocabulary therapy included targeting whole-word production, which is also a key feature of phonological recast intervention. Crosbie et al. reported that the whole-word, core vocabulary approach was associated with greater change in children with inconsistent speech as compared with phonological contrast intervention, suggesting that whole-word approaches can stabilize speech accuracy. Dodd and her colleagues have reported that core vocabulary intervention can be effective for improving SSD in a series of studies (e.g., Crosbie, Pine, Holm, &

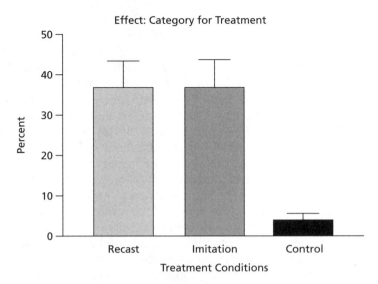

Figure 16.2. Results of a randomized clinical trial comparing phonemic recast and imitation approaches to speech treatment.

Dodd, 2006). The results of these studies also provide indirect support for the notion that phonological intervention can be based on lexical units in addition to the more traditional phonemic approaches that focus on individual speech sounds. Phonological recasts include lexical modeling of incorrectly produced words, integrating phonemic and lexical levels as is seen in natural speech production. That is, phonemic units are systematically included in the lexical modeling of correct phonemic production.

The third and strongest level of evidence includes a clinical trial designed to directly examine the effects of naturalistic speech intelligibility using recast intervention for children with severe speech and language impairments. In this study, Yoder, Camarata, and Gardner (2005) randomly assigned 52 preschoolers (*mean* chronological age in years = 3.65; *SD* = 0.71) with severe speech disorder (i.e., *mean* Time 1 percentile ranking on the Arizona Articulation Proficiency Scale [AAPS-R] = 2%, *SD* = 2), severely impaired expressive language (i.e., *mean* Time 1 percentile ranking on the Preschool Language Scale = 4%, *SD* = 3), typical nonverbal intelligence (*mean* Leiter = 104, *SD* = 15), and normal hearing to a recast treatment or to a control group. Recasts were associated with growth in speech intelligibility 8 months after the treatment ended in the children who began treatment with raw scores on the AAPS-R (a standardized measure of speech accuracy) less than 45 (Cohen's *d* for affected subgroup = .75; *p* = .03). In contrast, those children scoring higher than 45 on the AAPS-R at pretreatment did not demonstrate long-term speech intelligibility gains as compared with the control group. Intelligibility was measured on a conversational language sample with a staff member that was not the child's clinician and was blind as to group assignment. The results indicated that 1) recasts can affect long-term conversational intelligibility and 2) initial speech accuracy predicts response to recast treatment on intelligibility in preschoolers with severe speech and language impairment, with a higher number of speech errors being associated with significant increases in speech intelligibility at 8-month's follow-up.

Evidence for application to SSD in children with DS was provided by Camarata, Yoder, and Camarata (2006), who completed a multiple baseline single-subject design to investigate the effects of naturalistic speech intelligibility intervention in six participants with DS. They reported that naturalistic speech intervention was associated with significant growth in intelligibility in four of the six participants and that clear intervention effects could be confidently observed in two of these four children with DS who displayed growth during intervention. The study also included naturalistic language intervention for these children and reported significant growth for mean length of utterance (MLU) in five of the six children and clear intervention effects in two of these participants.

Evidence for application to children with autism was provided by Koegel et al. (1998), who compared imitation and drill to naturalistic speech intelligibility intervention in five children with autism. They reported significantly higher functional use of the targeted forms in generalized conversational context only in the naturalistic speech intelligibility condition. Similarly, Smith and Camarata (1999) employed a multiple baseline single-subject design to examine the impact of naturalistic speech intelligibility intervention in three children with autism and reported intervention effects in all three participants. The studies suggest that naturalistic speech intelligibility training can be effective in children with autism who also display significant speech disorder. The Koegel et al. study indicated that the naturalistic approach was associated with greater generalized improvements in speech intelligibility than the imitation and drill approach for children with autism.

PRACTICAL REQUIREMENTS

The practical requirements for a naturalistic approach to speech intelligibility intervention are relatively straightforward. Because this is a child-led approach (Fey, 1984), the clinician should set up the environment in such a manner that the child will naturally attempt to communicate. Although this means that the clinician should follow the child's lead, it also means that the clinician should practice environmental arrangement so that the child will be invited to attempt communication. In toddlers and preschoolers with severe SSD who are otherwise unimpaired, this can be relatively straightforward because they will often initiate at a relatively high rate despite an overall lack of intelligibility. Many children with DS also are relatively communicative so that the practical requirements are relatively straightforward. In contrast, children with autism by definition have a reduced motivation to engage in social interaction. Worse, those with severe SSD may be even less likely to attempt communication unless the environmental arrangement is strongly supportive. Therefore, for practical requirements, include toys and activities that are of interest to the individual child and result in communicative attempts as a platform for the word-level speech intelligibility recasts. This can be done in a traditional therapy setting, in a classroom, or in the home. Responders can include teachers (as in Smith & Camarata, 1999); clinicians (as in Yoder et al., 2006); and conceivably parents, older siblings, and in some cases, peers. From a practical standpoint, the only requirement for responding is following the child's attempt with a reasonably plausible guess as to the intended message, which then serves as a platform for the word-level model response from the communication partner.

Nature of Sessions

As noted previously, sessions can be completed in clinic, home, and classroom settings. Because the basic procedures follow naturalistic intervention principles, this treatment approach can be employed in any setting where spontaneous communication attempts occur. Moreover, speech intelligibility recasts are ubiquitous in typical interactions between parents and children. However, for children with severe SSD (e.g., children with DS), low intelligibility may make it difficult for untrained listeners to accurately respond to the child's initiations. Therefore, sessions should include systematic data collection by a trained listener such as an SLP so that teachers and/or parents can be oriented to the approach. Although some teachers and parents can be taught to listen for individual speech sounds and to respond with a phonemic recast required in naturalistic speech accuracy intervention, this can be difficult for some untrained listeners. However, it is often relatively simple to train relatively naïve listeners to respond using whole-word speech intelligibility responses. Therefore, at this time it is more likely that naturalistic intervention for speech intelligibility can be readily applied in different settings whereas naturalistic intervention for speech accuracy may be more limited to traditional one-to-one interaction in clinical settings. The exception to this is when parents and/or teachers can be taught to listen for individual target phonemes and respond appropriately using speech accuracy phonemic recast.

The actual sessions should include directed play that is responsive to the child's choice of activities and designed to facilitate initiations. Some children with relatively unintelligible speech may first be reluctant to attempt productions because they have experienced low success in their communication. However, by selecting engaging toys that are naturally interactive, children can usually be induced to attempt interpretable initiations. For example, toys that are engaging and that are sophisticated enough that they require the parent, teacher, or clinician to assist in the play are ideal for this approach. Such items include uninflated balloons (requiring assistance to inflate), spinning tops, engaging construction toys that the child cannot assemble without assistance, and games that inherently include back-and-forth communication. Even simple activities such as blowing bubbles wherein the child can request that the clinician, parent, or teacher blow the bubbles can be useful. As noted earlier, the suggestion here is not that the child be taught to blow bubbles in order to improve oral motor coordination in the hopes of improving speech production. Rather, the goal of these activities is to induce a child to attempt communication that can then be used as a platform for speech intelligibility recasts. The procedures for naturalistic speech accuracy and phonemic recast intervention are described by Camarata (1993, 1995, 1996). Essentially, the setting is the same as described previously with the exception that the environment is loaded to induce the child to attempt words that include the phonemic targets. So for example, if a target is [l], toys included in the setting will contain this target sound: Legos, lions, balloons, toy balls, and leopards are all possibilities. As with speech intelligibility training, the goal is to induce the child to attempt target words that contain /l/ so that the clinician can deliver the whole-word recast of the target phoneme.

Personnel

An advantage of the naturalistic speech intelligibility intervention is that it can readily be taught to untrained personnel, including teachers, parents, teachers' aides, and other family members, because no specific knowledge or experience with phonetic transcription for identifying individual errors is required to implement the intervention. Of course, a trained SLP is required to coordinate and monitor the implementation of the intervention. But, this approach can be readily transferred to other individuals in the child's life who frequently interact with him or her. Such a model is in keeping with the recommendations of McLeod and Bleile (2004) that intervention for SSD be extended to a child's functional environment in addition to traditional clinical settings.

Naturalistic intervention focusing on speech accuracy using phonemic recast requires a higher level of training for implementation. Some parents and teachers can be taught to quickly recognize errors in target phonemes and to deliver phonemic recast for individual sounds. This can be quite difficult if not impossible for some parents and teachers, however. Thus, the personnel needs for naturalistic speech accuracy intervention include fairly extensive direct involvement by a skilled SLP. If the approach is applied to more complex systems such as contrast therapy, which requires online monitoring of a number of diverse phoneme targets, then the skill level of the personnel implementing the intervention must be even higher and is likely beyond the capabilities of most parents or teachers. Therefore, the setting and personnel for these more complex phonological approaches using naturalistic phonemic recast is likely limited to traditional clinical settings with an SLP.

Dosage

There are no empirical studies addressing dosage. The literature includes primarily two or three weekly sessions conducted for 30 minutes to 1 hour in duration. Including parents in the program could increase the dose to daily sessions, or whenever naturally occurring opportunities for recast arise.

KEY COMPONENTS

The key components for naturalistic speech intelligibility intervention include a child initiation and an appropriate response from the adult. The materials and settings are quite flexible as long as these facilitate and support the child's initiations. When a child is unintelligible, a key component can be a relatively close set of materials or toys so that the clinician or parent has a reasonable idea of the meaning of the child's initiations. For speech accuracy, this approach requires that the child attempt the targeted phonemes so a key component of the approach is to include materials that will induce the child to attempt the phonemes the clinician is attempting to remediate. Traditional materials such as articulation cards depicting individual words containing phonemes can be used as long as a child will spontaneously name these pictures. That is, some children will readily name pictures whereas others require real objects and more engaging activities to induce communicative attempts. Note that imitative prompting and drill activities are not key components for this approach. Rather, a foundational component is that the child produces spontaneous word attempts followed by an adult recast that models correct production at the word level.

Nature of Goals

In naturalistic speech intelligibility training, goals are related to increases in functional intelligibility rather than improving articulation for individual phonemes. That is, goals are akin to those employed in improving speech intelligibility in children with severe hearing loss. Stated simply, the goal is to have the children more closely approximate the whole-word structure of the adult version so that even when a word is produced with phonemic errors it can be understood by the listener. This level of goal is broader than typically employed in speech intervention. However, it may be an important step toward achieving improved communication and incidentally provide access to the myriad of teaching and learning opportunities that are available in the ambient environment (Hart & Risley, 1995) but are missed or disrupted due to unintelligible child initiations. After a child's productions have become largely intelligible, then the focus of intervention can reasonably shift to increasing speech accuracy. Moreover, the approach is different than the traditional notion that unintelligible speech requires oral motor exercises and/or direct instruction on individual phonemes as a foundational step in training.

If naturalistic intervention procedures are applied to speech accuracy, then phonemic recasts can be delivered for any set of goals that are typically employed in speech intervention. For example, a traditional sound-by-sound approach can be used. That is, individual phonemes can be targeted using word-level phonological recast. However, the approach is not limited to a sound-by-sound approach. Phonological processes, phoneme splits, and specific contrasts can also be targeted. So for example, if the phonological process of liquid simplification (Shriberg & Kwiatkowski, 1988) is targeted, words that include /l/ and /ɹ/ are presented. These can also be presented along with similar words that the child is likely to produce in a homophonous fashion (see Weiner, 1981). Similarly, words that include specific targeted phonemic contrasts (as in Williams, 2005) can be presented. The actual targets can be selected to address essentially any phonemic goal or phonological model the clinician wishes to target.

Goal Attack Strategies

The primary goal attack strategy is simultaneous presentation of accuracy and intelligibility information delivered in a functional context. However, because the approach is readily adapted to speech accuracy goals and because the clinician has control of the materials used to induce initiations, sequential or cyclical attack strategies can be employed. That is, materials can be selected to focus on sequential target presentation or cyclical presentation. There is no a priori prohibition on using the approach to attack goals in the manner a clinician judges to be best suited to the individual.

Description of Activities

As with goal attack strategies, there is considerable latitude on the activities that can be used to deliver phonological recast intervention. The primary need is for activities that facilitate child initiations. These can include watching videos, playing with real objects, playing games, looking at cards from an articulation stimulus deck, reading books, and spontaneous conversation. The activities should induce the child to interact with the clinician.

Materials and Equipment Required

No special materials or equipment are required. Rather, the clinician should select materials that are of interest to the child and facilitate spontaneous, authentic functional interaction. Materials should be selected that support child initiations.

ASSESSMENT AND PROGRESS
MONITORING TO SUPPORT DECISION MAKING

In accord with best practice guidelines and evidence-based practice, it is essential that the effectiveness of the intervention be assessed and that progress be monitored. The evidence supporting naturalistic speech intelligibility training and naturalistic speech accuracy training clearly indicates that some children will not make significant progress using these approaches. Indeed, it is becoming increasingly clear that no single approach will be effective in all children with severe SSD. Therefore, it is crucial for the clinician to monitor the child's progress during and following intervention. Before treatment, a thorough speech evaluation is required and should include standardized testing and a spontaneous conversational speech sample. For speech intelligibility, an estimate of the child's overall intelligibility during the spontaneous sample is needed. Subsequent monitoring should be completed using similar materials and techniques so that any changes in speech intelligibility are not attributable to simply changing the context in which the sample is gathered. In addition, teachers and parents should be enlisted as external monitors of progress. Although they may not be sufficiently skilled to provide precise percent intelligibility data, parents and teachers can provide feedback on whether the child's successful communicative attempts are more frequent, less frequent, or unchanged. However, if teachers or parents are enlisted as intervention partners, the clinician should be aware that this may induce bias in their monitoring. This should not preclude getting feedback from these sources, but does suggest that the monitoring should include objective sources as well.

For speech accuracy, a comprehensive speech diagnostic session is also required in pretreatment. Depending on the goal attack strategies to be employed, this may also include a very detailed phonological analysis of the error patterns so that key phonemes can be selected. This approach lends itself to multiple baseline single-subject design if multiple targets are selected for treatment. Individual goals, if relatively independent, can be presented at different points during intervention to generate multiple baselines, which are then quite useful for monitoring progress. This approach was used in Camarata (1993). Moreover, speech accuracy can be systematically monitored using probe word lists relatively frequently. Constructing such a list may require a time investment prior to initiating intervention, but after this has been completed, collecting data to monitor progress on the targeted sounds and the expected patterns of generalization can be completed relatively efficiently. It is recommended that progress monitoring be completed not only in the clinical setting but also in the home and in the classroom to ensure that progress is generalized across settings and across communication partners.

CONSIDERATIONS FOR CHILDREN FROM
CULTURALLY AND LINGUISTICALLY DIVERSE BACKGROUNDS

It is well known that there are speech differences in linguistically diverse contexts. For example, f/th and d/th are common substitutions in African American English (AAE; Stockman, 2008) and should not be considered targets for remediation when using naturalistic speech accuracy intervention. Similarly, any phonological forms and/or pronunciation patterns from culturally or linguistically diverse groups that are typical for the group should not be viewed through the lens of SSD. Because naturalistic speech intervention has been developed in light of typical interactions between parents and children across cultures, other than the prohibition against selecting targets that are not evidence of SSD in a population, the approach can readily be applied to many different culturally and linguistically diverse individuals. Moreover, an advantage of using naturalistic speech intervention is that it is readily adaptable to a variety of settings and goals, including those that are appropriate in culturally and linguistically diverse populations.

Studies of naturalistic intervention have included individuals from culturally and linguistically diverse backgrounds, and the techniques are readily adaptable to speech intelligibility and/or speech accuracy goals in any group. Because the intervention is child-led such that the child has an active role in selecting materials and activities that form the basis of the intervention, the approach is flexible. In addition, because teachers and parents can easily be included in naturalistic speech intelligibility intervention, individuals from the child's cultural and linguistic background can be incorporated into the intervention. Indeed, the clinician may find that the parents and teachers are excellent source of ideas for materials and activities that engage the child. Rhymes, stories, books, photographs, and games from the ambient home and school environment should form the basis of the intervention and can be a direct link to the child's cultural and linguistic background.

CASE STUDIES

The case studies illustrating naturalistic speech intelligibility intervention are adapted from the data presented in Camarata, Yoder, and Camarata (2006), which included six children with DS and low intelligibility. The focus of this case presentation will include a child that demonstrated an intervention effect for naturalistic speech intelligibility training. In addition, a child demonstrating growth but not a clear intervention effect and a child who did not demonstrate growth (or, obviously, an intervention effect) are presented. These latter children are included to provide a model of how assessment and progress monitoring can be used to make clinical judgments on the effectiveness of the approach.

The three children in these cases were diagnosed with DS based on the results of physician report. Within the broad range of medical conditions evident in DS, the participants were in good health and had any major medical complications (e.g., heart defects) treated prior to enrollment in the speech treatment. In addition, the participants all had a negative history for cleft palate and passed an audiometric screening. The age range of these children was 4;3 to 7;4. The revised Leiter International Performance Scale (Roid & Miller, 1997) was administered to all participants. This is a standardized measure of nonverbal cognitive abilities that yields standard scores with a mean of 100 and a standard deviation of 15. The mean Leiter-R Score was 66.5 with a standard deviation of 5.0 for these participants, indicating that all three cases were below the normative average in terms of cognitive level.

The participants also demonstrated a mean standard score on the grammatical morphology subtest of the Test of Auditory Comprehension of Language, Third Edition (TACL-3, Carrow-Woolfolk, 2001) of 63.0 with a standard deviation of 10.5. In addition, the MLU was 1.38 with a standard deviation of .41, so all had some intelligible speech that could be coded for MLU. Percentage of utterances that were comprehensible was derived from baseline and intervention phase language samples. The actual percentage of communication units understood in a continuous speech sample were computed in the spontaneous samples (e.g., percentage of utterance attempts glossed) and may be among the most face-valid ways to quantify speech intelligibility (see Kwiatkowski & Shriberg, 1993). It was measured in a frequent speaking context for children with DS. Because such contexts are relatively uncontrolled, changes and treatment effects on this variable are arguably a conservative estimate. Initial speech-comprehensibility level was a mean of 46.56% with a standard deviation of 12.83, so less than half of the utterances were intelligible during spontaneous speech in baseline.

The children were enrolled in hour-long twice-weekly naturalistic speech intelligibility intervention sessions. These were conducted in a speech clinic with a certified SLP using child-led activities and broad speech intelligibility recast procedures. Spontaneous samples were collected weekly and plotted using traditional single-subject design procedures within a multiple baseline design. Note that stringent guidelines were employed to ensure a treatment effect was reliably observed. Intervention effect is defined as a clear increase following a stable baseline and minimal overlap between baseline and intervention phases. An intervention effect was seen in the data for child 3 ("SN") in Figure 16.3, whose data included a stable baseline, growth from baseline through intervention, and few overlapping points within baseline and intervention phases.

Growth that was not clear evidence of an intervention effect was defined as an increase in intelligibility from baseline to intervention, but because of an increasing trend in baseline and/or substantial overlap among data points, it is unclear whether the growth is attributable to intervention. An example of this is seen in child 1 ("GD") in Figure 16.3, whose data include an increasing baseline trend and substantial overlap across baseline and intervention phases. Finally, child 2 ("MEM") is an example of questionable or no growth during intervention. As seen in Figure 16.3, this child's intelligibility remained rather flat across baseline and intervention so that no substantial progress was observed during treatment.

STUDY QUESTIONS

1. What are the key elements of naturalistic speech intelligibility intervention?

2. How is this different than naturalistic speech intervention that focuses on speech accuracy?

3. Who are likely candidates for speech intelligibility intervention?

4. What is the difference between speech accuracy and speech intelligibility?

5. What adaptations to speech intervention are needed when treating children with autism who have severe SSD?

FUTURE DIRECTIONS

One may wonder why the case presentations included a child whose growth in speech intelligibility may or may not be attributable to the intervention (child one) and another

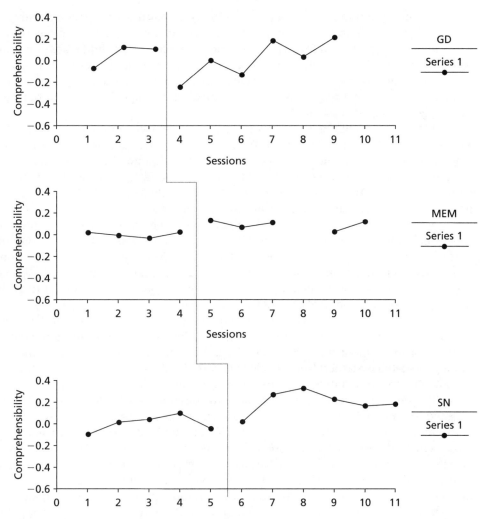

Figure 16.3. Results of multiple baseline evaluation of naturalistic speech intelligibility intervention in three cases of children with Down syndrome. *Key:* GD, child 1; MEM, child 2; SN, child 3.

who evidently did not improve while in treatment (child two) in addition to the case in which the treatment was evidently successful. This was done because it reflects the reality of treating children with severe SSD: No one treatment approach will always be success-ful. And, although a child may improve, it may not be clear this was due to the interven-tion. An important future direction for research will be to determine which pretreatment child characteristics are predictors of later success in different interventions. For ex-ample, Yoder, Camarata, Camarata, and Williams (2006) reported that auditory process-ing efficiency as measured using event-related potentials predicted comprehension of grammatical morphemes in children with DS. That is, a passive listening task that used electroencephalography to measure the listener's ability to detect phonemic differences in stop consonants was useful for predicting comprehension of morphophonemic units. This raises the question of whether overall auditory processing efficiency will predict a child's ability to detect differences in his or her productions as compared with the adult response during naturalistic speech intelligibility or naturalistic speech accuracy intervention. This kind of pretreatment ability may predict a child's potential response to different kinds of intervention for speech disorder. For example, a child whose auditory processing efficiency is relatively high may be able to more readily process the elements in recast intervention (see Nelson, 1989), whereas a child with relatively poor auditory processing efficiency may require more direct training on the differences in their productions as compared with the adult targets.

It should be emphasized that this is not to suggest that auditory processing training such as used in Fast ForWard (Scientific Learning Corporation, 1998) or Earobics (2000) is being recommended. These types of metalinguistic training have been shown to be no more effective than other more naturalistic and functional approaches to language intervention (see Camarata, 2008; Cohen et al., 2005; and Gillam et al., 2008). Thus, as with oral motor exercises, speech discrimination training is not viewed as a prerequisite skill for improving speech, and this approach is not being advocated herein. Rather, auditory processing efficiency is viewed in a similar light as degree of hearing loss as a potential predictor for SSD and response to speech intervention. Moreover, a future direction in research will be to determine whether individual talk characteristics predict response to intervention so that the clinician will have more detailed information as to which approaches are best suited to SSD in individual cases.

Because this is a relatively new approach to the problem of improving intelligibility in children with severe SSD, future directions include completing additional clinical trials in order to augment the current empirical basis for this approach. This includes extending the database to additional trials with preschoolers with severe SSD, children with DS, and children with autism who also display severe SSD. The question of whether naturalistic speech intervention is preferable to imitation and drill in stuttering remains untested to date and would also be an important future direction for research. Finally, many children with severe SSD also display significant language disorders including morphological skills. An intriguing direction for future research will be the integration of speech and language goals using naturalistic intervention procedures. Yoder et al. (2005) have taken the first step in this direction, and one can imagine that a real strength of the approach will be developing integrated intervention that highlights each child's individual speech and/or language goals as developmentally appropriate. After all, typically developing children learn both speech and language simultaneously within a naturalistic context with little or no direct instruction on metalinguistic aspects of morphology, syntax, or phonology so that one wonders whether intervention approaches can mimic the procedures parents employ while interacting with their children while extracting those features that are most facilitative of a child with disabilities' development.

SUGGESTED READINGS

Camarata, S. (1993). The application of naturalistic conversation training to speech production in children with speech disabilities. *Journal of Applied Behavior Analysis, 26,* 173–182.

Camarata, S., & Yoder, P. (2002). Language transactions during development and intervention: Theoretical implications for developmental neuroscience. *International Journal of Developmental Neuroscience, 20*(3–5), 459–465.

Camarata, S., Yoder, P., & Camarata, M. (2006). Simultaneous treatment of grammatical and speech-comprehensibility deficits in children with Down syndrome. *Down Syndrome Research and Practice, 11,* 9–17.

Yoder, P., Camarata, S., & Gardner, E. (2005). Treatment effects on speech intelligibility and length of utterance in children with specific language and intelligibility impairments. *Journal of Early Intervention, 28,* 34–49.

REFERENCES

Bellon-Harn, M., Hoffman, P., & Harn, W. (2004). Use of cloze and contrast word procedures in repeated storybook reading: Targeting multiple domains. *Journal of Communication Disorders, 37*, 53–75.

Bernthal, J.E., Bankson, N.W., & Flipsen, Jr., P. (2009). *Articulation and phonological disorders: Speech sound disorders in children.* (6th ed.). Boston: Pearson Education.

Bleile, K. (2003). *Manual of articulation and phonological disorders.* San Diego: Plural Publishing.

Buckley, S.J. (1993). Developing the speech and language skills of teenagers with Down's syndrome. *Down Syndrome: Research and Practice, 1*, 63–71.

Buckley, S. (2007). Shaping speech. *Down Syndrome: Research and Practice, 12*, 15.

Camarata, S. (1993). The application of naturalistic conversation training to speech production in children with speech disabilities. *Journal of Applied Behavior Analysis, 26*, 173–182.

Camarata, S. (1995). A rationale for naturalistic speech intelligibility intervention. In S.F. Warren & J. Reichle (Series Eds.) & M.E. Fey, J. Windsor, & S.F. Warren (Vol. Eds.), *Communication and language intervention series: Vol. 5. Language intervention: Preschool through the elementary years* (pp. 63–84). Baltimore: Paul H. Brookes Publishing Co.

Camarata, S. (1996). On the importance of integrating naturalistic language, social intervention, and speech-intelligibility training. In L. Koegel, R. Koegel, & G. Dunlap (Eds.), *Positive behavior support: Including people with difficult behavior in the community* (pp. 333–351). Baltimore: Paul H. Brookes Publishing Co.

Camarata, S. (2002). *Treating speech disorders in preschool children.* Paper presented at the Disabilities Conference, The Johns Hopkins University, Baltimore.

Camarata, S. (2003). Assessment of language and language disorders. In M. Wolraich (Ed.), *Disorders of development and learning* (3rd ed., pp. 49–60). Hamilton, Ontario, Canada: B.C. Decker.

Camarata, S. (2008). Fast ForWord does not significantly improve language skills in children with language disorders. *Evidence-Based Communication Assessment and Intervention, 2*, 96–98.

Camarata, S.M., & Nelson, K.E. (2006). Conversational recast intervention with preschool and older children. In S.F. Warren & M.E. Fey (Series Eds.) & R.J. McCauley & M.E. Fey (Vol. Eds.), *Communication and language intervention series: Treatment of language disorders in children* (pp. 237–264). Baltimore: Paul H. Brookes Publishing Co.

Camarata, S., Nelson, K.E., & Camarata, M. (1994). Comparison of conversational-recasting and imitative procedures for training grammatical structures in children with specific language impairment. *Journal of Speech and Hearing Research, 37*, 1414–1423.

Camarata, S., & Yoder, P. (2002). Language transactions during development and intervention: Theoretical implications for developmental neuroscience. *International Journal of Developmental Neuroscience, 20*, 459–467.

Camarata, S., Yoder, P., & Camarata, M. (2006). Simultaneous treatment of grammatical and speech–comprehensibility deficits in children with Down syndrome. *Down Syndrome Research and Practice, 11*, 9–17.

Carrow-Woolfolk, E. (2001). *Test of Auditory Comprehension of Language–Third Edition.* Austin, TX: PRO-ED.

Chapman, R. (1997). Language development in children and adolescents with Down syndrome. *Mental Retardation and Developmental Disabilities Research Reviews, 3*, 307–312.

Chapman, R. (2006). Language learning in Down syndrome: The speech and language profile compared to adolescents with cognitive impairment of unknown origin. *Down Syndrome: Research and Practice, 10*, 61–66.

Cohen, W., Hodson, A., O'Hare, A., Boyle, J., Durrani, T., McCartney, E., et al. (2005). Effects of computer-based intervention through acoustically modified speech (Fast ForWord) in severe mixed receptive-expressive language impairment: Outcomes from a randomized controlled trial. *Journal of Speech, Language, and Hearing Research, 48*, 715–729.

Crosbie, S., Holm, A., & Dodd, B. (2005). Intervention for children with severe speech disorder: A comparison of two approaches. *International Journal of Language and Communication Disorders, 40*, 467–491.

Crosbie, S., Pine, C., Holm, A., & Dodd, B. (2006). Treating Jarrod: A core vocabulary approach. *Advances in Speech-Language Pathology, 8*, 316–321.

Earobics. (2000). *Earobics* [Computer software]. Boston: Houghton Mifflin Harcourt Learning Technology.

Fenson, L., Dale, P., Reznick, J.S., Bates, E., Thal, D., Pethick, S., et al. (1994). Variability in early communicative development. *Monographs of the Society for Research in Child Development, 59*(5), i–185.

Fey, M. (1984). *Language intervention.* San Diego: College-Hill.

Fudala, J. (2001). *Arizona Articulation Proficiency Scale–Third Edition.* Los Angeles: Western Psychological Services.

Gillam, R., Frome Loeb, D., Hoffman, L., Bohman, T., Champlin, C., Thibodeau, L., et al. (2008). The efficacy of Fast ForWord language intervention in school-age children with language impairment: A randomized controlled trial. *Journal of Speech, Language, and Hearing Research, 51*, 97–119.

Goldman, R., & Fristoe, M. (2000). *The Goldman-Fristoe Test of Articulation–Second Edition.* Circle Pines, MN: American Guidance Service.

Haley, K., Camarata, S., & Nelson, K. (1994). Social valence in children with specific language impairment during imitation-based and conversation-based language intervention. *Journal of Speech and Hearing Research, 37*, 378–388.

Hanson, E., Yorkston, K., & Beukelman, D. (2004). Speech supplementation techniques for dysarthria: A systematic review. *Journal of Medical Speech-Language Pathology, 12*, 9–29.

Hart, B., & Risley, T.R. (1995). *Meaningful differences in the everyday experience of young American children.* Baltimore: Paul H. Brookes Publishing Co.

Ingram, D., & Ingram. K. (2001). A whole-word approach to phonological analysis and intervention. *Language, Speech, and Hearing Services in Schools, 32*, 271–283.

Kent, R. (1993). Speech-intelligibility and communication competence in children. In S.F. Warren & J. Reichle (Series Eds.) & A.P. Kaiser & D. Gray (Vol. Eds.), *Communication and language intervention series: Vol. 2. Enhancing children's communication: Research foundations for early language intervention* (pp. 223–242). Baltimore: Paul H. Brookes Publishing Co.

Koegel, R., Camarata, S., Koegel, L., Ben-Tal, A., & Smith, A. (1998). Increasing speech intelligibility in children with autism. *Journal of Autism and Developmental Disorders, 28*(3), 243–251.

Koegel, R.L., & Koegel, L.K. (2006). *Pivotal response treatments for autism: Communication, social, and academic development.* Baltimore: Paul H. Brookes Publishing Co.

Koegel, R., O'Dell, M., & Koegel, L. (1987). A natural language teaching paradigm for nonverbal autistic children. *Journal of Autism and Developmental Disorders, 17*, 187–200.

Kumin, L. (2001). Speech intelligibility in individuals with Down syndrome: A framework for targeting specific factors for assessment and treatment. *Down Syndrome Quarterly, 6*, 1–8.

Kwiatkowski, J., & Shriberg, L. (1993). Speech normalization in developmental phonological disorders: A retrospective study of capability-focus theory. *Language, Speech, and Hearing Services in Schools, 24*(1), 10–18.

Leddy, M. (1999). The biological bases of speech in people with Down syndrome. In J.F. Miller, M. Leddy, & L.E. Leavitt (Eds.), *Improving the communication of people with Down syndrome* (pp. 61–80). Baltimore: Paul H. Brookes Publishing Co.

Leonard, L., Camarata, S., Brown, B., & Camarata, M. (2004). Tense and agreement in the speech of children with specific language impairment: Patterns of generalization through intervention. *Journal of Speech, Language, and Hearing Research, 47*, 1363–1379.

Leonard, L., Camarata, S., Brown, B., & Camarata, M. (2008). The acquisition of tense and agreement in the speech of children with specific language impairment: Patterns of generalization through intervention. *Journal of Speech, Language, and Hearing Research, 51*, 120–125.

Leonard, L., Camarata, S., Pawlowska, M., Brown, B., & Camarata, M. (2006). Tense and agreement morphemes in the speech of children with specific language impairment during intervention: Phase II. *Journal of Speech, Language, and Hearing Research, 49*, 749–770.

Louko, L., Edwards, M.L., & Conture, E. (1990). Phonological characteristics of young stutterers and their normally fluent peers: Preliminary observations. *Journal of Fluency Disorders, 15*, 191–210.

McLeod, S., & Bleile, K. (2004). The ICF: A framework for setting goals for children with speech impairment. *Child Language Teaching and Therapy, 20*, 199–219.

Miller, J.F. (1999). Profiles of language development in children with Down syndrome. In J.F. Miller, M. Leddy, & L.A. Leavitt (Eds.), *Improving the communication of people with Down syndrome* (pp. 11–40). Baltimore: Paul H. Brookes Publishing Co.

Miller, J.F., Leddy, M. & Leavitt, L.A. (1999). *Improving the communication of people with Down syndrome.* Baltimore: Paul H. Brookes Publishing Co.

Nelson, K.E. (1987). Some observations from the perspective of the rare event cognitive comparison theory of language acquisition. In K.E. Nelson (Ed.), *Children's language* (Vol. 6, pp. 289–331). Mahwah, NJ: Lawrence Erlbaum Associates.

Nelson, K.E. (1989). Strategies for first language teaching. In M. Rice & R. Schiefelbusch (Eds.), *The teachability of language* (pp. 263–310). Baltimore: Paul H. Brookes Publishing Co.

Powell, T. (2008). The use of nonspeech oral motor treatments for developmental speech sound production disorders: Interventions and interactions. *Language, Speech, and Hearing Services in Schools, 39*, 374–379.

Roid, G.H., & Miller, L.J. (1997). *The Leiter International Performance Scale–Revised.* Los Angeles: Western Psychological Services.

Ruark, J., & Moore, C. (1997). Coordination of lip muscle activity by 2-year-old children during speech and nonspeech tasks. *Journal of Speech and Hearing Research, 40*, 1373–1385.

Ruscello, D. (2007). *Treating articulation and phonological disorders in children.* St. Louis: Mosby.

Ruscello, D. (2008). Nonspeech oral motor treatment issues related to children with developmental speech sound disorders. *Language, Speech, and Hearing Services in Schools, 39*, 380–391.

Scientific Learning Corporation. (1998). *Fast ForWord Language* [Computer software]. Berkeley, CA: Author.

Shriberg, L. (1980). An intervention procedure for children with persistent /r/ errors. *Language, Speech, and Hearing Services in Schools, 11*, 102–110.

Shriberg, L.D., Austin, D., Lewis, B., McSweeny, J., & Wilson, D. (1997). The percentage of consonants correct (PCC) metric: Extensions and reliability data. *Journal of Speech, Language, and Hearing Research, 40*(4), 708–722.

Shriberg, L.D., & Kwiatkowski, J. (1982). Phonological disorders III: A procedure for assessing severity of involvement. *Journal of Speech and Hearing Disorders, 47*, 256–270.

Shriberg, L., & Kwiatkowski, J. (1988). *Natural process analysis.* Baltimore: University Park Press.

Shriberg, L.D., Kwiatkowski, J., Best, S., Hengst, J., & Terselic-Weber, B. (1986). Characteristics of children with phonologic disorders of unknown origin. *Journal of Speech and Hearing Disorders, 51*(2), 140–161.

Smith, A., & Camarata, S. (1999). Using teacher-implemented instruction to increase language intelligibility of children with autism. *Journal of Positive Behavior Interventions, 1*(3), 141–151.

Stockman, I. (2008). Toward validation of a minimal competence phonetic core for African American children. *Journal of Speech, Language, and Hearing Research, 51*, 1244–1262.

Stoel-Gammon, C. (2001). Down syndrome phonology: Developmental patterns and intervention strategies. *Down Syndrome: Research and Practice, 7*, 93–100.

Swift, W. (1918). *Speech defects in school children.* Cambridge, MA: Riverside Press.

Tyler, A., Lewis, K., Haskill, A., & Tolbert, L. (2003). Outcomes of different speech and language goal attack strategies. *Journal of Speech, Language, and Hearing Research, 46*, 1077–1094.

Weiner, F. (1981). Treatment of phonological disability using the method of meaningful minimal contrast: Two case studies. *Journal of Speech and Hearing Disorders, 46*, 97–103.

Weismer, G., Kent, R.D., Hodge, M., & Martin, R. (1988). The acoustic signature for intelligibility test words. *Journal of the Acoustical Society of America, 84*, 1281–1291.

Weston, A., & Shriberg, L. (1992). Contextual and linguistic correlates of intelligibility in children with developmental phonological disorders. *Journal of Speech and Hearing Research, 35*, 1316–1332.

Williams, A.L. (2000). Multiple oppositions: Theoretical foundations for an alternative contrastive intervention approach. *American Journal of Speech-Language Pathology, 9*, 282–288.

Williams, A.L. (2005). A model and structure for phonological intervention. In S.F. Warren & M.E. Fey (Series Eds.), & A.G Kamhi & K.E. Pollock (Vol. Eds.), *Communication and language intervention series: Phonological disorders in children—Clinical decision making in assessment and intervention* (pp. 189–199). Baltimore: Paul H. Brookes Co.

World Health Organization. (2007). *International classification of functioning, disability and health: Children and youth version (ICF-CY).* Geneva: Author.

Yoder, P., Camarata, S., Camarata, M., & Williams, S. (2006). Association between differentiated processing of syllables and comprehension of grammatical morphology in children with Down syndrome. *American Journal on Mental Retardation. 111*, 138–152.

Yoder, P., Camarata, S., & Gardner, E. (2005). Treatment effects on speech intelligibility and length of utterance in children with specific language and intelligibility impairments. *Journal of Early Intervention, 28*, 34–49.

Yoder, P., & Warren, S.F. (1993). Can developmentally delayed children's language development be enhanced through prelinguistic intervention? In S.F. Warren & J. Reichle (Series Eds.) & A.P. Kaiser & D. Gray (Vol. Eds.), *Communication and language intervention series: Vol. 2. Enhancing children's communication: Research foundations for early language intervention* (pp. 35–62). Baltimore: Paul H. Brookes Publishing Co.

Parents and Children Together (PACT) Intervention

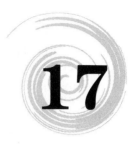

17

Caroline Bowen

ABSTRACT

Designed for poorly intelligible 3- to 6-year-olds, Parents and Children Together (PACT) is a family centered, broad-based intervention approach to developmental phonological disorder. PACT incorporates phonetic, phonemic, and perceptual targets; goals, procedures, and activities; and active participation of explicitly tutored caregivers. Theoretically coherent and empirically supported, it has five components: Parent Education, Metalinguistic Training, Phonetic Production Training, Multiple Exemplar Training, and Homework. Acknowledging the gradualness of phonological change in typical development, and the often problematic logistics of accessing adequate speech-language pathology services, PACT occurs in planned, individual, in-clinic therapy blocks and in breaks from therapy attendance during which tutored caregivers continue aspects of intervention. This chapter presents the theory and development of PACT, highlighting with examples its application in everyday practice.

INTRODUCTION

PACT was born of necessity and designed to be practicable. Over a 10-year period its feasibility was tried via clinical hypothesis testing under normal clinical conditions. Normal speech-language pathology clinical conditions in Australia at the time differed markedly among agencies and service delivery models, and still do. Throughout many parts of the world's largest island, waiting lists for understaffed, under-resourced publicly funded services were and are long. The services themselves were and are often scant, with some children waiting 18 months to 2 years for assessment that might turn out to be comprehensive or cursory, then only to receive just a few hours of intervention at best; and a so-called "home program" composed of a few worksheets to be administered by unsupervised, minimally supported parents or teachers' aides, with no relevant training, at worst.

This sorry state of affairs resembles the situation reported in the United Kingdom by Joffe and Pring (2008) and contrasts manifestly with what is available to families able to access unlimited speech-language pathology services in some public or private settings, or both. In the United States, for example, the law does not permit waiting lists for speech-language pathology intervention (Flipsen, 2009). With regard to private services for children with speech sound disorders (SSD), although some families may enjoy privileged circumstances, private clients vary enormously in their desire and capacity to access and pay for services, forcing an inevitable trade-off between both the depth of detail of assessment and the intensity of services on one hand, and the cost to the consumer on the other. Indeed, clinicians in private settings, working with low-, middle-, and single-income families struggling to pay fees, or with dual-income families reluctant to sacrifice too much time (e.g., due to career-path considerations), are often forced to budget the amount of speech evaluation, speech analysis, and speech-focused therapy delivered to particular children, while still endeavoring to provide effective intervention.

Part of the *motivation* for the development of PACT was, therefore, to devise an efficacious therapy that was cost efficient in therapist hours and practicable in terms of the real costs in time, money, and effort for families. In this sense PACT originated from a recurring clinical problem that led to a four-pronged practical clinical question. In what way would therapy outcomes be affected if children were seen

- For fewer clinical consultations within therapy blocks

- For fewer child–clinician contact hours overall

- For intervention split into therapy blocks (periods of therapy attendance) and therapy breaks (periods of nonattendance in which families would continue to apply skills and strategies learned during the blocks), alternating approximately every 10 weeks

- With primary caregivers, trained to collaborate as co-therapists for their own children

Meanwhile, the *inspiration* for the development of PACT was threefold. It came from linguistics theory and research in the form of published developments in clinical phonology (Grunwell, 1975; Ingram, 1976); family systems theory and therapy, particularly the structural and strategic models (for an accessible contemporary account see Bitter, 2009); and a growing appreciation in the 1990s within the profession of the tenets of family-centered services (see Chapter 20). The impetus to formally evaluate PACT arose from the need for accountability to the clients engaged in PACT therapy, and a responsibility to continuing professional development participants discovering it in speech-language pathology professional development workshops, as well as other colleagues keen to try it. Level IV evidence (American Speech-Language-Hearing Association, 2004) was available in the form of clinical experience, which suggested that the PACT approach was evoking phonological change and intelligibility gains over and above the expected effects of maturation. Stronger evidence than that was required however, because, in the words of Finn, Bothe, and Bramlett, "professionals should be wary about trusting their own clinical experience as the sole basis for determining the validity of a treatment claim" (2005, p. 182).

Evidence-based practice (EBP) is a process and a responsibility. It is commonly represented, with optimistic simplicity, as an equilateral triangle. The first point of the triangle signifies clinicians' dynamic engagement with scientific theory and research via the published literature and continuing education activity. The second point denotes their expert knowledge and skill bases and practical experience with their clients and their worlds. The third point represents their respect for their clients' beliefs, values, responsibilities, and priorities, and the *assets* (Kretzmann & McKnight, 1993) that *they* bring to the therapeutic encounter. The onus for *adopting* EBP rests with individual clinicians and cannot be imposed by professional associations, employers, legislators, or policy makers. Among the clinicians who do adopt it, probably very few play an active part in *constructing* the evidence apex of the EBP triangle. Nonetheless, for this clinician the imperative to step outside the comfortable clinician role and venture into research was irresistible because of the pressing need to evaluate PACT's efficacy, exploring the three Es of quality assurance—effectiveness, efficiency, and effects—articulated by Olswang (1998). Was PACT efficacious? Was it effective and valid: Did it work? How did its efficiency rate? Did it work as well as, or better than, traditional articulation therapies? And its effects— what changes did the therapy evoke? These questions, some of which remain incompletely addressed, prompted PACT's actualization as a formally tested intervention (Bowen, 1996a; Bowen & Cupples, 1998, 1999a).

TARGET POPULATIONS

Primary Populations

PACT is designed for 3- to 6-year-olds and arose from the desire for an intervention that families could access before their children with phonological impairment started school, potentially preempting or minimizing literacy acquisition difficulties (Bird, Bishop, & Freeman, 1995; Hesketh, Adams, Nightingale, & Hall, 2000).

Secondary Populations

PACT also has been used with other client populations with acceptable clinical outcomes, but it has not been formally evaluated (Bowen & Cupples, 2004). Across and within these populations, families and communicative milieus have represented a multicultural gamut of child-rearing practices, family structures, socioeconomic circumstances, parental educational attainment, and parental availability. Within our experience—and according to feedback from clinicians in several countries including Australia, Canada, France, Hong Kong, Malaysia, New Zealand, Norway, Singapore, the United Kingdom, and the United States—client groups have been preschool and younger school-age children (3–6 years old) with language processing and production issues and comorbid SSD; children up to age 10 with specific language impairment, and/or pragmatic difficulties, and/or cognitive challenges plus speech intelligibility issues; children fitted with cochlear implants; children with cleft palates; children with SSD at the high-functioning end of the autism spectrum; children diagnosed with Down syndrome, fragile X syndrome, and Williams syndrome; children from bilingual households; and children with childhood apraxia of speech (CAS; Bowen, 2009).

ASSESSMENT METHODS FOR DETERMINING INTERVENTION RELEVANCE

Assessment within the PACT approach, whether initial or ongoing, is integral to intervention. Because parents or primary caregivers play a key role in PACT intervention, it is desirable for them to understand the speech-language assessment process. Once audiology testing is complete; a history has been taken; and language, voice, and fluency have been screened, speech assessment begins with the administration and scoring of the Quick Screener (Bowen, 1996b, after Dean, Howell, Hill, & Waters, 1990) while parent(s) observe. The child's responses to the screener, usually administered as an engaging slide show on a laptop computer, are recorded using broad phonetic transcription and are analyzed for phonological processes and tentative *single-word* percentage of consonants correct (PCC) and percentage of vowels correct (PVC) estimates, in the parents' presence, and are discussed in the child's presence. Intelligibility ratings by parents and therapist are recorded on the Quick Screener data collection form (available with a processes analysis form; see Bowen, 1996b), single-word phonetic inventory is noted, and stimulability to two or three syllable positions is determined. Having parents present during screening and brief analysis gives them information about the clinician's theoretical orientation; namely, an interest in the child's *system* of sound contrasts, *intelligibility*, and *stimulability*. Including the child in discussions provides a demonstration, from the outset, that his or her own parents play a key role in the therapy process. Coupled with data from a 200-utterance conversational speech sample, gathered if possible and glossed if necessary during language screening, the Quick Screener usually provides sufficient information for a diagnosis (or at least a provisional diagnosis) of phonological impairment while alerting the clinician to associated difficulties. If needed, more detailed independent and relational analyses are performed at a later date, usually with caregivers observing. These procedures may incorporate standardized tests such as the Diagnostic Evaluation of Articulation and Phonology (DEAP; Dodd, Crosbie, Zhu, Holm, & Ozanne, 2002) or the Hodson Assessment of Phonological Patterns (HAPP-3; Hodson, 2004) to inform intervention planning and sometimes to accompany applications for funding of special support services at preschool or school, in addition to nonstandardized measures such as the Locke Speech Perception-Production Task (Locke, 1980) and imitative PCC (Johnson, Weston, & Bain, 2004).

THEORETICAL BASIS

Dominant Theoretical Rationale for the Intervention Approach

The principles underlying PACT are that phonemic change is motivated by homophony and enhanced through metalinguistic awareness of the sound system. Heightened perceptual saliency of contrasts makes new contrasts easier to learn (i.e., increases learnability), which also facilitates phonemic change. It embraces the threefold foundation of all minimal pair approaches: namely, 1) the modification of groups of sounds produced in error in a patterned way; 2) an emphasis on establishing feature contrasts rather than accurate sound production; and 3) making it explicit to the child that the function of phonology (phonemic contrasts) is communication, by working at word level, using naturalistic parent–child communicative contexts, and increasing the child's metaphonological awareness. Acknowledging the important role of families in children's development, PACT has five components: Parent Education, Metalinguistic Training, Phonetic Production Training, Multiple Exemplar Training, and Homework.

Rationale for Parent Education

We reasoned that collaborative engagement of well-informed parents would tap a special "therapeutic resource": namely, the people likely to spend the most time with the child and those most motivated and best situated to assist. Educating, guiding, and supporting parents would ensure that they used *their* time optimally with their efforts sufficiently focused on their child's unique intervention needs to promote new learning. Their involvement would enable fewer clinical consultations and contact hours and enhance the productivity of the breaks.

Rationale for Metalinguistic Training

The Metalinguistic Training component of PACT was inspired by a clinically focused article by Dean and Howell (1986) that gave voice to an innovative collection of ideas that eventually became Metaphon intervention (Dean et al., 1990). In it the authors explained how guided discussion and metalanguage could help children reflect on the phonetic properties or distinctive features of phonemes and syllable structure. Following Ingram (1976), PACT acknowledges three phonological levels: 1) underlying representation (the sound in the child's mind), 2) surface form (the way the child actually says the sound), and 3) the mapping rules or connections between the previous two. Working at phonological levels, PACT incorporates the principle that phonemic change is motivated by homophony, and a child's capacity to perceive, talk about, reflect on, and revise and repair homophonous productions is enhanced when his or her awareness of word/phoneme contrasts (e.g., *ship* and *sip* realized contrastively as /ʃɪp/ and /sɪp/, respectively) and phoneme collapses or homonymy (e.g., *ship* and *sip* realized homophonously as /sɪp/) are made overt. The suggestions of Dean and Howell were adopted and extended to allow metalinguistic awareness to be targeted in naturalistic, supportive clinic and home settings. This was done with the understanding that by drawing a child's attention to the communicative consequences of homophony and to sound and syllable properties, the probability of improving the accuracy of that child's knowledge of the system of phonemic contrasts grows, and the likelihood of spontaneous revisions and repairs (self-corrections) increases. In turn, the use of spontaneous revisions and repairs is fostered, particularly at home, by use of the "fixed-up-one routine" (discussed in the Metalinguistic Training section later in this chapter) and labeled praise.

Rationale for Phonetic Production Training

By definition, phonological therapy is directed at activating a child's underlying system for phoneme use and emphasizes achieving meaningful contrasts over achieving perfect phonetic execution, but at some point a child must learn how to produce the phonemes. Phonetic Production Training uses stimulability techniques (see Chapter 8) in which the therapist teaches a child to produce absent or distorted phones *beyond* the isolated level, or failing that, to produce approximations of consonants in the same sound class in CV and VC combinations.

Rationale for Multiple Exemplar Training

Multiple Exemplar Training involves auditory input and minimal contrasts therapy. The two aspects to auditory input are listening lists and thematic play based around therapy targets. With the listening lists, parent and therapist read to the child, without amplification, auditory input word lists of up to 15 words, or up to 7 word pairs or triplets, representing a target; or target and error; or target, error, and "foil." Thematic play involves playing games with and reading books to the child that give rise to frequent repetitions of targets. For example, when Bruno, age 4;2, was learning /f/ syllable-final word-final (SFWF) in one session, over the following week in Homework he listened to a comic-strip story about a gira*ff*e couple named Je*ff* and Ste*ph* (Bowen, 2009) and performed associated activities, played a game in which a super hero jumped o*ff* a roo*f*, and played with Smur*f*s all week. In minimal contrasts therapy a child sorts words pictured on cards according to their sound properties, in sessions and for Homework, and engages in homophony confrontation tasks. Suggestions for Multiple Exemplar Training procedures and activities are included in the Key Components section later in this chapter, but note that families are generally innovative in contriving comparable ones. The rationale for the Multiple Exemplar Training component is that the heightened perceptual saliency of contrasts, provided by the activities, increases the learnability of new contrasts.

Rationale for Homework

The Homework component provides children with practice, reinforcement, and opportunities to generalize new skills, and allows families to generalize teaching skills learned in therapy sessions. Engaging in activities independently, without the therapist, can potentially empower families and teachers to experiment with them, creating new learning opportunities in natural contexts. As parents' knowledge and awareness of speech acquisition processes increase and they gain in confidence, most will innovate and some will even initiate appropriate next steps in therapy. Because Homework guidelines are not dogmatic, the homework itself is conducive to internal development, so parents can tailor it to their family activities and the child's interests and preferences. It often takes on the family "stamp" in addition to the clinician's style, influencing the form of therapy sessions in a dynamic and interesting way, letting the adults involved construct activities a child really likes and is responsive to.

Rationale for the Blocks and Breaks Scheduling of Consultations

The breaks, we reasoned, would accommodate to the gradual nature of phonological acquisition in typical development, allow for some speech-language progress to occur in spurts and plateaus as it very often does, allow "space" for consolidation of new speech skills and make way for generalization, provide periodic respite from therapy, and allow families to refresh and regroup prior to therapy blocks (Bowen & Cupples, 2004).

Levels of Consequences Being Addressed

In an article about the scope of the International Classification of Functioning, Disability and Health for Children and Youth (ICF-CY; World Health Organization, 2007), Lollar and Simeonsson commented on the need for clear communication among members of treatment teams, observing that, "improvement in function is often the litmus test that society uses to evaluate the effectiveness of programs and treatments...assessment and classification of function are instrumental for characterizing the young person's lived experience" (2005, p. 323). Within the ICF Body Functions component, PACT impacts the primary ICF-CY domain b320 Articulation function in both assessment and intervention. The assessment process associated with PACT involves gathering baseline Articulation function data derived from Independent Analysis of a child's speech (e.g., vowel, consonant, phonotactic, and stress inventories and constraints) and Relational Analysis (e.g., PCC and PVC; percentage of occurrence of phonological processes), and intelligibility ratings, comparing the child's levels of function with normative data. In terms of Articulation function, the treatment process may involve production of vowels, consonants, tones, syllable shapes, and intelligible words and longer utterances. With regard to phonological (sound system) function, PACT is directed at functions of the reception and production of distinctive phonological units (phonemes and their features) that are linked to the child's ambient language, including recognition, representation, and processing of phonological information. Finally, in the area of discrimination function (ICF code b230), PACT involves sensory functions relative to spoken language such as the abilities to distinguish speech sounds from other sounds and distinguish phone from phone, word from word, and word from nonword. PACT also involves the Activities and Participation domain of the ICF with respect to its focus in assessment and intervention on speech and language in real contexts and acquiring speech sounds, syllables, prosody, stress, and intonation (enabling participation). Furthermore, with its emphasis on parent participation and developing children's capacity for self-monitoring, self-correcting, and metalinguistic functioning, PACT is concerned with Environmental factors and Personal factors, respecting McLeod and Bleile who wrote, "Probably the most important environmental factor relating to children with speech impairment is support and relationships. The incorporation of parental support into the intervention practices is frequently a key to success" (2004, p. 210).

Target Areas of Intervention

PACT targets speech perception and intelligibility in children with phonological disorder, and whether by default or by design, it also has an impact on morphosyntax and phonological awareness (particularly phonemic awareness) and hence literacy acquisition. It does so cognizant of the ICF goal-setting framework (McLeod & McCormack, 2007), taking into consideration the contributions of activities and participation in facilitating health and well-being, embracing those most relevant to children with SSD: namely, Communication (d3) including Conversation (d350); Learning and applying knowledge (d1); Interpersonal interactions and relationships (d7); and Community, social and, ultimately, civic life (d9).

As mentioned previously, PACT was not designed with children with CAS as the primary population. It has, however, been used in conjunction with integral stimulation therapy (Strand, Stoeckel, & Baas, 2006) and compatible techniques that follow the principles of motor learning (Schmidt & Lee, 2000) in treating children diagnosed with CAS. Within the area of children's SSD, the clinical characteristics, or symptoms, that CAS and phonological disorder may have in common include 1) consonant, vowel, and phonotactic inventory constraints; 2) omissions of segments and structures; 3) segmental errors; 4) altered suprasegmentals (prosody); 5) increased errors with utterance length and/or complexity; and 6) use of simple (but not complex) syllable and word shapes. In treating these common symptoms, with the overarching aim of improving intelligibility, specific goals might include the following:

1. Expanding the consonant inventory; promoting more accurate consonant production

2. Expanding the vowel inventory; promoting more accurate vowel production

3. Expanding the syllable shape inventory; promoting phonotactic accuracy

4. Expanding the word shape inventory; promoting more accurate word structures

5. Expanding the capacity to produce and differentiate strong and weak syllables

6. Promoting more varied and accurate use of phonotactic range in syllables and words

7. Promoting more effective use of suprasegmentals

8. Promoting generalization of new segments, syllable structures, word structures, and prosodic features to more challenging contexts

EMPIRICAL BASIS

Research Outcomes

There has been one efficacy study of PACT (Bowen, 1996a; Bowen & Cupples, 1999a, 1999b). The preschoolers in the efficacy study ranged in age from 2;11 to 4;9 at the commencement of treatment and had conversational PCCs between 27% and 70%. The severity of involvement (Shriberg & Kwiatkowski, 1982) of the 4-year-olds was mild-to-moderate (one participant), moderate-to-severe (three participants), and severe (five participants). The four 3-year-olds and one slightly younger child, age 2;11, were too young for severity ratings relative to conversational PCC, and their initial PCCs were 40%, 49%, 52%, 59%, and 67%, respectively. These values are displayed in Table 17.1. In the study, each child's major disability was at the phonological level, but as is so commonly the case with children with phonological impairment, the major disability was often accompanied by phonetic, auditory perceptual, and mild motor planning components, and some participants experienced, and were treated for, dysfluency during the speech intervention process.

A longitudinal matched groups design was used, composed of assessment, treatment, and reassessment or probe phases. In addition to the 14 children who received

Table 17.1. Parents and Children Together (PACT) efficacy study: Participant characteristics

Participant	Gender	Age	Percentage of consonants correct (PCC) and severity relative to PCC (Shriberg & Kwiatkowski, 1982)		Clinician severity rating (CSR) and severity relative to CSR (Bowen & Cupples, 1999b)		PPVT-R	MLUm
1	F	4;4	48	severe	3.75	moderate	115	5.30
2	F	4;8	50	moderate-severe	3.75	moderate	106	5.20
3	M	3;10	59	—	2.50	mild	105	4.50
4	F	4;2	41	severe	3.75	moderate	104	4.37
5	F	4;2	70	mild-moderate	2.75	mild	106	3.17
6	F	4;3	64	moderate-severe	2.75	mild	105	4.00
7	M	4;9	63	moderate-severe	3.25	moderate	127	4.00
8	F	2;11	40	—	2.75	mild	94	3.40
9	M	4;1	44	severe	3.50	moderate	91	4.30
10	M	4;3	27	severe	4.00	severe	97	3.64
11	F	3;10	52	—	3.25	moderate	99	3.50
12	F	4;5	35	severe	3.75	moderate	113	4.80
13	F	3;8	67	—	2.50	mild	114	4.00
14	F	3;11	49	—	2.75	mild	96	3.50

Key: PCC, percentage of consonants correct; CSR, clinician severity rating; PPVT-R, Peabody Picture Vocabulary Test–Revised (Dunn & Dunn, 1981); MLUm, mean length of utterance in morphemes; M, male; F, female.

treatment, treatment was withheld from eight well-matched children who participated as control participants. When the probe assessments were conducted, the treated children showed accelerated improvement in their productive phonology, compared with the untreated eight who did not. Standardized measures (e.g., the Peabody Picture Vocabulary Test–Revised [PPVT-R]; Dunn & Dunn, 1981) and objective observations (e.g., mean length of utterance in morphemes [MLUm], PCC, independent analysis, and relational analysis) as well as naturalistic probes (e.g., clinician severity rating) were used throughout. In the statistical analysis of the initial and probe clinician severity ratings (Bowen & Cupples, 1999b) for both groups, highly significant selective progress in the treated children only ($F(1,20) = 19.36$, $p < .01$) was evident. No such selective improvement was observed in either receptive vocabulary or MLUm, attesting to the specific effect of the therapy. The initial severity of the treated children's phonological impairments was the solitary predictor of the frequency and duration of consultations required for their speech patterns to fall within age-typical expectations. These initial severity ratings of the treated participants are displayed in Table 17.1 with the participant genders, ages, initial PCC, and severity increment where applicable (Shriberg & Kwiatkowski, 1982); initial clinician severity rating (Bowen & Cupples, 1999b); initial PPVT-R; and finally the MLUm at the commencement of treatment for each participant.

An exploration of its effectiveness (Bowen & Cupples, 1998) illustrating its practicability under conditions of everyday practice (Robey & Schultz, 1998) is provided in a case study of participant 1, Nina (Bowen & Cupples, 1998), and in a case study of participant 12, Ceri (Bowen & Cupples, 1999a). In addition, Bowen and Cupples (2004) detail an account of the participation of the children's families in optimizing intervention outcomes. Turning to the changes the therapy evoked, or its effects, Table 17.2 displays the characteristics of the treated children at their initial and probe assessments.

Finally, how did its efficiency rate; did it work as well as or better than traditional articulation therapies? To date, no formal comparisons between PACT and other interventions have been conducted. Clinical impressions suggest that it is efficient in reducing

Table 17.2. Initial and probe severity ratings and percentage of consonants correct (PCC)

Participant	Initial CSR	Probe CSR	Initial PCC	Probe PCC	Initial age (months)	Probe age (months)
1	3.75	2.25	48	84	52	63
2	3.75	1.50	50	90	56	67
3	2.50	1.00	59	97	46	52
4	3.75	2.50	41	88	50	62
5	2.75	1.00	70	100	50	57
6	2.75	1.00	64	100	51	61
7	3.25	1.75	63	94	57	68
8	2.75	2.00	40	86	35	45
9	3.50	1.00	44	84	49	58
10	4.00	3.25	27	65	51	62
11	3.25	1.00	52	94	46	53
12	3.75	1.00	35	97	53	63
13	2.50	1.00	67	100	44	47
14	2.75	1.00	49	96	47	56

Key: CSR, clinician severity rating.

Table 17.3. Levels of evidence for studies of treatment efficacy for Parents and Children Together (PACT)

Level	Description	References
Ia	Meta-analysis of > 1 randomized controlled trial	—
Ib	Randomized controlled study	—
IIa	Controlled study without randomization	Bowen & Cupples, 1999a, 1999b
IIb	Quasi-experimental study	—
III	Nonexperimental studies, i.e., correlational and case studies	Bowen & Cupples, 1998
IV	Expert committee report, consensus conference, clinical experience of respected authorities	Personal correspondence

Adapted from the Scottish Intercollegiate Guidelines Network (http://www.sign.ac.uk).

client–clinician face-to-face hours, but this must be weighed against the time parents spend and the analysis and therapy planning loads that fall to the clinician.

Summary of Levels of Evidence

See Table 17.3.

PRACTICAL REQUIREMENTS

Nature of Sessions

Children are seen individually, usually in a clinical, domiciliary, or school setting, once per week during therapy blocks. Treatment sessions are usually 50 minutes in duration. Within this time span, the child spends about 30–40 minutes alone with the therapist. At a minimum, parent participation at the clinic involves the parent joining the therapist and child for 20 minutes at the end of a session, or 10 minutes at the beginning and 10 minutes at the end. The maximal parent participation entails the parent being actively involved in a treatment triad with the child and therapist, for approximately half of the treatment session. These segments of parent participation require the child's continued involvement in order to demonstrate properly what should happen during Homework. A therapy session for Jacob, age 5;9, who was working to eliminate velar fronting provides an example of a typical 50-minute session. His father attended for the second half (25 minutes), as did his sister, age 3;0, who played quietly with toys, causing no distractions. Noting contrasts in PACT can represent error versus target, error versus targets, or correct versus target; in this instance the contrasts were presented as two minimal pair sets representing error-target (/t/ versus /k/ and /d/ versus /g/). This particular therapy session for Jacob consisted of

1. *Rhyming auditory bombardment* using five pictured, captioned minimal pairs (10 words; e.g., *key:tea, car:tar, call:tall, cape:tape, corn:torn*)

2. *Auditory bombardment rhyming cloze* with the same captioned pictures (e.g., Adult says, "*key* rhymes with..." and Jacob says, "*tea*," and so forth; note that Jacob said the word he could already say)

3. *Minimal contrasts task* requiring silent sorting of 10 cards into rhyming pairs (e.g., *gave:Dave, got:dot, gull:dull, game:dame, go:dough*)

4. *Judgment of correctness task* whereby the adult says, "You be the teacher and tell me if I say these words the right way or the wrong way" (e.g., *gull* versus *dull*)

5. *Fixed-up-one routine* for /k/ and /g/ (the particular routine used with Jacob can be found online at http://speech-language-therapy.com/tx-/fuo-velarfronting-k-vs-t-g-vs-d .pdf)

6. *Homophony confrontation* task (e.g., *key:tea, core:tore, call:tall*)

7. *Listening to an audio recording* of a "good" (funny) part of the preceding therapy session, providing an opportunity to laugh/praise and then to record the current week's listening list. Periodically audio recording the lists to be taken home provides input for child and provides a model for parent(s).

8. *Auditory bombardment* again with 15 single words (e.g., *gave, got, girl, gull, guard*) or minimal triplets instead of minimal pairs (e.g., *gave:Dave:shave, got:dot:shot, game:dame:shame, go:dough:show*) for novelty effect to increase saliency

9. *Homework explained, demonstrated, and rehearsed* by Jacob and his father, with discussion of targets to reinforce and how to reinforce them (parent education)

Personnel

The personnel involved in PACT are the child, primary caregiver(s), and the speech-language pathologist (SLP). Sometimes teachers become involved in Homework. The clinician helps all families to understand the therapy and encourages family members to become active participants in therapy sessions and to continue relevant activities at home. Using clinical judgment, the Parent Education components of PACT (Bowen & Cupples, 2004) are deployed according to need. For some families this may mean undertaking independent reading of information, including educative slide shows accessed from the Internet and run independently (e.g., on home computers), with follow-up discussion during which parents' questions are addressed and particular points clarified. Other families may require more support, and are talked through information sheets and watch individualized (for their child) PowerPoint presentations in the clinic that are carefully explained by the clinician. Some parents require very little explanation and learn most from observing and rehearsal; others require a lot of explanation, and can then carry out activities at home, but are shy with regard to parent-administered explicit practice in the clinic with the therapist watching. It has been found that parents' education level may have little bearing on how easily they understand concepts of sound patterns, modeling, labeled praise, reinforcement, revisions and repairs, progressive approximations, shaping, and gradualness of acquisition. This is difficult to explain, but understanding and working with these concepts appears to have much to do with whether a parent has an intuitive feel for the way language works and whether they are natural teachers. Parents with histories of similar problems to their child may bring a unique empathy to the situation, although some of them may have residual difficulties that affect their capacity to reflect on language function. Table 17.4 provides information on the degree of involvement in the efficacy study of family members in therapy overall.

Table 17.4. Participation in consultations and homework

Participant	Gender	Consultations	Mother only at consultation	Sibling(s) (occasions)	Homework with parent (times per week)	Percentage of homework with mother
1	F	27	27	5	18	100
2	F	32	26	2	12	60
3	M	12	12	11	24	50
4	F	36	28	35	12	60
5	F	15	15	14	8	100
6	F	19	18	17	24	80
7	M	24	21	2	12	20
8	F	24	23	3	12	50
9	M	22	22	21	12	100
10	M	54	54	2	12	85
11	F	14	06	13	6	0
12	F	23	23	1	24	100
13	F	10	06	3	24	50
14	F	21	21	2	12	100

Key: F, female; M, male.

Dosage

Therapy is administered in planned blocks and breaks. The first block and the first break are usually about 10 weeks each, after which the number of therapy sessions per block tends to reduce, with the period between blocks remaining constant at 10 weeks. During breaks, parents are asked to do no formal practice for 8 weeks. Two weeks prior to the next treatment block, they are asked to read the speech homework book with the child a few times and to do any activities the child is interested in doing. During the breaks, they continue to focus on providing modeling corrections, reinforcement of revisions and repairs, and metalinguistic activities, incidentally, as opportunities arise. They continue to use the strategies of modeling and reinforcement learned in the therapy block(s).

KEY COMPONENTS

Parent Education

Parents learn from the clinician techniques including modeling, recasting, encouraging the child's self-monitoring and self-correction, labeled praise, and providing auditory input via thematic play. The techniques are described for a lay readership in Bowen (1998), and the same information and slideshows are freely available at http://www.speech-language-therapy.com. The path education takes is responsive to parents' requirements, takes into account the principles of adult learning, and uses counseling and information-sharing techniques familiar to SLPs. Efforts are made to avoid overwhelming families with information at any point and to provide ample opportunity for them to rehearse new skills, question anything not understood, share their perspectives, and exercise choice. Parent education continues throughout therapy, simultaneously with other components, becoming less intensive as progress is made.

Metalinguistic Training

The child, parents, and SLP talk and think about speech and how it is organized to convey meaning, incorporating simple phonological awareness activities (see Chapter 10). Activities, at home and in therapy, involve sound picture associations (e.g., /ʃ/ means "be quiet"), phoneme segmentation for onset matching (*kookaburra* starts with /k/), awareness of rhymes and sound patterns between words (e.g., minimal pairs; near minimal pairs), rudimentary knowledge of the concept of *word*, understanding the idea of words *making sense*, awareness of the use of revision and repair strategies, judgment of correctness tasks (e.g., the puppy has a *coat* versus the puppy has a *tote*), and playing with lexical and grammatical innovations using morphophonological structures (e.g., *cup* versus *cups*, *climb* versus *climbed*). A 50:50 split between talking tasks versus thinking and listening tasks is recommended. The fixed-up-one routine is a metalinguistic technique that enables adults to talk simply to children about revisions and repairs. Scripts are provided to introduce them to the technique, and various versions of it are available (http://www.speech-language-therapy.com/tx-self-corrections.html) with an instructional slide show (http://www.speech-language-therapy.com/shows.html).

Phonetic Production Training

Using stimulability techniques (see Chapter 8) the therapist teaches the child how to make the sounds he or she has difficulty with, and parents work with the child at home with listening and talking games and activities, including production practice related to target sounds (observing the 50:50 split). Children are usually taught to produce target phonemes in two syllable positions, usually in the onset (syllable-initial word-initial [SIWI]) and coda (syllable-final word-final [SFWF]) positions. It is rarely necessary to train intervocalic stimulability; that is, syllable-initial within-word (SIWW) or syllable-final within-word (SFWW) or to train all vowel/diphthong contexts. For example, having taught /tʃu/ and /utʃ/ at syllable level, it is seldom necessary to teach /tʃu, tʃi, tʃɔ, tʃaɪ, tʃoʊ, tʃeɪ, tʃa/, and so forth, and /utʃ, itʃ, ɔtʃ, aɪtʃ, oʊtʃ, eɪtʃ, atʃ/, and so forth. Rather, the child proceeds straight from syllable to word level, having demonstrated the capacity to produce the phone in CV and/or VC contexts. Apart from introductory stimulability tasks that may be at individual sound and nonsense syllable level, PACT therapy is at *real* word level or above (see Bowen & Cupples, 2006, for discussion). Once a child is stimulable for a target, or is producing a passable approximation, or a phone in the same sound class, in syllables or words, therapy moves onto the phonemic level and all activities are *communication based* or *meaning based* and are at word level and beyond. Listening and talking games are used in the clinic and at home to provide production practice of a very small number of words: usually no more than six at a time, containing the target sound in a chosen syllable position, typically SIWI, but with SFWF as the usual starting point for fricatives because of the natural tendency for fricatives to emerge first in the coda position in typical acquisition. In the course of production practice, minimal pairs, minimal triplets, or sets of four stimuli, may be minimally, maximally, or multiply opposed. Phonetic Production Training is integrated with Multiple Exemplar Training.

Multiple Exemplar Training

Parent and therapist read word lists to the child, and the child learns to sort words according to their sound properties. Activities include

- *Point to the one I say:* The child points to pictures of the words, spoken in random order (e.g., *call, cop, tall, top*), or rhyming order (e.g., *call, tall, cop, top*) by the adult.

- *Put the rhyming words with these words:* The adult presents three to nine cards to the child (e.g., *seat, sell, sour*), and the child puts rhyming cards beside them (*sheet, shell, shower*).

- *Say the word that rhymes with the one I say:* The adult says words with the target phoneme, and the child says rhyming nontarget words (e.g., adult says *flat* and child says *fat;* adult says *slow* and child says *sew*).

- *Give me the word that rhymes with the one I say:* The adult says the nontarget word, and the child selects the rhyming word containing the target sound (e.g., adult says *pole*, and the child selects *foal*).

- *Tell me the one to give you:* The child says a word, and the adult responds to the word actually said. For example, a child pronounces *chip* as [tɪp] and is handed *tip*. The aim here is for the child to recognize a failure to communicate and attempt to revise production. This activity is not included in Homework.

- *You be the teacher; tell me if I say these words the right way or the wrong way:* The adult says words in rhyming or random order, or in sentences, and the child judges whether they have been said correctly.

- *Silly sentences:* The child judges whether a sentence is silly or not (e.g., "He *brote/broke* his crown").

- *Silly dinners:* In a variation of silly sentences the adult says what he or she wants for dinner, and the child judges whether it is a silly dinner ("I want *jelly/delly* for dinner").

- *Shake-ups and match-ups:* The child is presented first with four pictures representing contrasts, such as *tea:team* and *bee:beam*. The pairs are repeated to the child several times, then the cards are put in a container and shaken up. The child takes the cards and arranges them on the table "the same as they were before" (i.e., in pairs).

- *Find the two-step words:* The child sorts words with consonant clusters SIWI from contrasting words with singleton consonants SIWI (e.g., *plane:pain*).

- *Walk when you hear the two-steps:* The child finger-walks upon hearing a consonant cluster SIWI as opposed to a singleton consonant SIWI (e.g., the child walks for *true* but not *two*).

Homework

Homework comprises activities from the most recent session in 5- to 7-minute bursts, once, twice, or three times daily, one-to-one with an adult, in good listening conditions. Practice sessions can be as little as 10 minutes apart, the 50:50 split is observed, and parents are urged to make the homework regular, brief, naturalistic, and fun. Homework instructions and activities are contained in a homework book.

Nature of Goals

Pronunciation patterns are rule-governed and predictable, and this is the basis for all principles of phonological analysis and therapy (Bowen & Cupples, 1999a). The broad goal of PACT is to work at word level or above to promote phonological restructuring, thereby facilitating the emergence of intelligible speech. This is achieved by expanding a child's consonant, vowel, syllable-shape, syllable-stress, phonotactic, and suprasegmental repertoires and accuracy, and by promoting functional generalization of new segments, structures, and prosodic features to increasingly challenging contexts. Targets are selected using linguistic criteria taking into account motivational factors. Clinicians using PACT are encouraged to be flexible in choosing targets and feature contrasts and exercising clinical judgment, with constant reference to the growing evidence base and with consideration to the child's and the parents' attributes. For some children target selection is conservative and traditional, respecting developmental expectations and most phonological knowledge. For the right child, therapy targets may be nonstimulable, later developing, consistently in error, or supported by least phonological knowledge. Minimal and near-minimal pairs and triplets may be minimally or maximally opposed, and larger word sets may be multiply opposed (target versus up to four errors in one set). Intervention goals within PACT were summarized by Bowen and Cupples (1999a), as follows:

Basic Intervention Goals: 1) To facilitate cognitive reorganization of the child's phonological system, and his or her phonologically oriented processing strategies—a basic goal, or aim, unique to all phonological therapy approaches; and 2) To improve the child's intelligibility—a basic goal shared by traditional and phonological approaches.

Intermediate Intervention Goals: To target groups of sounds related by an organizing principle (phonological processes or phonological rules).

Specific Intervention Goals: To target a sound, sounds, or structures using horizontal strategies, targeting several sounds within a sound class or manner of production or syllable structure category, and/or targeting more than one process or deviation or structure simultaneously.

Target Selection

PACT has been shown to be appropriate for children with mild, moderate, and severe phonological impairment in terms of the Shriberg and Kwiatkowski (1982) severity scale. This means that the approach to target selection must be flexible, responsive to the needs of individual children, and evidence-based where possible. For children with mild involvement, more traditional target selection criteria *may* suffice. These criteria include working in developmental sequence; targeting readily stimulable phonemes for which the child has most knowledge via minimal meaningful contrasts using high-frequency (familiar) words; focusing on sounds that are inconsistently in error; and addressing deviations that are most destructive of intelligibility (e.g., widespread stopping of fricatives), most deviant from the norm (e.g., backing of alveolar stops), or that are socially or personally important to the particular child (e.g., Shaun, age 4;9, who called himself "Dawn," was being teased for having a girl's name, and wanted to tackle /ʃ/).

The 20 years or so of PACT's existence have seen remarkable changes in the way the profession has been encouraged to think more scientifically about target selection. Even with children with mild phonological impairment, outcomes may be enhanced by selecting targets relative to stimulability, or markedness theory, or the systemic function of phonemes within a given sound system, or distinctive feature contrasts, or sonority theory, or least phonological knowledge, or complexity, or lexical properties, or in fact any *combination* of these. Just as not all speech sound intervention approaches are ideal for every child, not all target selection strategies will be suitable for every child with a phonological disorder. By way of example, Tessa, age 5;10, with a phonetic inventory of 13 consonants, a PCC of 38%, and a high degree of homophony, met the criteria for a least-knowledge approach using high-frequency lexical targets. However, she was a timid participant who took few risks and whose hovering parents became highly critical of the clinician when anything presented looked "too hard" for Tessa. Tessa and her parents were not ready for the challenges of complex maximal oppositions or empty set feature contrasts for which she had least knowledge (demonstrated in videos by Williams, 2006, and in the DVD accompanying this book). As a trio, they were more suited initially to a softer, albeit less powerful, approach using unmarked, easily stimulable, inconsistently erred and early developing sounds, low-frequency words with low neighborhood density, and minimal feature contrasts. Once trust had built up, Tessa became more venturesome and her family less protective, and she was able to branch out and cope with multiply opposed word sets within the Multiple Exemplar Training component of PACT (see Chapter 3).

Goal Attack Strategies

Multiple goals are addressed in and across treatment sessions, within Homework, both sequentially and simultaneously and, rarely, cyclically. For example, Monique, age 5;1, worked on three goals in the fourth session of her second therapy block: namely, a stimulability/phonetic production goal to produce the voiced and voiceless affricates /dʒ/ and /tʃ/ in onset and coda position; a twofold phonological goal to recognize distinctions in input, and to mark distinctions in output at word and phrase level between the voiced and voiceless stop cognate pairs /p, b/, /t, d/, /k, g/; and a generalization goal to use the voiceless fricatives /f, s, ʃ/ but not /θ/ in conversation in untrained words.

Description of Activities

PACT includes stimulability and phonetic production activities for inventory expansion, sound–picture association games, scripted judgment of phonological correctness activities, scripted revision and repair activities, phoneme–grapheme correspondence tasks, lexical and grammatical innovation exercises, phoneme segmentation activities, rhyme completion games, and thematic play.

Materials and Equipment Required

The materials required include toys and vowel and consonant pictures on cards; a speech book, which can be an exercise book, ring binder, or scrapbook; drawing and other construction materials and equipment (e.g., crayons, scissors, glue); rewards; a computer to run educative slideshows and the Quick Screener; and an audio recorder to record therapy segments to take home. It is desirable but not essential for the family to own a com-

puter and an audio recorder. Suitable picture resources are available online (see http://
speech-language-therapy.com/freebies.htm).

ASSESSMENT AND PROGRESS
MONITORING TO SUPPORT DECISION MAKING

Initial assessment includes the administration of the Quick Screener while parents observe. This is followed by detailed independent and relational analyses, according to individual need (see Assessment Methods for Determining Intervention Relevance section
earlier in this chapter). It is usual to reassess, using the Quick Screener, with parent observation, at the beginning of each block (i.e., immediately after a break). This allows parents to observe any change, and they are usually excited to see what has happened to
their child's single-word PCC (and single-word PVC if applicable). If additional measures
are required, this may necessitate taking another language sample for phonological analysis, or the re-administration of the DEAP (Dodd et al., 2002), HAPP-3 (Hodson, 2004), or
the Speech Perception-Production Task (Locke, 1980), or an imitative PCC (Johnson et
al., 2004). Treatment planning after a break is in response to the outcome of reassessment. Typically children with phonological disorder only have required a mean of 21 clinical consultations over 101/2 months for their output phonology to fall within age expectations (Bowen & Cupples, 1999a). This means that many are ready for discharge at the
end of their second block (30 weeks after initial assessment) or immediately after their
second break (40 weeks after initial assessment). A small number need a third block,
fewer still need four, and there is no record of a child needing more than four. Children
with phonological disorder plus mild language or fluency difficulties have required about
the same volume of therapy for speech but may continue for longer to address nonspeech
goals. The decision to terminate or continue therapy, irrespective of progress, is made
jointly with parents.

CONSIDERATIONS FOR CHILDREN FROM
CULTURALLY AND LINGUISTICALLY DIVERSE BACKGROUNDS

In our experience (Bowen & Cupples, 2004) PACT has been effective in Australia with
English-learning children, in the 3- to 6-year age range for which it was designed, from
various cultural backgrounds including Chinese, Fijian, Indonesian, Japanese, Korean,
Lebanese, Malaysian, Sri Lankan, Tongan, and Thai. It has been our general observation
that Chinese, Malaysian, and Thai parents are more didactic and directive and less inclined to play when implementing PACT, preferring the clinician to be directive also;
whereas Pacific Islander parents are less direct and more playful. The form of PACT has
been different under different cultural conditions, but it is still workable. Beyond our experience, and according to feedback from colleagues, PACT's Parent Education has been
used extensively by SLPs with children with speech, language, voice, fluency, pragmatic,
and cognitive issues. For example the consumer slideshows (available from http://www
.speech-language-therapy.com/shows.html) and the fixed-up-one routine (available from
http://www.speech-language-therapy.com/tx-self-corrections.html) have been used in many
languages including Afrikaans, Bahasa Melayu, Cantonese, Egyptian Arabic, French, Por-

tuguese, Spanish, and Tamil. English- and French-speaking colleagues have reported widespread use of two books about PACT that were written for families and teachers (Bowen, 1998, 2007), and Bowen (2000) generated interest from French-speaking SLPs in France and Canada. It is currently undergoing evaluation in Portuguese, in Portugal.

CASE STUDY

In lieu of a case study, pertinent examples from the therapy of the author's clients (Bruno, age 4;2; Jacob, 5;9; Monique, 5;1; Shaun, 4;9; and Tessa, 5;10) have been included in this chapter. For detailed case studies, see accounts of Nina's therapy (Bowen & Cupples, 1998), Ceri's therapy (Bowen & Cupples, 1999a), and a hypothetical proposal of what therapy might have looked like for Jarrod (Bowen & Cupples, 2006).

STUDY QUESTIONS

1. For which age range and client group is PACT best suited?

2. What are the five components of PACT?

3. What is the typical duration and intensity of intervention in the first PACT therapy block?

4. How can the perceptual saliency of contrasts be highlighted for a child within PACT?

FUTURE DIRECTIONS

A valuable research goal would be to systematically examine the extent to which a family-centered approach such as PACT could be used with children from a variety of family situations. We have seen clinically that PACT can be used successfully in diverse situations, including single-parent families and families in which both parents work full time, and that PACT has proven effective with children from various cultural backgrounds. This anecdotal evidence might be strengthened if more systematic evidence for the generalizability of PACT were gathered. A second area lies in providing objective evidence of the value of parental involvement in PACT and other family-centered approaches to SSD. Finally, it would be interesting to systematically manipulate the components of PACT in order to streamline it and discard any superfluous aspects.

SUGGESTED READINGS

Bowen, C. (1998). *Developmental phonological disorders: A practical guide for families and teachers.* Melbourne, Australia: The Australian Council for Educational Research.

Bowen, C. (Ed.). (2009). *Children's speech sound disorders.* Oxford: Wiley-Blackwell.

Bowen, C., & Cupples, L. (2004). The role of families in optimizing phonological therapy outcomes. *Child Language Teaching and Therapy, 20,* 245–260.

For stimulating professional discussion of child speech development and disorders see http://health.groups .yahoo.com/group/phonologicaltherapy

REFERENCES

American Speech-Language-Hearing Association. (2004). *Evidence-based practice in communication disorders: An introduction* [Technical Report]. Table 1 retrieved May 28, 2008, from http://www.asha.org/docs/html/TR2004-00001-T1.html

Bird, J., Bishop, D.V.M., & Freeman, N.H. (1995). Phonological awareness and literacy development in children with expressive phonological impairments. *Journal of Speech and Hearing Research, 38*, 446–462.

Bitter, J.R. (2009). *Theory and practice of family therapy and counseling.* Belmont, CA: Brooks-Cole.

Bowen, C. (1996a). *Evaluation of a phonological therapy with treated and untreated groups of young children.* Unpublished doctoral dissertation, Macquarie University, Sydney, Australia.

Bowen, C. (1996b). *The Quick Screener.* Retrieved May 28, 2008, from http://www.speech-language-therapy.com/tx-a-quickscreener.html

Bowen, C. (1998). *Developmental phonological disorders: A practical guide for families and teachers.* Melbourne, Australia: The Australian Council for Educational Research.

Bowen, C. (2000). PACT: Collaboration avec les familles et les enseignants rééducation phonologique. *Rééducation Orthophonique, 203*(Septembre), 11–17.

Bowen, C. (2007). *Les difficultés phonologiques chez l'enfant: Guide à l'intention des familles, des enseignants et des intervenants en petite enfance*/Caroline Bowen; Rachel Fortin, traductrice et adaptatrice. Montréal, Québec, Canada: Chenelière-éducation.

Bowen, C. (Ed.). (2009). *Children's speech sound disorders.* Oxford: Wiley-Blackwell

Bowen, C., & Cupples, L. (1998). A tested phonological therapy in practice. *Child Language Teaching and Therapy, 14*(1), 29–50.

Bowen, C., & Cupples, L. (1999a). Parents and Children Together (PACT): A collaborative approach to phonological therapy. *International Journal of Language and Communication Disorders, 34*(1), 35–55.

Bowen, C., & Cupples, L. (1999b). A phonological therapy in depth. *International Journal of Language and Communication Disorders, 34*(1), 65–83.

Bowen, C., & Cupples, L. (2004). The role of families in optimising phonological therapy outcomes. *Child Language Teaching and Therapy, 20*(3), 245–260.

Bowen, C., & Cupples, L. (2006). PACT: Parents and Children Together in phonological therapy. *Advances in Speech-Language Pathology, 8*(3), 282–292.

Dean, E., & Howell, J. (1986). Developing linguistic awareness. *British Journal of Disorders of Communication, 21*, 223–238.

Dean, E., Howell, J., Hill, A., & Waters, D. (1990). *Metaphon.* Windsor, Berkshire, England: NFER Nelson.

Dodd, B., Crosbie, S., Zhu, H., Holm, A., & Ozanne, A. (2002). *Diagnostic Evaluation of Articulation and Phonology (DEAP).* London: Pearson PsychCorp.

Dunn, L.M., & Dunn, L.M. (1981). *Peabody Picture Vocabulary Test–Revised.* Circle Pines, MN: American Guidance Service.

Finn, P., Bothe, A., & Bramlett, R. (2005). Science and pseudoscience in communication disorders. *American Journal of Speech-Language Pathology, 14*, 172–186.

Flipsen, P., Jr. (2009). Severity and speech sound disorders: A continuing puzzle. In C. Bowen (Ed.), *Children's speech sound disorders* (pp. 65–68). Oxford, England: Wiley-Blackwell.

Grunwell, P. (1975). The phonological analysis of articulation disorders. *British Journal of Disorders of Communication, 10*, 31–42.

Hesketh, A., Adams, C., Nightingale, C., & Hall, R. (2000). Phonological awareness therapy and articulatory training approaches for children with phonological disorders: A comparative outcome study. *International Journal of Language and Communication Disorders, 35*, 337–354.

Hodson, B. (2004). *Hodson Assessment of Phonological Patterns* (3rd ed.). Austin, TX: PRO-ED.

Ingram, D. (1976). *Phonological disability in children.* London: Edward Arnold.

Joffe, V.L., & Pring, T. (2008). Children with phonological problems: A survey of clinical practice. *International Journal of Language and Communication Disorders, 43*(2), 154–164.

Johnson, C.A., Weston, A.D., & Bain, B.A. (2004). An objective and time-efficient method for determining severity of childhood speech delay. *American Journal of Speech-Language Pathology, 13*, 55–65.

Kretzmann, J.P., & McKnight, J.L. (1993). *Building communities from the inside out.* Chicago: Acta Publications.

Locke, J.L. (1980). The inference of speech perception in the phonologically disordered child. Part II: Some clinically novel procedures, their use, some findings. *Journal of Speech and Hearing Disorders, 45*, 445–468.

Lollar, D.J., & Simeonsson, R.J. (2005). Diagnosis to function: Classification for children and youths. *Journal of Developmental and Behavioral Pediatrics, 26*(4), 323–330.

McLeod, S., & Bleile, K. (2004). The ICF: A framework for setting goals for children with speech impairment. *Child Language Teaching and Therapy, 20*(3), 199–219.

McLeod, S., & McCormack, J. (2007). Application of the ICF and ICF-Children and Youth in children with speech impairment. *Seminars in Speech and Language, 28*, 254–264.

Olswang, L. (1998). Treatment efficacy research. In C. Frattali (Ed.), *Measuring outcomes in speech-language pathology* (pp. 134–150). New York: Thieme Publishers.

Robey, R.R., & Schultz, M.C. (1998). A model for conducting clinical-outcome research: An adaptation of the standard protocol for use in aphasiology. *Aphasiology, 12*, 787–810.

Schmidt, R.A., & Lee, T.D. (2000). *Motor control and learning: A behavioral emphasis* (3rd ed.). Champaign, IL: Human Kinetics.

Shriberg, L.D., & Kwiatkowski, J. (1982). Phonological disorders I: A diagnostic classification system. *Journal of Speech and Hearing Disorders, 47*, 226–241.

Strand, E., Stoeckel, R., & Baas, B. (2006). Treatment of severe childhood apraxia of speech: Treatment efficacy study. *Journal of Medical Speech Pathology, 14*, 297–307.

Williams, A.L. (2006). *Sound Contrasts in Phonology (SCIP)*. Eau Claire, WI: Thinking Publications.

World Health Organization. (2007). *International classification of functioning, disability and health: Children and youth (ICF-CY)*. Geneva: Author.

Enhanced Milieu Teaching with Phonological Emphasis for Children with Cleft Lip and Palate

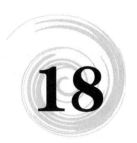

18

Nancy J. Scherer and Ann P. Kaiser

ABSTRACT

Enhanced milieu teaching with phonological emphasis (EMT/PE) is a naturalistic intervention paradigm designed to simultaneously facilitate vocabulary and speech sound production for young children who show both language and speech production impairments. This program is adapted for children with cleft lip and palate who show early vocabulary and speech sound disorders (SSD). The program is based on enhanced milieu teaching (EMT), a language intervention program with considerable empirical evidence. This language program has been augmented with speech recasting to prompt speech production simultaneously within the targeted vocabulary. EMT/PE includes all the components of EMT including environmental arrangement and traditional milieu teaching. The traditional milieu teaching prompts of model, mand-model, time delay, and incidental teaching are supplemented with speech recasts.

INTRODUCTION

EMT is a naturalistic, conversation-based model of early language intervention that uses child interest and initiations as opportunities to model and prompt language use in everyday contexts (Kaiser, 1993). The effects of EMT have been documented over a wide range of language targets, including vocabulary and word combinations across many groups of children with language, behavior, or cognitive impairments (Hancock & Kaiser, 2006; Kaiser, Hancock, & Hester, 1998; Kaiser, Hancock, & Trent, 2007; Kaiser, Ostrosky, & Alpert, 1993). EMT/PE extends the prompting strategies of EMT to include speech recasting. Speech recasts are a subtype of recasts that target correct phonological production in response to the child's incorrect pronunciation (Camarata, 1993; Yoder, Camarata, & Gardner, 2005). This chapter focuses on using EMT/PE to teach vocabulary targets and correct sound production conjointly as part of an integrated naturalistic intervention for young children with cleft palate.

TARGET POPULATIONS AND ASSESSMENTS FOR DETERMINING INTERVENTION RELEVANCE

Primary Population

EMT/PE is designed for children with cleft lip and/or palate who are in the early stages of vocabulary acquisition and show developmental impairments in both speech sound production and lexical development. This program is also likely to be appropriate for other populations of young children with concomitant language delays and phonological impairments that are not structurally based.

Characteristics that are associated with positive response to intervention (Scherer & Kaiser, 2007) include the following: 1) verbal imitation skills, indicating a child's attempt to imitate at 75% approximated correct on a 10-item word probe (in which "approximated correct" means that intelligible attempts were considered correct imitations); 2) production of 5–10 word approximations reported by parents; 3) mean length of utterances (MLUs) between 1.0 and 2.5; and 4) repaired cleft lip/palate.

Assessment Methods for Determining Intervention Relevance

Assessment to determine whether EMT/PE is likely to be appropriate for a child should include a combination of standardized measures of receptive and expressive language, parent report of child vocabulary and imitation skills, single word expressive naming, a spontaneous language sample, and oral mechanism examination (Peterson-Falzone, Trost-Cardamone, Karnell, & Hardin-Jones, 2006). Table 18.1 summarizes the assessment tools used for this intervention.

The standardized language tests and MLU from the language sample provide a comparison with peers as well as an estimate of language level. Measures of lexical development from a parent report inventory (the MacArthur-Bates Communicative Development Inventories [CDIs]; Fenson et al., 2007) and language sample (number of total and different words used in the sample) provide estimates of vocabulary size and diversity. These measures provide a baseline level of performance and are used in the target word selection process. Speech sound measures should include single words and connected speech contexts. Single words are best elicited in a naming activity with objects or pictures. The object naming activities may be embedded within play for very young children, whereas picture naming may be used for children who can respond to a picture-naming task. The goal of the single-word naming activity is to sample consonants in at least initial and final word contexts.

PEEPS: Profile of Early Expressive Phonological Skills (Williams & Stoel-Gammon, 2008) is a new assessment of phonology in a picture-naming task developed for children in the early stages of phonological development. Analysis of children's production of single words should include both independent and relational measures of phonological development, including consonant inventory, percentage of consonants correct (PCC) (Shriberg, Austin, Lewis, McSweeny, & Wilson, 1987), developmental and compensatory errors, and positional constraints. Ratings of nasal emission on consonant production during the speech sample provide a baseline measure of resonance. Resonance ratings may change as the child's experience with word production increases. Instrumental assessment of resonance is not conducted until children have consistent use of words on

Table 18.1. Pre- and postintervention assessment

Assessment area	Measures
Receptive/expressive language functioning	Receptive and expressive standard scores for age
	MLU from language sample
Lexical development	Language sample (SALT)
	Total number of words
	Number of different words
	Parent questionnaire (CDIs)
	Vocabulary size
Speech sound development	Single word naming/connected speech
	Consonant inventory
	PCC
	Developmental/compensatory error analysis
	Speech resonance rating
Oral mechanism status	Presence of palatal fistulae

Key: MLU, mean length of utterance; SALT, Systematic Analysis of Language Transcripts; CDI, MacArthur-Bates Communicative Development Inventories; PCC, percentage of consonants correct.

request and sufficient developmental maturity to comply with the procedures. The assessment should be repeated following intervention in order to examine change on the speech measures.

THEORETICAL BASIS

Dominant Theoretical Rationale for the Intervention Approach

EMT/PE is based on EMT and adapted to include speech recasting to enhance children's correct phonological production. Thus, this section discusses the theoretical basis of EMT as it was developed to teach vocabulary and grammar to young children. This section also briefly considers the theoretical bases for recasting phonological features because this process is included in the adaptation of EMT specifically for children with phonological delays.

Enhanced Milieu Teaching

EMT procedures derive from three distinct theoretical perspectives on early language learning: behavioral, developmental-social interactionist, and parents as speech and language facilitators. EMT is grounded in behavioral principles for prompting, reinforcing, modeling, and shaping new language. Imitation and production practice with feedback are essential child behaviors for learning in this framework. Embedded in the four milieu prompting procedures (model, mand-model, time delay, and incidental teaching) are strategies for shifting control of the child responses from imitation (model), to responses to questions and mands (mand-model), to the child initiating requests and comments (time delay and incidental teaching). The behavioral paradigm dictates what will be taught in EMT: specific targets that are functional in the child's immediate environment.

Selection of targets in EMT is, however, driven by both functional and developmental considerations. A general developmental sequence for semantic and syntactic forms is followed in selecting targets for the early stages of learning (e.g., Brown's stages I–IV), and specific lexical items (e.g., nouns, verbs, modifiers) are typical words for early language learners. Traditionally, child targets are vocabulary, semantic, and early syntactic classes. The specific examples taught are those that are immediately functional in the child's environment. For children with cleft lip and/or palate, it is important to maintain this functional perspective while also selecting words on the basis of their sound composition.

The behavioral perspective dictates a strong interest in critical phases of learning: acquisition, generalization, and maintenance. EMT embodies the core principles for promoting generalization that were first outlined by Stokes and Baer (1977), including teaching multiple exemplars, teaching with multiple trainers, teaching in multiple settings, loose training (allowing natural variations in stimuli and reinforcers to occur), and training specifically to promote generalization to functional contexts. For children with cleft lip and/or palate, generalized changes in patterns of sound production across linguistic and social contexts may be challenging. Thus, it may be particularly important for children with cleft lip and/or palate to use multiple contexts (e.g., play in clinic with clinician, routines at home with parent) and multiple exemplars (words with sounds in varying positions, words composed of sounds both within and outside the children's initial repertoires, and words embedded in varied phrases and sentences).

A second theoretical strand in EMT is a social interactionist perspective on the learning of language through meaningful communicative interactions (Bruner, 1975). From this perspective, language is learned in the context of social interaction, particularly interactions between children and their caregivers. The responsiveness of the caregiver to the child's communicative attempts provides a framework in which models of new language (without prompts to imitate), occurring contiguously with the child's focus of attention and actions, support the child's learning new forms and meanings. Language learning in this model is driven by the social purpose of communication. The adult plays a critical role in reading the child's intentions and providing language that maps the child's interests and focus. EMT emphasizes reciprocity, turn taking, following the child's lead in play and conversation, semantically contingent (meaningful) feedback, and expansions of child utterances to model more complete forms. Developmental studies have shown these interactional strategies to be associated with optimal language learning in typical mother–child dyads (Moerk, 1992). It is relatively easy to blend procedures derived from behavioral and social interactionist perspectives because both perspectives maintain the importance of modeling language in context to promote acquisition of meaning and forms (Hancock & Kaiser, 2006). Consistent with the social interactionist perspective and emphasis on language use in everyday, functional contexts, EMT frequently includes parents as language facilitators (Hancock & Kaiser, 2002). Both behavioral and developmental social interactionist theories support the involvement of primary caregivers in child language intervention. The behavioral perspective emphasizes that language is learned when it is functional for communication; such learning occurs in environments that provide both stimuli (e.g., contexts, setting events, specific social communicative events) and contingencies for a child's attempts to communicate. Generalization is promoted when the stimuli and consequence of language occur in the natural environment; thus, parents in everyday settings are likely to use naturally occurring stimuli (events, objects, interaction) to teach language, and the child is likely to be reinforced by the functional consequences of his or her communication. In the social interactionist perspective, the ongoing interactions between child and parent provide social meaning, physical proximity, and an affective relationship that will be supportive of language learning. Parents are ideal teachers because of their likely responsiveness to child communicative attempts, their ability to closely monitor child communicative attempts based on proximity to the child, and their ability to provide language that elaborates those attempts. In typical learners, parent linguistic modeling and responsiveness to communication shapes early language development; thus, a social interaction perspective on early intervention places parents in the key role as teachers of new language in the context of ongoing parent–child interactions (Kaiser et al., 1998).

Recasting Phonological Forms

In a social interactionist perspective, language acquisition is facilitated when adult input is verbally responsive and closely matches the content and structure of the child's productions (Snow, 1994). Adult recasting of child utterances into their correct form is a parental response process that enhances broad aspects of language performance (Camarata, 1993, 1995, 1996). Recasts are 1) contingent upon the child's spontaneous utterance; 2) share the referential context and central meaning of the platform utterance; 3) reformulate constituents found in the platform utterance; and 4) provide an immediate contrast between an adult form and the form of the platform utterance, frequently correcting the child's form (Conti-Ramsden, Hutcheson, & Grove, 1995; Fey, Krulik, Loeb, & Proctor-Williams, 1999; Nelson & Welsh, 1998).

TARGET AREAS OF INTERVENTION

EMT/PE intervenes in vocabulary and speech sound production simultaneously.

EMPIRICAL BASIS

Research Outcomes

The effects of naturalistic language interventions implemented by parents, teachers, and clinicians have been systematically examined in more than 50 studies spanning the last 30 years. Five variations of naturalistic teaching have been developed and tested: 1) traditional milieu teaching (MT); 2) responsive interaction (RI); 3) EMT; 4) blended EMT and behavior intervention; and 5) EMT/PE, as discussed in this chapter. EMT is a hybrid of the MT and RI approaches and will be discussed as part of the EMT/PE approach. The blended EMT and behavioral approaches are not discussed here but a description is provided in Hancock, Kaiser, and Delaney (2002). The synthesis of these approaches is ideal for parent implementation because it builds responsiveness within the parent–child relationship while providing the child with specific support for language production. The EMT/PE model makes specific adaptations to EMT to promote concurrent learning of language and speech forms. Parents learn strategies for modeling language, prompting functional communication, and recasting phonological forms within a naturalistic teaching paradigm.

Milieu Teaching

MT is a conversation-based model of early language intervention that uses child interest and initiations as opportunities to model and prompt language use in everyday contexts (Hart & Rogers-Warren [Kaiser], 1978). Experimental applications of MT typically have included four sequential steps: 1) arranging the environment to increase the likelihood that the child will initiate communication with the adult; 2) selecting specific language targets appropriate to the child's skill level; 3) responding to the child's initiations with prompts for elaborated language consistent with the child's targeted skills; and 4) functionally reinforcing the child's communicative attempts by providing access to requested objects, continued adult interaction, and feedback in the form of expansions and confirmations of the child's utterances (see Kaiser, Yoder, & Keetz, 1992, for a partial review).

The authors' model of MT extended and specified the incidental teaching model of Hart and Risley (1968, 1975) to include four related procedures: 1) elicitive model, 2) mand-model, 3) time delay, and 4) incidental teaching. In an early efficacy study, Alpert and Kaiser (1992) investigated the effects of teaching six mothers of preschoolers with language impairments to use these four milieu language training procedures. The children participating in the study were all boys between the ages of 35 and 51 months who had at least a 10-month expressive delay (range of 11–27 months) at the beginning of the study. In addition, four of the six boys had a severe articulation disorder. A multiple baseline design across pairs of mother–child dyads and within each dyad across milieu techniques was used to evaluate the effects of training. All mothers learned the milieu procedures; all children in the study increased their use of total and spontaneous targets during their mothers' implementation of the MT procedures. All mothers used MT during home observation sessions. Mothers also generalized use of these techniques to two nontraining situations (domestic chore and "television on") and showed acceptable levels of maintenance 3 months after training was completed. Comparison of child language behaviors at baseline and maintenance showed improvements in three areas for four of the six children. Specifically, average monthly gains in MLU exceeded or were approximately equal to the increase predicted for typically developing children, the number of total words produced and the number of novel words produced more than doubled, and the number of the children's communicative requests increased. Two of six children did not show clinically significant gains on these developmental measures (which were collected by an adult not involved in training). The findings of this study suggested that mothers could be taught to correctly apply milieu language teaching procedures and that use of these procedures may have a positive effect on children's acquisition of new vocabulary, early syntactic/semantic forms, and appropriate use of requests.

Responsive Interaction

RI includes a set of behaviors (e.g., following the child's lead, responding to the child's verbal and nonverbal initiations, providing meaningful semantic feedback, expanding the child's utterances) that maintain the child's interest in the conversation and provide linguistic models slightly in advance of the child's current language (Kaiser & Delaney, 2001). MT can be compared with RI in a series of studies with parents and teachers. In one of the early efficacy studies, Kaiser, Alpert, Fischer, Hemmeter, Tiernan, and Ostrosky (1990) compared the effects of parent-implemented RI with parent-implemented MT on children's language outcomes. Thirty-six preschool-age children with developmental disabilities and their parents were randomly assigned to either the RI condition ($n = 18$) or MT ($n = 18$). Parents in both groups completed 24 individualized sessions, with similar child language targets taught in the RI and MT interventions. The majority of parents reached preset criterion levels for the strategies taught in their assigned intervention group. No main effects for intervention type were observed; children in both groups showed improvements in language skills from pre- to posttesting. Children at the lower end of the language continuum (MLU < 1.8) appeared to respond better to the MT intervention, whereas children at the upper end of the language continuum (MLU > 3.0) responded somewhat better to the RI intervention.

In one of the later efficacy studies, Kaiser and colleagues (1996) evaluated the effectiveness of parent-implemented RI on the language and communication skills of preschool children with disabilities. Twelve parents participated in individual training sessions. A multiple baseline design across groups of families was used to evaluate the parents' use of the intervention strategies and the effects of the intervention on the children's language skills. Results indicated that all parents learned to use the procedures after 20 sessions in the clinic and generalized their use of the procedures to interaction sessions conducted in the home. Although there was variability in child outcomes, positive effects were observed for all children. Maintenance sessions conducted with 9 of the 12 parents 6 months after the end of training indicated that all of these parents maintained their use of the procedures. In addition, seven of the nine children who participated in the maintenance sessions were observed to use their targeted language spontaneously at levels comparable to or higher than the levels achieved during intervention. All parents indicated that they were highly satisfied with their participation in the intervention and the effects of the intervention on their children's language and communication skills.

Enhanced Milieu Teaching With Phonological Emphasis

EMT/PE adapts the EMT model to provide support for phonological change simultaneously with language. Both language (vocabulary) and speech targets are identified and used to determine target words for intervention. The EMT components discussed previously facilitate the target vocabulary use, and speech recasting is added to the EMT prompting options to provide correction strategies for target sounds. Two preliminary studies have explored the effects of EMT/PE on the early speech development of children with cleft lip and/or palate. Scherer (1999) investigated the effects of EMT/PE provided by speech-language pathologists on the speech sound development of three toddlers with cleft palate using a multiple baseline design. Extensive pre- and postintervention assessment described the hearing, general receptive and expressive language, vocabulary, MLU, speech sound inventories, and speech sound accuracy used by the children in a spontaneous language sample. Following the EMT/PE intervention, the children increased their vocabulary use. In addition, the children increased their sound inventories and speech sound accuracy without intervention directly on speech sounds. A reduction in compensatory articulation error use was reported for one child (Scherer, 1999).

A second study compared focused stimulation and EMT/PE in an alternating treatment design with two toddlers with cleft lip and palate (Scherer, 2006). This study also compared the role of lexical selectivity on the acquisition of vocabulary containing sounds within the children's sound inventory compared with words outside their inventory during these two interventions. The study showed that EMT/PE was more effective in eliciting words containing sounds outside the children's sound inventories than focused stimulation. Both interventions facilitated increased sound inventories at about the same rate. These intervention studies yielded substantial preliminary information regarding the intervention procedures that had the most beneficial outcome for speech production.

Compensatory articulation errors are of particular concern in children with cleft lip and/or palate because once habituated, these patterns are particularly resistant to intervention at older ages (Kuehn & Moller, 2000; Peterson-Falzone, Hardin-Jones, & Karnell, 2001). Broadly defined, these are sounds made by shifting the place of articulation posteriorly in the vocal tract. Studies of early vocal development have described a range of compensatory articulation patterns including glottal stops, velar and pharyngeal fricatives, posterior nasal fricatives, and nasal substitutions (Chapman, Hardin-Jones, Schulte, & Halter, 2001; Morris & Ozanne, 2003; O'Gara & Logemann, 1988; Salas-Provance, Kuehn, & Marsh, 2003; Trost, 1981). Golding-Kushner (2001) estimated that at least 25% of preschool-age children with cleft lip and/or palate undergo speech therapy for compensatory errors, with glottal stops being the most frequent form of compensatory error.

Research examining the impact of early intervention on the development of compensatory articulation patterns is limited. Scherer, D'Antonio, and McGahey (2008) reported that 50% of the toddlers in their study showed some use of glottal stop substitutions, and 35% of the children used glottal stop substitutions consistently in their speech. Broen, Doyle, and Bacon (1993) reported a single case study in which intervention was conducted to increase the use of consonants across the manner categories of nasal and stop consonant groups (m, b, p, n, t, d, ŋ, k, g). Although the study showed an increase in nasal and stop consonants, an increase in use of glottal stops was also observed during intervention.

In addition to the SSD characteristic of children with cleft lip and/or palate, studies of early language development indicate that these children show delays in onset of first words and early expressive vocabulary development (Broen, Devers, Doyle, Prouty, & Moller, 1998; Chapman, Hardin-Jones, & Halter, 2003; Jocelyn, Penko, & Rode, 1996; Olson, 1965; Scherer, D'Antonio, & Kalbfleisch, 1999). The presence of both vocabulary and speech impairments suggests an interaction between limited sound production and early vocabulary development. Two studies have examined the relationship between sound production and lexical learning in children with cleft lip and/or palate. Estrem and Broen (1989) assessed the speech characteristics of five young children with cleft lip and/or palate and five children without clefts during acquisition of their first 50 words. The children with cleft lip and/or palate produced more words beginning with nasals, vowels, and glides and produced fewer words beginning with oral stop consonants than the children without clefts, suggesting a relationship between lexical choice and speech sound production limitations. Scherer (1999) explored the relationship between lexical selectivity and SSD in an intervention study. She found that young children with cleft lip and/or palate learned words with sounds that were within their consonant inventories faster than words with sounds that were outside their inventories. Together these preliminary studies suggest that children with cleft lip and/or palate display speech sound limitations during the first year of life that may impact early vocabulary learning.

Intervention models to date for children with cleft lip and/or palate have emphasized articulation approaches that intervene directly in the production of speech sounds (Peterson-Falzone et al., 2001; Peterson-Falzone et al., 2006). Historically, the approach used most frequently was the sound-by-sound approach that treated one sound at a time in a sequential manner from isolated sound to syllable, word, phrase, sentence, and conversation levels (Golding-Kushner, 2001; Peterson-Falzone et al., 2001). This sound-by-sound approach has persisted despite the availability of phonological approaches that would address multiple sounds simultaneously (Van Demark & Hardin, 1986). In a study by Pamplona, Ysunza, and Espinosa (1999), a sound-by-sound approach was compared with a multiple sound approach, and the multiple sound approach resulted in a shorter course of intervention. However, the effectiveness of either approach in eliminating compensatory articulation patterns has not received much attention in the literature and may account for the restricted use of phonological approaches for young children with cleft lip and/or palate. From the data reported in early studies (Broen et al., 1993; Van Demark & Hardin, 1986), it appears that children could have reduced their compensatory articulation use but did not maintain that success following the studies. One such exception was a study conducted by Pamplona, Ysunza, Gonzalez, and Ramirez (2004) in which they compared responses to a multiple sound approach and language intervention. Both interventions were equally effective in reducing compensatory articulation use in terms of length of intervention; however, the language intervention resulted in better maintenance over a 3-month interval.

Summary of Levels of Evidence

The modification of EMT with phonological emphasis using speech recasts is a recent adaptation of EMT. A randomized pilot study of EMT/PE and a community-based intervention is currently under way by the authors. Table 18.2 summarizes the levels of evidence for the research reviewed in the preceding section.

PRACTICAL REQUIREMENTS

Data from the existing intervention literature for young children with cleft lip and/or palate suggests the following optimal conditions for early speech and language intervention: 1) target both speech and language, particularly vocabulary, 2) deliver intervention in transactions with the child that promote functional use of language in meaningful interactions, 3) provide models of lexicon that facilitate phonological advancement through modeling and recasting, 4) increase feedback to the child resulting in correct lexical and phonological production, 5) increase child production practice, and 6) have parents deliver intervention across settings beyond the traditional clinical setting in functional communicative activities that promote generalization and maintenance with sufficient intensity to accelerate development. When these conditions are met, children

Table 18.2. Levels of evidence for studies of treatment efficacy for enhanced milieu teaching with phonological emphasis

Level	Description	References
Ia	Meta-analysis of > 1 randomized controlled trial	—
Ib	Randomized controlled study	—
IIa	Controlled study without randomization	Scherer (1999); Scherer, D'Antonio, & McGahey (2008)
IIb	Quasi-experimental study	—
III	Nonexperimental studies, i.e., correlational and case studies	Scherer & Kaiser (2007)
IV	Expert committee report, consensus conference, clinical experience of respected authorities	Kaiser (2004, personal communication)

Adapted from the Scottish Intercollegiate Guidelines Network (http://www.sign.ac.uk).

with cleft lip and/or palate may overcome the impact of their early impairments faster and reduce the likelihood that they will habituate early compensatory articulation production. Determining an optimal early intervention program is a next step toward increasing the efficacy of early speech and language interventions for children with cleft lip and/or palate.

Nature of the Sessions and Personnel

For Clinicians

Clinicians must have experience delivering EMT/PE methods in order to reliably execute the program components and train parents. A basic understanding and experience implementing generic naturalistic intervention programs is beneficial. For clinicians who have used naturalistic intervention methods, EMT/PE components will be familiar, but the authors feel that attention to several components of the program is warranted. First, it is important to maximize target word exposure. Selecting and updating target words once the child has achieved the criterion performance is important to promote generalization. Data collection and graphing of child responses provide important feedback regarding the implementation of the EMT/PE components. In addition, some clinicians may maintain use of prompting to elicit imitation longer than is necessary. It is important to transition from strategies that prompt elicited imitation to strategies that facilitate spontaneous production. It is recommended that clinicians administer EMT/PE procedures with three children in order to gain sufficient experience with procedures to optimize training effectiveness and enhance credibility with parents.

For Parents

The EMT/PE procedures are implemented using the therapist–parent model developed by Kaiser (1993; Kaiser et al., 1998, 2007). In this model, the clinician provides intervention to the child from the beginning of the intervention phase. Concurrently, the parent observes the trainer sessions, learns the naturalistic teaching procedures, practices them in the clinic with coaching from the clinician, and generalizes his or her newly learned skills to the home setting. The parent's generalized teaching is presumed to affect the child's functional use of language at home, resulting in better generalization and developmental outcomes.

Parents are taught to implement components of EMT/PE during individual sessions in the clinic, corresponding with the trainer-implemented intervention sessions. Parents are taught using a variety of techniques and modalities including standardized written and verbal information; modeling through clinician demonstration; role playing; videotapes; verbal, written, and graphic feedback; viewing videotapes of previous sessions; and evaluations of child progress (Hemmeter & Kaiser, 1994; Kaiser & Hancock, 2000). A typical daily intervention schedule is provided in Table 18.3.

Dosage

The sequence of introducing EMT/PE to parents is based on the well-defined EMT training sequence for parents that takes 20–36 sessions (depending on parent pretreatment skills) to reach criterion on all components of the program (see Table 18.3; Camarata, 1993; Hancock & Kaiser, 2006; Kaiser et al., 1998; Kaiser & Hancock, 2003).

Table 18.3. Organization of intervention sessions and parent training sessions

Typical session schedule	0–10 minutes: Review home assignments and strategies or introduce new strategy
	10–30 minutes: Clinician demonstrates strategy with the child
	30–45 minutes: Parent practices strategy with clinician coaching
	45–50 minutes: Clinician provides feedback and guidelines for home interactions
Sequence of content in parent training sessions	1. Orienting child to target words and using play routines as a context for child learning
	2. Choosing materials and arranging the environment to promote engagement and requesting
	3–4. Talking at the child's level and modeling of target words
	5. Using phonological recasts to respond to target words
	6. Providing choice making to facilitate target words
	7. Using expansions at the child's target level
	8. Incidental teaching 1: using models after requests
	9. Incidental teaching 2: using mand-model after child requests
	10. Time delay
	11. Putting it all together: balancing responsiveness and milieu teaching
	12–20. Practice teaching targets, increasing parent fluency, and promoting generalization to home

KEY COMPONENTS

The components of EMT/PE include the key components of EMT, which involve arranging the environment to foster engagement and scaffolding the adult interactions with the child to encourage balanced conversational turn taking. Production of specific target vocabulary and other communicatively appropriate forms is facilitated using prompts as developed in the MT prompting procedures (model, mand-model, time delay, incidental teaching [Hancock & Kaiser, 2006]). In EMT/PE, the selection of target words is critical because it integrates both vocabulary and speech sound production goals. EMT/PE includes two elements to facilitate speech production goals: 1) a phonetic awareness component to promote awareness of phonetic placement associated with phonological targets and 2) use of phonological recasting to provide correct, contrasting models of speech production.

Nature of Goals: Target Vocabulary Selection

Target words are selected to reflect both vocabulary and phonological targets. To select these words, a consonant inventory is developed, then target words are selected from the CDIs (Fenson et al., 2007). The consonant inventory is established based on the results of a spontaneous language sample using the criteria of two uses to credit the sound within the child's inventory (Stoel-Gammon, 1989). Target words are identified that include sounds within and outside the children's sound inventory (i.e., not used in the speech sample). Using words with sounds within and outside their current inventory ensure that children will have some early success in speech production as well as opportunities to hear specific contrasts between existing sounds (usually nasals) and new sound targets (oral consonants). The word set based on sounds within the children's sound inventory (WI) includes words containing consonants within the inventory and syllable structures documented in the language sample. The second word set includes words with at least one consonant outside the children's sound inventory (OI) and syllable structures documented in the language sample. Positional constraints evident in the consonant inventory are avoided when selecting the first WI and OI target sounds. Later, positional constraints are addressed in the target words if they have not changed as a result of the intervention. Probes for production of the target words are collected routinely before and after the interactional play portion of the intervention.

Phonetic Awareness

Some children may need additional activities outside the EMT/PE intervention session to acquaint them with phonetic placement. Activities to promote new consonant production and oral airflow may include play activities to stimulate sounds (e.g., animal noises or motor noises [i.e., babababa]), gestures plus sounds (e.g., *shhhhh* to request quiet), and limited activities to direct oral airflow, such as limited use of low resistance blowing toys (e.g., bubbles, whistles, horns/flutes). Plugging the nose may assist the child to direct the airstream through the mouth.

Speech Recasts

This strategy provides a cue to the child to modify substitution or omission errors within naturalistic interaction. Recasting is the repetition of the child's utterance using correct grammatical and/or phonological forms (Camarata, 1995; Camarata & Nelson, 2006). Speech recasts are those recasts that provide correct phonological information in response to a child's incorrect production. For example, the child may say [ba] for *ball*, and the adult would provide a speech recast by responding with, "Ball. You want the ball?" The effectiveness of speech recasts has been described within naturalistic conversational intervention for preschool children with speech and language impairments (Camarata, 1993; Yoder et al., 2005). Scherer (1999), Scherer and Kaiser (2007), and Scherer, D'Antonio and McGahey (2008) have applied speech recasts to children younger than 3 years of age with organic speech disorders by embedding speech recasts into the EMT model. The EMT procedures, especially environmental arrangement and responsive interaction, provide the foundation for child engagement. If the child initiates with target vocabulary, then expansions are used to provide models of greater linguistic complexity. If the child does not use target vocabulary or produces the vocabulary with phonological errors, then corrective prompts are used to facilitate vocabulary or speech targets.

Goal Attack Strategies: Vocabulary Facilitation

Environmental Arrangement

Environmental arrangement is designed to increase the child's engagement with the physical setting, which then can provide more frequent opportunities for the adult to communicate with the child, elicit communicative responses, model appropriate language forms, and respond contingently to the child's verbal and nonverbal communication attempts. Parents are taught to select toys and materials that are of interest to the child, to engage in play with the child with the toys and materials, and to match and elaborate the child's play schemes as a means of promoting and enhancing the child's engagement with the environment.

Three environmental strategies to select, arrange, and manage materials have been shown to increase the likelihood that children will show interest in the environment and make communicative attempts (Kaiser et al., 2007). The goal of these strategies is to engage the child in activities that promote vocalizations and word attempts. These strategies provide a context for prompting vocabulary as well as facilitating spontaneous production attempts that can be recast by the adult to include phonologically correct models. Table 18.4 provides a description of environmental strategies to select, arrange, and manage materials to increase the likelihood the child will initiate and maintain communicative interaction.

Responsive Interaction

In the RI component of EMT, emphasis is placed on developing a conversational style of interaction that promotes balanced turn taking between adult and child while providing models of appropriate language. The basic RI strategies include the interactional compo-

Table 18.4.   Principles of environmental arrangement

Selecting materials	Select toys/materials that are high preference and interesting to the child.
	Select toys with multiple parts (e.g., Legos, Mr. Potato Head) or add-ons (e.g., add the barnyard animals to water play) to extend topics for conversation.
	Select toys that require assistance opening (e.g., playdough) or putting together (e.g., a train track) to promote requesting.
	Select toys/tasks that require turn taking with the child (e.g., throwing and catching a ball, hiding and finding an object). Nonverbal turn taking provides a foundation for verbal turn taking (balanced conversation).
Arranging materials	Limit the number of materials/toys available to the child at any one time. Limiting materials helps the child attend to the toys he or she is playing with rather than being overwhelmed by too many toys. It also may provide an opportunity for the child to request additional materials.
	Have some toys in the child's view but out of reach (e.g., on a high shelf or in plastic containers up on a counter).
	Keep toys in containers that the child will need assistance opening.
Managing materials	Be a gatekeeper. Place yourself between the child and the materials or keep some portion of the materials in your control.
	Seat the child in a highchair or in a location that limits his or her easy access to toys.
	When the child seems to start losing interest, add in materials to keep the play going. Be creative as you mix toys and materials that may not generally go together. For example, add food coloring to water play or have the barnyard animals go through the car wash made for the Matchbox cars.
	When the child does not receive all of the toys or materials at once, there is an opportunity for the child to request more. For example, give him or her two Lego blocks instead of the whole container of Legos.
	Provide incomplete toy sets. You can also provide an opportunity for the child to communicate with you by not providing all the materials he or she might need for an activity. For example, you could give the child a jar of bubbles without a wand so that he or she will need to ask for the material.
	Provide opportunities for unexpected events. For example, if you put Mr. Potato Head's arm where his eye goes, your child may use language to tell you that it is wrong or to move it to the right location.

nents of responsiveness (e.g., responding to every child communication attempt, responding to the meaning of child utterances with related comments or questions), following the child's lead in play and conversation, facilitating turn taking, and matching and extending the child's topic. Language modeling strategies include passive techniques to match the child's linguistic level, imitate or mirror the child's words and actions, and systematically expand the child's utterances while maintaining child meanings.

Milieu Teaching Procedures

The third component of EMT includes the milieu prompting procedures embedded within episodes. The four core MT procedures (i.e., elicitive modeling, mand-model, time delay, and incidental teaching procedures) are used in sequence to provide a least-to-most supportive hierarchy.

Modeling

Elicitive modeling may be considered the most fundamental MT strategy. Following the establishment of joint attention, the adult presents a verbal model of target language that is related to the child's immediate interest. The adult prompts the child's production of the model with "Say [target word]." If the child imitates the model correctly, he or she receives immediate positive feedback (which includes an expansion of the child's response) and the object of interest. If the child does not respond to the initial model or responds with a partial, incorrect, or unrelated response, the adult establishes joint attention again and presents the model a second time (a corrective model). If the child responds with an unintelligible response, a speech recast is provided (discussed under Mand-Model Procedure). If the child does respond to the corrective model, the adult simply models the desired verbal response and then gives the object to the child.

Mand-Model Procedure

This procedure begins with a verbal prompt in the form of a real question (e.g., "What do you want?"), a choice (e.g., "Would you like the car or ball?"), or a mand to verbalize (e.g., "Tell me what you want"). If the child responds with a target vocabulary word, the adult acknowledges the child's response and provides the requested object. If the child does not respond or gives an incorrect response, the adult models the desired target vocabulary. By arranging the environment and presenting choices among interesting objects or activities, the adult makes the child's language immediately functional. Modeling and mand-model procedures provide a means of structuring a child's responses to facilitate the use of target vocabulary. However, it is also important to provide opportunities for the child to initiate conversation in order to foster spontaneous use of the target vocabulary. The time delay procedure (discussed in the following section) was developed to establish child initiation instead of relying on models and mands as cues for vocabulary (Halle, Baer, & Spradlin, 1981; Halle, Marshall, & Spradlin, 1979).

Time Delay

Once joint attention has been established, the adult waits for the child to initiate communication. If the child initiates but does not use his specific targets, other strategies (e.g., mands, models) can be used as follow-up prompts to elicit specific vocabulary forms.

Time delay can be an important bridging strategy for helping children who rely on prompts to move toward more independent and spontaneous use of language.

Incidental Teaching

Incidental teaching was developed to encourage children to use elaborated language in conversational interaction. The environment is arranged to promote requesting objects and assistance; ideally, the environmental arrangement includes contrasting features that make use of specific vocabulary necessary for adequate communication and for improving conversational skills. For children with cleft lip and/or palate, these strategies provide opportunities for generalization of vocabulary and speech production targets into conversational use when the child makes a request and the adult responds by modeling, manding, or delaying for a more elaborated response or for a targeted vocabulary response. A child's attempts to produce targeted vocabulary can then be recast to model the correct phonology. The child's ability to request verbally or nonverbally and the ability to imitate target forms are the only prerequisite skills for incidental teaching.

Description of Activities

EMT/PE occurs in functional play and activities of daily living both in the clinic and in the home. Each 5- to 10-minute activity is selected to promote optimal opportunity to facilitate the target words and to maintain interaction between the adult and the child.

ASSESSMENT AND PROGRESS MONITORING TO SUPPORT DECISION MAKING

Pre-Post Intervention Data

Pre- and postintervention assessment is important to compare the child's performance to age-matched peers and to provide benchmarks for progress. Baseline information regarding the child's speech, language, and resonance characteristics is critical for diagnosis and a thorough description of the child's speech and language performance. Standardized speech and language tests, such as the Preschool Language Scale-4 (PLS-4; Zimmerman, Steiner, & Pond, 2002), provide a comparison to an age-matched peer group for both receptive and expressive language. In addition, measures of vocabulary size, use, and independent and relational measures of phonology are warranted to provide baseline performance and determine intervention targets (Stoel-Gammon, 1992, 1998). The authors use the MacArthur-Bates CDIs (Fenson et al., 2007) to measure vocabulary size and a language sample to estimate vocabulary use in a routine communicative setting. Total number of words and total number of different words are calculated from a 30-minute play interaction with a parent and an object naming activity consisting of words controlled for place and manner of production. The play interaction is analyzed using Systematic Analysis of Language Transcripts (SALT; Miller & Chapman, 2007). The two language sample vocabulary measures provide an indication of how often the child is attempting words and the diversity of these words.

Phonology is assessed through an independent measure—sounds used without reference to the adult sound system—such as a consonant inventory. Following phonetic transcription of the sample, consonants produced are grouped by manner and place of articulation. A sample consonant inventory is provided in Appendix 18A. Two relational measures are conducted to assess sound errors relative to the adult system. A general measure, PCC (Shriberg et al., 1987), is used to assess speech sound accuracy. In addition, an error analysis is conducted to identify consonant substitutions, deletions, and omissions for the sample used to calculate PCC. Percent compensatory error use is also calculated, as is percent nasal substitution, because these two error patterns may be particularly problematic in young children with cleft lip and/or palate (Scherer, D'Antonio, et al., 2008). Finally, nasal emission is transcribed for the consonants produced in the sample.

Session Data

Observational data collected during each session includes measures of both the child's communication (vocabulary and phonological correctness) and adult use of the EMT/PE strategies. During sessions, it is important to indicate if the child uses targets as spontaneous initiations, responses to prompts, or imitations of the adult's language. In addition, probes using pictures may be administered before or after the interaction sessions to measure child acquisition of targets under more controlled conditions. Trial-by-trial data are collected in response to picture probes of target words. Child measures of target vocabulary and phonology include the frequency of imitative and spontaneous target word use and PCC for target words, percent nasal and compensatory substitutions, and percent developmental errors (consisting of all other substitutions and omissions). A sample analysis spreadsheet for examining children's performance in interactions and in probes is provided in Appendix 18B. Adult administration of the EMT/PE procedures during the intervention is also important to monitor. Data on the use of the procedures in daily sessions informs the clinician about the supports being provided to the child. For example, if the goal for the child is to move from responding to initiation, it would be important to see the adult using time delay and incidental teaching frequently during the interaction rather than relying on modeling and mand-models that facilitate responding. Even clinicians who are experienced with EMT require this feedback to adjust their implementation during the course of intervention. The EMT implementation checklist (see Figure 18.1) is a means of assessing the adult's use of EMT procedures from a videotaped clip of the session.

Generalization Data

Other areas of data collection include gaining information about the child's use of the target words inside and outside of the therapy setting, especially in the home environment. Home visits to facilitate parent training and assess the home environment provide insight into obstacles to generalization (e.g., parent does not understand the child's communication attempts, parent is prompting the child without waiting for the child to indicate interest). Alternatively, parents are often willing to provide videotaped excerpts of the child's play interaction at home. In addition, a weekly questionnaire regarding target words and sounds can be carefully structured and then used to help parents observe and report about their child's communication. Information regarding generalization of the targets at home is valuable to the clinician when determining the type of EMT prompting that should be emphasized or the amount of parent training that should be provided. For

Enhanced Milieu Teaching Implementation Checklist

	Not Observed	Poor	Adequate	Good	Excellent
1. Environmental arrangement					
Play area is well organized	1	2	3	4	5
Selection of activities is appropriate	1	2	3	4	5
Length of activities is appropriate	1	2	3	4	5
Arrangement encourages engagement	1	2	3	4	5
Activities are available	1	2	3	4	5
2. Clinician style and affect					
Clinician responds quickly to child	1	2	3	4	5
Clinician is warm and positive	1	2	3	4	5
Clinician listens to child	1	2	3	4	5
Clinician often at child's eye level	1	2	3	4	5
3. Enhanced milieu teaching					
Clinician engages in conversation with child	1	2	3	4	5
Clinician talks at child level	1	2	3	4	5
Clinician responds to content of child talk	1	2	3	4	5
Clinician expands child utterances	1	2	3	4	5
Clinician talks about what child is doing	1	2	3	4	5
Clinician balances turns with child	1	2	3	4	5
Clinician engages in child's activity	1	2	3	4	5
Clinician prompts language at target levels	1	2	3	4	5
Clinician prompts in response to child's requests	1	2	3	4	5
Clinician follows through on prompts for language	1	2	3	4	5
4. Circle prompting techniques observed					
• Model	1	2	3	4	5
• Mand	1	2	3	4	5
• Time delay (wait)	1	2	3	4	5
• Incidental teaching	1	2	3	4	5
• Recast	1	2	3	4	5
5. Summary of observation					
Opportunities for modeling	1	2	3	4	5
Quality of interaction	1	2	3	4	5
Levels of prompting	1	2	3	4	5
Positive responding to child	1	2	3	4	5
Child's behavior well managed	1	2	3	4	5
Child participation	1	2	3	4	5

Figure 18.1. Enhanced milieu teaching implementation checklist.

example, a child who is not generalizing targets may require more support outside of the therapy setting; for example, by increasing levels of parent training.

CONSIDERATIONS FOR CHILDREN FROM CULTURALLY AND LINGUISTICALLY DIVERSE BACKGROUNDS

When using EMT with different cultural and linguistic groups, we must consider the intersect between the cultural or linguistic group and 1) specific EMT strategies; 2) specific EMT behavioral outcomes; and 3) the venue for EMT intervention, including toys and materials used in the play-based interaction.

Enhanced Milieu Teaching Strategies

EMT is anchored in a responsive, contingent adult–child interaction. When considering the appropriateness of applying an EMT intervention within any culture, it would be important to consider the norms for such responsiveness within that culture. Considering the culture's norms around behaviors that are foundational to responsiveness, such as eye contact, touch, and physical closeness, would be especially important. If the professional is unfamiliar with a culture, observing naturally occurring parent–child interactions within that culture may provide valuable information. The families with whom we are working have some baseline rate of the strategies we are trying to teach, but we are often asking them to implement the strategies more frequently or more systematically than they are using them in their natural interactions. A cultural informant independent from the parent may also provide some helpful information allowing the professional to determine the appropriateness of EMT strategies within that culture and if what is being observed with the parent may be individual variation within that culture.

Enhanced Milieu Teaching Outcomes

A second consideration when determining the appropriateness of EMT for members of a specific cultural/linguistic group involves the language forms targeted for the EMT intervention. Successful language outcomes of EMT are often driven by the extent to which the adult can model and elicit developmentally appropriate targets for individual children. One implicit requirement in implementing EMT successfully is that adults must be relatively competent in the language in which they will teach children. Competence includes sufficient vocabulary and grammatical knowledge to make the adjustments needed when talking at the child's targeted language level. This can be an issue when the parent's first language is not English, or when parents have learning or language-related difficulties. The authors have had parents who were English speakers who were not metalinguistically sophisticated enough to be able to teach their child's specific targets. These parents had difficulty when children's targets were longer than three words (e.g., agent–action–preposition–object). Although these parents did learn to increase their responsiveness and globally expand their children's utterances, they had difficulty modeling specific linguistic structures and sometimes giving systematic corrective feedback. It is important, regardless of cultural background or first language, to determine whether a parent's language competence will support teaching specific linguistic targets beyond a three-word level.

Enhanced Milieu Teaching Venue

Because EMT intervention generally occurs within a play context, it is important for an interventionist to select culturally appropriate toys and materials. Often this may mean supplementing existing toys so that there are more culturally appropriate choices. For example, when working with African American families, use of African American dolls and culturally appropriate hair products for a hairdressing play scheme may be appropriate. Open communication with parents and cultural informants can be helpful in determining creative and appropriate ways to supplement toys and materials or to choose familiar activities. In addition, in some cultures, sustained play with a child does not occur in the home. Although the goal of EMT is use across everyday environments, initially teaching and practicing EMT skills is easiest using play as a context. It is important to discuss the rationale for this approach with parents, ask them to participate in play during training, and encourage them to create a comfortable context at home to practice the EMT strategies.

It is also important to systematically ask every parent to provide written and informal verbal feedback about teaching procedures, materials and toys, and expectations for practice at home, as there is much to be learned about adapting EMT for families from varied cultures.

CASE STUDY

B.F. is a 24-month-old with velocardiofacial syndrome. He had an isolated cleft palate, which was repaired at 18 months of age. His intervention began at 9 months of age and was conducted on a weekly basis until after palatal surgery, when it increased to twice weekly. On preintervention assessment, B.F. showed a receptive-expressive language delay (standard score of < 50 on both subscales on the PLS-4). He was using one word occasionally at home as reported by the parents on the CDIs. A second preintervention session was conducted to administer a picture/object naming activity to provide more opportunities to assess speech production that occurred in the language sample. B.F.'s speech was characterized by a small consonant inventory (two consonants) and a high use of nasal (45%) and compensatory (35%) substitutions, particularly glottal stops. His language sample contained no word use and few vocalizations, which consisted primarily of vowels, nasals, and glottal stops. Communicative attempts were limited.

Given the limited vocalizations, targets initially included increasing communicative intents and vocalizations and simultaneously increasing the use of oral consonants with reduction in nasal and glottal substitutions. Responsive interaction and environmental arrangement strategies were used initially to increase communicative attempts and vocalizations. These strategies were used until B.F. began using single words. Vocal play activities were supplemented with nasal occlusion to facilitate oral airflow.

B.F.'s frequency of word attempts increased from an occasional word per session to 50–60 words per session. Figures 18.2 and 18.3 display progress on nasal and stop consonant use across one semester.

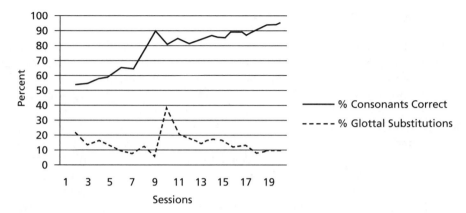

Figure 18.2. Progress with words containing nasal consonants.

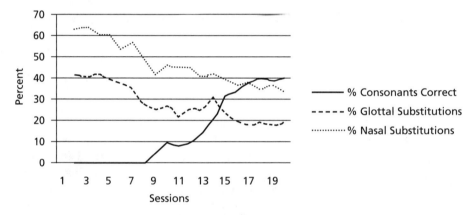

Figure 18.3. Progress with words containing oral stop consonants.

STUDY QUESTIONS

1. EMT/PE facilitates which two communicative components?

   a. verb tenses and speech sounds

   b. vocabulary and speech sounds

   c. communicative functions and speech sounds

   d. semantic relations and speech sounds

2. Generalization of goals into routine communicative interaction is enhanced through

   a. target word selection

   b. clinician use of speech recasting

    c.   parent training

    d.   transcribing data

3.   EMT/PE fosters speech development in children with cleft palate through

    a.   expansion of consonant inventories

    b.   prevention of habituation of compensatory articulation errors

    c.   reduction of phonological processes

    d.   both a and b

    e.   all of the above

FUTURE DIRECTIONS

EMT has considerable research to support its efficacy for parents and children with a variety of disabilities; however, the simultaneous targeting of both language and speech sounds is a new direction. Although there are a small number of studies supporting the use of EMT/PE, additional studies are needed to 1) compare EMT/PE to other techniques, such as focused stimulation or simple imitation training; 2) examine the long-term outcomes of the intervention on the development of both language and speech; 3) explore the use of parent-plus-therapists models of intervention that have been successful with EMT; and 4) examine the use of additional strategies (using multiple trainers, teaching sets of related targets across settings, arranging multiple environments to provide practice opportunities) for increasing generalization of correct sound production across settings and activities. For children with cleft lip and/or palate, research is needed to explore the application of EMT/PE primarily by parents as well as to evaluate methodology for integrating speech recasts into the EMT prompts. In addition, EMT/PE should be explored with other populations of children who demonstrate both speech and language impairments. Of particular interest are children with phonological impairments who frequently have concomitant language delays, children on the autism spectrum, and children with global developmental delays.

SUGGESTED READINGS

Kaiser, A.P., & Grim, J.C. (2005). Teaching functional communication skills. In M. Snell & F. Brown (Eds.), *Instruction of students with severe disabilities* (pp. 447–488). Upper Saddle River, NJ: Pearson.

Kaiser, A.P., Hancock, T.B., & Trent, J.A. (2007). Teaching parents communication strategies. *Early Childhood Services: An Interdisciplinary Journal of Effectiveness, 1,* 107–136.

Kaiser, A.P., & Trent, J.A. (2007). Communication intervention for young children with disabilities: Naturalistic approaches to promoting development. In S. Odom, R. Horner, M. Snell, & J. Blacher (Eds.), *Handbook of developmental disabilities* (pp. 224–246). New York: Guilford Press.

Scherer, N.J., D'Antonio, L., & McGahey, H. (2008). Early speech intervention for children with cleft palate. *Cleft Palate-Craniofacial Journal, 45*(1), 18–31.

Scherer, N.J., & Kaiser, A. (2007). Early intervention in children with cleft palate. *Infants & Young Children, 20,* 355–366.

REFERENCES

Alpert, C.L., & Kaiser, A. (1992). Training parents as milieu language teachers. *Journal of Early Intervention*, *16*(1), 31–52.

Broen, P.A., Devers, M.C., Doyle, S.S., Prouty, J.M., & Moller, K.T. (1998). Acquisition of linguistic and cognitive skills by children with cleft palate. *Journal of Speech, Language, and Hearing Research*, *41*, 676–687.

Broen, P.A., Doyle, S.S., & Bacon, C. (1993). The velopharyngeally inadequate child: Phonologic change with intervention. *Cleft Palate-Craniofacial Journal*, *30*(5), 500–507.

Bruner, J.S. (1975). From communication to language: A psychological perspective. *Cognition*, *3*(3), 255–287.

Camarata, S. (1993). The application of naturalistic conversation training to speech production in children with speech disabilities. *Journal of Applied Behavioral Analysis*, *26*, 173–182.

Camarata, S.M. (1995). A rationale for naturalistic speech intelligibility intervention. In S.F. Warren & J. Reichle (Series Eds.) & M.E. Fey, J. Windsor, & S.F. Warren (Vol. Eds.), *Communication and language intervention series: Vol. 5. Language intervention: Preschool through the elementary years* (pp. 63–84). Baltimore: Paul H. Brookes Publishing Co.

Camarata, S.M. (1996). On the importance of integrating naturalistic language, social intervention, and speech intelligibility training. In L. Koegel, R. Koegel & G. Dunlap (Eds.), *Positive behavioral support*. Baltimore: Paul H. Brookes Publishing Co.

Camarata, S.M., & Nelson, K.E. (2006). Conversational recast intervention with preschool and older children. In S.F. Warren & M.E. Fey (Series Eds.) & R.J. McCauley & M.E. Fey (Vol. Eds.), *Communication and language intervention series: Treatment of language disorders in children* (pp. 237–264). Baltimore: Paul H. Brookes Publishing Co.

Chapman, K., Hardin-Jones, M., & Halter, K.A. (2003). Relationship between early speech and later speech and language performance for children with cleft palate. *Clinical Linguistics and Phonetics*, *17*(3), 173–197.

Chapman, K., Hardin-Jones, M., Schulte, J., & Halter, K.A. (2001). Vocal development of 9-month-old babies with cleft palate. *Journal of Speech, Language, and Hearing Research*, *44*, 1268–1283.

Conti-Ramsden, G., Hutcheson, G.D., & Grove, J. (1995). Contingency and breakdown: Children with SLI and conversations with mothers and fathers. *Journal of Speech and Hearing Research*, *38*, 1290–1320.

Estrem, T., & Broen, P.A. (1989). Early speech production of children with cleft palate. *Journal of Speech and Hearing Research*, *32*, 12–23.

Fenson L., Marchman, V.A., Thal, D.J., Dale, P.S., Reznick, J.S., & Bates, E. (2007). *MacArthur-Bates Communicative Development Inventories* (CDIs; 2nd ed.). Baltimore: Paul H. Brookes Publishing Co.

Fey, M., Krulik, T., Loeb, D., & Proctor-Williams, K. (1999). Sentence recast use by parents of children with typical language and children with specific language impairment. *American Journal of Speech-Language Pathology*, *8*, 273–286.

Golding-Kushner, K. (2001). *Therapy techniques for cleft palate speech and related disorders*. San Diego: Singular.

Halle, J.W., Baer, D.M., & Spradlin, J.E. (1981). Teachers' generalized use of delay as a stimulus control procedure to increase language use in handicapped children. *Journal of Applied Behavior Analysis*, *14*, 387–400.

Halle, J.W., Marshall, A.M., & Spradlin, J.E. (1979). Time delay: A technique to increase language use and facilitate generalization in retarded children. *Journal of Applied Behavior Analysis*, *12*, 431–440.

Hancock, T.B., & Kaiser, A.P. (2002). The effects of trainer-implemented enhanced milieu teaching on the social communication of children who have autism. *Topics in Early Childhood Special Education*, *22*(1), 39–54.

Hancock, T.B., & Kaiser, A.P. (2006). Enhanced milieu teaching. In S.F. Warren & M.E. Fey (Series Eds.) & R.J. McCauley & M.E. Fey (Vol. Eds.), *Communication and language intervention series: Treatment of language disorders in children* (pp. 203–236). Baltimore: Paul H. Brookes Publishing Co.

Hancock, T.B., Kaiser, A.P., & Delaney, E.M. (2002). Teaching parents of high-risk preschoolers strategies to support language and positive behavior. *Topics in Early Childhood Special Education*, *22*(4), 191–212.

Hart, B.M., & Risley, T.R. (1968). Establishing the use of descriptive adjectives in the spontaneous speech of disadvantaged preschool children. *Journal of Applied Behavior Analysis*, *1*, 109–120.

Hart, B.M., & Risley, T.R. (1975). Incidental teaching of language in the preschool. *Journal of Applied Behavior Analysis*, *8*, 411–420.

Hart, B.M., & Rogers-Warren, A.K. (1978). Milieu teaching approaches. In R.L. Schiefelbusch (Ed.), *Bases of language intervention* (Vol. 2, pp. 193–235). Baltimore: University Park Press.

Hemmeter, M.L., & Kaiser, A.P. (1994). Enhanced milieu teaching: Effects of parent-implemented language intervention. *Journal of Early Intervention*, *18*, 269–289.

Jocelyn, L., Penko, M.A., & Rode, H.L. (1996). Cognition and hearing in young children with cleft lip and palate and in control children: A longitudinal study. *Pediatrics, 97*(4), 529–534.

Kaiser, A.P. (1993). Parent-implemented language intervention: An environmental system perspective. In S.F. Warren & J. Reichle (Series & Vol. Eds.) & A.P. Kaiser & D.B. Gray (Vol. Eds.), *Communication and language intervention series: Vol. 2. Enhancing children's communication: Research foundations for intervention* (pp. 63–84). Baltimore: Paul H. Brookes Publishing Co.

Kaiser, A.P., Alpert, C.L., Fischer, R., Hemmeter, M.L., Tiernan, M., & Ostrosky, M. (1990, October). *Analysis of the primary and generalized effects of milieu and responsive-interaction teaching by parents.* Paper presented at the annual meeting of the Division of Early Childhood, Albuquerque, NM.

Kaiser, A.P., & Delaney, E.M. (2001). Responsive conversations: Creating opportunities for naturalistic language teaching. *Young Exceptional Children Monograph Series No. 3,* 13–23.

Kaiser, A.P., & Hancock, T.B. (2000, April). *Supporting children's communication development through parent-implemented naturalistic interventions.* Presented at the 2nd Annual Conference on Research Innovations in Early Intervention (CRIEI), San Diego.

Kaiser, A., & Hancock, T. (2003). Teaching parents new skills to support their young children's development. *Infants & Young Children, 16,* 9–17.

Kaiser, A., Hancock, T., & Hester, P. (1998). Parents as cointerventionists: Research on application of naturalistic language teaching procedures. *Infants & Young Children, 10,* 46–55.

Kaiser, A.P., Hancock, T., & Trent, A. (2007). Teaching parents communication strategies. *Early Childhood Services, 1,* 107–136.

Kaiser, A., Hemmeter, M.L., Ostrosky, M., Fischer, R., Yoder, P., & Keefer, M. (1996). The effects of teaching parents to use responsive interaction strategies. *Topics in Early Childhood Special Education, 16,* 375–406.

Kaiser, A.P., Ostrosky, M.M., & Alpert, C.L. (1993). Training teachers to use environmental arrangement and milieu teaching with nonvocal preschool children. *The Journal for the Association for Persons with Severe Disabilities, 18*(3), 188–199.

Kaiser, A.P., Yoder, P.J., & Keetz, A. (1992). Evaluating milieu teaching. In S.F. Warren & J. Reichle (Series & Vol. Eds.), *Communication and language intervention series: Vol. 1. Causes and effects in communication and language intervention* (pp. 9–47). Baltimore: Paul H. Brookes Publishing Co.

Kuehn, D.P., & Moller, K.T. (2000). Speech and language issues in the cleft palate population: The state of the art. *Cleft Palate-Craniofacial Journal, 37,* 348.

Miller, J., & Chapman, R. (2007). *Systematic analysis of language transcripts.* Madison, WI: University of Wisconsin.

Moerk, E.L. (1992). *A first language taught and learned.* Baltimore: Paul H. Brookes Publishing Co.

Morris, H., & Ozanne, A. (2003). Phonetic, phonological, and language skills of children with a cleft palate. *Cleft Palate-Craniofacial Journal, 40*(5), 460–470.

Nelson, K.E., & Welsh, J.A. (1998). Progress in multiple language domains by deaf children and hearing children: Discussions with a rare event transactional model of language delay. In S.F. Warren & J. Reichle (Series Eds.) & R. Paul (Vol. Ed.), *Communication and language intervention series: Vol. 8. Exploring the speech-language connection* (pp. 179–225). Baltimore: Paul H. Brookes Publishing Co.

O'Gara, M., & Logemann, G. (1988). Phonetic analysis of the speech development of babies with cleft palate. *Cleft Palate Journal, 25*(2), 122–134.

Olson, D.A. (1965). *A descriptive study of the speech development of a group of infants with unoperated cleft palate.* Unpublished doctoral dissertation, Northwestern University, Evanston, IL.

Pamplona, M.C., Ysunza, A., & Espinosa, J. (1999). A comparative trial of two modalities of speech intervention for compensatory articulation in cleft palate children: Phonologic approach versus articulatory approach. *International Journal of Pediatric Otorhinolaryngology, 49,* 21–26.

Pamplona, M.C., Ysunza, A., Gonzalez, M., & Ramirez, P. (2004). Naturalistic intervention in cleft palate children. *International Journal of Pediatric Otorhinolaryngology, 68,* 75–81.

Peterson-Falzone, S.J., Hardin-Jones, M.A., & Karnell, M.P. (2001). *Cleft palate speech* (3rd ed.). St. Louis: Mosby.

Peterson-Falzone, S.J., Trost-Cardamone, J., Karnell, M., & Hardin-Jones, M. (2006). *The clinician's guide to treating cleft palate speech.* St Louis: Mosby.

Salas-Provance, M.B., Kuehn, D.P., & Marsh, J.L. (2003). Phonetic repertoire and syllable characteristics of 15-month-old babies with cleft palate. *Journal of Phonetics, 31*(1), 23–38.

Scherer, N.J. (1999). The speech and language status of toddlers with cleft lip and/or palate following early vocabulary intervention. *American Journal of Speech Language Pathology, 8,* 81–93.

Scherer, N.J. (2006) *Early intervention and parent training models for young children with clefts.* International Conference on Treatment of Speech Disorders in Individuals with Cleft Lip and Palate, Loma Linda University, Loma Linda, CA.

Scherer, N.J., D'Antonio, L., & Kalbfleisch, J. (1999). Early speech and language development in children with velocardiofacial syndrome. *American Journal of Medical Genetics, 88,* 714–723.

Scherer, N.J., D'Antonio, L., & McGahey, H. (2008). Early speech intervention for children with cleft palate. *Cleft Palate-Craniofacial Journal, 45*(1), 18–31.

Scherer, N.J., & Kaiser, A. (2007). Early intervention in children with cleft palate. *Infants & Young Children, 20,* 355–366.

Scherer, N.J., Williams, A.L., & Proctor-Williams, K. (2008). Early and later vocalization skills in children with and without cleft palate. *International Journal of Pediatric Otorhinolaryngology, 72,* 827–840.

Shriberg, L., Austin, D., Lewis, B., McSweeny, J., & Wilson, D. (1987). The percentage of consonants correct (PCC) metric: Extensions and reliability data. *Journal of Speech, Language, and Hearing Research, 40,* 708–722.

Snow, C. (1994). Parent–child interaction and the development of communicative ability. In R.L. Schiefelbusch & J. Pikar (Eds.), *The acquisition of communicative competence* (pp. 69–107). Baltimore: University Park Press.

Stoel-Gammon, C. (1989). Prespeech and speech development of two late talkers. *First Language, 9,* 207–224.

Stoel-Gammon, C. (1992). Prelinguistic vocal development: Measurements and predications. In C.A. Ferguson, L. Menn, & C. Stoel-Gammon (Eds.), *Phonological development: Models, research, implications* (pp. 439–456). Timonium, MD: York Press.

Stoel-Gammon, C. (1998). The role of babbling and phonology in early linguistic development. In S.F. Warren & J. Reichle (Series Eds.) & A.M. Wetherby, S.F. Warren, & J. Reichle (Vol. Eds.), *Communication and language intervention series: Vol. 7. Transitions in prelinguistic communication* (pp. 87–110). Baltimore: Paul H. Brookes Publishing Co.

Stokes, T.F., & Baer, D.M. (1977). An implicit technology of generalization. *Journal of Applied Behavior Analysis, 10*(2), 349–367.

Trost, J.E. (1981). Articulatory additions to the classical description of the speech of persons with cleft palate. *Cleft Palate Journal, 18,* 193–203.

Van Demark, D.R., & Hardin, M. (1986). Effectiveness of intensive articulation therapy for children with cleft palate. *Cleft Palate Journal, 23,* 215–224.

Williams, A.L., & Stoel-Gammon, C. (2008). *PEEPS: Profiles of Early Expressive Phonological Skills.* Unpublished assessment tool.

Yoder, P., Camarata, S., & Gardner, E. (2005). Treatment effects on speech intelligibility and length of utterance in children with specific language and intelligibility impairments. *Journal of Early Intervention, 28,* 34–49.

Zimmerman, I.L., Steiner, V.G., & Pond, R.E. (2002). *Preschool Language Scales* (4th ed). San Antonio, TX: Pearson PsychCorp.

Manner	Place	
	#_____	_____#
Nasals	m n	
Stops	b ?	?
Fricatives		
Affricates		
Glides	w j	
Laterals		

EMT	No. of words	No. of correct consonants	Total consonants	PCC (%)	No. of nasal substitutions	Nasals (%)	No. of comp substitutions	Comp errors (%)	No. of dev errors	Dev errors (%)
Within inventory targets										
boot	10	15	20	75	2	10	3	15	0	0
soap	6	12	12	100	0	0	0	0	0	0
pig	9	14	18	77.78	0	0	2	11.11	2	11.11
top	9	14	18	77.78	0	0	2	11.11	2	11.11
Total	**34**	**55**	**68**	**80.88**	**2**	**2.94**	**7**	**10.29**	**4**	**5.88**
Outside inventory targets										
cookie	10	10	20	50	0	0	10	50	0	0
zoo	8	6	8	75	2	25	0	0	0	0
sheep	8	14	16	87.50	0	0	2	12.50	0	0
duck	11	9	22	40.91	4	18.18	2	9.09	0	0
Total	**37**	**39**	**66**	**59.09**	**6**	**9.09**	**14**	**21.21**	**0**	**0**

Key: EMT, enhanced milieu teaching; PCC, percentage of consonants correct; Comp, compensatory; Dev, developmental.

PROMPT

A Tactually Grounded Model

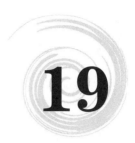

Deborah A. Hayden,
Jennifer Eigen, Anne Walker, and Lisa Olsen

ABSTRACT

PROMPT (Prompts for Restructuring Oral Muscular Phonetic Targets), a tactually grounded, sensory-motor, cognitive-linguistic intervention model, is explored as an approach, system, and technique in the treatment of children with speech production disorders. PROMPT may be used for children as young as 2 years who have sensory, motor, and phonological impairments. The PROMPT Conceptual Framework and the Motor Speech Hierarchy are described as assessment and intervention frameworks that help clinicians develop a holistic communication focus that centers on motor speech control for speech and language development. The function of tactual systems and use of tactile input are explained with relevance to their importance in early childhood motor and speech development, the neurological support they provide in developing speech production, and why clinicians need to consider using focused tactile input in intervention.

INTRODUCTION

This chapter briefly explains the PROMPT model and its philosophical grounding on the interactive and dynamic nature of communication from which all domains must be considered in intervention (Hayden, 2004, 2006). PROMPT assumes that audition and somatosensory information (including tactile-kinesthetic-proprioceptive input) are equally important in the development and organization of motor speech behavior. These two distinguishing characteristics identify PROMPT as a dynamic and tactually grounded approach.

TARGET POPULATIONS AND ASSESSMENTS FOR DETERMINING INTERVENTION RELEVANCE

Primary Populations

Children who benefit from PROMPT are

1. Children who have typical cognitive and social skills but evidence mild-to-severe oromotor delays/disorders and motor speech difficulties. These include children with persistent articulation and/or phonological errors (Chumpelik [Hayden] & Sherman, 1984; Houghton, 2003).

2. Children with mild-to-severe sensory-motor impairments that affect their speech. These include children with hearing impairment (with or without cochlear implants) and children diagnosed with childhood apraxia of speech (CAS). PROMPT has also been reported to be effective for supporting initiation, transition, and timing of speech movements in motor planning for children with fluency disorders (Chumpelik [Hayden] & Sherman, 1984; Square, Goshulak, Bose, & Hayden, 2000).

3. Children with speech impairment who are diagnosed with disorders affecting the physical, sensory-motor, and cognitive domains. This group includes children with cerebral palsy (CP), Down syndrome, attention deficit disorder (ADD)/attention-deficit/hyperactivity disorder (ADHD), and developmental dysarthria, as well as pervasive developmental disorders (PDD) or autism spectrum disorder (ASD; Rogers et al., 2006; Sherman & Chumpelik [Hayden], 1981).

In summary, children for whom PROMPT is appropriate must have an articulation, motor speech or speech production disorder affecting execution, planning, fluency, or prosody. As well, the child must be able to attend to or be taught to attend to a single task for at least a few moments, engage in joint attention with another, and demonstrate verbal or nonverbal intent to communicate. Therefore it is generally recommended for use with children from 2 years or older, but may be used with children as young as 18 months.

PROMPT Assessment Considerations

In the PROMPT approach, a holistic assessment of the entire child is recommended across all developmental domains (Physical-Sensory, Cognitive-Linguistic, and Social-Emotional) to determine relative strengths and weaknesses and identify the best context for speech intervention. A communication focus allows the clinician to embed all goals and motor objectives within a larger functional communication framework.

In general, dynamic assessment techniques, as well as criterion-referenced or standardized test instruments may be used to determine the child's overall cognitive-linguistic and social-emotional functioning. Two recommended measures are The Vineland Social-Emotional Early Childhood Scales (Sparrow, Balla, & Cicchetti, 1998), which is used to obtain basic information about the child's cognitive and social skills, and a parent questionnaire (Carswell et al., 2000). The parent questionnaire helps determine how the parent believes the child is progressing in areas important to the child's societal functioning. Next, a formal articulation or phonological test, such as the Diagnostic Evaluation of Articulation and Phonology (DEAP; Dodd, Hua, Crosbie, Holm, & Ozanne, 2007), is used to determine what type of errors are present in the child's speech.

A PROMPT assessment must also include the System Analysis Observation (SAO) checklist (Hayden, 2008). The SAO is an observational checklist that assesses seven aspects of speech subsystem control and development (i.e., tone; breath support and valving; mandibular, labial-facial, lingual, sequenced actions; and prosody). The SAO includes both a structural observation at rest and a dynamic movement, or in spontaneous speech production, assessment of how the various speech subsystems have developed and are interacting.

The motor speech hierarchy (MSH; Hayden, 2004), shown in Figure 19.1, uses information from the SAO and was created to describe the interactive nature and development of the motor speech subsystems. It has been validated using objective measures (Square, Hayden, Ciolli, & Wilkins, 1999), kinematic data (Green, Moore, Higashikawa, & Steeve,

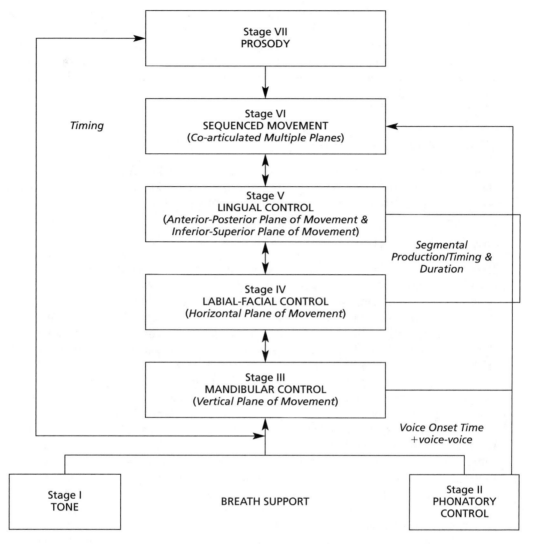

Figure 19.1.   Motor speech hierarchy. (Hayden [1986]; adapted and reprinted with permission.)

2000), and visual tracking data (Smith, 2004; Smith & Zelaznik, 2004). The SAO and MSH suggest where breakdowns in the speech subsystems are occurring and to what degree the speech subsystems have differentiated or begun to develop independence with finely graded control. Once the level of speech subsystem control has been determined, developmentally appropriate motor action sets or syllables can be identified and priorities within the speech subsystems delineated for intervention. The PROMPT lexicon is also developed through this process. Similar to the SAO, the MSH is divided into the seven stages named previously. These stages are also referred to as motor speech subsystems, parameters, and/or priorities (See Hayden, 2004, for a detailed description.)

To assess a child's motor system and response to various types of input (i.e., auditory, visual, tactual), the Verbal Motor Production Assessment for Children (VMPAC; Hayden & Square, 1999), which is based on the MSH model, may be used. This assessment tool uniquely evaluates motor speech subsystem development in three main areas: 1) global motor control, 2) focal oro-motor control, and 3) verbal and nonverbal sequencing of motor movements.

THEORETICAL BASIS

This section presents theories considered critical to PROMPT and related to PROMPT intervention. All of these ideas are interrelated and suggest how PROMPT uses somatosensory input to work toward interactive verbal communication.

Dynamic Systems Theory

Dynamic Systems Theory (DST) considers motor development as a process of self-organization arising from interactions among multiple factors, such as skeletal structure, brain development, and environmental conditions. Harnessing and controlling the many degrees of freedom involved in these interactions is essential in the development of motor control for speech. For example, in order to develop lingual independence for productions such as *snake*, the jaw must be able to reduce its range and grade its movement (Schoner & Kelso, 1988; Thelen, 2004; Thelen et al., 1993).

Fogel and Thelen (1987) also suggested that development may be understood as a temporal series of attractor states; that is, muscle biasing conditions or states in which one motor pattern or type of motor pattern is dominant. Such states create stability within a complex system. Development occurs through phase shifts in which there is a transition from one attractor state to another. Phase shifts arise as a result of multiple interactions between intrinsic and extrinsic factors, such as an individual's physical development, the level of experience with a skill, environmental conditions, or the nature of the task. From this theoretical position, speech development is determined by a dynamic system influenced by interactions among both internal and external factors. Following this view, PROMPT works by enabling the child to move from less efficient attractor states through phase shifts to more efficient attractor states in order to help produce the most efficient and flexible motor control for the development of speech.

Neuronal Group Selection Theory

Neuronal Group Selection Theory (NGST) provides both a theoretical foundation and neurobiological underpinning to DST and strongly suggests that somatosensory input is necessary, especially in the early stages of typical motor and motor speech development or when learning a new motor skill. NGST enhances DST by helping explain the nature of the central nervous system (CNS) and its role in motor speech development (Guenther, 2006; Sporns & Edelman, 1993). NGST posits that neuronal groups are the basic functional units of selection, which are arranged in maps representing the body surface or visual space, which are anatomically coupled via long-range connections throughout the cortex (Pearson, Finkel, & Edelman, 1987).

In NGST, brain circuitry is considered plastic, responsive to environmental changes, and is determined by the selection of somatosensory inputs (Kass, 2004). NGST suggests that after several successful attempts at a task, modified pathways are formed, which reorganize previous sensory maps. Neural connections are strengthened when they are involved in the successful generation of movement, resulting in natural selective shaping. It is also hypothesized that this selection is used for discrimination and categorization of sensory inputs and integrates both sensory and motor behavior, thereby producing adaptive behavior (Monfils, Plautz, & Klein, 2005). The neural connections that are formed are reciprocal and provide integration across multiple sensory and motor areas.

Reentry, or recursive reciprocal signaling, then appears to be necessary for integrating multiple sensory and motor pathways in the brain. The maps created via the sensory receptors influence the appropriate execution of motor movement and reciprocally, accurate, articulate, and functional motor movement influences somatosensory selection. Also recognized within NGST are the multiple degrees of freedom that a motor system exhibits. *Degrees of freedom* refers to the amount of movement necessary across spatial planes, but within a limited framework, to achieve motor equivalence or a target movement. In order to handle this redundancy of motor movement or multiple degrees of freedom, it is proposed that the motor system is organized into classes of movement actions. This phenomenon, although producing a class of similar but not identical trajectories that nevertheless lead to the same outcome or target, has been described as motor equivalence (Abbs & Cole, 1987; Hebb, 1949). In other words, each articulator works with multiple muscle groups and articulators to achieve a target. These actions are not produced in isolation and involve a number of interactions that may be more realistically thought of as classes of motor action sets.

A prime supposition of NGST is that there must be spontaneous generation of a number of different primary movement patterns during early development that are produced with sufficient variability. It is suggested that most synergies emerge after early sensory-motor practice subsequent to postnatal development and underlie well practiced actions, such as walking, or reaching. These changes are thought to reflect both structural (biomechanical) changes and neural development (Jackson, 1958; Kent, 2004). The second supposition is that these movements must be sensed by the organism and have differential effects on the environment. Finally, NGST implies that the preceding steps (using sensory inputs) will produce synaptic change in various global mappings, thereby leading to successive and adaptive change of the motor behavior. NGST suggests the idea that dynamic tactual input is important in changing motor speech action sets or patterns of movement for speech production. It suggests that providing appropriately tailored somatosensory feedback that leads to intelligibility for functional purposes will alter existing neuronal maps to form new maps. Thus, NGST provides a neural explanation for DST and suggests that both the organism and the environment, or external manipulating events, can contribute to the development of flexible motor behavior.

Central Nervous System Maturation and Structural Changes in Early Development

As early as 1953, Jackson proposed that CNS maturation proceeds in "ascending development in a particular order" (Jackson, 1958, p. 46). His theory of CNS maturation acknowledged that early reflexes, developed in utero and after birth, provide a stable and basic repertoire of movement patterns that enable the infant to survive and interact with the environment. He suggested that in the typical infant, these reflexes are somewhat flexible. As maturation occurs, the development of higher cortical centers provides an inhibitory influence allowing movement patterns to gain even more flexibility and come under conscious control. He indicated that CNS activity evolved from the most simple, most automatic, and most organized toward the most complex, least organized, and least automatic. Kent (Kent, 2004; Kent & Vorperian, 2007), realizing the interactive nature of speech development, described the biological basis for speech and suggested that the infant goes through successive remodeling and maturation of both structural and CNS systems. While Jackson looked at the innate changes brought about by CNS maturation, Kent called attention to the interaction of the physical, sensory-motor, and cognitive changes to the development of speech and language.

Jackson's theory of evolution and dissolution reminds the clinician using PROMPT that early reflexes provide the initial or primary movement patterns with which the infant contacts his or her world and begins the diversification of multiple action sets. It is therefore critical that the clinician using PROMPT evaluate the client's developmental stage and assess how much independence of movement may be achieved, ranging from reflex actions to consciously controlled motor behaviors. Kent's work further reminds us that the development of the organism has a distinct relationship to the development of sound production. If normal development within the musculoskeletal system does not occur within the expected time periods, it may impede, to greater or lesser degrees, the ability of the motor speech system to develop adequate motor abilities for speech and, therefore, language.

Motor Learning Theories

Schema theory was originally discussed by Head (1926a, 1926b) as early as 1920. He proposed that creating a motor memory or "schema" involved the process of extracting core elements from motor experiences and that these elements reflect rules that have led to success in performing a given action. Bellezza (1987) proposed that these same features characterized successful speech schemas and that the rules underlying successful speech schemas encompassed core properties of one's experience that could be tested continually and redefined by other experiences of a similar nature. Similar to NGST, schemas, as Bellezza proposed them, become more effective with greater repetition and through a wider variety of experiences with a similar activity. In this way the schemas become more dynamic and usable. In other words, patterns that require less effort and lead continually to more success are easiest to learn, particularly when they revolve around meaningful events involving real-world objects and routines (Fletcher, 1992; Nelson, 2004).

Schmidt (1975) suggested four steps that must occur for a child to learn a motor skill. First, the initial proprioceptive conditions (or postural pretuning) for the movement must be met. Second, the child must be able to pull forward the motor plan. Third, the child must be able to recognize if the motor plan was correct or faulty by comparing sensory stimuli (e.g., proprioceptive, kinesthetic, auditory) and, finally, the success of the response in relation to the intended outcome evaluated. Both *recall* memory, necessary for generating motor commands, and *recognition* memory, critical for evaluating and comparing the response-produced feedback to derive error information, are needed. Motor learning theory, as described previously, is constantly used by clinicians who use PROMPT. Not only can the motor actions be shaped by using different amounts and types of tactual input, but the ways in which these actions are practiced (e.g., massed or distributed practice; Schmidt & Bjork, 1992; Schmidt & Wrisberg, 2000) can be naturally embedded in age-appropriate activities or routines. Schema Theory and Motor Learning Theory remind the clinician who uses PROMPT that speech requires many different elements in both sensory and motor production in order to be successful. It also requires that the child have frequent opportunities to practice the motor actions repetitively and then embed them within generalized action schemas. In all these events, the child must be able to remember and recall a movement sequence or action set and be able to compare and contrast them in order to change motor outcomes.

In summary, PROMPT's theoretical position is consistent with the idea that somatic selection (i.e., the dynamic and active feel of a movement or coordinated action; Guenther, 2006; Nasir & Ostry, 2006; Sporns & Edelman, 1993) plays a critical role in cognitive function and in the development of coordinated movement. Specifically, tactual input is used to effect somatosensory change and promote motor speech accuracy while the motor skill is simultaneously linked to cognitive and socially relevant communicative content. From this base, active touch is considered especially important for the development of motor action sets; that is, groups of coordinated muscle actions forming the basis for syllable production and leading to the development of connected speech. Further, PROMPT acknowledges the complex interrelationship among the Physical-Sensory, Cognitive-Linguistic, and Social-Emotional domains, and the critical interaction among these domains in the development of motor speech control (Hayden, 2004, 2006).

Level of Consequences Being Addressed

The PROMPT approach provides clinicians with tools to assess and treat motor speech disorders from a structural/functional, activity limitations/inclusion, and participation perspective to achieve effective functional communication. This model addresses all aspects of the World Health Organization's (WHO's) International Classification of Functioning, Disability and Health (ICF) framework (WHO, 2001). PROMPT's conceptual framework reflects the relationship between the environment and the individual, as shown in Figure 19.2. Bidirectional arrows acknowledge that impairment in any one of the domains affects functioning in the other domains in a nonlinear manner.

EMPIRICAL BASIS

PROMPT was initially devised as an approach for speech production disorders and *was not* designed *specifically* for children with speech sound disorders. To date, investigations of PROMPT have focused on how its use of tactual input aids the child or adult in developing, rebalancing, or accessing motor targets of a linguistic nature. Of the nine studies, three have appeared in peer-reviewed journals, one resulted in a master's thesis, four have appeared in peer-reviewed conference proceedings, and one is in preparation for publication. Only studies involving intervention with children by a treating clinician who has had at least some PROMPT training or has met fidelity in the method have been included (see Table 19.1).

The first exploratory (case) study focusing on PROMPT (Sherman & Chumpelik [Hayden], 1981) studied the effects of PROMPT along with behavioral methods for a nonverbal 8-year-old child with ASD and concomitant severe cognitive and behavioral impairments. Prompted stimuli initially included 10 CV and CVC words that could be used by the child with caregivers to indicate basic needs and wants. As the child attained 85%

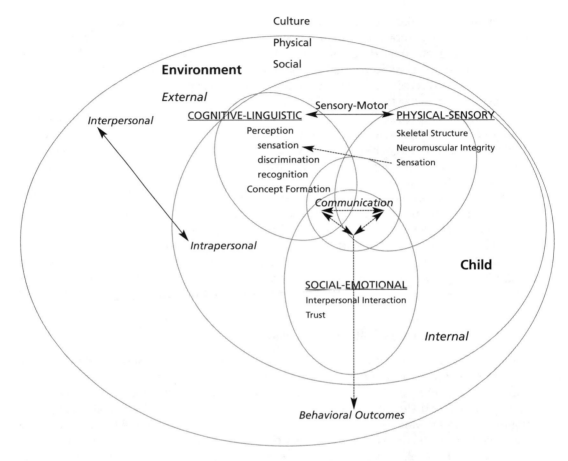

Figure 19.2. PROMPT conceptual framework. From Hayden, D.A. [2000]. *Bridging PROMPT technique to intervention manual*. Santa Fe, NM: The PROMPT Institute; reprinted by permission.)

accuracy over three sessions, new words were added until the end of the 32-session intervention block (2 sessions per week for 16 weeks). Words achieving the 85% criterion could not drop below 75% accuracy or they were added back into the PROMPT condition. All words, in the active and inactive condition, were probed 10 times during each session and were scored online as correct or incorrect by two behavioral therapists. Three measures of agreement of scored responses across the two scorers ranged from 87% to 93%. Results indicated that over the 4-month period, the child acquired 30 intelligible words after no previous interventions had been successful. Staff and caregivers also noted a reduction in problem behavior. At a 6-month follow-up, the parents reported the child's continued use of about 25 trained words, as well as a continued reduction in the frequency of problem behaviors.

In 1984, Chumpelik (Hayden) and Sherman investigated PROMPT's efficacy with two groups of four male participants with severely impaired speech—one group with typical cognition and the other with moderate-to-severe cognitive impairment, as determined using the Wechsler Intelligence Scale for Children–Fourth Edition (WISC-IV; Wechsler, 2002). Both groups were given traditional auditory-visual (AV) intervention using an integral stimulation approach and PROMPT using a multiple baseline across behaviors design. Each child was administered a probe testing all English phonemes and selected words and phrases. Each phoneme, word, and phrase had been rated by five speech-language pathologists (SLPs) on a 1–4 scale for earliest-to-latest to acquire and easiest-to-hardest to teach. Six error sounds were then selected for each child. Two phonemes were randomly assigned from level one, and three from each of levels two, three, and four for each child. Two nonsense words were constructed for each child from the individual phonemes in their training sets; one word with two phonemes (CV, VC) and one with three phonemes (CVC).

A complete session incorporated 50 trials on each sound and nonsense word. A maximum of 400 trials was presented to each child, with fewer trials used if the child met a criterion of 2 days of 45 correct productions. Fifty trials were presented on the first sound; 50 were then presented on the next, and so forth until 50 trials had been presented on all stimuli. The order of presentation of 50 trial blocks was determined randomly, except that the penultimate block always included the two-phoneme nonsense word and the last block always included the three-phoneme nonsense word. Intervention was administered twice weekly, over a 12-week period, by two SLPs trained in both methods. Each participant began intervention on the first sound with PROMPT while all other phonemes were presented with AV. Once the first sound reached criterion, the next sound was treated using PROMPT and so forth until all stimuli were completed. All 8 participants demonstrated improvement in their randomly selected phoneme and nonsense target words with PROMPT. Although participants with typical cognitive and motor skills demonstrated greater progress in the PROMPT condition than in the AV condition, the children with cognitive impairment demonstrated change only with the addition of PROMPT.

Table 19.1. Levels of evidence for PROMPT intervention

Level	Description	References
Ia	Meta-analysis of > 1 randomized controlled trial	—
Ib	Randomized controlled study	—
IIa	Controlled study without randomization	Chumpelik (Hayden) & Sherman (1984); Rogers et al. (2006); Square, Chumpelik [Hayden], Morningstar, & Adams (1986); Square et al. 2000
IIb	Quasi-experimental study	Houghton (2003); Square, Chumpelik (Hayden), & Adams (1985)
III	Nonexperimental studies, i.e., correlational and case studies	Bose, Square, Schlosser, & van Lieshout (2001); Freed, Marshal, & Frazier (1997); Sherman & Chumpelik (Hayden) (1981)
IV	Expert committee report, consensus conference, clinical experience of respected authorities	—

Adapted from the Scottish Intercollegiate Guidelines Network (http://www.sign.ac.uk).

Studies of PROMPT's Effectiveness with Children

Square et al. (2000) measured PROMPT's effectiveness in treating *children with oro-motor and sequencing impairments*. The participants were six males (ages 4;2 to 4;6) with unintelligible speech who had made minimal progress in traditional therapy. Standardized tests of phonological, motor, language, and social skills were administered before and after intervention. A multiple probe design across behaviors was used to evaluate effects of PROMPT on auditory perceptual and visual speech movement accuracy across two similar sets (A-B) of lexical items. Set A focused on jaw and labial-facial control; set B on lingual control. Motor goals were selected by two investigators for each child based on observations of his speech performances on the VMPAC and a storytelling task. The intervention goals were prioritized using the MSH.

A list of 40 words was generated for each child—20 words were treated and 20 were used to probe generalization. Words were randomly assigned to the training and probe conditions but were matched according to the corresponding motor goals and movement parameters. The 20 trained lexical items were grouped into two sets of behaviors for each child; set A and set B. In each set, there were two subsets of words—one devoted to jaw movements and one to lip movements. The teaching criterion was a maximum of 15 training sessions for each set.

During intervention and maintenance phases, probes were taken every 2–3 sessions. A group intervention paradigm, with four children in each group, was conducted twice per week for 1.5 hours over 12 weeks, or a total of 36 hours intervention time. Sessions followed the same routine: who is here, show and tell, floor time, and storytelling with embedded PROMPT lexicons/motor goals for each child. All children then moved to the table for paper and coloring tasks while one child received individual work. After individual work, the children participated in a story retell or reenactment requiring responses from the children. The PROMPT intervention resulted in significant perceptually improved speech on both auditory and visual measures across both training sets and on untrained or similar words.

Children with severe persistent sound system disorders were studied by Houghton (2003). Five children, ages 3;9 to 9;8 (mean age [MA] 6;0) participated in the study. All children had received a minimum of 1 year of therapy (range 1;1 to 4;0) using a phonological approach and had reportedly made minimal gains. Determination of phonemes to be targeted was established using the Fisher-Logemann Test of Articulatory Competence (Fisher & Logemann, 1971) over three consecutive sessions. Percentage of consonants correct (PCC) was calculated according to Shriberg and Kwiatkowski's (1982) procedure for assessing severity of involvement. A second SLP scored 46.6% of randomly selected samples. Inter-rater reliability for the PCC was 96.8%. Four phonemes that had never been articulated correctly on the test were studied. Two phonemes were selected that differed by more than one feature, for example /ʧ/ versus /g/, and one phoneme was selected that differed by only one feature, for example /p/ versus /b/, to examine within-class generalization. A fourth unrelated phoneme was chosen to act as a control sound. For the two target phonemes, two CV words, two CVC or CVCC words, and one functional phrase containing the target phoneme were developed for training. In the intervention phase, 10 trials for each word/phrase were elicited each session until 80% accuracy was attained on two consecutive sessions, or a total of 8 sessions were completed. Sessions were conducted two times per week for 20–40 minutes. In intervention, each target word/phrase was presented with an auditory model and an accompanying visual stimulus picture. Only the target phoneme was scored for accuracy. If the phoneme was judged to be accurate perceptually, it was scored as correct. If not, the child was instructed to wait while the SLP provided a surface prompt of the word/phrase. The child was then required to produce the word while the SLP simultaneously prompted in the word/phrase. One child failed to complete intervention and a second child was unable to adhere to the intervention protocol. Of the three remaining participants, each showed an overall increase in control over production of target phonemes, although in some instances there was an irregular profile of acquisition. Spontaneous speech samples taken at the completion of the intervention phase revealed that five of the six trained phonemes significantly increased in accuracy of production in both trained and untrained words in conversational speech. Evidence of within-class generalization also occurred for three participants, whereas their untrained phonemes remained at 0% accuracy.

A study conducted by Rogers et al. (2006) compared the effectiveness of the Denver Treatment Model (Rogers & Lewis, 1989) and PROMPT with *nonverbal autistic children 2–4 years of age*. This single-subject, multiple-probe design across behaviors examined these interventions for 10 nonverbal autistic boys ages 24–50 months of age, with five children randomly assigned to each type of intervention. Data for only eight children (four in each group) are described here because one child in each group made no changes. All children met the diagnostic criteria for autism on the Autism Diagnostic Observation Schedule (ADOS; Lord, Rutter, DiLavore, & Risi, 1999), the Autism Diagnostic Interview–Revised (ADI-R; Lord, Rutter, & Le Couteur, 1994), and the *Diagnostic and Statistical Manual of Mental Disorders, Fourth Edition* (DSM-IV; American Psychiatric Association, 2000); used five or fewer words per day; had a ratio IQ $\geq$ 35; and had a then-current nonverbal developmental level of 15 months. Previous time in intervention for the children ranged from 380–3,400 hours. Standardized test data were collected pre- and postintervention, then 3 and 6 months later; in addition, random 10-minute probes of each intervention session were obtained. Intervention coding of the random 10-minute samples of each session was scored by two reliable observers for the number of words (or approximations)/phrases produced, as well as function and level of independence. All four children in the PROMPT condition acquired words over the 12-week intervention period. The high and moderate responders (MA 23–28 months) increased word output from less than five words per day to more than 2,000 words per hour and 90 words per hour, respectively, and were found to use approximately 100–160 phrases per hour by the end of the 12-week intervention period. The low responders (MA > 13–14 months), who had averaged no more than three words per day, averaged 10–20 words per hour by the end of the 12-week intervention period. All children made expressive language gains on the Mullen Scales of Early Learning (Mullen, 1995). The two high responders made a total of 30 months' gain in expressive language. All but one child made receptive language gains. The two high responders achieved approximately 20 months' receptive gain over a 4-month period. Analysis of individual participants' data revealed that children made changes in both intervention conditions. Interestingly, for children using PROMPT, it appeared to be most effective for those autistic nonverbal children who were in early linguistic stages (e.g., 24 months) or had motor involvement as well as autism and had made little or no change with other intervention methods.

PRACTICAL REQUIREMENTS

PROMPT involves work on motor practice embedded into activities involving social interaction and activities of daily living, making sessions a positive and motivating experience for the child, the family, and the clinician. It does not require that families spend large sums of money for frequent and intensive services, with a significant impact having been demonstrated when intervention is administered once or twice per week for 12–16 weeks (Houghton, 2003; Rogers et al., 2006; Square et al., 2000). However, recommended intervention frequency depends on the nature and severity of the presenting disorder. In general, if a child presents with mild-to-moderate cognitive impairments, PROMPT is recommended for a maximum of twice per week in a pull-out condition. For children with moderate-to-severe cognitive impairments, PROMPT would be most effective in the context of a functional environment such as a home, preschool, or classroom. Regardless of the intervention frequency, professionals should begin to see changes in a child's motor speech control and/or language production within four to eight sessions. The rate of change will depend on the level of impairment across domains and the skill level of the clinician. PROMPT can be administered in a group setting as well as in individual sessions. The length of most individual sessions is 30–60 minutes, whereas group sessions can be up to 90 minutes to 2 hours in duration.

Involvement of individuals in the child's environment is another essential component of PROMPT. Support can be recruited from team members, family members, and peers in order to help a child carry over his or her PROMPT lexicon. These people do not need to be trained in PROMPT; instead, they can provide additional, functional opportunities for carryover.

Because PROMPT is administered during functional activities, no specific materials are required. Materials such as toys, books, and academic resources in a typical intervention room, home, or classroom can be used. In addition PROMPT can be implemented during activities of daily living, such as bath time or snack time. For some children, it may be appropriate to send home a book with pictures or words or a game-like activity representing the PROMPT lexicon to aid the family in creating opportunities for carryover. Nonetheless, some materials have been specifically designed for PROMPT, including computer software, stimulus cards, and a web site with additional resources that are available through the SmarTalk web site (http://www. smartalk.info).

Because PROMPT is a holistic framework that requires knowledge of neuromotor principles, including the direct actions, placements, and the amount of contraction and timing changes within and across speech subsystems, becoming a PROMPT-certified SLP requires extensive training, taking 1½ to 2 years and entailing two courses and two self-study projects. In addition, a self-study PROMPT Certification Project is required. (See the PROMPT Institute's web site, http:// www.promptinstitute.com, for details.)

KEY COMPONENTS

This section explains the core intervention elements of PROMPT therapy within the PROMPT conceptual framework (see Figure 19.2).

Assessment of Global Domains for Intervention Planning

In order to execute an effective PROMPT program, a clinician should use the Global Domain Profile (Hayden, 2002) to organize the informal and formal assessment data to determine the child's strengths and weaknesses within and across domains. A PROMPT evaluation is structured around critical questions that examine the Cognitive-Linguistic, Social-Emotional, and Physical-Sensory domains. For a detailed description of questions within each domain, see Hayden (2004).

The most critical domain for planning the motor speech aspect of PROMPT is the Physical-Sensory domain. Assessment in this domain requires the clinician to evaluate skeletal structure; general neuromotor control; specific motor subsystem control; the processing of auditory, visual, and tactual sensory input; and the interaction between structure and function, as described in the assessment considerations section of this chapter.

Determination of a Communication Focus and the Uses of PROMPT

Following the Global Domain Assessment, a Communication Focus for intervention is selected. The Communication Focus helps the clinician and the parents/caregivers determine the communicative priorities for the child and provides a context in which to embed motor, language, cognitive, and social interaction objectives. The Communication Focus should center on a specific area of a child's life that will be improved with the intervention (e.g., play skills, interactive routines, self-help skills).

PROMPT can then be used in one of three ways. The first use, to develop an interactive focus/awareness for oral communication, is for minimally verbal children. The second is to develop an association between simultaneous dynamic tactual and auditory input to specific words or concepts. The third use of PROMPT would be to develop, rebalance, or restructure speech subsystems at the sound, word, or phrase level.

Selection and Implementation of Priorities and Motor-Phoneme Targets

After thorough assessment using the SAO and MSH, three motor speech subsystems are selected as the focal priorities for change and must be kept in mind in all intervention activities. Within the three prioritized stages, the clinician determines which motor subsystem should receive the most input, or which plane of movement(s) will be targeted first. To change speech production, the lowest levels need to be developed or refined before independence can be expected at higher levels (Hayden & Square, 1999). The first priority is often the lowest stage that is not functioning adequately. However, the clinician must determine which priority will provide the most stabilizing factor for change.

Priorities are supported primarily through the use of auditory-tactual input consisting of four different PROMPT types (see Table 19.2). In PROMPT, the refinement of motor actions occurs though successive shaping. Shaping involves the reinforcement of each intermediate response that more closely resembles the desired response. Steps used in this process usually entail the following sequence, but may use different PROMPT types, typically applied in varied combinations depending on the child's cognitive and motor resources. For example, the clinician maps in the pattern (i.e., the syllable, word or phrase) while the child is passive, then the clinician either repeats the same pattern or chooses

Table 19.2. PROMPT types

Type of PROMPT	Definition of tactual support	Component in Schema Theory (Schmidt, 1975) that is taught
Parameter PROMPT	Broad-based support for one parameter (e.g., jaw support, broad rounding)	Initial proprioceptive conditions
Surface PROMPT	Information in one dimension to an articulator to signal place, timing, and transition	Motor plan or basic phonetic sequence
Complex PROMPT	Information in more than one plane of movement in order to construct a holistic representation of a motor-phoneme	Motor plan for a single sound
Syllable PROMPT	Combination of Parameter and Surface PROMPT to guide the holistic shape of a syllable and ease the motor load for a child	Initial proprioceptive conditions and motor plan or basic phonetic sequence

From Hayden, D.A. (2004). PROMPT: A tactually grounded treatment approach to speech production disorders. In I. Stockman (Ed.), *Movement and action in learning and development: Clinical implications for pervasive developmental disorders* (pp. 255–297). San Diego: Elsevier/Academic Press; reprinted with permission.

an easier variant of the motor pattern and prompts this again while the child participates. Then, depending on the child's accuracy of response, the clinician may repeat the above or reduce the motor pattern further for the child to succeed. The child then says the word again and is verbally reinforced.

As mentioned, a clinician who uses PROMPT is always mindful of motor learning principles, such as including both massed and distributed practice (Skelton, 2004). For example, massed practice may require a child to use the word *up* for each block used to build a tower with blocks. In distributed practice, the targeted word should be embedded within other naturalistic and interactive activities (e.g., cars going *up* and down ramps in a garage) or within a phrase (e.g., using a farm with stairs each animal can go up: *cow up, sheep up*). Each PROMPT type provides a different amount of support; they all help a child with one of the four critical elements of learning new motor action sets (Schmidt, 1975). In addition, as mentioned previously, surface PROMPTs can be mapped in before or after the production to help the child recognize if the motor plan was correct or faulty and to evaluate the outcome as compared with the targeted movement. The different PROMPT types are summarized in Table 19.2.

In PROMPT, phonemes are referred to as motor-phonemes because they represent the schema used to plan and execute the production of a sound. The term *motor-phoneme* reflects an individual's dynamic movements that produce the acoustic equivalents used to build words and phrases. A clinician identifies approximately 10 motor-phonemes as part of intervention planning. These phonemes, which are selected from the three priorities previously discussed, must also be able to be combined to produce functional words (i.e., motor action sets) in the prioritized areas. For example, if the first priority of intervention is mandibular control, the clinician may be working to help the child establish typical jaw excursion or reduced lower boundary action during speech production. Motor-phonemes such as /ɑ/ as in *hot* and /æ/ as in *hat* would be selected so that the child would learn to use them with less jaw opening, thereby promoting initial back tongue contraction. Parameter and surface PROMPTs would be helpful at this stage.

The selected motor-phonemes are then combined to form syllables, word approximations, and words that are referred to as the PROMPT lexicon. It is critical that the words in a child's lexicon be both motorically achievable and functional so that the improved motor speech control can be used in everyday interactions with parents, caregivers, and/or peers. In addition, for children with impairments in the cognitive-linguistic and/or social-emotional domains, the lexicon can be used to develop skills within these domains. Another important consideration when determining the PROMPT lexicon is to select words that are cognitively and semantically appropriate for the mental age of the child. As a child's motor speech and language skills develop, the words in the lexicon can be combined for use in phrases. In addition, carrier phrases can be developed in the same plane of movement as the targeted word, thereby reducing the motor load for the child.

Establishing Long-Term Goals and Short-Term Objectives

Next, the clinician who uses PROMPT writes at least three broad, language-based long-term goals that embody the Communication Focus, work to rebalance a child's functioning across the three domains, and address the three priorities through the selected motor-phonemes and lexicon. Long-term goals help guide a child's intervention for 6–12 months. For example, if a child's Communication Focus is play skills, one long-term goal may be, "During constructive activities, the child will use verbal communication to name the parts or request additional pieces" (Hayden, 2006). Up to three specific objectives that identify the observable behaviors are then developed for each long-term goal, including the rebalancing or development of motor speech skills to be learned in intervention. PROMPT short-term objectives may be focused in the Cognitive-Linguistic, Social-Emotional, or Physical-Sensory domains. An essential component of PROMPT is that the clinician embeds motor learning into language objectives that work to strengthen weaknesses in any domain. When writing the objectives, the therapist must continue to think about what skills should be developed in each domain while also addressing the child's motor speech control by including words and phrases from the planned lexicon. Examples of short-term objectives are illustrated in the case study later in this chapter and demonstrate how a PROMPT therapist can embed motor priorities in a language-based activity to help develop improved phonological, language, and motor speech skills. Generally, depending on the individual child's disability, short-term objectives are written so that they may be achieved within a relatively short time (i.e., within 1 week to 1 month).

Intervention Sessions

PROMPT sessions include 1) three to four activities, routines, or scripts that reflect the Communication Focus and can be expanded over time; 2) long-term goals and short-term objectives that embed the PROMPT lexicon and MSH priorities; 3) turn-taking between the clinician and child; 4) the use of various levels of PROMPTs to either develop interaction, associate sensory to cognitive-linguistic information, or rebalance, develop, or organize motor speech control; and 5) mass and distributed practice. Portions of a PROMPT session are shown in the accompanying DVD for this book.

ASSESSMENT AND PROGRESS
MONITORING TO SUPPORT DECISION MAKING

Depending on the presenting disorder, there are several ways to monitor intervention progress and make decisions. First, standardized testing, such as the VMPAC (Hayden & Square, 1999) or the DEAP (Dodd et al., 2007), is administered at least three times during the 16-week intervention to see how underlying systems are responding and changing or how motor behavior is being refined. Second, target word sets, selected after determining the MSH priorities for each of the three motor speech subsystems, form the basis or core PROMPT lexicon for intervention and are monitored weekly for change.

Third, a set of untrained probe words can be administered approximately every second or third session throughout intervention. This frequent probing serves to help the clinician 1) monitor the original and changing MSH intervention priorities and ensure that those motor priorities are being met, 2) evaluate how the motor actions (stages) are developing and if they are generalizing to untrained word forms, and 3) support decisions about when to change the level or relevance of the priorities. For example, the first priority may be Stage III, Mandibular. After working on vertical plane movements within words, the child may achieve smooth opening and closing phases with good grading and appropriate range. Then, this priority may drop into third place where it is only monitored and the new highest priority may now become Stage IV, Labial-Facial. If the child achieves 80% accuracy on an untrained probe word set over three consecutive probe sessions, a new motor speech subsystem priority is selected.

The achievement of long-term goals related to the overall Communication Focus and objectives also provides evidence of progress. The following language skills are also monitored on an ongoing basis: syntax and morphology, use of communicative functions, mean length of utterance, and responsiveness to recasts. Finally, as suggested in Schema Theory, recall and recognition memory are checked to see if the child can monitor and self-correct his or her own speech production. This aspect is extremely important because the presence of such skills suggests that the child may no longer need tactile input to make a change in motor actions and can rely solely on auditory, visual, and cognitive-linguistic information to continue learning.

CONSIDERATIONS FOR CHILDREN FROM
CULTURALLY AND LINGUISTICALLY DIVERSE BACKGROUNDS

The fundamental principles underlying PROMPT mean that it is inherently flexible and easily adaptable across speech and language systems internationally. PROMPT training manuals (Hayden, 2006, 2008) have been translated into French, German, Dutch, Spanish, Cantonese, and Singlish. Instructional training programs have also been presented to teach PROMPT to SLPs within their home country in the context of their own practice.

Because PROMPT views speech as a linked motor skill, translating it into other languages requires systematic analysis of the multidimensional aspects of speech sound production, as well as how physiological and linguistic development interact to determine first words and early semantic–syntactic relationships in that language. There appear to be universal articulatory preferences in the babble and early speech of young children across languages, which are driven predominantly by oscillating movements of the mandible in combination with static postures of the lips and tongue (McNeilage & Davis,

2000). Early communicative intents and words then appear to be shaped in relation to this developing vocal repertoire (Smith & Goffman, 2004). Therefore not only is the PROMPT technique modified in terms of the tactual cues used, but variations also occur in terms of initial lexicon choices in therapy. Because speech production practice in PROMPT is embedded within functional contexts for the child, intervention involves key members of the child's community, including but not limited to caregivers, teachers, and peers, and communication foci reflect the conversational style and pragmatics of the child's language. Consequently, PROMPT can be used by clinicians working with children who speak other languages who have a speech sound disorder, as well as with bilingual children who have either a speech sound disorder or difficulty with sounds present in their new, but not their first, language.

CASE STUDY

ZR was a 6-year-old boy with severe speech difficulties in the presence of average cognition and receptive language skills. Early developmental history was unremarkable apart from delayed speech and expressive language milestones, with his first intelligible words reported at $2^1/_2$ years of age. ZR's past intervention included 12 months of weekly or biweekly individual and group-based speech pathology programs through a community health service and 6 months of weekly, individual speech therapy at school. Sessions ranged from 30–45 minutes in length and focused on improving production of single target sounds within a traditional articulation hierarchy. Visual symbols and cued articulation were used to support sequencing within words and phrases. ZR's parents reported only limited gains in speech intelligibility following these interventions. ZR was in first grade at a local public school when first considered for PROMPT.

Global Domains Analysis

ZR was an engaging child who was experiencing academic difficulties and some social isolation at school due to his poor speech intelligibility. He presented with significant difficulties maintaining attention to tasks and he struggled to filter relevant from irrelevant stimuli in the environment. In learning situations, ZR was eager to please but impulsive and highly distractible, requiring consistent structure and clear boundaries in order to self-manage his behavior.

Systems Analysis Observation

ZR presented with normal skeletal structure and dentition; however, functioning of individual speech subsystems was significantly impaired. He presented with mild low tone throughout his body. Phonatory control and breath support for speech were adequate although he experienced difficulty in timing the closure of the velopharyngeal port in connected speech resulting in resonance issues. Mandibular movements were poorly graded, often too wide and ballistic in nature. Independent lip movement could only be achieved in combination with high front or back vowels, and no individual lip movement was evident. Overall, labial-facial musculature showed poor retraction and protrusion in connected speech. Lingual

Table 19.3. Example of an activity

Communication focus	Academic skills
Goal	In academic tasks, ZR will label consonants by name and sound and be able to orally segment and blend sounds in CVC words.
Activity	Phonological awareness Bingo game
Objective: physical-sensory	In a Bingo game, ZR will demonstrate reduced jaw movement with controlled jaw gradation when identifying single CVC words on his board on 10 of 12 occasions (e.g., *map, hop, bob*).
Objective: cognitive-linguistic	In a Bingo game, ZR will orally blend sounds to identify simple CVC words with a picture cue on 10 of 12 occasions.

movements were accomplished through jaw release with significant recruitment of labial-facial musculature in order to facilitate adequate contraction. Due to these considerable lower-level issues, ZR exhibited significant difficulty sequencing movements across planes, and his prosody was also severely compromised.

Baseline Measures

Baseline data were collected for target words to be used in therapy, and untrained probe words were chosen in order to detect change across untrained vocabulary. Probe words were matched across priority areas (i.e., Mandibular, Labial-Facial, and Lingual control). At the commencement of therapy, ZR's baseline accuracy rates across parameters for target and control stimuli were 27% and 23%, respectively (see Table 19.3 for example activity).

Probe Data

After 3 weeks and six 30-minute sessions, probe data were collected. Accuracy rates across parameters for target and control stimuli had improved to 47% and 40%, respectively. These results reflected improved grading of jaw movements across both target and control stimuli; however, lingual contractions were still broad for the productions of /t/, /d/, and /n/, and bilabial productions used whole lip rather than the medial one third of labial surface. Objectives were then revised to reflect these new targets: *independent lip movement and anterior tongue separation.*

Results of Intervention

ZR's skills were reassessed after 12 weeks of intervention (see Table 19.4). The SAO revealed improved jaw grading, refined labial-facial movements, and true anterior tongue separation. Excessive recruitment of labial-facial movement was still evident for untrained consonants. In addition, lingual contractions for mid-back and back sounds required further development and integration. ZR's parents commented that unfamiliar listeners could understand more of his speech and it was the first time they had heard him produce words accurately. They also reported that ZR was beginning to show more interest in reading and was keeping up with his peers across most literacy areas. Further therapy was recommended.

Table 19.4. Results of intervention

Assessment tool	Pretest results		Posttherapy results	
Verbal Motor Production Assessment for Children (VMPAC; Hayden & Square, 1999)	Global motor control:	90%	Global motor control:	100%
	Focal oro-motor control:	40%	Focal oro-motor control:	67%
	Sequencing:	22%	Sequencing:	65%
	Connected speech:	35%	Connected speech:	65%
	Speech characteristics:	66%	Speech characteristics:	80%
Percentage of phonemes correct (PPC)	Assessed using 60 SmartCards	26%	Assessed using 60 SmartCards	65%
Sutherland Phonological Awareness Test–Revised (SPAT-R; Neilson, 2003)	Total score: 12 of 60 Percentile: 15th Below average for Grade 1		Total score: 30 of 60 Percentile: 63rd Average range for Grade 1	
Clinical Evaluation of Language Fundamentals–Fourth Edition (CELF-4; Semel, Wiig, & Secord, 2003)	Receptive language score: 106 Expressive language score: 61		Word structure subtest standard score: 3 → 5	
Wechsler Intelligence Scale for Children–Fourth Edition (WISC-IV; Wechsler, 2002)	Performance intelligence quotient (PIQ): 42nd percentile Average for age		Not reassessed	

STUDY QUESTIONS

1. What are ZR's strengths and weaknesses across the global domains?

2. Based on your assessment data and your conversations with the family/caregivers, in what interactive Communication Focus would you choose to embed the motor speech goals?

3. Using the SAO and MSH, how is the client's motor–speech system functioning and what are the three initial priorities for therapy?

4. Which motor-phonemes, words, and phrases have you chosen to target as the first priority?

5. What type of prompts will you use to support the motor-to-language connection (i.e., parameter, syllable, complex, or surface) and why?

FUTURE DIRECTIONS

Future studies are underway to examine how priorities are selected within the MSH and how these priorities directly affect progress and change in articulation and phonological abilities. At the time of this writing, two studies are investigating these areas; one study in preparation for publication examined the effectiveness of PROMPT therapy for children with CP presenting with motor speech disorders. This particular study examined both kinematic tracking of articulator changes and how the MSH influenced goal selection and intervention priorities. A second study focusing on the efficacy of PROMPT in treating CAS is being proposed.

Many aspects of PROMPT continue to need efficacy research. First, studies to determine the effect of adding tactual information to support speech actions are needed—

especially in children with CAS, motor speech disorders, and hearing impairment (with and without cochlear implants). These studies in particular need to be supported by kinematic and/or visual tracking instrumentation and combine both instrumental and subjective/perceptual data sets. Two such studies are in progress at the time of this writing.

Another area of investigation involves the frequency of prompting (i.e., the dosage) needed to be most effective; this should be determined for different speech production disorders. Research is also warranted to examine changes across functional domains, even those that are not being directly targeted (e.g., receptive language or improved peer relationships). These changes are often reported and documented in clinical practice. Finally, clinical trials need to be conducted to determine the most efficient interventions for various speech disorders. These could include both phonological and motor-based interventions and measure both language and speech processes.

SUGGESTED READINGS

Hayden, D.A. (1994). Differential diagnosis of motor speech dysfunction in children. Developmental apraxia of speech: Assessment. *Clinics in Communication Disorders, 4*(2), 118–147, 162–174.

Hayden, D.A. (2004). PROMPT: A tactually grounded treatment approach to speech production disorders. In I. Stockman (Ed.), *Movement and action in learning and development: Clinical implications for pervasive developmental disorders* (pp. 255–297). San Diego: Elsevier/Academic Press.

Hayden, D.A. (2006). The PROMPT model: Use and application for children with mixed phonological-motor impairment. *Advances in Speech-Language Pathology, 8*(3), 265–281.

REFERENCES

Abbs, J.H., & Cole, K.J. (1987). Neural mechanisms of motor equivalence and goal achievement. In S.P. Wise (Ed.), *Higher brain functions: Recent explorations of the brain's emergent properties* (pp. 15–43). New York: John Wiley & Sons.

American Psychiatric Association. (2000). *Diagnostic and statistical manual of mental disorders, fourth edition.* Washington DC: Author.

Bellezza, J.K. (1987). Mnemonic devices and memory schemas. In M.A. McDaniel & M. Pressley (Eds.), *Imagery and related mnemonic processes* (pp. 34–55). New York: Springer-Verlag.

Bose, A., Square, P.A., Schlosser, R., & van Lieshout, P. (2001). Effects of PROMPT therapy on speech motor function in a person with aphasia and apraxia of speech. *Aphasiology, 15*(8), 767–785.

Carswell, A., Polatajko, H., Law, M., Baptiste, S., McColl, M., Pollock, N., et al. (2000). *Canadian Occupational Performance Measure: Workbook companion to training video.* Ottawa: CAOT Publications ACE.

Chumpelik (Hayden), D.A., & Sherman, J. (1984). [The efficacy of the PROMPT system in the treatment of developmental apraxia]. Unpublished raw data.

Dodd, G., Hua, Z., Crosbie, S., Holm, A., & Ozanne, A. (2007). *Diagnostic Evaluation of Articulation and Phonology (DEAP).* San Antonio, TX: Pearson Psych-Corp.

Fisher, H.B., & Logemann, J.A. (1971). *The Fisher-Logemann Test of Articulation Competence.* Chicago: Riverside.

Fletcher, S.G. (1992). *Articulation: A physiological approach.* San Diego: Singular.

Fogel, A., & Thelen, E. (1987). Development of early expressive and communicative action: Reinterpreting the evidence from a dynamic systems perspective. *Developmental Psychology, 23*, 747–761.

Freed, D.B., Marshal, R.C., & Frazier, K.E. (1997). Long term effectiveness of PROMPT treatment in a severely apraxic-aphasic speaker. *Aphasiology, 11*(4/5), 365–342.

Green, J.R., Moore, C., Higashikawa, M., & Steeve, R.W. (2000). The physiologic development of speech motor control: Lip and jaw coordination. *Journal of Speech, Language, and Hearing Research, 43*, 239–256.

Guenther, F.H. (2006). Cortical interactions underlying the production of speech sounds. *Journal of Communication Disorders, 39*, 350–365.

Hayden, D.A. (1986). *The motor-speech treatment hierarchy.* Unpublished manuscript, Toronto.

Hayden, D.A. (2000). *Bridging PROMPT technique to intervention manual.* Santa Fe, NM: The PROMPT Institute.

Hayden, D.A. (2002). *Bridging PROMPT technique to intervention manual.* (rev.ed.). Santa Fe, NM: The PROMPT Institute.

Hayden, D.A. (2004). PROMPT: A tactually grounded treatment approach to speech production disorders. In I. Stockman (Ed.), *Movement and action in learning and development: Clinical implications for pervasive developmental disorders* (pp. 255–297). San Diego: Elsevier/Academic Press.

Hayden, D.A. (2006). The PROMPT model: Use and application for children with mixed phonological-motor impairment. *Advances in Speech-Language Pathology, 8*(3), 265–281.

Hayden, D. (2008). *P.R.O.M.P.T. prompts for restructuring oral muscular phonetic targets, introduction to technique: A manual.* Santa Fe, NM: The PROMPT Institute.

Hayden, D.A., & Square, P. (1999). *Verbal Motor Production Assessment for Children* (VMPAC). San Antonio, TX: Pearson PsychCorp.

Head, H. (1926a). *Aphasia and kindred disorders of speech* (Vol. I). London: Cambridge University Press.

Head, H. (1926b). *Aphasia and kindred disorders of speech* (Vol. II). London: Cambridge University Press.

Hebb, D.O. (1949). *The organization of behavior: A neuropsychological theory.* New York: John Wiley & Sons.

Houghton, M.A. (2003, September). *The effect of the PROMPT system of therapy on a group of children with severe persistent sound system disorders.* Presentation to the School of Health and Rehabilitation Sciences, University of Queensland.

Jackson, J.H. (1958). Evolution and dissolution of the nervous system. In J. Taylor (Ed.), *Selected writings of John Hughlings Jackson* (Vol. 2, pp. 45–75). New York: Basic Books.

Kass, J.H. (2004). Plasticity of somatosensory and motor systems in developing and mature primate brains. In I. Stockman (Ed.), *Movement and action in learning and development: Clinical implications for pervasive developmental disorders* (pp. 75–93). San Diego: Academic Press.

Kent, R.D. (2004). Models of speech motor control: Implications from recent developments in neurophysiological and neurobehavioral science. In B. Maassen, R.D. Kent, H.F.M. Peters, P.H.M. Van Lieshout, & W. Hulstijn (Eds.), *Speech motor control in normal and disordered speech* (pp. 1–28). Oxford, England: Oxford University Press.

Kent, R.D., & Vorperian, H.K. (2007). In the mouths of babes: Anatomic, motor, and sensory foundations of speech development in children. In R. Paul (Ed.), *Language disorders from a developmental perspective: Essays in honor of Robin S. Chapman* (pp. 55–82). Mahwah, NJ: Lawrence Erlbaum Associates.

Lord, C., Rutter, M., DiLavore, P., & Risi, S. (1999). *Autism Diagnostic Observation Schedule–WPS Edition.* Los Angeles: Western Psychological Services.

Lord, C., Rutter, M., & Le Couteur, A. (1994). Autism Diagnostic Interview–Revised: A revised version of a diagnostic interview for caregivers of individuals with possible pervasive developmental disorders. *Journal of Autism and Developmental Disorders, 24,* 659-685.

McNeilage, P., & Davis, B. (2000, April). On the origin of internal structure of word forms. *Science, 288,* 527.

Monfils, M., Plautz, E., & Klein, J. (2005). In search of the motor engram: Motor map plasticity as a mechanism for encoding motor experience. *The Neuroscientist, 11*(5), 471–483.

Mullen, E.M. (1995). *Mullen Scales of Early Learning.* Circle Pines, MN: American Guidance Service.

Nasir, S., & Ostry D. (2006, March). *An examination of somatosensory precision requirements of speech production.* Paper presented at the Thirteenth Biennial Conference on Motor Speech: Motor Speech Disorders and Motor Speech Control, Austin, TX.

Neilson, R. (2003). *Sutherland Phonological Awareness Test–Revised.* Wollongong, Australia: Author.

Nelson, K. (2004). The event basis of conceptual and language development. In I. Stockman (Ed.), *Movement and action in learning and development: Clinical implications for pervasive developmental disorders* (pp. 117–139). San Diego: Academic Press.

Pearson, J.C., Finkel, L.H., & Edelman, G.M. (1987). Plasticity in the organization of adult cerebral cortical maps: a computer simulation based on neuronal group selection. *Journal of Neuroscience, 7,* 4209–4223.

Rogers, S.J., Hayden, D., Hepburn, S., Charlifue-Smith, R., Hall, T., & Hayes, A. (2006). Teaching young nonverbal children with autism useful speech: A pilot study of the Denver Model and PROMPT interventions. *Journal of Autism and Developmental Disorders, 36*(8), 1007–1024.

Rogers, S.J., & Lewis, H. (1989). An effective day treatment model for young children with pervasive developmental disorders. *Journal of the American Academy of Child and Adolescent Psychiatry, 28,* 207–214.

Schmidt, R.A. (1975). A schema theory of discrete motor skill learning. *Psychological Review, 82*(4), 225–260.

Schmidt, R.A., & Bjork, R.A. (1992). New conceptualizations of practice: Common principles in three paradigms suggest new concepts in learning. *Psychological Science, 3,* 207–217.

Schmidt, R.A., & Wrisberg, C. (2000). *Motor learning and performance.* Champaign, IL: Human Kinetics.

Schoner, G., & Kelso, J.A.S. (1988). Dynamic pattern generation in behavioral and neural systems. *Science, 239,* 1513–1520.

Semel, E., Wiig, E.H., & Secord, W. (2003). *Clinical Evaluation of Language Fundamentals–Fourth Edition.* San Antonio, TX: Pearson PsychCorp.

Sherman, J., & Chumpelik (Hayden), D.A. (1981). [Tactile cueing with non-verbal autism]. Unpublished raw data.

Shriberg, L.D., & Kwiatkowski, J. (1982). Phonological disorders III: A procedure for assessing severity of involvement. *Journal of Speech and Hearing Disorders, 47,* 256–270.

Skelton, S.L. (2004). Motor-skill learning approach to the treatment of speech-sound disorders. *CSHA, 34*(1), 8–9, 16.

Smith, A. (2004). Speech motor development: Integrating muscles, movements and linguistic units. *Journal of Communication Disorders, 39,* 331–349.

Smith, A., & Goffman, L. (2004). Interaction of motor and linguistic factors in the development of speech production. In B. Maassen, R.D. Kent, H.F.M. Peters, P.H.M. Van Lieshout, & W. Hulstijn (Eds.), *Speech motor control in normal and disordered speech* (pp. 225–252). New York: Oxford University Press.

Smith, A., & Zelaznik, H. (2004). Development of functional synergies for speech motor coordination in childhood and adolescence. *Developmental Psychology, 45*(1), 22–33.

Sparrow, S., Balla, D., & Cicchetti, D.C. (1998). *Vineland Social-Emotional Early Childhood Scales.* Circle Pines, MN: American Guidance Service.

Sporns, O., & Edelman, G. (1993). Solving Bernstein's problem: A proposal for the development of coordinated movement by selection. *Child Development, 64*(4), 960–981.

Square, P., Hayden (Chumpelik), D., & Adams, S. (1985). Efficacy of the PROMPT system for the treatment of acquired apraxia of speech. In R. Brookshire (Ed.), *Clinical aphasiology conference proceedings* (pp. 319–320). Minneapolis, MN: BRK Publishers.

Square, P., Hayden (Chumpelik), D., Morningstar, D., & Adams, S. (1986). Efficacy of the PROMPT system for the treatment of acquired apraxia of speech. In R. Brookshire (Ed.), *Clinical aphasiology conference proceedings* (pp. 221–226). Minneapolis, MN: BRK Publishers.

Square, P.A., Goshulak, D., Bose, A., & Hayden, D.A. (2000, February). *The effects of articulatory subsystem treatment for developmental neuromotor speech disorders.* Paper presented at the Tenth Biennial Conference on Motor Speech Disorders and Speech Motor Control, San Antonio, TX.

Square, P.A., Hayden, D.A., Ciolli, L., & Wilkins, C. (1999, November). *Speech motor performances of children with moderate to severe articulation disorders.* Paper presented at the American Speech-Language-Hearing Association conference, San Francisco.

Thelen, E. (2004). The central role of action in typical and atypical development: A dynamic systems perspective. In I. Stockman (Ed.), *Movement and action in learning and development: Clinical implications for pervasive developmental disorders* (pp. 49–73). San Diego: Elsevier/Academic Press.

Thelen, E., Corbetta, E., Kamm, K., Spencer, J.P., Schneider, K., & Zernicke, R.F. (1993). The transition to reaching: Mapping intention and intrinsic dynamic. *Child Development, 64,* 1058–1098.

Ward, R., Leitao, S., & Strauss, G. (2009). The effectiveness of PROMPT therapy for children with moderate-to-severe speech disorders associated with cerebral palsy. *Developmental Medicine & Child Neurology, 51*(Suppl. 5), 76.

Wechsler, D. (2002). *Wechsler Intelligence Scale for Children–Fourth Edition.* San Antonio, TX: Pearson PsychCorp.

World Health Organization. (2001). *International classification of functioning, disability and health.* Geneva: Author.

Family-Friendly Intervention

Nicole Watts Pappas

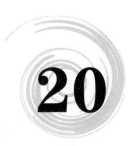

20

ABSTRACT

The family-friendly approach to speech intervention provides a model for interacting with and engaging families using any speech intervention approach. It can be used with children of all ages and with all types of speech sound disorders (SSD). This model provides both a framework for interacting with families and specific strategies for engaging families in all aspects of the intervention process including preassessment planning, assessment, intervention planning, intervention provision, and the evaluation of intervention. It is based on family-centered practices, which promote positive relationships between families and speech-language pathologists (SLPs).

INTRODUCTION

In the past few decades, family involvement in speech-language pathology and other allied health interventions for young children has increased. International policy now mandates family participation in pediatric allied health intervention (Edwards, Millard, Praskac, & Wisniewski, 2003; Franck & Callery, 2004). In addition, models of best practice encourage early intervention (EI) professionals to view families as partners in the intervention process (Crais, Poston Roy, & Free, 2006). This has created an imperative for SLPs to work closely with the families of their pediatric clients, endeavoring to involve them in both intervention provision and planning. However, some SLPs lack confidence and feel their university training has not prepared them for this role (Watts Pappas & McLeod, 2009b). This lack of confidence may be particularly prevalent in SLPs' feelings about intervention for SSD. SLPs have reported experiencing more difficulty involving parents in intervention for SSD than for other areas of communication such as language or stuttering (Watts Pappas & McLeod, 2009b). However, to meet the requirements of legislation and best practice, family involvement in SSD intervention is necessary.

TARGET POPULATIONS

The family-friendly approach to speech intervention is not specific to children of any particular age, cultural or linguistic background, or form of SSD. Instead, it can be used in conjunction with any intervention approach for children with SSD that involves families in some aspect of the intervention (Watts Pappas & McLeod, 2009b). Many speech intervention approaches describe family involvement as part of their technique. For example, the cycles approach (Hodson & Paden, 1991), the psycholinguistic approach (Stackhouse, Pascoe, & Gardner, 2006), and the nonlinear approach (Bernhardt, Stemberger, & Major, 2006) all include family involvement. In these approaches, family involvement predominantly consists of home practice activities involving the child. Other approaches to speech intervention, such as PROMPT (Hayden, 2006), Parents and Children Together (PACT; Bowen & Cupples, 2006), and core vocabulary (Dodd, Holm, Crosbie, & McIntosh, 2006) involve families to an even greater extent, recommending incorporation of family priorities in goal setting and family participation in intervention sessions. The family-friendly approach can be used with any of these approaches to most effectively facilitate their involvement in the way stipulated in the individual approach. The family-friendly approach also encourages SLPs to consider individual families' views and priorities and provide service that is empowering, supportive, and respectful to clients and their families (Watts Pappas, McLeod, & McAllister, 2009).

THEORETICAL BASIS

Dominant Theoretical Rationale for the Intervention Approach

Children's speech development is influenced not only by inherent qualities but also by their interaction with significant others in their world (Bronfenbrenner, 1979). Family members therefore exert a strong influence on children's speech acquisition. Family demographics such as socioeconomic status, family structure, parents' education levels, and family history of speech impairment may play an influential role in the child's communicative environment (Felsenfeld, McGue, & Broen, 1995; Hoff & Tian, 2005). For example, Campbell et al. (2003) established that low maternal education levels were positively associated with speech impairment. Because of the family's impact on children's speech acquisition, intervention that involves the family may be more effective than intervention that treats the child in isolation.

Policy makers and experts now recognize the importance of the family in intervention for young children. The World Health Organization's International Classification of Functioning, Disability and Health for Children and Youth (ICF-CY; World Health Organization [WHO], 2007) considers a child's difficulties not only at the traditional levels of body structure and function but also in the way a child's difficulties and their environment impact on his or her ability to participate in the activities of daily life (McLeod & McCormack, 2007). Family involvement in assessing, planning, and providing intervention may allow environmental factors and the child's activities and participation in daily life to be more successfully incorporated into a child's intervention.

Legislation in the provision of services to young children has also reflected the move toward more family-centered models of service. Traditionally, speech-language pathology and other allied health services were delivered in a therapist-centered manner, with families allowed little opportunity to participate in their child's intervention (Crais, 1991). However, campaigning by parents and resultant changes in policy and legislation have led to the adoption of models of service delivery that incorporate increased family involvement and power. In the United States, the Education for all Handicapped Children Act of 1975 (PL 94-142; Turnbull & Turnbull, 1982) and later the Individuals with Disabilities Education Act (IDEA) of 1990 (PL 101-476; Wehman, 1998) mandated family involvement in decision making about their child's intervention. Similar policy changes occurred in the

United Kingdom, with government policy mandating the use of family-centered practices in intervention for children from 1991 (Franck & Callery, 2004). The family-centered philosophy of EI promotes partnerships between families and professionals and is flexible to adapt to the differing needs, cultures, and beliefs of individual families (Rosenbaum, King, Law, King, & Evans, 1998). Family-centered models of care and intervention focus on families' developing competence rather than dependence on professionals (Dunst, 2002) and represent a more respectful and appropriate way of providing services to young children and their families (Crais, 1991).

The family-friendly approach to speech intervention is based on the family-centered philosophy of practice, with a focus on providing respectful, supportive, and empowering services to clients and their families (Watts Pappas et al., 2009). In the family-centered approach, professionals are required to follow the families' lead even if they disagree with family decisions. However, in the family-friendly approach to speech intervention, SLPs use their expertise to guide the intervention process, thereby fulfilling their responsibility to provide evidence-based and effective intervention to the child. Table 20.1 illustrates the differences between family-centered and family-friendly practice.

The family-friendly model was created as a result of longitudinal in-depth interviews with parents of children undergoing intervention for SSD. The needs and experiences of these families as well as the findings of other studies of families' perceptions of EI have been integrated to form the family-friendly approach to SSD intervention (Watts Pappas & McLeod, 2009b). Not only a philosophy of care, family-friendly speech intervention provides specific strategies to assist SLPs to more effectively work with families in a way that maximizes the outcomes for the child and meets the requirements of legislation.

Target Areas of Intervention

In the family-friendly approach to speech intervention, the manner in which the SLP interacts with the family and the strategies they use to motivate and facilitate the family's involvement are the targets of the intervention. It is designed to be used in tandem with other speech intervention approaches; therefore, specific speech sound processes are not targeted per se. Rather, the approach can be used to complement a multitude of intervention approaches, which may target many different areas of speech sound production.

Table 20.1. Comparison of family-centered and family-friendly models of intervention

Model	Family involvement in intervention provision	Family involvement in intervention planning	Primary decision maker	Primary client
Family-centered	Varies according to family's wishes	Varies according to family's wishes	Family	Usually the family (varies according to family's wishes)
Family-friendly	Families supported to be involved in the intervention if required	Varies according to family's wishes	Professional	Usually the child (varies according to family's wishes)

From Watts Pappas, N., McLeod, S., & McAllister, L. (2009). Models of practice used in SLPs' work with families. In N. Watts Pappas & S. McLeod (Eds.), *Working with families in speech-language pathology* (pp. 1–38). San Diego: Plural Publishing; adapted by permission.

EMPIRICAL BASIS

As professionals, we believe that working with families in intervention for SSD is important. For example, 98% of SLPs who participated in a survey conducted by Watts Pappas, McLeod, McAllister, and McKinnon (2008) agreed that involving parents in speech intervention was essential to the effectiveness of the intervention. SLPs also translate this belief into practice. Studies of family involvement in speech intervention indicate that the majority of clinicians report they involve families in SSD intervention in some way (Joffe & Pring, 2008; McLeod & Baker, 2004; Watts Pappas et al., 2008). For example, Watts Pappas and colleagues found that 95% of SLPs reported they asked parents to provide home activities to their child, and Joffe and Pring reported that 76.5% of the SLPs they surveyed used parental involvement as a therapy strategy for SSD. Considering assessment practices, Skahan, Watson, and Lof (2007) found that 87% of SLPs reported family involvement in the assessment process. However, is there empirical evidence to confirm the reported beliefs and practices of SLPs with regard to family involvement?

Many effective intervention approaches for SSD involve families as part of their treatment regimens (Bernhardt et al., 2006; Bowen & Cupples, 2004; Dodd et al., 2006; Hodson & Paden, 1991). For example, the PACT approach, which involves a significant amount of parental participation, has been demonstrated to be more effective than no intervention (Bowen & Cupples, 1998). However, although these approaches have been demonstrated to be effective, it is not known whether they would be just as effective without parental involvement.

Although no recent studies have examined the relative impact of family involvement in speech intervention, from the late 1950s to the early 1990s, a number of experimental studies were conducted that investigated the impact of various forms of family participation on speech intervention outcomes (Broen & Westman, 1990; Eiserman, McCoun, & Escobar, 1990; Fudala, England, & Ganoung, 1972; Sommers, 1962; Sommers et al., 1964; Tufts & Holliday, 1959; see Table 20.2). These studies explored a range of methods of parental involvement including parental attendance at intervention sessions, participation in intervention sessions, provision of home activities, and parents acting as the primary providers of intervention for their child. The studies were all conducted using traditional or minimal pair intervention approaches (see Watts Pappas, McLeod, McAllister, & Simpson, 2005, for a full review). Five of the six studies were randomized controlled trials in which the children were randomly allocated into the different treatment conditions (Eiserman et al., 1990; Fudala et al., 1972; Sommers, 1962; Sommers et al., 1964; Tufts & Holliday, 1959). All of these studies used blinded examiners to assess the children pre- and postintervention. The study conducted by Broen and Westman (1990) involved two groups of children—an experimental group and a contrast group who received no intervention during the period of the study. However, the children were not randomly allocated into these two conditions, with children in the experimental group showing appreciably poorer speech skills than those in the control group.

Although the studies were primarily randomized controlled trials, they could also be categorized as efficacy studies of parental involvement in intervention (level 2), with the amount of parental involvement required to achieve the outcomes unlikely to be achieved in the conditions of everyday practice (see Table 20.2). However, some studies could be described as studies of effectiveness (level 3) in which the type and frequency of parental involvement could be achieved in everyday practice. Overall, the findings of the studies indicated that parental involvement in the provision of home activities (when parents are

Table 20.2. Levels of evidence for studies of treatment efficacy for involving families in intervention

Level	Description	References
Ia	Meta-analysis of > 1 randomized controlled trial	—
Ib	Randomized controlled study	Eiserman et al. (1990); Fudala et al. (1972); Sommers (1962); Sommers et al. (1964); Tufts & Holliday (1959)
IIa	Controlled study without randomization	Broen & Westman (1990)
IIb	Quasi-experimental study	—
III	Nonexperimental studies, i.e., correlational and case studies	—
IV	Expert committee report, consensus conference, clinical experience of respected authorities	—

Adapted from the Scottish Intercollegiate Guidelines Network (http://www.sign.ac.uk).

trained to provide them) and parental attendance at intervention sessions can improve intervention outcomes for children with SSD.

Other studies demonstrated that trained parents can provide intervention to their child that is just as effective as intervention provided by an SLP (Eiserman et al., 1990; Fudala et al., 1972). For example, in a study of forty 3- to 5-year-old children with SSD, children whose parents provided them with a home program made just as much progress as children attending group intervention sessions with the SLP. However, intensive training and support (visits from the SLP every 2 weeks) was provided to the parents to conduct these programs.

In summary, SLPs' anecdotal beliefs and practices regarding family involvement in intervention for SSD appear to have empirical justification. Family involvement in SSD intervention can improve outcomes. However, to achieve these outcomes parents need to be provided with adequate support and training to act in this role. When families are involved in intervention without training and support they may find participation difficult, causing frustration for both the parent and the child (Watts Pappas & McLeod, 2009a). In fact, many studies of parents' perceptions of their involvement in allied health intervention have demonstrated that they can find it difficult and time consuming (Case-Smith & Nastro, 1993; Hinojosa & Anderson, 1991). Incorrectly conducted home practice may be detrimental rather than helpful to the child's progress in speech production, even leading to the child's production of a new error sound (Gardner, 2006).

Families also need to be motivated to participate in intervention. If parents are not inclined to be involved, then their provision of home activities or attendance at sessions is unlikely to impact positively on outcomes. Some families may report doing home activities even when they are not (Hinojosa & Anderson, 1991). SLPs need to ensure a relationship with the family that allows honest discussion of difficulties. To gain the benefits of family involvement, SLPs need to possess the skills to both engage families in the intervention and train them for effective involvement. Family-friendly speech intervention provides SLPs with strategies to achieve these aims.

A family-friendly intervention approach may also improve family satisfaction with service. Studies of families' perceptions of general EI services indicate that families prefer family-centered services (Law et al., 2003) and professionals who are respectful, supportive, and good communicators (Carrigan, Rodger, & Copely, 2001). Many parents are eager to be involved in speech intervention (Broen & Westman, 1990; Eiserman et al., 1990; Watts Pappas & McLeod, 2009a) but need to feel adequately supported to do so.

PRACTICAL REQUIREMENTS

To use family-friendly practice in SSD intervention, SLPs need to take the time and be flexible enough to allow individual family involvement (Watts Pappas & McLeod, 2009b). They should also hold a belief in the importance of treating families with respect and sensitivity and "think the best of families" (McWilliam, Tocci, & Harbin, 1998, p. 279). A number of studies have asked families to list the qualities that they find of most value in their health professionals. These qualities form the key skills required by SLPs to use the family-friendly approach to speech intervention. It is important to note that the majority of these studies were conducted in English-speaking countries and may represent primarily Western approaches to professional/family collaboration. However, the family-friendly approach is flexible, so the SLP can respond to the needs and beliefs of families from different cultures and ethnic groups.

Some of the most common relational skills reported by families as desirable include

Being approachable and friendly: Not surprisingly, families value professionals who are approachable and friendly as opposed to being condescending or rude (Baxter, 1989; MacKean, Thurston, & Scott, 2005; Watts Pappas & McLeod, 2009a). Many parents also want professionals who genuinely care about their child and family. When the professional establishes a positive, trusting relationship with the family and makes them feel comfortable, parents may be more likely to be honest with that professional. Establishing warm, welcoming relationships with families may also increase their motivation to be involved in the intervention (Baxter, 1989).

Respecting parents' ideas and opinions: Parents value professionals who they feel listen carefully to their concerns and respect their input to their child's care (Washington & Schwartz, 1996). When families feel that their opinions are disregarded by professionals, this can lead to frustration and negative feelings about that professional (Baxter, 1989; Case-Smith & Nastro, 1993; Glogowska & Campbell, 2000). For example, some parents interviewed in a study conducted by Baxter described their frustration at "having what we said brushed aside so as not to prolong the interview" (p. 265). When a professional listens to families' ideas and opinions, this can establish the family's trust in that professional. It also allows the professional to access the family's expertise about the child.

Communicating effectively: Families perceive that one of the key roles of the professional is to provide them with information. The professional's ability to communicate clearly and without jargon is therefore an important component in a family's satisfaction with their health professional. Families have reported that they want their professional to keep them informed about their child's intervention, sharing information in a timely, open, and honest fashion (Baxter, 1989; Carrigan et al., 2001; MacKean et al., 2005; Washington & Schwartz, 1996; Watts Pappas & McLeod, 2009a).

Establishing a positive rapport with the child: The professional's ability to engage the child in intervention has been found to be a very important component in establishing a positive and trusting relationship with the child's family. Parents want intervention to be a positive experience for their child and therefore value professionals who they feel genuinely like and can establish a positive rapport with their child (Baxter, 1989; Carrigan et al., 2001; Case-Smith & Nastro, 1993; MacKean et al., 2005). To some families, the professional's relationship with the child is as important, if not more important than their relationship with the parent (Case-Smith & Nastro, 1993; Watts Pappas & McLeod, 2009b). By engaging the child in the intervention, the parent's involvement and commitment to the intervention can also be engaged.

Nature of Sessions

The nature of the sessions provided in the family-friendly approach is determined by the speech sound intervention approach used by the SLP. In general, however, the family-friendly approach suggests that families attend both assessment and intervention sessions. If that is not possible, time for unrushed meetings with the family needs to be provided. If convenient for the family, home-based sessions are recommended for younger children.

Personnel

Not surprisingly, the family plays a major role in intervention planning and provision in the family-friendly approach. Family represents not only a child's parents but also other members of a child's extended family, including grandparents, siblings, aunts/uncles, foster parents, cousins, and family friends. The way in which family members are trained and engaged is the cornerstone of the family-friendly intervention approach for SSD and will be described in the key components section later in this chapter. In line with the approach's philosophy to provide holistic intervention to the child, other people who interact frequently with the child (e.g., child care teachers, coaches, friends) may also play a part in intervention. The SLP's role is to guide the intervention process and coordinate the different people involved in the child's intervention.

Dosage

Dosage of intervention is determined by the speech intervention approach used in conjunction with the family-friendly approach.

KEY COMPONENTS

The key principles of family-friendly practice are establishing positive relationships with families and children; respecting families' ideas, opinions, and individuality; communicating effectively; being sensitive and responsive to the individual needs of families; considering the child in the context of their family; supporting and encouraging family members to be involved in the intervention; and providing professional guidance and expertise to lead the intervention process (Watts Pappas et al., 2009). The key components of family-friendly practice can be used to guide interacting with and engaging families at each step of the intervention process. These steps include preassessment planning, assessment, assessment feedback, intervention planning, intervention, and evaluation of services.

Preassessment Planning

The assessment is often a family's first introduction to speech-language pathology or other EI services. They may be unsure of what an SLP does and what to expect from their initial appointment. Families may have varying prior experiences of EI for their child, and different cultural backgrounds may also impact on parents' initial expectations of and feelings about speech-language pathology services (Marshall, 2000). In some instances, families may have experienced various difficulties accessing the service, such as lengthy wait times, difficulty obtaining a referral, or disagreement within the family over the need for EI. The parents and the child may therefore experience some anxiety about their initial appointment. As one parent commented about her child's initial speech-language pathology assessment: "I was a nervous wreck...'cos I didn't honestly know what to expect when I got there" (Glogowska & Campbell, 2000, p. 398). To decrease potential anxiety and facilitate the assessment process, preassessment planning can focus on three purposes:

1. To provide families with information regarding the assessment process so as to allay any anticipatory anxiety they may be experiencing.

2. To begin the establishment of a positive relationship between the family and the professional who will be conducting the assessment.

3. To utilize the family's expertise about the child to more successfully evaluate the child's skills and increase the relevancy of the assessment to the child and family.

Creating a good first impression with families can lead to the establishment of a positive family/professional partnership for the intervention process. If parents or other family members are not able to attend the assessment appointment, preassessment planning allows the SLP to discuss the assessment with the family. Although family-friendly practice is flexible and can be adapted to suit the needs of individual families and limitations of different services, some basic components of preassessment planning will now be discussed.

The clinician conducting the assessment initially makes telephone contact with the family to organize a mutually convenient time and location for the assessment. To encourage family involvement and use their expertise about the child, family attendance at assessment sessions is recommended if possible. To tailor the assessment to the family's concerns, the SLP asks the family member to describe his or her major concerns regarding the child's communication, then plans an assessment that will answer the family's questions. Preassessment planning can also take place at a separate, face-to-face appointment with family members (usually the parents) and the SLP if time commitments of both the family and SLP allow.

During preassessment planning, the SLP provides the family with information about what will happen during the assessment session, including a description of possible assessment tasks, the people who will be present, information that will be requested from the family, and the length of the assessment. Parents are given the option to invite other family members or family friends to the assessment. They will be asked if they are comfortable talking about the child's difficulties in his or her presence. If not, a separate appointment or telephone interview is made to gain background information.

The family is asked about the child's temperament, behavior, likes and dislikes, and possible reaction to the assessment session. This lets the SLP plan an assessment that will provide the best opportunity to evaluate the child's abilities. If the child had been previously assessed, the family is asked about that assessment and what aspects of it were helpful or unhelpful. To put the child at ease and stimulate SLP/child discussion when the assessment will not be conducted at the child's home, the SLP may suggest that the family bring along some of the child's favorite toys or books. Other adaptations to the assessment environment or participants can also be explored. For example, the child may be more verbal around siblings or more likely to participate in a play-based rather than a table-based assessment task.

To increase involvement in the assessment process, the SLP may ask the family to begin collecting information before the assessment. This may take the form of writing down the child's utterances or speech errors or asking for input from others in the child's environment. The Speech Participation and Activity Assessment of Children (SPAA-C; McLeod, 2004), a questionnaire-based assessment, is a useful tool for accessing family members' and friends' knowledge of the child's communication skills in different settings. The SPAA-C also includes a section addressing children's perceptions of their own talking. This assessment tool can be sent to the family to complete ahead of time. Active family involvement in assessment tasks can enable the SLP to obtain information about the child's communication skills in a variety of settings.

After the preassessment interview, an information pack can be sent or given to the family. This can contain information regarding the assessment location, the SLP's contact information, the proposed time and date of the assessment, and other possible details, such as parking information and a photo of the SLP. It can also contain information about speech-language pathology services and a book to read to younger children about the upcoming assessment session. Giving families information about what will happen at the assessment session will help put them at ease, hopefully paving the way for a collaborative and trusting SLP/family relationship.

Assessment to Support Decision Making

Various assessments to evaluate a child's speech sound production exist. The decision of which assessment tasks to use with a child may be influenced by the resources at the SLP's disposal, their knowledge base, usual practice, the age of the child, the difficulties the child presents with, and the intervention approach the SLP wishes to use. In the family-friendly approach to assessment, the assessment tasks are planned according to the family's concerns, and the child is considered holistically, including how he or she communicates in a variety of settings. Family members are provided with the opportunity to be involved in the assessment—by providing information regarding their child, giving advice regarding the conduct of the assessment, participating actively in the collection of information about their child, and evaluating the results of the assessment. Some of the key components of a family-friendly assessment will now be described. As family-friendly practice is flexible, these components may be adapted to meet the needs of individual families.

The way that the SLP and other staff members interact with the family is important to their feelings of comfort. The SLP should endeavor to be friendly and approachable when first meeting the family, and respectful and sensitive when interviewing the parents about their child. Establishing a good rapport with the child is also an important way to put parents at ease. Of similar importance is the attitude of other staff members, such as administration staff, who should be welcoming and sensitive to the family.

At the beginning of the assessment session, the SLP introduces him- or herself to the family and the child. The SLP ensures he or she is on time for the appointment or apologizes if delayed, showing respect for the family's time. Making an effort to ensure that appointments run on time can make a great difference to the families' initial feelings about EI (Baxter, 1989).

First, the SLP briefly reviews the agreed plan for the session. The family is invited to suggest changes to the proposed assessment. Information about the child's history is taken from family members in a respectful manner, being sensitive to the family's feelings. Information is gathered regarding the child's strengths and weaknesses and the impact of his or her communication skills on the child's participation in the activities of his or her daily life. If possible, the SLP assesses the child's communication skills in additional settings, such as at school.

If the family has completed checklists or assessment tools for their child prior to the assessment session, the findings of these assessments are then discussed. If family members are involved in the assessment, the SLP should acknowledge the importance of the family's input and consider it in the assessment. The SLP then describes the assessment tasks that will be used and how these tests will answer the family's questions about the child's communication skills. Providing information about the tests can aid the family's understanding of the assessment report (Donaldson, McDermott, Hollands, Copley, & Davidson, 2004) and make them feel more comfortable during the assessment session, as for example, when the assessment task requires failure on a number of items before the test is discontinued. For assessments that do not allow family members to prompt the child, they are encouraged to write down observations about the child's performance to discuss at the end of the assessment.

Family members are invited to sit with the child while the assessment is being conducted if they wish or to leave if they believe the child will perform better without them present. The family can help identify factors that may affect the child's performance and suggest how these performance variables may be overcome. For some assessment tasks, it may be useful for family members to be actively involved. For example, if children are not cooperative with an oro-motor assessment, they may perform some activities for their parent rather than the SLP. The SLP can also use the parents' knowledge about the child's motivation and attention throughout the assessment.

During the assessment, the principles of dynamic assessment are used. Dynamic assessment focuses not only on what the child can't do but what they can be taught to achieve (Law & Camilleri, 2007). The child's abilities to perform tasks with various levels of prompting are assessed. In speech-sound assessment this may take the form of assessing a child's stimulability for a sound using gestural, verbal, or physical prompts or manipulating the linguistic environment, number of presentations, or reinforcements given (Glaspey & Stoel-Gammon, 2007). Specific stimulability assessments are available (see Glaspey & Stoel-Gammon for a review) or the SLP can incorporate dynamic assessment into existing assessment tasks. The family may also have attempted to help the child say certain sounds at home. At this point they may be able to demonstrate strategies that they have found to be useful. The use of dynamic assessment can not only guide intervention planning but also highlight the child's strengths and abilities rather than focusing only on his or her weaknesses.

At the completion of the assessment, the SLP asks the family if they have any questions or concerns. They are also asked about their perception of their child's performance during the assessment tasks and whether they felt that the performance was typical of the child. Some brief initial assessment feedback is given to the family to avoid leaving the family unsure of their child's performance until they are provided with formal feedback. The SLP then organizes a session with the family in which to provide formal verbal and written feedback about the assessment results and plan the management of the child's difficulties with the family.

Assessment Feedback

The communication of assessment findings to the family is an important task that should be conducted with sensitivity and thoroughness. Although professionals perform this activity frequently, for individual families this information is critical to themselves and their child. An assessment can often highlight and confirm concerns about the extent of a child's difficulties, thereby upsetting family members. Providing assessment feedback in a timely, unrushed, sensitive, and caring manner, as well as in a way that is easily understood by the family, is therefore of great importance.

In the family-friendly approach to speech intervention, assessment feedback is provided to families face to face if possible. The family is invited to attend an appointment without the child to discuss assessment findings and plans for future management. The assessment feedback should include a discussion of the information regarding the child's functioning that is contained in a report that they are given to take home as well as the formulation of an intervention plan for the child and family. The family is given the option of inviting other family members or friends to attend the assessment feedback meeting if they wish.

At this meeting it is important to make the family feel welcome, especially if a number of professionals are providing feedback, which may feel imposing to families. If a number of professionals are attending the meeting, make sure that they are not seated across the table from family members. Seating at a round table is more inclusive and conducive to a collaborative discussion between family members and professionals. Using name tags including both the person's name and his or her profession can help the family keep track of the variety of professionals who may have seen their child. Providing drinks such as tea or coffee can, in some cases, make the family feel more welcome and create a less formal atmosphere. The time allocated for the assessment feedback session should be sufficient for the family to ask questions and feel unrushed. Professionals should remember to use language that is free of jargon or acronyms and is easy to understand.

The SLP reads through the report provided to the family, checks for understanding and agreement with the findings, and answers any questions. As Crais (1993) noted, if family members' and professionals' views about the results of the assessment differ, families may be less likely to follow through with recommendations.

The Assessment Report

Providing a report of the assessment ensures families have the information they need to make informed choices regarding their child's intervention. When families are unable to attend assessment or intervention sessions, reports may act as one of the primary methods of communication between the SLP and family. Even when parents attend an assessment feedback session, they may have difficulty remembering the information they are told, so reports provide a record of assessment results that can be referred to later and shared with others. Failure to receive adequate feedback about assessment results can cause the family to feel disempowered.

The style and content of the report should be carefully considered. Traditionally, SLP reports have been written for other professionals, rather than for families. These reports often contain jargon and can be difficult for family members to understand. For example, Donaldson and colleagues (2004) conducted a study of parents' satisfaction with occupational therapy and SLP reports in a university EI clinic. They found that many parents found the reports difficult and frustrating to read.

Reports that are difficult to understand can potentially exclude families from the assessment process, denying them information about their child (Donaldson et al., 2004). In the family-friendly approach to speech intervention, the report is written specifically with the family's understanding in mind and is individualized to cater to each family's needs. If professional terms are used, then explanations need to be provided. Terms such as *devoicing*, *stimulability*, *phonological processes*, and *oro-motor* can be confusing for parents, and their use should be avoided.

The information included in the report should also be considered. In the family-friendly approach to speech intervention, first and foremost the report is written to answer the family's questions. The report may also contain the following information:

- Information regarding the assessments conducted and the child's performance on those assessments, including information about how the child's skills compare to other children of the same age (if appropriate). Specifically in relation to SSD, parents report they want information about which sounds their child produces in error (Watts Pappas & McLeod, 2009b). Tables and the use of real examples can be helpful in outlining speech sound errors.

- Information regarding the practical implications of the child's difficulties. What does the child's performance on the assessment suggest about his or her likely performance on functional tasks? Are the child's difficulties remediable? How long will the child require intervention? How will the child's difficulties affect him or her in the future? For example, many children presenting with SSD may also experience difficulty with literacy. When necessary, this information is provided in the report along with plans for managing that possible difficulty.

- Information regarding the child's strengths as well as his or her weaknesses.

- Information about how the child responded to learning new skills based on dynamic assessment, such as his or her stimulability for error sounds and the cues that were most helpful in eliciting these new skills.

- Information about the child's communication in a variety of settings and activities.

- The families' input to the assessment.

- Possible options for intervention targets.

- Practical strategies that the family and others may use to help the child.

- Information regarding services the family may be able to access.

Through the report and assessment feedback session, the family can be offered a variety of helpful information. When family members are given assessment feedback, they are asked if they agree with the findings of the assessment and are given the opportunity to suggest changes to the report.

Intervention Planning

Nature of Goals

To make the intervention relevant to the child and family, family involvement in intervention planning is essential and makes it more likely that parents will be supportive of and motivated to be actively involved in the intervention provision. Although some families may be happy to follow the SLP's general recommendations for the type of intervention required, their input into aspects of the intervention plan can be useful.

After discussing the assessment report and answering any family questions about its contents, the child's intervention plan (which may take the form of an individualized education program or an individualized family service plan) is created with both SLP and family input. The family is asked what their major goals are for the child and what they would like to achieve from intervention. They are also asked about any previous intervention and what aspects of the intervention they found helpful or unhelpful. The family expectations of their involvement in the intervention and family/SLP roles are discussed. Some families may be difficult to engage in intervention provision due to an initial mismatch between the SLP and family expectations of involvement. If time is spent initially discussing the importance of family involvement, families may be more willing to actively participate in their child's intervention.

The SLP presents possible options for the child's intervention. Although the SLP retains leadership of this process, the families' choices regarding sound targets or other aspects of intervention are considered and included when possible. When several options are appropriate, the family is provided with information to enable them to make an informed choice. If the family's wishes cannot be accommodated because of service limitations or because they would be detrimental to the child's progress, reasons for this are respectfully explained to the family. This is different from family-centered practice in which the SLP follows the family's wishes even if he or she does not professionally agree with their decision (Brown, Humphrey, & Taylor, 1997). In keeping with the holistic focus of the approach, goals for intervention not only focus on speech sound production but also on the child's participation in activities of daily life. For example, education could be provided to teachers and students at the child's school about their difficulties. Other service delivery factors, such as the timing of intervention sessions and the type and duration of intervention, are also discussed.

The intervention plan is written down, including the expected roles of both the SLP and the family. Both the family and the SLP keep a copy of this plan. The family is reassured that they can request that intervention goals be reevaluated during the intervention. Involving the family in intervention planning gives them a sense of ownership over the process, making them more motivated to be involved and increasing their satisfaction with proposed goals and activities.

Goal Attack Strategies

The goal attack strategies used are determined by the individual speech intervention approach that is used in conjunction with family-friendly practice.

Intervention

Many intervention approaches have been demonstrated to ameliorate children's speech impairment effectively (Baker, 2006). This book provides a review of a number of different SSD intervention approaches that vary in how they involve families. The family-friendly approach to speech intervention can be used in conjunction with any intervention approach that involves families as part of its intervention regimen.

Description of Activities

The first section of the intervention session focuses on relationship building, such as inquiring about the family's week, before moving on to specific speech-sound activities. If sessions are held outside the home, family members including other children are made to feel welcome. Parents are particularly appreciative when provision is made for siblings (Edwards et al., 2003; Watts Pappas & McLeod, 2009a). Some siblings may be able to be involved in intervention activities. By incorporating siblings within the intervention session (when possible) the SLP can gain an understanding of the environment that the parent works in with the child at home and can give the parent strategies to manage the practice with siblings present. Inclusion of siblings also values and highlights the important input that they can have in their brother's or sister's lives (Barr, McLeod, & Daniel, 2008).

Seat placement in the intervention session is important because it provides nonverbal cues about the family's expected involvement (or noninvolvement) in the intervention session. In the family-friendly approach, the parent is invited to sit with the child and the SLP. This gives the parent a sense of involvement in the intervention and allows for easy communication with the SLP throughout the session.

If home practice activities have been given, the SLP first asks the parent about his or her experiences conducting these with the child at home. Enquiring about home activities demonstrates to the parent and the child that these activities are valued and also allows the SLP to problem-solve with the parent regarding any problems he or she experienced. Depending on the intervention approach, the SLP may then ask the parent to demonstrate how he or she conducted the activities with their child at home so that the SLP can determine if the parent is conducting the activities correctly and can give appropriate feedback. Because demonstrating in front of the SLP may be a source of potential anxiety for the parent, the SLP should provide positive comments regarding the parent's involvement and be sensitive when providing constructive feedback.

The SLP then outlines the plan for the rest of the intervention session, discussing the planned intervention activities and goals with the parent. At this stage, the parent may suggest changes to the proposed intervention activities or provide advice regarding ways in which the SLP can most successfully engage the child in the intervention activities. The parent may give information regarding the child's favorite activities or toys and provide guidance regarding the child's temperament on different days. In addition, because individual parents and families will have unique skills and attributes to bring to the child's intervention, they can often suggest innovative ideas. As Hinojosa and Anderson commented in their reflection on their interviews of parents of children with cerebral palsy: "We were fascinated by the mothers' creative skills in their ability to adapt home activities and routines to address their children's therapeutic goals" (1991, p. 277). In this section of the intervention session, the SLP and parent both use their individual expertise and skills to plan and conduct the intervention activities collaboratively.

Next, the SLP demonstrates the intervention activities to the child. At the same time, he or she continues to interact with the family member, describing the reasoning behind tasks or strategies and using family input to most successfully engage the child. This may make the family feel more confident about home practice. Furthermore, families may feel uneasy if they do not know the purpose of intervention activities. For example, in a parent interview study, one parent reported feeling concerned when her SLP used hand gestures to cue her child to produce sounds. Not knowing the reason for the hand gestures the parent commented, "I thought he was going deaf." She went on to say, "Don't expect that they [the parents] will know what you [the SLP] are doing" (Watts Pappas, 2007, p. 238).

If the parents wish, they can be actively involved in providing intervention. First, the SLP demonstrates the activity. Then both the parent and the SLP take turns providing the intervention to the child. In this way the parent is given a repeated model of the intervention as well as an opportunity for direct practice. Such collaboration can allow the SLP to provide feedback to the parent, the child to become comfortable with having the parent conduct therapy, and the parent to become more confident in working with the child. Intervention progresses in a collaborative fashion with both the parent and SLP feeling comfortable to suggest changes.

At the end of each intervention session, the SLP spends time discussing how the family felt the session went and what they might focus on in the next session. If home activities are provided, the SLP discusses those with the parent at this time. Allowing time for discussion at the end of the session allows the parent to provide input to the intervention program and the SLP to provide information to the parent. Parents appreciate being kept updated about their child's progress and being given an opportunity to speak with the SLP.

Home Practice

In many speech sound intervention approaches, families are provided home activities. These can be an essential component of the intervention, providing additional practice and intervention in different settings. Many SLPs believe that home practice can make an important contribution to overall progress (Watts Pappas et al., 2009). However, benefits from home practice depend on the types of activities being performed and whether these activities are being performed correctly. The two components of successful home practice, therefore, are motivation and effective parent training.

Despite its frequent use by SLPs (Watts Pappas et al., 2009), home practice is often provided without appropriate family training and support, thus making it a source of frustration and distress for both the parents and the child. For example in the study conducted by Hinojosa and Anderson, one parent reflected on the EI home activities she was provided in this way: "She [the SLP] would give me an incredible amount of work to do. . . There was no physical human way I could do it" (1991, p. 275).

Families need to be considered individually when providing home practice activities, with the SLP needing to be flexible to adapt activities to each family, their abilities, and daily routine. The SLP first discusses the family's routines and ability to do activities with the child at home so that activities are provided that can fit into daily routines. The activities may utilize games and toys from the home, or activities and games may be provided. Parents often report that children can be uncooperative with homework. Providing games and activities to assist the parent in motivating the child is therefore an essential component of successful homework completion. Families themselves can often suggest excellent ways in which home activities can fit into their daily routine and innovative ways in which sound targets can be practiced. Utilizing the family's knowledge of their own abilities and home environment can increase the actual implementation and success of home practice.

Both Bowen and Cupples (1998) and Gardner (2006) described useful models of training parents to work with their child at home. In the PACT approach to speech intervention, Bowen and Cupples described using PowerPoint to provide parents with information via slideshows. They covered specific techniques such as "modelling, recasting, encouraging self-modelling and self-correction...using labelled praise and providing focused auditory input" (p. 284). Gardner described a similar program entitled "Talking About Speech," created from an examination of the specific skills that SLPs use to work with children with SSD. This program also teaches family members the skills to elicit sounds from children, such as modeling and imitation, encouraging self-correction, teaching correct productions, giving praise, and stepping down support. These methods supplement those described previously in which families participate and receive instruction. Providing information in written, visual, and verbal forms is also useful. If families do not attend intervention sessions, then a video of the session may help families work with the child at home.

Besides enhancing intervention outcomes, a family's involvement in their child's intervention can be a positive experience providing a sense of achievement (Watts Pappas, 2007). As one parent in the Watts Pappas study reflected: "I achieved something, I helped Jacob achieve something, we did it" (2007, p. 254). Using the principles of family-friendly practice to engage and support families to be involved in speech intervention may make the family participation elements of individual intervention approaches more effective and increase the acceptability of those intervention techniques to families.

Evaluation of Intervention

Family involvement in the evaluation of intervention can improve services, making them more responsive to children's and families' needs (Carrigan et al., 2001). In the family-friendly approach to speech intervention, families are encouraged to participate in evaluation of the intervention both during and at the completion of the intervention process. During intervention provision, the SLP consistently communicates with the family about how they feel the intervention is progressing. If the child is old enough, they may also be involved in evaluation. Formal family evaluation occurs when a block of intervention is completed or the family exits the service. The SLP discusses with the family their feelings about the intervention outcomes and asks them to identify ways in which the intervention and the service worked well or could be improved. Families could also be given the opportunity to fill out an anonymous questionnaire or participate in an interview conducted by another staff member. Regular evaluation of services by the child and their family is an essential element of family-friendly practice, ensuring service that is congruent with family needs.

CONSIDERATIONS FOR CHILDREN FROM CULTURALLY AND LINGUISTICALLY DIVERSE BACKGROUNDS

In increasingly multicultural societies, SLPs and clients often come from different cultural and linguistic backgrounds (Crais et al., 2006). However, most SSD intervention research has been conducted within a Western cultural framework. Beliefs about speech, interactions with children, and perceptions about accessing intervention differ from culture to culture. Families from different cultures may interact with their children in very different ways than families from a mainstream Western community. The likelihood that a family will access intervention, and their views of intervention, may also be culturally dependent (Marshall, 2000). Because the family-friendly approach focuses on adapting intervention for individual families, it is well suited for use with children and families from different cultural and linguistic backgrounds.

CASE STUDY

Caiden (age 3;7) was referred for SLP services at a community health center by his parents, Stephen and Kelly. Prior to the assessment the SLP called Kelly and asked about her concerns. Kelly indicated that she felt Caiden was bright and that his understanding of language was good for his age but that his speech was "holding him back." She was concerned that Caiden's speech difficulties were making it difficult for him to form friendships. Kelly also wanted to know how long it would take for his problem to be remediated and whether he would be "right" prior to entering school. The SLP then described the specific assessments she planned to administer to answer Kelly's questions. From Kelly's description of her concerns, the SLP planned to assess Caiden's expressive language, speech sound production, and phonological awareness skills. The SLP ascertained that Kelly was comfortable speaking about Caiden's difficulties in front of him. The SLP then asked Kelly about Caiden's likes and dislikes and how he would possibly react to the assessment situation.

Kelly attended the assessment appointment with her mother, Sandra, and Caiden. When Kelly, Sandra, and Caiden arrived, the SLP introduced herself and showed them to the room in which the assessment would take place. She then briefly reviewed the plan for the assessment session and asked Kelly and Sandra whether they would like to suggest any changes. After taking background information about Caiden in a respectful and sensitive manner, the SLP asked about the assessment tasks that Kelly had completed at home with Caiden. The results indicated that although Caiden was very social with adults, he tended to play alone in child care and became frustrated when not understood by other children.

The SLP described the tests she would use to assess Caiden. She highlighted that for some of the assessments, it would be important not to provide Caiden with any prompts so that his performance could be compared with others of the same age. However, she gave both Sandra and Kelly some paper to write down anything about Caiden's performance that they would like to discuss with the SLP. Kelly and Sandra were invited to sit with Caiden while the assessment took place. Caiden's speech sound production in words, the consistency of his production, his oro-motor skills and his stimulability for error sounds were then assessed. At the completion of the assessment the SLP quickly scored the results and gave Kelly and Sandra some information about Caiden's performance. Most significantly, Caiden presented with a moderate-to-severe inconsistent SSD (Dodd et al., 2006). The SLP provided this information in a simple and clear way and checked for Kelly and Sandra's understanding. She included information about Caiden's strengths and reassured the family that his difficulties could be addressed with intervention. She also asked Kelly and Sandra whether they agreed with the findings.

Next Kelly and her husband Stephen attended an assessment feedback session. The SLP welcomed Stephen and Kelly, offered them a beverage, and provided them with a draft of Caiden's report for discussion and potential modification. The SLP then went through the report with them. The report was written in lay language and focused on answering the questions posed by Kelly at the pre-assessment planning meeting. The report also included suggestions for home and child care. The SLP then discussed intervention options with Caiden's parents. The local clinic would be able to offer Caiden 16 intervention sessions initially. Information about other options for intervention, such as sessions offered by private SLPs, was also provided. Stephen and Kelly were given an information sheet about SSD and expressive language delay as well as information about a local support group for parents of children with various forms of speech impairment.

Stephen and Kelly indicated they would like to access intervention at the center. The SLP then discussed possible intervention goals. Caiden's parents indicated they were more concerned about Caiden's speech sound production than his expressive language and would prefer a focus on that difficulty. The SLP accepted the parents' priority for work on speech sounds by her and the family, but suggested that some expressive language activities could be provided for child care. Kelly and Stephen felt that this was a good idea. By focusing on the family's priorities the SLP made the intervention more relevant to them and increased the likelihood they would follow her recommendations. Considering the inconsistency of Caiden's speech, the SLP suggested use of the core vocabulary approach (Dodd et al., 2006) and discussed the parents' expectations of their own involvement in the intervention. At the end of the session the SLP gave the parents a copy of the plan that they had created during the session. The family would choose the 50 target words for the intervention the following week and email the SLP with the list of words so corresponding picture cards could be made before the first session. The number and length of the intervention sessions was discussed. As the core vocabulary technique suggests, intervention sessions would be provided twice weekly (Dodd et al., 2006).

At intervention sessions, Kelly was invited to sit at the table with Caiden and the SLP and actively participate in the sessions. Sessions usually began with a general discussion of how the family was and the activities they had engaged in during the week. Initially, the home activities that Caiden was provided with at the previous session would be reviewed and his mother would be asked to demonstrate one of them to determine if she were giving the activities correctly. How Kelly found working on the activities at home with Caiden was also discussed. As outlined in the core vocabulary approach in the first session of the week, Caiden would pull the 10 target words for the week out of a bag. The session then focused on providing Caiden with visual and descriptive cues to facilitate his production of those words. In the second intervention session, games and activities were used to help Caiden practice these words a number of times in the session. Once the SLP had demonstrated an activity, Kelly was invited to take turns to give the activity to Caiden with the SLP. The SLP provided feedback respectfully and sensitively to Kelly about her provision of intervention. In addition, the SLP sought Kelly's advice about how to approach particular activities with Caiden. The intervention proceeded collaboratively with both parties offering their particular expertise and skills to ensure the intervention was successful. At the end of every session the SLP spent some time discussing the session and Caiden's progress with Kelly, then introduced home activities for the week.

At the end of the intervention block, Caiden's speech was reassessed using the same assessment used at the initial assessment. The consistency of his speech on both the words targeted in therapy and nontargeted words had improved from 75% to 25% inconsistency. He also had added three sounds to his phonemic inventory. These sounds were reported by his parents to be used consistently in conversation. Caiden's parents were involved in evaluating Caiden's progress by providing information on his use of the target words in conversation and obtaining information about his intelligibility from communication partners in other settings. They were also asked how they felt about the intervention. They reported that although they found it hard to attend the clinic twice a week and implement the activities at home, they felt the intervention had been "well worth it." They felt that Caiden was now more easily understood and noted that improvements in his speech had been commented on by others. Stephen and Kelly were also provided with a questionnaire requesting feedback and designed to help improve future service to Caiden and other families.

STUDY QUESTIONS

1. How could the SLP prepare the family for the assessment?

2. In what ways could the family be involved in the assessment process?

3. How could the SLP respond to the family's differing priorities for intervention?

4. How could the family be involved in the intervention?

5. How can the SLP support the family to work with the child at home?

FUTURE DIRECTIONS

Current best practice and legislation mandate family involvement in intervention for speech impairment and other difficulties. The family-friendly approach to speech intervention provides a proposed framework for interacting with families to most appropriately and successfully engage them in intervention. Further research needs to be conducted to identify whether the family-friendly practice approach to speech intervention can improve intervention outcomes of and family satisfaction with existing approaches to SSD.

SUGGESTED READINGS

Gardner, H. (2006). Training others in the art of therapy for speech sound disorders: An interactional approach. *Child Language Teaching and Therapy*, *22*(1), 27–46.

Watts Pappas, N., & McLeod, S. (2009). Working with families of children with speech impairments. In N. Watts Pappas & S. McLeod (Eds.), *Working with families in speech-language pathology* (pp. 189–228). San Diego: Plural Publishing.

REFERENCES

Baker, E. (2006). Management of speech impairment in children: The journey so far and the road ahead. *Advances in Speech-Language Pathology, 8*(3), 156–163.

Barr, J., McLeod, S., & Daniel, G. (2008). Siblings of children with speech impairment: Cavalry on the hill. *Language, Speech, and Hearing Services in Schools, 39*(1), 21–32.

Baxter, C. (1989). Parent-perceived attitudes of professionals: Implications for service providers. *Disability, Handicap and Society, 4*(3), 259–269.

Bernhardt, B.H., Stemberger, J., & Major, E. (2006). General and nonlinear intervention perspectives for a child with a resistant phonological impairment. *Advances in Speech-Language Pathology, 8*(3), 190–206.

Bowen, C., & Cupples, L. (1998). A tested phonological therapy in practice. *Child Language Teaching and Therapy, 14,* 29–50.

Bowen, C., & Cupples, L. (2004). The role of families in optimizing phonological therapy outcomes. *Child Language Teaching and Therapy, 20*(3), 245–260.

Bowen, C., & Cupples, L. (2006). PACT: Parents and Children Together in phonological therapy. *Advances in Speech-Language Pathology, 8*(3), 282–292.

Broen, P.A., & Westman, M.J. (1990). Project parent: A preschool speech program implemented through parents. *Journal of Speech & Hearing Disorders, 55,* 495–502.

Bronfenbrenner, U. (1979). *The ecology of human development.* Cambridge, MA: Harvard University Press.

Brown, S., Humphry, R., & Taylor, E. (1997). A model of the nature of family-therapist relationships: Implications for education. *The American Journal of Occupational Therapy, 51*(7), 597–603.

Campbell, T.F., Dollaghan, C.A., Rockette, H.E., Paradise, J.L., Feldman, H.M., Shriberg, L.D., et al. (2003). Risk factors for speech delay of unknown origin in 3-year-old children. *Child Development, 74*(2), 346–357.

Carrigan, N., Rodger, S., & Copley, J. (2001). Parent satisfaction with a pediatric occupational therapy service: A pilot investigation. *Physical and Occupational Therapy in Pediatrics, 21*(1), 51–76.

Case-Smith, J., & Nastro, M. (1993). The effect of occupational therapy intervention on mothers of children with cerebral palsy. *The American Journal of Occupational Therapy, 47*(9), 811–817.

Crais, E. (1991, September). Moving from "parent involvement" to family-centered services. *American Journal of Speech-Language Pathology, 1,* 5–8.

Crais, E. (1993). Families and professionals as collaborators in assessment. *Topics in Language Disorders, 14*(1), 29–40.

Crais, E., Poston Roy, V., & Free, K. (2006). Parents' and professionals' perceptions of family-centered practices: What are actual practices vs. what are ideal practices? *American Journal of Speech-Language Pathology, 15,* 365–377.

Dodd, B., Holm, A., Crosbie, S., & McIntosh, B. (2006). A core vocabulary approach for management of inconsistent speech disorder. *Advances in Speech-Language Pathology, 8*(3), 220–230.

Donaldson, N., McDermott, A., Hollands, K., Copley, J., & Davidson, B. (2004). Clinical reporting by occupational therapists and speech pathologists: Therapists' intentions and parental satisfaction. *Advances in Speech-Language Pathology, 6*(1), 23–38.

Dunst, C.J. (2002). Family-centered practices: Birth through high school. *The Journal of Special Education, 36*(3), 139–147.

Education for All Handicapped Children Act of 1975, PL 94-142, 20 U.S.C. §§ 1400 *et seq.*

Edwards, M., Millard, P., Praskac, L., & Wisniewski, P. (2003). Occupational therapy and early intervention: A family-centred approach. *Occupational Therapy International, 10*(4), 239–252.

Eiserman, W., McCoun, M., & Escobar, C. (1990). A cost-effectiveness analysis of two alternative program models for serving speech-disordered preschoolers. *Journal of Early Intervention, 14*(4), 297–317.

Felsenfeld, S., McGue, M., & Broen, P.A. (1995). Familial aggregation of phonological disorders: Results from a 28-year follow-up. *Journal of Speech and Hearing Research, 28,* 1091–1107.

Franck, L.S., & Callery, P. (2004). Re-thinking family-centred care across the continuum of children's healthcare. *Child: Care, Health & Development, 30*(3), 265–277.

Fudala, J.B., England, G., & Ganoung, L. (1972). Utilization of parents in a speech correction program. *Exceptional Children, 1,* 407–412.

Gardner, H. (2006). Training others in the art of therapy for speech sound disorders: An interactional approach. *Child Language Teaching and Therapy, 22*(1), 27–46.

Glaspey, A., & Stoel-Gammon, C. (2007). A dynamic approach to phonological assessment. *Advances in Speech-Language Pathology, 9*(4), 286–296.

Glogowska, M., & Campbell, R. (2000). Investigating parental views of involvement in pre-school speech and language therapy. *International Journal of Language and Communication Disorders, 35*(3), 391–405.

Hayden, D. (2006). The PROMPT model: Use and application for children with mixed phonological-motor impairment. *Advances in Speech-Language Pathology, 8*(3), 265–281.

Hinojosa, J., & Anderson, J. (1991). Mothers' perceptions of home treatment programs for their preschool children with cerebral palsy. *American Journal of Occupational Therapy, 45,* 273–279.

Hodson, B.W., & Paden, E.P. (1991). *Targeting intelligible speech: A phonological approach to remediation* (2nd ed.). Austin, TX: PRO-ED.

Hoff, E., & Tian, C. (2005). Socioeconomic status and cultural influences on language. *Journal of Communication Disorders, 38,* 271–278.

Individuals with Disabilities Education Act (IDEA) of 1990, PL 101-476, 20 U.S.C §§ 1400 *et seq.*

Joffe, V., & Pring, T. (2008). Children with phonological problems: A survey of clinical practice. *International Journal of Language and Communication Disorders, 43*(2), 154–164.

Law, J., & Camilleri, B. (2007). Dynamic assessment and its application to children with speech and language learning difficulties. *Advances in Speech-Language Pathology, 9*(4), 271–272.

Law, M., Hanna, S., King, G., Hurley, P., King, S., Kertoy, M., & Rosenbaum, P. (2003). Factors affecting family-centred service delivery for children with disabilities. *Child: Care, Health and Development, 29,* 357–366.

MacKean, G., Thurston, W., & Scott, C. (2005). Bridging the divide between families and health professionals' perspectives on family-centred care. *Health Expectations, 8,* 74–85.

Marshall, J. (2000). Critical reflections on the cultural influences in identification and habilitation of children with speech and language difficulties. *International Journal of Disability, Development and Education, 47*(4), 355–369.

McBride, S., Brotherson, M., Joanning, H., Whiddon, D., & Demmitt, A. (1993). Implementation of family-centered services: Perceptions of families and professionals. *Journal of Early Intervention, 17*(4), 414–430.

McLeod, S. (2004). Speech pathologists' application of the ICF to children with speech impairment. *Advances in Speech-Language Pathology, 6,* 75–81.

McLeod, S., & Baker, E. (2004). Current clinical practice for children with speech impairment. In B.E. Murdoch, J. Goozee, B.M. Whelan, & K. Docking (Eds.), *Proceedings of the 26th world congress of the International Association of Logopedics and Phoniatrics.* Brisbane, Australia: University of Queensland.

McLeod, S., & McCormack, J. (2007). Application of the ICF and ICF-Children and Youth in children with speech impairment. *Seminars in Speech and Language, 28,* 254–264.

McWilliam, R.A., Tocci, L., & Harbin, G.L. (1998). Family-centered services: Service providers' discourse and behavior. *Topics in Early Childhood Special Education, 18,* 206–221.

Rosenbaum, P., King, S., Law, M., King, G., & Evans, J. (1998). Family-centred service: A conceptual framework and research review. *Physical and Occupational Therapy in Pediatrics, 18,* 1–20.

Skahan, S.M., Watson, M., & Lof, G.L. (2007). Speech-language pathologists' assessment practices for children with suspected speech sound disorders: Results of a national survey. *American Journal of Speech-Language Pathology, 16,* 246–249.

Sommers, R.K. (1962). Factors in effectiveness of mothers trained to aid in speech correction. *Journal of Speech-Hearing Disorders, 27,* 178–186.

Sommers, R.K., Furlong, A.K., Rhodes, F.E., Fichter, G.R., Bowser, D.C., Copetas, F.G., et al. (1964). Effects of maternal attitudes upon improvement in articulation when mothers are trained to assist in speech correction. *Journal of Speech and Hearing Disorders, 29*(2), 126–132.

Stackhouse, J., Pascoe, M., & Gardner, H.(2006). Intervention for a child with persisting speech and literacy difficulties: A psycholinguistic approach. *Advances in Speech-Language Pathology, 8*(3), 293–315.

Tufts, L.C., & Holliday, A.R. (1959). Effectiveness of trained parents as speech therapists. *Journal of Speech and Hearing Disorders, 24,* 395–401.

Turnbull, A.P., & Turnbull, H. (1982). Parent involvement in the education of handicapped children: A critique. *Mental Retardation, 20,* 115–122.

Washington, K., & Schwartz, P. (1996). Maternal perceptions of the effects of physical and occupational therapy services on caregiving competency. *Physical and Occupational Therapy in Pediatrics, 16*(3), 33–54.

Watts Pappas, N. (2007). *Parental involvement in intervention for speech impairment.* Unpublished doctoral dissertation, Charles Sturt University, Bathurst, Australia.

Watts Pappas, N., & McLeod, S. (2009a). Parents' perceptions of their involvement in pediatric allied health intervention. In N. Watts Pappas & S. McLeod (Eds.), *Working with families in speech-language pathology* (pp. 73–110). San Diego: Plural Publishing.

Watts Pappas, N., & McLeod, S. (Eds.). (2009b). Working with families of children with speech impairments. In *Working with families in speech-language pathology* (pp. 189–228). San Diego: Plural Publishing.

Watts Pappas, N., McLeod, S., & McAllister, L. (2009). Models of practice used in SLPs' work with families. In N. Watts Pappas & S. McLeod (Eds.), *Working with families in speech-language pathology* (pp. 1–38). San Diego: Plural Publishing.

Watts Pappas, N., McLeod, S., McAllister, L., & McKinnon, D.H. (2008). Parental involvement in speech intervention: A national survey. *Clinical Linguistics and Phonetics, 22*(4), 335–344.

Watts Pappas, N., McLeod, S., McAllister, L., & Simpson, T. (2005). Partnerships with parents in speech intervention: A review. In L. Brown & C. Heine (Eds.), *Pro-

ceedings of the Speech Pathology Australia national conference (pp. 62–73). Melbourne: Speech Pathology Australia.

Wehman, T. (1998). Family-centered early intervention services: Factors contributing to increased parent in-volvement and participation. *Focus on Autism and Other Developmental Disabilities, 13*(2), 80–86.

World Health Organization. (2007). *International classi-fication of functioning, disability and health: Children and youth (ICF-CY)*. Geneva: Author.

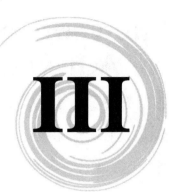

III

Interventions for Achieving Speech Movements

Interventions for Achieving Speech Movements

Rebecca J. McCauley, Sharynne McLeod, and A. Lynn Williams

T his overview provides a summary of four interventions that primarily focus on helping children with speech sound disorders (SSD) produce movements required to achieve appropriate speech production:

- Visual feedback therapy with electropalatography (EPG; Chapter 21)

- Vowel intervention (Chapter 22)

- Developmental dysarthria intervention (Chapter 23)

- Nonspeech oral motor intervention (Chapter 24)

With their overall focus on helping children produce speech movements, the approaches in this section are often undertaken as adjuncts to interventions such as those discussed in earlier sections of this book (e.g., nonlinear phonology [Chapter 13] and motor learning theory [Chapter 12]). Sometimes they are adopted because problems with movements critical for speech production are anticipated based on a child's diagnosis. For example, when the child is diagnosed with cerebral palsy or another medical condition that is often associated with a sensorimotor speech disorder, difficulties in establishing movement patterns will be anticipated from the beginning. For other children, these approaches are turned to when other frequently less technologically demanding approaches prove unproductive or have reached a plateau in their effectiveness.

Despite the differences involved, as in the previous two sections, comparisons across these interventions were undertaken with respect to the following 10 factors: client age, primary client populations, key intervention agents, key components, broad goals, basis of target selection, level of focus, session type, technology and/or materials required, and key codes from the *International Classification of Functioning, Disability and Health: Children and Youth Version* (ICF-CY; World Health Organization [WHO], 2007). Table III.1 provides a comparative summary of these 10 factors across the four intervention approaches. Before discussing each of these factors, however, it is again important to summarize each approach with regard to the available levels of evidence (LOE).

LEVELS OF EVIDENCE

As in the previous two sections, authors in this section used the Scottish Intercollegiate Guideline Network (SIGN; http://www.sign.ac.uk) as a common framework for characterizing the scientific evidence available for each intervention approach. Table III.2 provides a summary of the authors' findings.

This table looks and is in fact a bit different from those in earlier sections because of two of the four interventions. First, in Chapter 21, Gibbon and Wood did not individually discuss the very large number of studies that have been published regarding EPG (in fact, more than 150 existed as of 2003 [Gibbon, 2003]). Instead, they characterized those studies as low in quality, falling at Levels III (nonexperimental studies) and IV (expert committee reports, consensus conferences, or clinical experience of respected authorities). This is indicated in the Table III.2 by the asterisk in the relevant cells.

Second, in Chapter 24, Clark selected the studies included in the LOE table because they focused on children's SSD and had recently been included in a systematic review of nonspeech oral motor exercises (McCauley, Strand, Lof, Schooling, & Frymark 2009, in press). Like Gibbon and Wood, Clark had been faced with quite a large number of possible studies to discuss but chose a different strategy for dealing with them. Obviously, the basis for selection she used departs from those used for other interventions, because studies reviewed for all of the other interventions (except EPG) were *primarily* for their support of the reviewed intervention and only secondarily based on their associated LOE. Interestingly, Clark reported four studies that fell close to the highest LOE (Level Ib: randomized controlled studies) and was the only author in this section to report such well-designed studies, indicative of research that might be described as suggestive of effectiveness, rather than simply exploratory or suggestive of efficacy. Nonetheless, Clark interpreted the results of those studies as providing little support for oral motor exercises. This pairing of higher credibility research and negative findings highlights the importance of con-sidering not simply the LOE provided by studies conducted for an intervention but also the studies' results. Thus, as in earlier section overviews, readers are cautioned here to always consider the broader context in which summary data such as an LOE table are presented.

The departures represented in Table III.2 (compared with those in earlier section overviews) make it hard to interpret as an overall indicator of the nature of research available to support interventions targeting the achievement of speech movements. Perhaps it is safest to say that studies in this area appear at all points along the continuum from those representing what are usually considered the earliest stage of research, that is, nonexperimental studies (Levels III and IV), to those suggesting more mature studies that can provide greater support for an intervention's efficacy (Levels Ia and b and IIa and b).

COMPARATIVE FACTORS

Client Age

Most of the interventions in Section III are better suited to older children and may also be useful for adults. This is because of the interventions' degree of intrusiveness (e.g., use of bite blocks, palatal plates) and their requirements for understanding instructions related to the exploration of movement alternatives and interaction with instrumentation, as well as their demands for high amounts of practice. In particular, visual feedback therapy with EPG is specified as appropriate for school-age children, and nonlinear phonology and articulatory visual feedback is specified for children and adults. Although many of the general comments made in the chapter on intervention for children with developmental dysarthria are applicable to such children of any age (and age is not specified by the au-

Table III.1. Characteristics of speech interventions for approaches featured in Section III

Intervention approach (chapter)	Client age	Primary client populations	Key intervention agents	Key components	Broad goals
Visual feedback therapy with electropalatography (EPG) (21)	Children (typically school-age) and adults	Children with SSD with errors due to lingual placement, with dentition adequate for secure EPG placement and without significant cognitive or motor impairments; frequently used with children with cleft palate	SLPs with specialized training in EPG	Real-time and static displays of tongue activity provided through the EPG system; practice organized to take motor learning into account	Improve intelligibility by improving tongue placement and tongue-palate contacts
Vowel intervention (22)	Children and adults	Children or adults with persistent speech impairment involving vowels that is due to hearing impairment or unknown causes	SLPs with experience in ultrasound, supported by caregivers	Ultrasound to provide visual feedback on articulation combined with treatment strategies and goal setting based on nonlinear phonology	Improvement of vowel production by improving tongue position and movements

Basis of target selection	Level of focus	Session type	Technology and/or materials required	Key ICF-CY codes[a]
Targets that are considered achievable based on tongue positions observed using EPG	Speech production for lingual targets	Individual sessions	EPG hardware and software as well as a custom-made palatal plate	b320: Articulation Functions
Target vowels and vowel features selected based on nonlinear phonological theories as well as the client's ability to handle multiple target types simultaneously, his or her need for consonant and word structures, and functionality (frequency in common words)	Production of spoken vowels	Individual sessions	Ultrasound equipment and audio-visual recording equipment	b320: Articulation Functions

(continued)

Table III.1. *(continued)*

Intervention approach (chapter)	Client age	Primary client populations	Key intervention agents	Key components	Broad goals
Developmental dysarthria (DD) intervention (23)	Children	Children with DD whose attempts at lingual consonants are accompanied by weakness or excessive movement of the mandible; for example, those with cerebral palsy, congenital conditions affecting the cranial nerves, and early onset muscular dystrophy	SLPs supported by family and caregivers	Bite block use followed by phonemic practice received the most attention and is the focus of entries in this table; however, two other interventions are briefly described (i.e., intensive voice treatment and phonetic placement via electromyography)	Increase control of speech muscles, thereby increasing intelligibility in children with DD
Nonspeech oral motor intervention (24)	Children	Children with SSD, especially those with sensorimotor impairments, including children with Down syndrome, cerebral palsy, or tongue thrust	SLP, SLPA, and/or parents, depending on the specific intervention approach	Variable depending on the specific intervention; for example, practice with bite block, continuous positive airway pressure (CPAP)	Normalizing sensorimotor function of the speech mechanism

Key: SLP, speech-language pathologist; SLPA, speech-language pathology assistant; SSD, speech sound disorders.
[a]Within the ICF-CY, Articulation Functions includes phonological functions.

Basis of target selection	Level of focus	Session type	Technology and/or materials required	Key ICF-CY codes[a]
Unsuccessful attempts to produce clear, well-differentiated alveolar and velar consonants	Production of lingual consonants	Individual sessions that are intensive but short-term	Bite block and associated materials for its safe use	b320: Articulation Functions; b2304: Speech Discrimination; d330: Speaking
Variable depending on theoretical basis of the specific intervention approach; empirical bases for selection are absent	Underlying sensorimotor physiology of the oral musculature	Individual	Numerous materials are available, but generally unsupported by empirical evidence	b320: Articulation Functions; b749: Additional muscle Functions; b279: Additional sensory functions

Table III.2. Number of published research studies pertaining to each level of evidence for speech interventions targeting the achievement of speech movements identified by chapter authors in Section III

Intervention approach (chapter)	Ia: Meta analysis of > 1 randomized controlled trial	Ib: Randomized controlled study	IIa: Controlled study without randomization	IIb: Quasi-experimental study	III: Non-experimental study	IV: Expert report, consensus conference, clinical experience of respected authorities
Visual feedback therapy with electropalatography (21)	0	0	0	0	*a	*a
Vowel intervention (22)	0	0	2	7	0	0
Developmental dysarthria intervention (23)	0	0	0	0	2	2
Nonspeech oral motor intervention (24)	0	4	2	2	5	4
TOTAL	0	4	4	9	7	6

*a Although a large number of studies were cited, none was described in detail for empirical support of the intervention; instead the authors characterized them as a group as falling primarily at Levels III and IV.

thor), school-age children appear to be those most commonly included in research on this topic.

Primary Client Populations

The four interventions in this section are intended for use with children with SSD of unknown etiology, particularly for such children who have failed to respond to other interventions. These interventions are also intended for children with medical diagnoses that are frequently associated with SSD, such as severe hearing loss (Chapter 22), especially diagnoses associated with pediatric motor speech disorders. Examples of this second set of diagnoses include Moebius syndrome, early-onset muscular dystrophy (Chapter 23), Down syndrome (Chapter 24) and cerebral palsy in which speech muscles are affected (Chapters 23 and 24).

Key Intervention Agents

For interventions in Section III, a speech-language pathologist (SLP) with specialized training is recommended as the key intervention agent for the two interventions that involve the use of sophisticated technology (visual feedback therapy with EPG and nonlinear phonology and articulatory visual feedback). Parents and caregivers are mentioned as having a supportive role in vowel intervention, intervention for developmental dysarthria, and nonspeech oral motor treatment. With regard to oral motor exercises, Clark asserts that the person functioning as key intervention agent depends upon the purpose for which the exercises are used. When the purpose is directing the child's attention to relevant articulators, the SLP or SLP assistant serve as key intervention agents, whereas when the purpose is strengthening, the parent may assume that role after training.

Key Components

The four interventions that target the achievement of speech movements use either augmented sensory feedback or altered movement patterns to elicit improved movement, followed by practice conducted under more typical speaking conditions in order to facilitate generalization. Two of the chapters in this section make use of precise visual feedback (Chapters 21 and 22), and two restrict movement of one articulator (the jaw) in order to trigger changes in movement in another (the tongue) (Chapters 23 and 24). Visual information (through EPG in Chapter 21 and ultrasound in Chapter 22) is used to augment intrinsic feedback mechanisms to help clients modify their tongue movements to more closely resemble those used in more well-formed speech productions. In the second two chapters in this section, a bite block is used to restrict mandibular contributions to movements for speech production, thereby promoting changes in habitual lingual movements that can then be shaped to achieve more accurate speech sound production. Readers will recall that these last chapters reported approaches encompassing several related interventions. In Chapter 23, use of a bite block received greater attention than other interventions that were mentioned, but in Chapter 24, it is only briefly mentioned among others. Other interventions in Chapter 24 involve quite a variety of activities designed to normalize sensorimotor function of the speech mechanism. Although the literature describes the use of movements outside of speech (nonspeech oral motor exercises), the chapter author prefers their use within the integrated and specific movement patterns associated with speech.

Broad Goals

The basic goal of interventions in this section is to improve speech production by helping children achieve speech movements. Only two chapters indicate that improved intelligibility is expected to result as well, although it seems safe to infer that all four share that expectation.

Basis of Target Selection

Interventions in this section use a variety of strategies for target selection, many of which reflect the child's ability at the start of intervention to approximate movements underlying specific speech sounds. Targets for visual feedback therapy with EPG are chosen because they are considered achievable based on movement patterns initially observed using EPG. For nonlinear phonology and articulatory visual feedback, targets are selected based on nonlinear phonologic theory, the client's ability to handle several types of targets simultaneously, patterns of missing sounds, and the functionality of potential sound targets (e.g., their frequency, especially in functional words). Targets for the use of a bite block as part of interventions for developmental dysarthria are selected when assessment suggests that the child is unable to produce well-differentiated alveolar and velar consonants. Finally, because of the number of interventions encompassed within oral motor exercises, target selection is equally varied and frequently not well defined (e.g., when strength is targeted, but only subjective methods of detecting weakness are used).

Level of Focus

Most of the interventions in Section III focus on production of individual sounds: lingual targets (Chapter 21), spoken vowels (Chapter 22), and lingual consonants (Chapter 23). These speech sounds are often elicited in isolated syllables or words. In contrast, however, oral motor exercises (Chapter 24) are sometimes used to focus on movements of the oral musculature outside of speech (see Table III.1).

Session Type

Interventions in this section occur predominantly within individual sessions. These may be intensive and short-term, as they are in interventions for children with developmental dysarthria using a bite block to help with initial elicitation of improved movement patterns.

Technology and/or Materials Required

Clearly, technology is critical when implementing visual feedback therapy with EPG and nonlinear phonology and articulatory visual feedback, which uses ultrasound. The equipment and software used for these interventions are quite expensive, but in Chapter 21, Gibbon and Wood describe methods that can be used to make EPG more readily available, and similar methods might also be adopted to promote use of ultrasound. The use of a bite block is vital for the specific approaches that make use of it in interventions for developmental dysarthria and oral motor exercises. Methods for preparing bite blocks are described in some detail in Chapter 23.

Key Codes from the *International Classification of Functioning, Disability and Health: Children and Youth Version*

As mentioned in the previous two sections, authors categorized outcomes using the ICF-CY (WHO, 2007). In that system, codes identify whether outcomes target Body Structure, Body Functions, and/or Activities and Participation. Interventions in this section address the ICF-CY code that targets Articulation Functions (b320: "Functions of the production of speech sounds"; WHO, 2007, p. 71), which falls under Body Function. Both of the complex interventions in the last two chapters included other outcomes. The second code listed for interventions for developmental dysarthria addresses Speech Discrimination, which also falls under Body Function, and the third code listed for that intervention is the only code listed for this group that targets Activities and Participation, specifically by targeting "speaking." In fact, probably all of these interventions imply such a target. As the ICF-CY (WHO, 2007) is used more widely, we might expect increased consistency in how they are applied and a greater likelihood that they will be considered during intervention development, thereby avoiding the post hoc categorizations required of authors in this book.

REFERENCES

Gibbon, F. (2003). The contribution of EPG to the diagnosis of childhood apraxia of speech. In L.D. Shriberg & T.F. Campbell (Eds.), *Proceedings of the 2002 Childhood Apraxia of Speech Research Symposium.* Carlsbad, CA: Hendrix Foundation.

McCauley, R.J., Strand, E.A., Lof, G., Schooling, T., & Frymark, T. (2009). Evidence-based systematic review: Effects of nonspeech oral motor exercises on speech. *American Journal of Speech-Language Pathology,* *18*(4), 343–360.

World Health Organization. (2007). *International classification of functioning, disability and health: Children and youth version.* Geneva: Author.

Visual Feedback Therapy with Electropalatography

Fiona E. Gibbon and Sara E. Wood

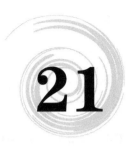

ABSTRACT

Electropalatography (EPG) is an instrumental technique that detects the tongue's contact against the hard palate during speech and creates a visual display of the resulting patterns. This chapter focuses on EPG as a visual feedback device in therapy for children with speech sound disorders (SSD). Tongue–palate contact information is rich in detail and as a result it can be used for diverse research and clinical purposes. Examples of clinically relevant information contained in EPG data are place of articulation, lateral bracing, groove formation, timing of tongue movements, and coarticulation. Furthermore, the technique records measurable amounts of contact for sound targets that are frequently produced as errors by children with SSD (e.g., /s/, /ʃ/, /tʃ/). These features make EPG valuable for both diagnosis and therapy. During EPG therapy, children's abnormal articulation patterns are revealed to them on the computer screen, and they can use this dynamic visual feedback display to help them produce normal contact patterns. An attractive property of EPG as a therapy device is that the visual display is relatively intuitive. This means that children can understand the link between the speech sounds they hear and the associated contact patterns displayed on the screen. There is now an extensive literature on the benefits of using EPG in therapy, but the quality of evidence would improve by conducting large clinical trials in the future.

INTRODUCTION

Investigating the actions of the tongue during speech poses particular challenges. The difficulties are due to the tongue's inaccessible location within the mouth, its sensitivity, the unique properties of its internal structure, and the speed and complexity of its movements. EPG is a technique designed for just this purpose, in other words, to record tongue movements during speech. EPG (also termed *palatometry* and *dynamic palatometry*) in fact only records one aspect of tongue activity—the location and timing of tongue contacts against the hard palate (Gibbon, 2008; Hardcastle & Gibbon, 1997; Hardcastle, Gibbon, & Jones, 1991). Compared with other instruments available for investigating tongue movements in speech, EPG is both safe and relatively convenient to use. Safety is an ob-

Some of the material for this article has been adapted from previous articles and book chapters written by the authors, and we therefore acknowledge the contribution of co-authors and funding bodies. We are grateful to Joanne Cleland for helpful comments on an early draft of the chapter.

vious necessity and convenience is highly desirable when designing instrumental techniques for use with clinical populations. The focus of this chapter is on using EPG for visual feedback therapy, but in preparing the ground for later discussions, there follows a description of the EPG technique and an explanation of its important role in diagnosis.

EPG—the Technique

A number of different EPG systems have emerged in research and clinical use over the past 40 years. A British system—the EPG3 system developed at the University of Reading—has been used in the majority of studies conducted by researchers in Europe and Hong Kong (Hardcastle et al., 1991; Hardcastle & Gibbon, 1997). A new Windows version of the Reading EPG has been developed at Queen Margaret University, Edinburgh (WinEPG, Articulate Instruments Ltd, 2008). In the past, the Kay Elemetrics Palatometer was used in research carried out in the United States (Fletcher, 1983), although there is now a new EPG system developed by Logmetrix (Schmidt, 2007). In Japan, the Rion EPG system was the one most widely used until it was discontinued (Fujimura, Tatsumi, & Kagaya, 1973). All EPG systems share some common general features but differ in details such as the construction of the EPG plates, number and configuration of sensors, and hardware/software specifications (Gibbon & Nicolaidis, 1999; Hardcastle & Gibbon, 1997).

A prerequisite for EPG therapy is manufacturing a special plate, which resembles a dental plate. Each one is custom-made to ensure a perfect fit, and when properly constructed it should fit securely and comfortably against the roof of the mouth. Although relatively expensive to construct, one advantage of having them custom-made is that they can be tailored to fit individuals with unusually shaped hard palates (e.g., children with cleft palate, children with Down syndrome), dental anomalies, dentures, or dental braces. Figure 21.1(a) shows a Reading EPG plate for a typical speaker. The figure shows how the 62 sensors are arranged in a standard configuration of eight horizontal rows placed according to identifiable anatomical landmarks (Hardcastle et al., 1991). The sensors are spaced so that the distance between the front four rows is half that of the back four rows. The high concentration of sensors in the alveolar region allows crucial aspects of tongue-tip articulation, such as grooving during sibilant productions, to be recorded in detail. In the posterior region, the sensors extend to the junction of the hard and soft palates and in the lateral margins they extend to the gingival border.

Individual wires from each sensor emerge from the posterior region of the plate in two bundles, exiting at the corners of the speaker's mouth. The EPG plate and a handheld electrode (providing a small current) are connected to an external processing unit or a multiplexer, which is in turn connected to a computer. A circuit is completed when the tongue surface contacts any of the sensors and the resulting pattern of contact is displayed on a computer monitor. Figure 21.1(b) shows a single EPG palatogram, with row numbers 1–8 indicated. Palatograms are schematic displays, which are standard for every speaker regardless of individual differences in the shape and size of the EPG plate. Figure 21.1(b) indicates how the schematic palatograms broadly correspond to the phonetic regions of the palate (i.e., alveolar, postalveolar, palatal, and velar) and to the relevant active articulators (i.e., tongue tip and tongue body).

The most recent version of EPG software, the WinEPG system (Articulate Instruments Ltd, 2008), can sample at different rates, although usually the EPG is set at 100 Hz with simultaneous sampling of the acoustic signal at 22,050 Hz. The EPG data are displayed as sequences of two-dimensional representations of tongue–palate contact, re-

(a)

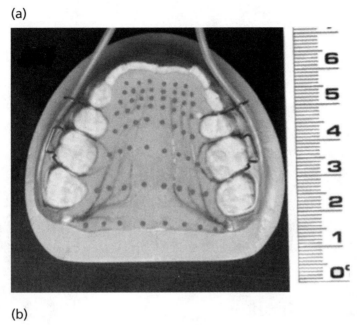

(b)

Normal	Row		
0 0 0 0 0 0	1	Alveolar	Anterior
0 0 0 . . 0 0 0	2		(tongue
0 . . . . . 0 0	3	Post-alveolar	tip/blade)
0 0	4		
0 0	5		
0 0	6	Palatal	Posterior
0 0	7		(tongue
0 0	8	Velar	dorsum)

Figure 21.1. A Reading EPG (artificial) plate for a typical speaker placed on top of a plaster impression of the upper palate and teeth is shown in (a). A single EPG frame, showing a typical contact pattern for alveolar stops /t/, /d/, and /n/ is shown in (b), along with the EPG frame row numbers, the phonetic regions of the palate, and the part of the tongue that makes contact with these regions.

ferred to as palatograms or EPG frames. The EPG data can be stored and analyzed using the Articulate Assistant software (Wrench, 2007). Figure 21.2 shows a dynamic sequence of EPG frames for an alveolar stop /t/ produced by a typically developing 12-year-old child. The figure shows individual palatograms, which are numbered and read from left to right. In this printout, the frames occur at 10 ms intervals, and tongue contact is indicated by filled black squares along the eight horizontal rows.

Figure 21.2(a) illustrates contact patterns for the alveolar plosive /t/ in the phrase *a toolshed*. During the stop closure phase (frames 72–80), there is contact along the lateral margins combined with closure across the palate in the alveolar region. This combination of lateral and alveolar contact gives rise to the so-called *horseshoe shape*, which is a characteristic pattern for normal alveolar stops /t/, /d/, and /n/. The closure phase of /t/ in Figure 21.2(a) is followed by the release phase, which starts at frame 81. Notice that an

(a)

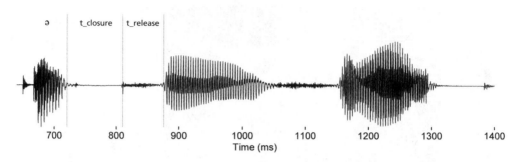

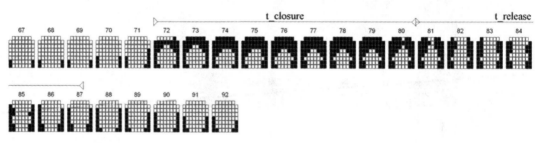

(b)

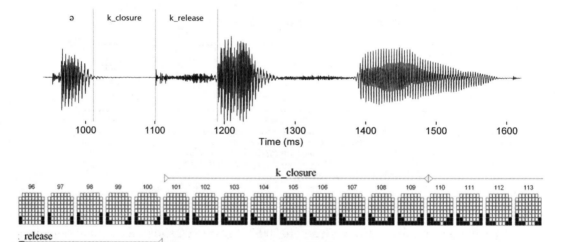

Figure 21.2. EPG printouts for (a) /t/ in *a toolshed* and (b) /k/ in *a kettle* produced by a typically developing 12-year-old boy. These are full, dynamic EPG printouts, where the top of individual palatograms represents the alveolar region, and the bottom is the velar region located at the junction between the hard and soft palates. The sampling interval is 10 msec.

/s/-like configuration occurs fleetingly at the start of the release. The patterns for the alveolar stop are in contrast to those for the velar stop in Figure 21.2(b), which shows a /k/ target in the phrase *a kettle* spoken by the same typically developing child. Here, the palatograms during the closure period (frames 102–109) have contact along the posterior lateral margins and closure in the velar region.

Figure 21.2 illustrates how the sounds /t/ and /k/ are associated with visually distinct, recognizable EPG patterns. In fact, EPG records characteristic patterns in typical speakers for all English lingual phoneme targets, which include /t/, /d/, /k/, /g/, /s/, /z/, /ʃ/, /ʒ/, /tʃ/, /dʒ/, the palatal approximant /j/, nasals /n/, /ŋ/, and the lateral /l/ (for reports of typical adult EPG patterns, see Gibbon, Yuen, Lee, & Adams, 2007; Hardcastle & Gibbon, 1997; Liker & Gibbon, 2008; Liker, Gibbon, Wrench, & Horga, 2007; McLeod, Roberts, & Sita, 2006; McLeod & Singh, 2009). Hardcastle and Gibbon (1997) presented idealized static EPG patterns, which have proved to be useful reference frames, although they are not based on recorded data. McLeod and Singh (2009) presented comprehensive coverage of EPG patterns for typical and disordered speakers.

Although studies have identified characteristic patterns for consonant targets, typical speakers vary in the overall amount of contact they produce. Gibbon, Yuen, et al. (2007) conducted a study on typical alveolar stops (i.e., /t/, /d/, and /n/) and found that some speakers had more than twice as much contact as other speakers. This held true despite the finding that all speakers produced characteristic horseshoe-shaped patterns for these targets. Studies of typical velars (Liker & Gibbon, 2008), bilabials (Gibbon, Lee, & Yuen, 2007), and affricates (Liker et al., 2007) reached a similar conclusion, namely that some speakers had two or three times more contact than others. One explanation for this variation is that the amount of contact relates to inter-speaker differences in palatal shape. More specifically, individuals with flatter palates tend to have higher overall amounts of contact than those with more steeply arched palates (Hiki & Itoh, 1986). There are other possible explanations, however. It may be the case that the amount of contact reflects speakers' long-term jaw and tongue settings. In other words, speakers produce high amounts of contact when they articulate because they have high habitual settings. Likewise speakers with low amounts of contact have low settings. Another possible explanation is that the degree of articulatory effort exerted by speakers influences the amount of contact. Here, speakers with higher overall amounts of contact exert more tongue–palate pressure, as a result of increased effort, compared with speakers with lower amounts of contact. Although the precise relationship between speaker characteristics (e.g., anatomy, articulatory settings, speech style) and EPG data is unknown at present, clinicians need to assess whether these characteristics are influencing the EPG patterns produced by children with SSD.

Varying patterns of contact are registered during bunched and retroflex varieties of /r/; relatively close vowels, such as /i/, /ɪ/, /e/, /u/, and /ʊ/; and rising diphthongs, such as /eɪ/, /aɪ/, /oɪ/, /aʊ/, and /əʊ/. There is usually minimal contact during open vowels, such as /ɑ/ and /ɒ/. Equally, consonants that have their primary constriction either further forward than the most anterior row of sensors (e.g., dentals, bilabials) or further back than the most posterior row of sensors (e.g., velars in the context of open vowels, uvulars, pharyngeals, glottals) show limited contact. Some EPG contact occurs during these consonant sounds, however, when they occur in the context of relatively close vowels, rising diphthongs (Gibbon, Lee, et al., 2007), or complex clusters (Zharkova, Schaeffler, & Gibbon, 2009).

The richness of spatial and temporal detail available in the full dynamic EPG printouts has already been described and illustrated in Figure 21.2. However, these full printouts can be unwieldy because of the sheer amount of information contained in them. In order to make the information more manageable and for the purposes of statistical processing, it is useful to reduce the data to single numerical indices. These indices may be based on preselected frames or even just a single frame (e.g., frame of maximum contact during a stop or fricative) that has been extracted from the full printout. Indices are now available that allow researchers to quantify important aspects of EPG contact patterns, such as place of articulation, amount of contact, symmetry, and variability (see Gibbon & Nicolaidis, 1999, for a review). Indices are invaluable when differentiating typical from disordered patterns and when measuring subtle differences between similar contact patterns. To illustrate the latter point, a study of typical speakers revealed that oral stops (/t/, /d/) had significantly more contact than the nasal stop /n/ (Gibbon, Yuen, et al., 2007). These oral and nasal targets all exhibited similar horseshoe-shaped EPG patterns, so any differences that existed were subtle and measurable only by statistical analysis of numerical values derived from contact indices.

EPG—Its Role in Diagnosis

In clinical practice, EPG assessment data is always used in conjunction with more routinely available assessment procedures for diagnostic purposes. The objective data from EPG is valuable when used alongside subjective data from auditory-impressionistic transcriptions. Although transcription is the most widely and routinely used method for assessing disordered speech, it has well-recognized limitations (Heselwood & Howard, 2008; Kent, 1996). One drawback is that a transcriber can only infer what the visually inaccessible articulators such as the tongue are doing during speech. Such inferences are based on an accumulation of complex cues contained in the acoustic signal. Examples of EPG data presented in later sections will show that inferences about tongue articulation, specifically about placement, can be misleading when based on perceptual judgments alone. Another limitation is that a linear notation system, such as transcription, is not able to measure speech motor control, which may be impaired in some children with speech disorders.

In contrast to transcribed data, EPG gives direct information about important features of tongue articulation (e.g., place of articulation, lateral bracing, groove formation) and can measure some key aspects of motor control, such as speed, spatial (i.e., positional) accuracy, and consistency of movement, as well as differential control of apical, lateral, and posterior regions of the tongue (Gibbon, 1999). Therefore, direct objective measures derived from EPG data make it possible to identify abnormal articulations and speech motor impairments. These measurements can be used for diagnostic purposes as well as for quantifying subtle changes in tongue behavior due to factors such as the normal speech maturational process, disease progression, or the effects of therapeutic intervention. EPG data therefore complements transcription data.

Researchers have devised a variety of EPG classification schemes in order to capture the types of EPG error patterns produced by individuals with speech disorders. Hardcastle and Gibbon (1997) suggested that EPG patterns could be classified broadly as follows: 1) those that have predominantly abnormal spatial configurations of tongue–palate contact (e.g., complete tongue–palate contact), 2) those that have abnormal timing (e.g., long durations), and 3) those that are normal in terms of spatial configuration and timing but occur in an abnormal location (e.g., substitutions). Gibbon (2004) devised a classification scheme for abnormal EPG patterns that occur in the speech of children with cleft palate. These studies give numerous illustrations of the different types of error patterns, but the most frequently occurring EPG error pattern, the spatial distortion, is illustrated in Figure 21.3. The EPG data shown in Figure 21.3 are from four children ages 8–15 years; three had distorted spatial patterns associated with articulation disorders and one had normal patterns associated with typical speech development. The patterns are for the /ʃ/ target extracted from the phrase *a shop*. All /ʃ/ targets produced by the children with disorders were heard by listeners as lateral fricatives [ɬ].

Figure 21.3(a) shows that the child with typical speech produced /ʃ/ with lateral contact and an anterior groove configuration. These two features (lateral contact and anterior groove) are absent from the patterns produced by the children with speech disorders. For example, one child (Figure 21.3[b]) made extensive contact across most of the palate, similar to an undifferentiated gesture (Gibbon, 1999, and described later in the chapter), during the production of this sound. Another child had a pattern rather like that of an alveolar stop (Figure 21.3[c]) but with some asymmetry and incomplete lateral seal on the right side. The incomplete seal indicates where air was escaping into the buccal cavity during the lateral fricative. The third child had contact predominantly in the palatal and velar regions of the palate (Figure 21.3[d]). Here there is evidence of a groove in the posterior region of the palate, indicating that air could be escaping centrally as well as laterally during this child's productions of lateral fricatives. Figure 21.3 shows that children can have substantially different articulations for errors that are represented with the same phonetic symbol, in this case [ɬ]. The perceptual consequences of the different articulation errors were apparently too subtle for listeners to detect.

Although EPG data and transcription provide complementary information, data from the two sources can conflict. An example is the phenomenon of *covert contrast*, in which instrumentally measurable differences between target phonemes oppose evidence from listeners' perceptions of phonological neutralization. These differences are measurable from EPG data but are not detected reliably by the human ear (see Gibbon, 2002, for a review of instrumental studies of covert contrast). Kornfeld captured the point in stating "adults do not always perceive distinctions that children make" (1971, p. 462). Instances of conflicting, also called divergent, information are important in facilitating new insights into diagnosis. For instance, the presence of covert contrasts has been interpreted as evidence that a child has phonological and articulatory knowledge about that contrast (Gibbon, 2002; Gibbon & Scobbie, 1997).

Another type of articulation error, called an *undifferentiated gesture* (Gibbon, 1999), involves tongue–palate contact that lacks clear differentiation between the tongue tip, the tongue body, and the lateral margins of the tongue. As shown in Figure 21.2, typically developing children produce alveolar stops /t/ and /d/ with finely controlled tongue actions, which combine lateral bracing with an upward movement of the tongue tip to the alveolar ridge. Velar stops /k/ and /g/ have an upward movement of the tongue body, which rises until it reaches the posterior region of the hard palate. In contrast to typical alveolar or velar articulations, undifferentiated gestures involve placement that is not confined to the anterior/lateral regions of the palate for alveolars or the posterior region for velars. Instead, contact extends across the whole of the palate. Thus, undifferentiated gestures involve simultaneous alveolar, palatal, and velar placement.

Examples of undifferentiated gestures are shown in Figure 21.3(b), and in the case study of Lisa described at the end of the chapter. Lisa produced undifferentiated gestures for specific targets, namely postalveolar fricative /ʃ/, /ʒ/ and affricate /tʃ/, /dʒ/ targets. Some children, however, produce undifferentiated gestures for a much wider range of lin-

(a)

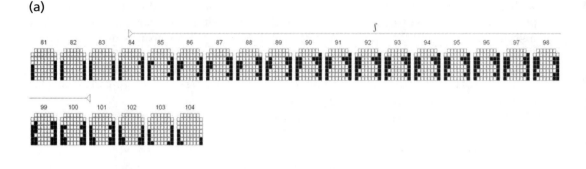

(b)

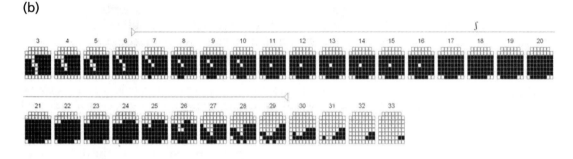

(c)

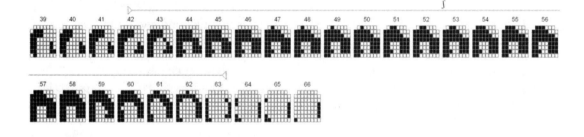

(d)

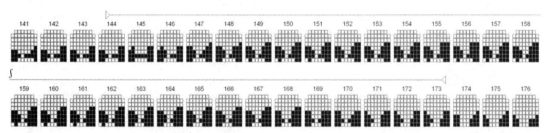

Figure 21.3. EPG printouts for four children's productions of /ʃ/ in *a shop*. (a) shows a printout from a 12-year-old boy with typical speech. (b), (c), and (d) show contact patterns for three school-age children with SSD. Each child exhibits different EPG patterns, although all were heard by listeners as lateral fricatives [ɬ].

gual targets. The widespread occurrence of undifferentiated gestures in a child's speech is interpreted as reflecting that the child has poor coordination between the tongue tip and the tongue body. Furthermore, it reflects a lack of lateral anchorage or bracing, suggesting an overall instability of tongue movement control (Gibbon, 1999). Children who produce undifferentiated gestures across-the-board for lingual targets often have speech features that are frequently reported in the literature as being characteristic of childhood apraxia of speech (Gibbon, 2003a).

As well as having simultaneous alveolar, palatal, and velar contact, undifferentiated gestures often have a different place of articulation at the onset and at the release of closure (Gibbon & Wood, 2002). Gibbon and Wood found that the majority of children who produced undifferentiated gestures had perceptually variable placement for lingual stops. They suggested that an abnormal shift in tongue placement during the closure phase, termed *drift*, can lead to conflicting acoustic cues for place of articulation. Drift has been reported to occur in a wide range of speech disorders, including cleft palate (Gibbon, Ellis, & Crampin, 2004; Hardcastle, Morgan Barry, & Nunn, 1989; Howard, 2004) and phonological disorders (Gibbon, 1999). A perceptual experiment used computer-generated speech stimuli to investigate the effect of drift on perceptual judgments about lingual place of articulation (Gibbon & Mayo, 2008). The results showed that listeners were significantly more inconsistent when asked to judge placement of stimuli with conflicting cues compared with stimuli with congruent cues. The presence of undifferentiated gestures may explain why some children present with inconsistent speech disorder (Dodd, 1995), which involves extensive perceptual variability in placement for lingual stops.

EPG Assessment—Pre- and Posttherapy

An EPG assessment precedes visual feedback therapy because goals of intervention are derived largely from an analysis of pretherapy data. In addition to an EPG recording, a comprehensive clinical assessment of children's speech and language skills is essential before proceeding with EPG therapy; any etiological or maintaining factors need to be fully explored. As part of a pretherapy EPG assessment, it is usual to record a standard word list designed to elicit a range of consonants and consonant sequences in a variety of phonetic contexts. (Appendix 21A shows the CLEFTNET word list as an example.) Standard word lists provide a screen of children's articulation repertoire or inventory. Initial observations of EPG data from a standard word list usually lead to further recordings that probe specific areas of difficulty. Examples of additional probes include

- Multiple exemplars of problematic targets—Word lists should focus specifically on problematic sounds, eliciting multiple examples in a variety of different phonetic contexts, including different vowel environments, syllable positions, clusters, and multisyllabic words.

- Nonspeech tasks, such as diadochokinetic rates—EPG can measure precisely the speed and accuracy of tongue movements for the alveolar (e.g., /t/) and velar (e.g., /k/) articulations included in maximum performance tasks.

- Imitation versus spontaneous productions—EPG can quantify whether children's articulations are more accurate during imitation compared with spontaneous productions, or vice versa.

- Minimal pairs that listeners judge to be neutralized in children's speech—These can be elicited in order to determine whether children are producing covert contrasts.

- Connected speech—Sentences or spontaneous speech can be elicited to reveal whether children are using normal connected speech processes.

- Variability—Multiple repetitions of the same word provide EPG data about articulatory variability of children's productions.

The speech materials are recorded using high-quality audio tape facilities, ideally in a sound-proofed studio. It is customary to record some speech material on two occasions, once with and once without the EPG plate in situ. The purpose is to estimate whether the EPG plate is affecting the perceptual quality of the child's habitual speech. EPG assessments are usually undertaken on a minimum of three occasions: the first one taking place before the start of EPG therapy; the second on completion of therapy; and a third on a follow-up occasion, usually 3 months or more after the completion of therapy. If it is practical to do so, it is useful to make short EPG recordings of words containing target sounds at the start of every EPG therapy session. This allows the clinician to monitor progress on a regular basis and to show children their own patterns recorded from previous sessions. Demonstrating improvements in EPG patterns from previous therapy sessions can motivate children and reminds them of therapy goals.

TARGET POPULATIONS

Due to the specialist nature of the technique and the cost of buying equipment and making plates, EPG therapy is usually only offered to children in situations in which other more widely available intervention options have failed. Children referred for EPG therapy are therefore usually of school age, with complex as well as apparently intractable speech difficulties. These hard-to-treat children often have poor self-image and esteem, and they can lack confidence due to previous failures. Many have additional literacy difficulties. For these reasons, children undergoing EPG therapy are not typical of children with SSD reported in the literature, who tend to be younger and have not experienced failure to the same extent as those for whom EPG is recommended. Developing new and effective interventions for older children with persisting SSD is challenging and one of the most neglected research areas in speech therapy (Smit, 2004).

The pediatric populations that could potentially benefit from EPG therapy include children with speech disorders affecting lingual consonants and high vowels. EPG therapy is not suitable for speech difficulties that are due to abnormal functioning of articulators other than the tongue, such as the lips or velum; these difficulties will need a different approach. Targets that are suitable for EPG therapy are those that register measurable amounts of tongue palate contact. Gibbon and Paterson (2006) conducted a survey of a large group of children and adults who had undergone EPG therapy. They found that /s/ was by far the most frequently targeted sound in EPG therapy. The postalveolar fricative, /ʃ/, and alveolar plosives /t/ and /d/ were also frequent targets, with just less than half the group having EPG therapy for these sounds. A somewhat surprising finding was the frequency with which the velar sounds /k/ and /g/ were targets in EPG therapy. Almost one third of the group had EPG therapy for errors affecting velar targets, although Gibbon, McNeill, Wood, and Watson (2003) discussed the potential pitfalls of using EPG therapy for these sounds. In contrast, the survey showed that clinicians never used EPG to remediate errors affecting the retroflex /ɻ/ or vowels.

The target pediatric population for EPG therapy is consequently large because almost all speech disorders in children affect sounds that are articulated with the tongue. This is true regardless of the underlying cause (e.g., sensory, language, structural, motor, developmental, or cognitive impairments). Although the target population is sizeable, at the present time EPG therapy is not available to most children with speech disorders. Apart from children in the UK with cleft palate who can access the national CLEFTNET initiative (Lee, Gibbon, Crampin, Yuen, & McLennan, 2007), this type of therapy is only available to those living close to specialist EPG centers.

Visual feedback therapy is potentially beneficial for children with speech difficulties that arise from diverse etiologies and that affect lingual articulation. From this large group, children with functional articulation disorders (including phonological disorders) or cleft palate are most frequently selected for EPG therapy. A study by Gibbon and Paterson (2006) found that out of 60 individuals who received EPG therapy over a 10-year period in Scotland, the overwhelming majority were school-age children with either functional articulation disorders or cleft palate. Although they have different etiologies, these populations are similar insofar as both can give rise to intractable forms of articulation difficulties. Furthermore, targets that register measurable amounts of tongue–palate contact are vulnerable to errors in both groups (Smit, Hand, Freilinger, Bernthal, & Bird, 1990). Finally, these errors, when they occur in older children, are unlikely to resolve spontaneously and are notoriously resistant to speech therapy (Noordhoff, Huang, & Wu, 1990).

ASSESSMENT METHODS FOR DETERMINING INTERVENTION RELEVANCE

Due to the underlying principles of EPG and the strategy of using visual feedback in therapy, two hard-and-fast criteria apply when selecting children. One is that they have abnormal articulation that affects lingual targets and the other is that children have sufficient visual acuity to see the contact patterns displayed on the screen. In addition, clinicians consider the inherent practical and procedural demands of the technique when selecting children for EPG therapy.

Age is one factor that is taken into account when selecting children for EPG therapy. EPG is not normally used with young children, toddlers, or infants, although in Japan, EPG has been used with preschool children with cleft palate (Yamashita, Michi, Imai, Suzuki, & Yoshida, 1992). Elsewhere, EPG is rarely offered as a therapy option for children until they are older than the age of 6 years. Younger children are often not considered for EPG therapy because they may still benefit from other more widely available, and less expensive, intervention approaches. Furthermore, using visual feedback is a relatively demanding form of therapy, requiring children to understand the links between tongue activity and the visual display and to develop conscious control of fine-grain tongue movements. Lastly, success of EPG therapy depends at least in part on a high level of motivation and attention. These cognitive, motor, and psychological prerequisites mean that EPG is not considered an appropriate therapy option for preschool children or children with severe forms of learning or motor disorders.

An additional procedural consideration is that children need to wear the plate during EPG assessment and therapy. For this to be constructed, the child needs to visit a dentist for a dental impression. Most children tolerate having the impression made and the plate's presence in the mouth once it has been manufactured, but some are hypersensitive in this region and therefore may not be suitable candidates for EPG therapy. Children need adequate dentition to retain the plate in the mouth during therapy, which needs to take place at a time in their life when minimal changes in dentition are expected. Changes in dentition during the EPG therapy, such as those due to growth or orthodontic treatment, can result in the plate becoming unusable or at least uncomfortable to wear. This situation is undesirable and can lead to EPG therapy being terminated prematurely. For these reasons, decisions about when to offer EPG therapy are best made in collaboration with dentists or orthodontists.

THEORETICAL BASIS

Dominant Theoretical Rationale for the Intervention Approach

At the heart of EPG therapy is its facility to provide real-time visual feedback of tongue activity. This moment-to-moment (i.e., real-time) feedback makes EPG unique and distinct from other approaches to therapy for children with SSD. In relation to speech disorders, Shuster, Ruscello, and Smith (1992) have suggested that biofeedback is effective in situations in which details about the articulation of target sounds are difficult to describe to children. The position of the tongue and its movements during speech are exceptionally difficult to describe, making EPG a particularly valuable intervention tool.

Under normal circumstances, individuals do not have precise knowledge or awareness about how their tongues are moving when they speak. Although tongue movements are consciously controlled, they are executed automatically. The internal cues (e.g., tactile, kinesthetic) associated with tongue movements are too subtle for children to perceive clearly or accurately. Although perception of these cues is not a prerequisite to normal speech production or to its acquisition in typically developing children, nevertheless, EPG therapy derives its effectiveness from enabling children to develop conscious control of the internal cues associated with tongue activity.

The predominant theoretical approach underpinning EPG therapy is that it adheres to principles of motor learning (see Strand, 1995, and Strand & Skinder, 1999, for discussion of these principles). A central tenet of motor learning is to provide learners with knowledge of results, which EPG does in the form of visual feedback of tongue–palate contact. In EPG therapy, children use the visual feedback continuously in the early stages of learning new articulation patterns. As therapy progresses, clinicians gradually reduce the external feedback by withdrawing the visual display. The aim at this stage is for children to learn to rely more and more on internal cues (e.g., auditory and kinesthetic), rather than visual cues, when producing new articulation patterns. Reliance on internal cues is equally necessary when generalizing new articulation skills into everyday speech.

Another key component of motor learning is that children are given opportunities for repetitive and intensive practice. In the context of EPG therapy, practice is used to establish accurate and consistent motor programs for new articulation patterns. EPG therapy sessions therefore frequently contain repetitive drill activities in some form. Furthermore, the portable EPG units described in the Assessment Methods section were designed specifically so that children could benefit from regular practice between clinical sessions. A final element of motor learning requires grading the motor complexity of tasks so that new articulation patterns are presented first in simple monosyllables (e.g.,

CV, VC). More demanding monosyllable structures (e.g., CVC, CCV, VCC) follow, then disyllabic and polysyllabic structures are gradually introduced. Grading complexity in this way is evident in many well-established therapy approaches, such as traditional articulation therapy (Van Riper & Emerick, 1984) and the Nuffield Dyspraxia Programme (see Chapter 7) (Connery, 1994).

EPG therapy provides children with visual feedback about their own tongue movements. This information is not available under normal circumstances and it can be revelatory. The following paragraph, written by a 12-year-old boy undergoing EPG therapy, illustrates the impact that this information can have on a child:

> It [EPG] has helped me a lot with my speech and confidence. Before [EPG therapy] I couldn't distinguish between the sounds I heard other people make and the way I was trying to repeat them. I really thought I was doing it the same. It surprised me to hear myself on tape, but I still didn't realize what I was doing wrong. Now with the help of EPG, I can see what is happening inside my mouth and where I am putting my tongue, so I know where I am going wrong. I had fallen into some bad habits which I am gradually beginning to eliminate. EPG helps me to try and place my tongue in the right place for the right sound.

An assumption born out in EPG therapy studies (see Empirical Basis section) is that improving articulation patterns has a direct beneficial effect on speech intelligibility. Vocal tract movements are organized as motor schemas (see Square, 1999) and improving function of one component, such as the tongue, can have far-reaching benefits on the functioning of other articulators, such as the velum, located elsewhere in the vocal tract. An example is when improved articulation co-occurs with a simultaneous reduction in abnormal nasal emission in children with cleft palate. Reduced emission after EPG therapy has been noted to occur when compensatory errors, termed *posterior nasal fricatives*, are eliminated as a result of EPG therapy and replaced by anterior oral fricatives. Dent, Gibbon, and Hardcastle (1992) reported on a 9-year-old child with a cleft palate who produced /s/ and /z/ targets as posterior nasal fricatives. EPG therapy was successful in establishing near normal EPG patterns for these sounds, which were judged as alveolar oral fricatives without accompanying nasal emission.

In terms of the International Classification of Functioning, Disability and Health (ICF; World Health Organization, 2001), visual feedback therapy is focused directly at the level of impairment of Body Functions. Specifically, EPG therapy aims to improve the physiological functioning of the tongue during speech. Although focusing on Body Functions, clinicians who use EPG recognize the importance of a holistic approach, acknowledging the full range of difficulties experienced by children with speech disorders.

EMPIRICAL BASIS

There is a substantial literature reporting EPG therapy for children with SSD. Gibbon (2003b) found that out of 150 research papers on the clinical applications of EPG, half investigated cleft palate or functional articulation disorders, with a substantial number reporting neurological disorders and hearing impairment. Speech disorders in children arising from a wide range of etiologies have been investigated, including functional articulation and phonological disorders (Carter & Edwards, 2004; Dagenais, Critz-Crosby, & Adams, 1994; Gibbon & Hardcastle, 1987; McAuliffe & Cornwell, 2008), cleft palate (Fujiwara, 2007; Gibbon & Hardcastle, 1989; Hardcastle et al., 1989; Michi, Suzuki, Yamashita, & Imai, 1986; Whitehill, Stokes, & Man, 1996; Yamashita et al., 1992), neurological disorders

(Gibbon & Wood, 2003; Hardcastle, Morgan Barry, & Clark, 1987), hearing impairment (Bacsfalvi, Bernhardt, & Gick, 2007; Dagenais & Critz-Crosby, 1991; Nicolaidis, 2004), and Down Syndrome (Gibbon et al., 2003).

Although a large number of EPG therapy studies exist, there are limitations in the quality of the evidence about effectiveness. In terms of levels of clinical evidence, the quality is low, at levels III or IV according to the Scottish Intercollegiate Guidelines Network (SIGN) Guidelines (SIGN, 2008). Most are nonanalytic studies (e.g., case reports, case series) or expert opinion, reporting a small number of children as single cases or small groups. Such studies are useful as descriptive accounts of therapy for that individual, but it is not possible to generalize the results. Another limitation of current studies is that none so far has included an adequate control group. Lee, Law, and Gibbon (2008) conducted a Cochrane review of studies on EPG therapy for individuals with cleft palate and concluded that there is no evidence from randomized trials to support or refute the effectiveness of EPG in speech therapy and that there is a need for high-quality, randomized trials to be undertaken in the future. By linking all the specialist cleft palate centers throughout the United Kingdom together—as in the CLEFTNET network—it becomes realistic, as well as desirable, to conduct larger scale research projects than has been possible in the past (Lee et al., 2007).

PRACTICAL REQUIREMENTS

Some practical requirements of EPG therapy, such as how EPG plates are constructed, have already been discussed. Some important additional comments are included here.

EPG plates are custom-made and relatively costly to construct, although new cheaper types are now under development (Wrench, 2007). Children therefore need to learn to take care of plates and become familiar with inserting and removing them before and after therapy sessions. There is also the issue of adaptation to the plate. Most adults with normal speech adapt in a short period to wearing the plate, allowing them to speak naturally with it in place (McAuliffe, Lin, Robb, & Murdoch, 2008; McLeod & Searl, 2006). Children also need time to become accustomed to wearing their plate before EPG therapy can begin. Some find that wearing and speaking with it in place is strange or even uncomfortable at first. A sign of insufficient adaptation to the plate is excessive salivation. Children will usually adapt gradually, increasing the time they wear the plate, until they can wear it comfortably for about 2 hours at a time. Once this is achieved, they are ready for the pretherapy EPG recording, and therapy sessions can begin. Most children adapt within a few days.

Speech-language pathologists (SLPs) are familiar with using computers as part of their clinical practice and in general do not have difficulties learning how to use the clinical functions of EPG. SLPs need to develop skill and confidence in using EPG, however, and can develop these by attending training workshops. An ideal context for clinicians to learn how to use EPG is as part of a collaborative network, such as CLEFTNET (Lee et al., 2007). The CLEFTNET initiative represents a novel form of EPG service delivery—it links the cleft palate centers throughout Scotland to Queen Margaret University, Edinburgh, through an electronic network. EPG data collected in specialist cleft palate centers throughout the UK are sent to Edinburgh, where experts conduct detailed analysis leading to a precise diagnosis of each individual's specific articulation difficulty. Therapy guidelines are drawn up based on the EPG analysis and sent to the specialist clinicians who provide therapy for the children. The initiative provides regular workshops and ready access to technical support. The project also analyzes and archives EPG data sent electronically from the participating centers. EPG materials for use by those involved in the project were developed including new speech material for EPG recordings (see Appendix 21A), an EPG brochure, information sheets, individual consent forms, and EPG data analysis reports. Regular 2-day EPG workshops are organized, taking the form of self-directed hands-on tutorials with the WinEPG software (Articulate Instruments Ltd, 2008), lectures about the clinical use of EPG, and clinical case discussions.

KEY COMPONENTS

Description of Activities

During a typical EPG therapy session, a child and a clinician sit side by side in front of a computer screen, as shown in Figure 21.4. New versions of software give the clinician flexibility in terms of the amount of information and the content of the EPG screen displays. Usually the screen shows dynamic (i.e., real-time) and static displays alongside each other, as in Figure 21.4. EPG has the facility for two multiplexers to be connected, one for the child and one for the clinician, with a switch to toggle between the two. When the clinician is connected, it is possible to demonstrate normal contact patterns on the dynamic display. When children are connected to the EPG equipment, they can see their own tongue contact patterns. It is also possible to capture or *freeze* a target pattern onto the static display. A target pattern for a velar articulation is shown on the right-hand side of the computer screen in Figure 21.4. Prerecorded target static patterns can be stored in the computer and retrieved when needed.

At the beginning of intervention with EPG, the clinician demonstrates typical EPG patterns and explains to the child, using appropriate terminology, the relationship between tongue patterns (as displayed on the EPG screen) and the resulting speech sounds. The clinician also ensures that the child understands how the visual display relates to his or her own tongue and hard palate. Although visual feedback of tongue articulation makes EPG intervention unique, clinicians use a variety of other standard intervention strategies (e.g., modeling, demonstrating, cuing, reinforcing) alongside feedback within therapy sessions.

The target EPG pattern that the child attempts to copy in therapy resembles a normal pattern. The word *resembles* is emphasized here because it is necessary for the pattern that the child attempts (the therapy target pattern) to be tailored for each child. The clinician identifies appropriate therapy target patterns based on the shape of the child's palate, knowledge of typical patterns, and whether the target pattern results in a perceptually accurate speech sound. Some children with abnormally shaped palates produce a perceptually accurate /s/ with a wide anterior groove. In these cases, the /s/ therapy target pattern may resemble a typical /s/, but with a wider groove than would be expected in a typical speaker. Therapy targets are rarely precisely defined in terms of individual sensors that must, or must not, be contacted. Instead, targets are defined in terms of having important elements of typical contact patterns, such as an anterior groove for /s/ or contact in the posterior region for /k/. Furthermore, therapy targets need to be flexible in terms of amount of contact, given the extensive individual differences in the amount of contact produced by typical speakers for all lingual sounds. During therapy sessions, the clinician is careful to ensure that speech sounds associated with therapy target patterns are perceptually accurate.

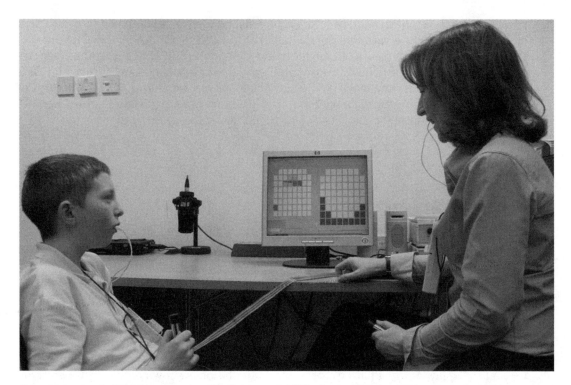

Figure 21.4. A typical EPG therapy session. The clinician and child both wear EPG plates and are connected to the computer display. The EPG pattern on the right shows a static therapy target for a typical velar sound, /k/. The child is attempting to copy this velar pattern. The display on the left is "live" (i.e., real time), giving the child moment-to-moment visual feedback of his attempts to produce the velar pattern.

Children with strongly habituated error patterns can find learning new articulations difficult. A useful strategy in eliminating entrenched patterns is first of all to introduce new patterns in the absence of other speech features, such as airstream or voicing (Hardcastle et al., 1991). In these situations, the child is encouraged to articulate silently, focusing on achieving a consistently accurate target EPG pattern, with appropriate airstream and voicing added at a later stage. Once new patterns are stable and consistent, visual feedback is gradually withdrawn. A first step is removing visual feedback from the child but keeping the EPG plate in situ. This is possible by arranging the computer screen so that the clinician can see it but the child cannot, or alternatively by unplugging the EPG plate. The former option has the advantage that the clinician is able to check that the child can maintain the correct contact pattern without visual feedback. At a still later stage, the goal is for the child to articulate a perceptually accurate sound after the plate is removed from the mouth.

ASSESSMENT METHODS

Making clinical decisions, such as identifying therapy goals and their sequencing, is the responsibility of the clinician. Decisions are based on the conceptual framework that the clinician adopts and the assessment results for individual children. For example, a clinician adopting a phonological orientation might introduce new articulation patterns in terms of how they function as systematic and rule-governed aspects of language. For a child who exhibits the phonological process of backing alveolar targets to velar place of articulation, /t/ may be introduced alongside /k/, perhaps within minimal pairs, in order to emphasize the alveolar-velar phonological contrast and to avoid overgeneralization.

Goal selection is usually straightforward for children with articulation difficulties affecting only a few targets, such as lateralization of sibilant targets. Goal selection is more complex for children with multiple articulation errors. In these cases, a clinician may focus EPG therapy on developing an underlying skill, such as speech motor control. A goal of therapy here may be to increase overall tongue stability; this is appropriate for children with evidence of undifferentiated gestures. A number of researchers have suggested that control of the lateral margins of the tongue is essential for normal speech production because lateral anchorage gives stability to the whole of the tongue (Fletcher, 1992; Stone, Faber, Raphael, & Shawker, 1992). One way to increase tongue stability is to establish reliable patterns of lateral contact for lingual consonants, such as /t/, /d/, and /n/, and this may be an intervention goal for some children. As a final example, a clinician may aim to increase consistency in tongue–palate contact patterns in children demonstrating a high amount of variability. A limited number of targets may be introduced during initial stages of therapy, with a greater range of targets introduced once earlier targets are consistently articulated.

Researchers and clinicians in the CLEFTNET project developed a systematic way of determining EPG therapy goals (see Lee et al., 2007, for details and a case illustration). Goals were formulated on the basis of a summary of an EPG analysis of pretherapy assessment data. An analysis report included a table summarizing children's EPG patterns for each target phoneme, with error patterns classified according to a scheme developed by Gibbon (2004). This is followed by a set of therapy guidelines and EPG printouts illustrating the child's error patterns. Setting therapy goals in CLEFTNET is based on identifying any correct as well as incorrect patterns. Patterns that are variable, notably those produced correctly in some phonetic contexts but not others, are identified. Goals are selected in which a pattern is achievable and already in the individual's articulation repertoire.

Analysis of pretherapy EPG data often reveals *facilitative contexts*, which involve placing the target in specific phonetic environments so that components of a preceding or following sound facilitate production of that target (Kent, 1982). The concept of facilitative contexts has a long tradition in speech therapy (e.g., McDonald, 1964), although its application in EPG therapy is unique in identifying contexts that facilitate specific tongue–palate contact patterns. The case study of Lisa presented at the end of the chapter illustrates how a facilitative context was identified and used successfully in EPG therapy.

In order to identify potential facilitative contexts, it is necessary first of all to assess the full range of articulations in an individual's repertoire. The next step is to identify contexts in which the child can already spontaneously produce articulation features (e.g., alveolar placement, lateral contact, velar placement, an alveolar groove). These contexts are then used to facilitate articulations that are incorrectly produced (e.g., retracted placement, minimal EPG contact, no anterior groove). For example, some children with cleft palate are able to articulate the nasal stop /n/ with a typical horseshoe-shaped pattern but have abnormally retracted placement for the oral stops /t/ and /d/. Facilitation is possible because /t/, /d/, and /n/ all have similar EPG patterns in typical speakers. The idea is to use a child's correct (i.e., /n/) productions to facilitate correct productions of articulation errors (i.e., /t/, /d/). This is achieved by placing correct and incorrect articulations next to each other in adjacent contexts, such as in m*int t*ea, wi*nd*y, and so forth. In these sequences, for successful production of /t/ and /d/, the child needs to hold constant the alveolar placement (facilitated by /n/) during production of the following /t/ or /d/.

The main aim of intervention when using EPG for visual feedback therapy is to enhance children's speech intelligibility by improving articulation patterns for lingual targets. To achieve this aim, children first need to modify abnormal articulations using visual feedback, then retain newly learned articulations without feedback, and finally use newly learned articulation in everyday speaking situations. The process of monitoring progress for children in EPG therapy involves shifting the emphasis away from learning new articulation patterns with the aid of visual feedback to using them spontaneously outside the clinic setting. Achieving carryover of newly learned skills is challenging for many children. Gibbon and Paterson (2006) found that although most children undergoing EPG therapy had improved articulation to some extent, most experienced difficulties generalizing to everyday speech. These authors concluded that clinicians need to adopt specific strategies to promote generalization and maintenance when using EPG in therapy. Davis and Drichta (1980) reached a similar conclusion when they reviewed earlier biofeedback techniques used in the clinical management of speech disorders; they highlighted the need to demonstrate in future research that skills learned in the clinical setting were carried over into other speaking situations.

In the past, the frequency and location of EPG therapy sessions were determined by practical considerations, such as the distance to be travelled in order to attend therapy. Frequent practice of new articulation patterns using EPG for feedback was often impossible for those living at a distance, and therapy was sometimes discontinued because it was too far for children to attend on a regular basis. A device that has proved successful in overcoming this practical difficulty has been the EPG portable training unit (Fujiwara, 2007; Gibbon, Stewart, Hardcastle, & Crampin, 1999; Jones & Hardcastle, 1995). The major design features of these units are that they are small, comparatively inexpensive, lightweight, and simple to operate. The portable units allow visual feedback therapy to take place close to, or in, children's homes, so increasing opportunities for practice and avoiding the need to travel long distances for therapy sessions (see Figure 21.5).

A wide range of factors can affect rate of progress in intervention for SSD, and this applies equally to visual feedback therapy with EPG. The case study of Lisa, described at the end of the chapter, is an example of a child for whom EPG therapy was successful after only seven clinic sessions. It remains unclear why some children respond positively to EPG therapy after just a few sessions, whereas others require many sessions over an extended period before making any tangible progress (Dent, Gibbon, & Hardcastle, 1995; Gibbon & Paterson, 2006; McAuliffe & Cornwell, 2008; Michi et al., 1986). Irrespective of the number of sessions required to succeed, all children need sufficiently high levels of attention and motivation to learn new articulation patterns, to practice them until they become automatic, and then to use them outside the clinic setting. In terms of attention and motivation, an advantage of computer-mediated procedures, such as EPG, is that some children are more inclined to persist with tasks when performance is measured objectively (i.e., by a computer) rather than when it is judged by another person (i.e., the clinician; Volin, 1991). A factor likely to facilitate generalization is plenty of support from family, friends, teachers, and others in the child's life. These people play an important role in providing encouragement and opportunities for children undergoing EPG therapy to practice new articulations in everyday life.

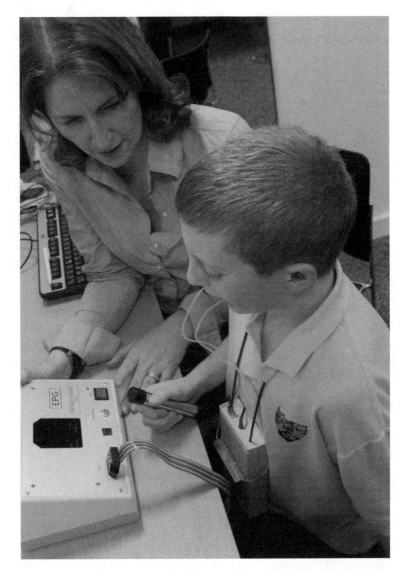

Figure 21.5. A child receiving visual feedback therapy with a portable training unit.

Many factors can affect progress in EPG intervention, but we lack knowledge about the most critical variables for predicting and maximizing progress. A study by Carter and Edwards (2004) found that it was difficult to predict which children out of a group of 10 with functional disorders would make maximum improvement in EPG therapy. Baker and Bernhardt (2004) discussed a number of variables that can affect response to therapy for SSD. These factors include those to do with the child (e.g., age, type and severity of speech disorder, degree of motivation), intervention (time in therapy, therapy approach), and therapist characteristics (e.g., ability to motivate child, experience in intervention). Although any of these factors may affect progress in EPG therapy, the precise impact of any one of these on an individual's progress is difficult to determine.

CONSIDERATIONS FOR CHILDREN FROM CULTURALLY AND LINGUISTICALLY DIVERSE BACKGROUNDS

The importance of normative EPG data from children's own linguistic background has been highlighted already, and clinicians need to be aware of regional variations when judging whether a child's tongue–palate contact patterns are typical or abnormal. Knowledge of regional variation is equally important in determining target patterns for children to emulate during therapy. There is already an extensive literature on typical EPG patterns, and although most report data from adults, an increasing number report data from typically developing children (Cheng, Murdoch, Goozée, & Scott, 2007; Fletcher, 1989). Fletcher reported EPG data from nine children with typical speech development, ages 6–14 years. A general finding for all lingual consonants was that amount of contact decreased as children got older. This decrease in contact was paralleled by relatively fine-grained articulatory adjustments, such as a shift to a more posterior placement as children grew and an overall reduction in the length of midsagittal contact of lingual targets. Fletcher interpreted these findings to show that during the school years articulation accuracy and precision continued to develop.

Many lingual targets, consonants, and vowels that register measurable amounts of tongue–palate contact show variation depending on regional, cultural, and linguistic backgrounds (see McLeod, 2007). One example in which children's backgrounds need careful consideration is in their use of glottal stops. Glottal stops can be used in place of voiceless plosive /t/, and sometimes also /p/ and /k/ in typical speakers; this is observed in many varieties of English and is part of normal English speech in specific phonetic contexts (Wells, 1982). The EPG patterns associated with the targets /t/ or /k/ will be entirely different from those associated with glottal stops. It is therefore critical when interpreting EPG patterns to distinguish between glottal stops that are a normal part of everyday speech from those that are abnormal due to, for example, compensatory articulations in cleft palate speech or as abnormal substitutions in phonological disorder or childhood apraxia of speech.

CASE STUDY

Lisa, a 9-year-old girl, was referred for EPG therapy because of distortions affecting sibilant targets /s/, /z/, /ʃ/, /ʒ/, /tʃ/, and /dʒ/. Lisa had an unusual history of speech development insofar as she produced a variety of different distortions for sibilant targets during the preschool period. At the age of 18 months, her mother noticed that Lisa produced /s/ in the word *soap* with a nasal quality. At 3;1, an assessment by an SLP revealed that Lisa realized all sibilant targets with *phoneme-specific nasality* (Peterson-Falzone & Graham, 1990). This abnormal nasality was functional—velopharyngeal abnormality was ruled out at this time based on an oral examination by an otolaryngology consultant, combined with perceptual evidence of adequate oral pressure for all obstruent sounds, apart from attempts at sibilant targets.

By 4;7, Lisa's speech had changed spontaneously (she had not received any intervention during the preschool years) but remained problematic; there were now two different types of distortions evident for sibilant targets. Alveolar sibilants /s/ and /z/ were still realized with phoneme-specific nasality, but /ʃ/, /ʒ/, /tʃ/, and /dʒ/ targets were now lateral fricatives and affricates. At this stage, Lisa received therapy using a traditional approach in order to eliminate the abnormal nasality affecting /s/ and /z/ targets. Therapy was partially successful; nasality was eliminated, but these targets became interdental fricatives instead. These various distortions affecting sibilants—namely nasality, lateralization, and interdental placement—could have been associated with an early conductive hearing loss. A loss was identified when Lisa was 3 years old and consisted of a 40 dB loss in the right ear and a 20 dB loss in the left ear. The hearing loss had resolved by the time Lisa was 4;0.

Lisa was referred for EPG therapy when she was 9 years old. From a perceptually based phonetic transcription made at this time, it was evident that her speech had not improved spontaneously since she had been assessed 5 years previously; /s/ and /z/ were consistently interdental fricatives, and /ʃ/, /ʒ/, /tʃ/, and /dʒ/ were consistently lateral fricatives and affricates. Lisa perceived her speech difficulty as serious and viewed it as having a detrimental effect on her quality of life and as limiting her participation in some activities. Prior to undergoing EPG therapy, an SLP attempted to modify Lisa's distorted productions using traditional methods, with no success.

Figure 21.6 shows Lisa's pretherapy EPG patterns for sibilant targets alongside patterns from a typically developing child of a similar age. These are composite EPG frames taken at the temporal midpoint during words containing fricatives, affricates, and stops (from the CLEFTNET word list, Appendix 21A, Section D, Minimal Pairs). The left column in Figure 21.6 shows the typical child's patterns for /s/, /ʃ/, /tʃ/, and /t/ (for the affricate, the stop /t'/ component is shown separately from the fricative /ʃ'/ component). As can be seen from the next column in the figure, pretherapy EPG data showed that Lisa's patterns for /s/ and /z/ were abnormal, involving minimal tongue–palate contact and only a few sensors showing contact in the periphery of the palate. These EPG patterns fit with listeners' perceptual impressions of interdental placement. Her EPG patterns for /s/ and /z/ contrasted dramatically with her EPG patterns for the lateralized distortions of /ʃ/, /ʒ/, /tʃ/, and /dʒ/ targets; these had extensive contact across the palate similar to undifferentiated gestures described by Gibbon (1999).

Excessive amounts of contact have been noted to occur during lateralized distortions of sibilant targets, although as Figure 21.3 demonstrates, much variation occurs in the articulation patterns that can underlie this type of articulation error. It is noteworthy that Lisa's EPG patterns for /tʃ/ and /ʃ/ were similar in having extensive contact across the palate. A final observation is that Lisa had normal tongue contact for /t/, suggesting that she had developed independent control of the lateral and apical regions of the tongue. Lisa's normal articulations of /t/ were additionally relevant in providing a potentially facilitative context for /s/. Recall that normal /t/ articulations show an /s/-like groove at the start of closure release (see frame 81 in Figure 21.2[a]).

Lisa had seven once-weekly EPG therapy sessions with an SLP based in her local community clinic. In addition to these clinic-based sessions, Lisa was also given a portable training unit, which allowed her to practice at home on her own or with the help of her mother. Therapy aimed to correct her abnormal articula-

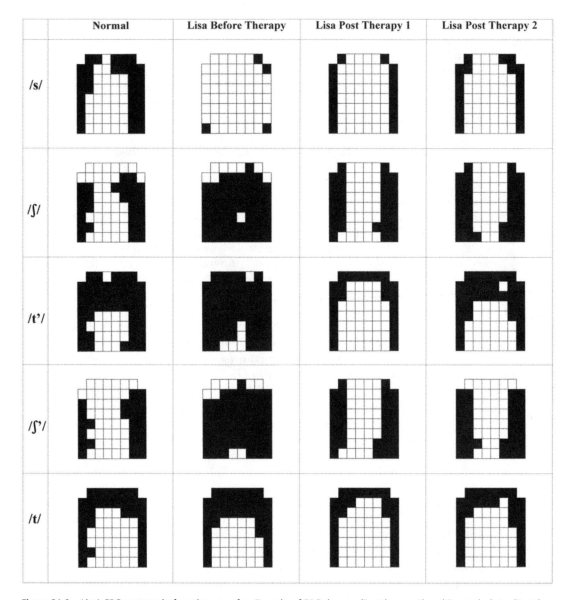

Figure 21.6. Lisa's EPG patterns before therapy, after 7 weeks of EPG therapy (Posttherapy 1) and 3 months later (Posttherapy 2). Patterns for a typically developing child of the same age are in the left column for comparison. The figure shows patterns for /s/, /ʃ/, /tʃ/, and /t/ (for the affricate, the stop /t'/ component is shown separately from the fricative /ʃ'/ component). These are composite EPG frames, taken at the midpoint of the target sounds, with sensors contacted >50% registered as black squares.

tions of all sibilant targets. The focus of the initial sessions was to ensure that Lisa understood how sibilant targets were articulated in typical speakers. The link between articulation and the visual display on EPG was explained. Terms such as *side contact*, *horseshoe shape*, and *groove* were introduced. The clinician and Lisa discussed the differences between EPG printouts of normal patterns and Lisa's own printouts. They agreed on the aims of therapy.

During these early sessions, the clinician used the EPG visual feedback display to demonstrate typical EPG patterns and for Lisa to gain confidence using the technique. The first target for therapy was /s/, which was selected on the basis that a facilitative context had been identified. This meant that she could already produce a normal /s/-like configuration, albeit for a different target (i.e., at the release of /t/). Lisa felt encouraged by her discovery that she could already produce key features of articulations that had proved so difficult previously. She was able to modify /t/ patterns quite easily using visual feedback so that they contained an anterior, central groove for /s/ when prolonging the release of /t/ (e.g., *tssssss*) and in facilitative contexts such as in words containing /ts/ (e.g., *hats*). Importantly, the fricative that Lisa produced when prolonging the release phase of /t/ was judged perceptually as a normal /s/.

Once Lisa could produce normal EPG patterns consistently for /s/ targets, they generalized readily to /z/ targets. Later sessions focused on producing normal tongue contact patterns for /ʃ/, /ʒ/ and then /tʃ/, /dʒ/. Using visual feedback, Lisa was able to modify her now normal /s/ articulation in order to produce the more retracted and wider groove that is characteristic of /ʃ/. In each session, visual feedback was provided until Lisa could produce target patterns consistently, at which point the feedback was withdrawn by covering the screen or unplugging the EPG plate. Once Lisa could produce target patterns without visual feedback, she was encouraged to remove the plate and practice without it in situ.

After seven sessions of EPG therapy, Lisa could produce typical EPG patterns (see posttherapy patterns in Figure 21.6) for all sibilant targets, and these were judged as perceptually normal. She continued to receive traditional therapy for several months following EPG therapy to help her to carry over these newly learned articulation patterns into everyday speech. The final column in Figure 21.6 demonstrates that Lisa maintained progress when a third EPG recording was made 3 months later. (This case study was adapted from Hailstone [2003].)

STUDY QUESTIONS

1. Describe typical tongue–palate contact patterns for /s/ and /t/. In what ways are the EPG patterns for these two sounds 1) similar and 2) different?

2. How does EPG differ from the other intervention approaches to SSDs?

3. How can an analysis of EPG patterns assist in 1) diagnosis and 2) devising therapy goals?

4. What are the key features of portable training units? Under what circumstances would an SLP consider using a portable EPG unit?

FUTURE DIRECTIONS

Gibbon (2007) proposed that, instead of children using the EPG display to provide biofeedback of their own tongue movements, they could actively engage in observing articulation patterns produced by another speaker to enhance their learning of new articulation patterns. This *observation window* would consist of the live (i.e., real-time) EPG display. This form of therapy would involve the child observing the dynamic display of contact patterns produced by the clinician during speech. There are good theoretical reasons why observing another speaker's motor actions might enhance the effectiveness of articulation therapy. For example, visual information is a central component of therapy in the integral stimulation approach developed by Strand and Skinder (1999). Integral stimulation, recently renamed *dynamic temporal and tactile cueing* (Strand, Stoeckel, & Baas, 2006), requires that the child imitates utterances modeled by the clinician, with an important component being that children focus their visual attention on the clinician's face. The tongue's actions are hidden from view under normal circumstances, however. It may be that information about the clinician's tongue activity contained in an *observation window*, such as the EPG display, may facilitate therapy by providing details about articulation that are not normally available.

Some support for the beneficial role that observation plays in enhancing motor behavior comes from the theory of mirror neurons (Rizzolatti & Arbib, 1998). These specialized neurons make it possible for people to enhance their learning of complex motor skills by watching the performance of others. Kent (2002) suggested potential applications of the theory of mirror neurons to speech pathology, outlining that this theory provides compelling reasons why additional visual information facilitates the accuracy of motor performance. One practical advantage of this approach is that it does not require that children have individual EPG plates constructed. This idea requires investigation in future research.

SUGGESTED READINGS

Gibbon, F.E. (1999). Undifferentiated lingual gestures in children with articulation/phonological disorders. *Journal of Speech, Language, and Hearing Research, 42*, 382–397.

Gibbon, F.E. (2008). Instrumental analysis of articulation in speech impairment. In M. Ball, M. Perkins, N. Müller, & S. Howard (Eds.), *Handbook of clinical linguistics* (pp. 311–331). Oxford, England: Wiley-Blackwell.

Gibbon, F.E., & Paterson, L. (2006). A survey of speech and language therapists' views on electropalatography therapy outcomes in Scotland. *Child Language Teaching and Therapy, 22*, 275–292.

REFERENCES

Bacsfalvi, P., Bernhardt, B.M., & Gick, B. (2007). Electropalatography and ultrasound in vowel remediation for adolescents with hearing impairment. *Advances in Speech-Language Pathology, 9*, 36–45.

Baker, E., & Bernhardt, B. (2004). From hindsight to foresight: Working around barriers to success in phonological intervention. *Child Language Teaching and Therapy, 20*, 287–318.

Carter, P., & Edwards, S. (2004). EPG therapy for children with long-standing speech disorders: Predictions and outcomes. *Clinical Linguistics and Phonetics, 18*, 359–372.

Cheng, H.Y., Murdoch, B.E., Goozée, J.V., & Scott, D. (2007). Electropalatographic assessment of tongue-to-palate contact patterns and variability in children, adolescents, and adults. *Journal of Speech, Language, and Hearing Research, 50*, 375–392.

Connery, V. (1994). The Nuffield Dyspraxia Programme: Working on the motor programming of speech. In J. Law (Ed.), *Before school: A handbook of approaches to intervention with pre-school language impaired children* (pp. 125–141). London: AFASIC.

Dagenais, P.A., & Critz-Crosby, P. (1991). Consonant lingual-palatal contacts produced by normal-hearing and hearing-impaired children. *Journal of Speech and Hearing Research, 34*, 1423–1435.

Dagenais, P.A., Critz-Crosby, P., & Adams, J.B. (1994). Defining and remediating persistent lateral lisps in children using electropalatography: Preliminary findings. *American Journal of Speech-Language Pathology, 3*, 67–76.

Davis, S.M., & Drichta, C.E. (1980). Biofeedback: Theory and application to speech pathology. In N.J. Lass (Ed.), *Speech and language: Advances in basic research and practice* (pp. 283–286). New York: Academic Press.

Dent, H., Gibbon, F., & Hardcastle, W. (1992). Inhibiting an abnormal lingual pattern in a cleft palate child using electropalatography. In M.M. Leahy & J.L. Kallen (Eds.), *Interdisciplinary perspectives in speech and language pathology* (pp. 211–221). Dublin, Ireland: School of Clinical Speech and Language Studies.

Dent, H., Gibbon, F., & Hardcastle, W.J. (1995). The application of electropalatography to the remediation of speech disorders in school aged children and young adults. *European Journal of Disorders of Communication, 30,* 264–277.

Dodd, B. (Ed.). (1995). *Differential diagnosis and treatment of children with speech disorder.* London: Whurr.

Fletcher, S. (1983). New prospects for speech by the hearing impaired. In N. Lass (Ed.), *Speech and language: Advances in basic research and practice* (pp. 1–42). New York: Academic Press.

Fletcher, S.G. (1989). Palatometric specification of stop, affricate and sibilant sounds. *Journal of Speech and Hearing Research, 32,* 736–748.

Fletcher, S.G. (1992). *Articulation: A physiological approach.* San Diego: Singular.

Fujimura, O., Tatsumi, I.F., & Kagaya, R. (1973). Computational processing of palatographic patterns. *Journal of Phonetics, 1,* 47–54.

Fujiwara, Y. (2007). Electropalatography home training using a portable training unit for Japanese children with cleft palate. *Advances in Speech-Language Pathology, 9,* 65–72.

Gibbon, F.E. (1999). Undifferentiated lingual gestures in children with articulation/phonological disorders. *Journal of Speech, Language, and Hearing Research, 42,* 382–397.

Gibbon, F. (2002). Features of impaired motor control in children with articulation/phonological disorders. In F. Windsor, L. Kelly, & N. Hewlett (Eds.), *Investigations in clinical linguistics and phonetics* (pp. 299–309). London: Lawrence Erlbaum Associates.

Gibbon, F. (2003a). The contribution of EPG to the diagnosis of childhood apraxia of speech. In L.D. Shriberg & T.F. Campbell (Eds.), *Proceedings of the 2002 Childhood Apraxia of Speech Research Symposium.* Carlsbad, CA: Hendrix Foundation.

Gibbon, F.E. (2003b, August). Using articulatory data to inform speech pathology theory and clinical practice. *Proceedings of the 15th International Congress of Phonetic Sciences* (pp. 261–264). Barcelona, Spain: Causal Productions.

Gibbon, F.E. (2004). Abnormal patterns of tongue–palate contact in the speech of individuals with cleft palate. *Clinical Linguistics and Phonetics, 18,* 285–311.

Gibbon, F. (2007, November). *EPG and mirror neurons.* Presentation at CLEFTNET study day, Edinburgh.

Gibbon, F. (2008). Instrumental analysis of articulation in speech impairment. In M. Ball, M. Perkins, N. Müller, & S. Howard (Eds.), *Handbook of clinical linguistics* (pp. 311–331). Oxford, England: Wiley-Blackwell.

Gibbon, F.E., Ellis, L., & Crampin, L. (2004). Articulatory placement for /t/, /d/, /k/ and /g/ targets in school age children with speech disorders associated with cleft palate. *Clinical Linguistics and Phonetics, 18,* 391–404.

Gibbon, F., & Hardcastle, W. (1987). Articulatory description and treatment of "lateral /s/" using electropalatography: A case study. *British Journal of Disorders of Communication, 22,* 203–217.

Gibbon, F., & Hardcastle, W. (1989). Deviant articulation in a cleft palate child following late repair of the hard palate: A description and remediation procedure using electropalatography. *Clinical Linguistics and Phonetics, 3,* 93–110.

Gibbon, F., Lee, A., & Yuen, I. (2007). Tongue–palate contact during bilabials in normal speech. *Cleft Palate-Craniofacial Journal, 44,* 87–91.

Gibbon, F.E., & Mayo, C. (2008, November). *Adults' perception of conflicting acoustic cues associated with EPG-defined undifferentiated gestures.* Poster session presented at the 5th International EPG symposium, Edinburgh.

Gibbon, F.E., McNeill, A.M., Wood, S.E., & Watson, J.M.M. (2003). Changes in linguapalatal contact patterns during therapy for velar fronting in a 10-year-old with Down's syndrome. *International Journal of Language and Communication Disorders, 38,* 47–64.

Gibbon, F., & Nicolaidis, K. (1999). Palatography. In W.J. Hardcastle & N. Hewlett (Eds.), *Coarticulation in speech production: Theory, data, and techniques* (pp. 229–245). Cambridge, England: Cambridge University Press.

Gibbon, F.E., & Paterson, L. (2006). A survey of speech and language therapists' views on electropalatography therapy outcomes in Scotland. *Child Language Teaching and Therapy, 22,* 275–292.

Gibbon, F.E., & Scobbie, J.M. (1997). Covert contrasts in children with phonological disorder. *Australian Communication Quarterly, Autumn,* 13–16.

Gibbon, F., Stewart, F., Hardcastle, W.J., & Crampin, L. (1999). Widening access to electropalatography for children with persistent sound system disorders. *American Journal of Speech-Language Pathology, 8,* 319–334.

Gibbon, F.E., & Wood, S.E. (2002). Articulatory drift in the speech of children with articulation/phonological disorders. *Perceptual and Motor Skills, 95,* 295–307.

Gibbon, F.E., & Wood, S.E. (2003). Using electropalatography (EPG) to diagnose and treat articulation disorders associated with mild cerebral palsy: A case study. *Clinical Linguistics and Phonetics, 17,* 365–374.

Gibbon, F., Yuen, I., Lee, A., & Adams, L. (2007). Normal adult speakers' tongue–palate contact patterns for alveolar oral and nasal stops. *Advances in Speech-Language Pathology, 9,* 82–89.

Hailstone, L. (2003). *The assessment and treatment of sibilant distortions using electropalatography: A case study.* Unpublished honors project, Queen Margaret University College, Edinburgh.

Hardcastle, W.J., & Gibbon, F. (1997). Electropalatography and its clinical applications. In M.J. Ball & C. Code (Eds.), *Instrumental clinical phonetics* (pp. 149–193). London: Whurr.

Hardcastle, W.J., Gibbon, F.E., & Jones, W. (1991). Visual display of tongue–palate contact: Electropalatography in the assessment and remediation of speech disorders. *British Journal of Disorders of Communication, 26,* 41–74.

Hardcastle, W.J., Morgan Barry, R.A., & Clark, C.J. (1987). An instrumental phonetic study of lingual activity in articulation-disordered children. *Journal of Speech and Hearing Research, 30,* 171–184.

Hardcastle, W., Morgan Barry, R., & Nunn, M. (1989). Instrumental articulatory phonetics in assessment and remediation: Case studies with the electropalatograph. In J. Stengelhofen (Ed.), *Cleft palate: The nature and remediation of communicative problems* (pp. 136–164). Edinburgh: Churchill Livingstone.

Heselwood, B., & Howard, S. (2008). Clinical phonetic transcription. In M. Ball, M. Perkins, N. Müller, & S. Howard (Eds.), *Handbook of clinical linguistics* (pp. 318–399). Oxford, England: Wiley-Blackwell.

Hiki, S., & Itoh, H. (1986). Influence of palate shape on lingual articulation. *Speech Communication, 5,* 141–158.

Howard, S. (2004). Compensatory articulatory behaviours in adolescents with cleft palate: Comparing the perceptual and instrumental evidence. *Clinical Linguistics and Phonetics, 18,* 313–340.

Jones, W., & Hardcastle, W.J. (1995). New developments in EPG3 software. *European Journal of Disorders of Communication, 30,* 183–192.

Kent, R.D. (1982). Contextual facilitation of correct sound production. *Language, Speech, and Hearing Services in Schools, 13,* 66–76.

Kent, R.D. (1996). Hearing and believing: Some limits to the auditory-perceptual assessment of speech and voice disorders. *American Journal of Speech-Language Pathology, 5,* 7–23.

Kent, R. (2002). Speech motor models and developments in neurophysiological science: Recent developments. In B. Maassen, W. Hulstijn, R. Kent, H. Peters, & P. Van Lieshout (Eds.), *Speech motor control in normal and disordered speech* (pp. 1–3). Nijmegen, The Netherlands: Vantilt.

Kornfeld, J.R. (1971). *Theoretical issues in child phonology.* Papers of the 7th Regional Meeting, Chicago Linguistic Society (pp. 454–468). Chicago: University of Chicago.

Lee, A., Gibbon, F., Crampin, L., Yuen, I., & McLennan, G. (2007). The national CLEFTNET Project for individuals with cleft palate. *Advances in Speech-Language Pathology, 9,* 57–64.

Lee, A., Law, J., & Gibbon, F. (2008). *Electropalatography for articulation disorders associated with cleft palate.* London: John Wiley & Sons.

Liker, M., & Gibbon, F. (2008). Tongue–palate contact patterns of velar stops in normal adult English speakers. *Clinical Linguistics and Phonetics, 22,* 137–148.

Liker, M., Gibbon, F., Wrench, A., & Horga, D. (2007). Articulatory characteristics of the occlusion phase of /t/ compared to /t/ in adult speech. *Advances in Speech-Language Pathology, 9,* 101–108.

McAuliffe, M.J., & Cornwell, P. (2008). Intervention for lateral /s/ using electropalatography (EPG) biofeedback and an intensive motor learning approach: A case report. *International Journal of Language & Communication Disorders, 43,* 219–229.

McAuliffe, M.J., Lin, E., Robb, M.P., & Murdoch, B.E. (2008). Influence of a standard electropalatography artificial palate upon articulation: A preliminary study. *Folia Phoniatrica and Logopaedica, 60,* 45–53.

McDonald, E.T. (1964). *Articulation testing and treatment: A sensory motor approach.* Pittsburgh, PA: Stanwix House.

McLeod, S. (Ed.). (2007). *The international guide to speech acquisition.* Clifton Park, NY: Thomson Delmar Learning.

McLeod, S., Roberts, A., & Sita, J. (2006). Tongue/palate contact for the production of /s/ and /z/. *Clinical Linguistics and Phonetics, 20,* 51–66.

McLeod, S., & Searl, J. (2006). Adaptation to an electropalatography palate: Acoustic, impressionistic, and perceptual data. *American Journal of Speech-Language Pathology, 15,* 192–206.

McLeod, S., & Singh, S. (2009). *Speech sounds: A pictorial guide to typical and atypical speech.* San Diego: Plural Publishing.

Michi, K., Suzuki, N., Yamashita, Y., & Imai, S. (1986). Visual training and correction of articulation disorders by use of dynamic palatography: Serial observation in a case of cleft palate. *Journal of Speech and Hearing Disorders, 51,* 226–238.

Nicolaidis, K. (2004). Articulatory variability during consonant production by Greek speakers with hearing impairment: An electropalatographic study. *Clinical Linguistics and Phonetics, 18,* 419–432.

Noordhoff, M.S., Huang, C.S., & Wu, J. (1990). Multidisciplinary management of cleft lip and palate in Taiwan. In J. Bardach & H.L. Morris (Eds.), *Multidisciplinary management of cleft lip and palate* (pp. 18–26). Philadelphia: W.B. Saunders.

Peterson-Falzone, S.J., & Graham, M.S. (1990). Phoneme-specific nasal emission in children with and without physical anomalies of the velopharyngeal mechanism. *Journal of Speech and Hearing Disorders, 55,* 132–139.

Rizzolatti, G., & Arbib, M.A. (1998). Language within our grasp. *Trends in Neuroscience, 21*, 188–194.

Schmidt, A.M. (2007). Evaluating a new clinical palatometry system. *Advances in Speech-Language Pathology, 9*, 73–81.

Scottish Intercollegiate Guidelines Network. (2008). *SIGN 50: A guideline developers handbook.* Edinburgh: NHS Quality Improvement Scotland.

Shuster, L., Ruscello, D.M., & Smith, K.D. (1992). Evoking [r] using visual feedback. *American Journal of Speech-Language Pathology, 1*, 29–34.

Smit, A.B. (2004). *Articulation and phonology resource guide for school-age children and adults.* Clifton Park, NY: Thomson Delmar Learning.

Smit, A.B., Hand, L., Freilinger, J., Bernthal, J.B., & Bird, A. (1990). The Iowa articulation norms project and its Nebraska replication. *Journal of Speech and Hearing Disorders, 55*, 779–798.

Square, P.A. (1999). Treatment of developmental apraxia of speech: Tactile-kinesthetic, visual and rhythmic methods. In A.J. Caruso & E.A. Strand (Eds.), *Clinical management of motor speech disorders* (pp. 149–186). New York: Thieme.

Stone, M., Faber, A., Raphael, L.J., & Shawker, T.H. (1992). Cross-sectional tongue shape and linguopalatal contact patterns in [s], [ʃ], and [l]. *Journal of Phonetics, 20*, 253–270.

Strand, E. (1995). Treatment of motor speech disorders in children. *Seminars in Speech and Language, 16*, 126–139.

Strand, E.A., & Skinder, A. (1999). Treatment of developmental apraxia of speech: Integral stimulation methods. In A.J. Caruso & E.A. Strand (Eds.), *Clinical management of motor speech disorders in children* (pp. 109–148). New York: Thieme.

Strand, E.A., Stoeckel, R., & Baas, B. (2006). Treatment of severe childhood apraxia of speech: A treatment efficacy study. *Journal of Medical Speech-Language Pathology, 14*, 297–307.

Van Riper, C., & Emerick, L. (1984). *Speech correction: An introduction to speech pathology and audiology.* Englewood Cliffs, NJ: Prentice Hall.

Volin, R.A. (1991). Microcomputer-based systems providing biofeedback of voice and speech production. *Topics in Language Disorders, 11*, 65–79.

Wells, J.C. (1982). *Accents of English I: An introduction.* Cambridge, England: Cambridge University Press.

Whitehill, T.L., Stokes, S.F., & Man, Y.H.Y. (1996). Electropalatography treatment in an adult with late repair of cleft palate. *Cleft Palate-Craniofacial Journal, 33*, 160–168.

World Health Organization. (2001). *International classification of functioning, disability and health (ICF).* Geneva: Author.

Wrench, A. (2007). Advances in EPG palate design. *Advances in Speech-Language Pathology, 9*, 3–12.

Wrench, A. (2008). Articulate Assistant User Guide (Version 1.17) and WinEPG Installation and Users Manual (Revision 1.15). Edinburgh, Scotland: Articulate Instruments Ltd.

Yamashita, Y., Michi, K., Imai, S., Suzuki, N., & Yoshida, H. (1992). Electropalatographic investigation of abnormal lingual-palatal contact patterns in cleft palate patients. *Clinical Linguistics and Phonetics, 6*, 201–217.

Zharkova, N., Schaeffler, S., & Gibbon, F.E. (2009). Adult speakers' tongue–palate contact patterns for bilabial stops within complex clusters. *Clinical Linguistics and Phonetics, 23*(12), 901–910.

Appendix 21A CLEFTNET Speech Word List

A. Repetition

Repeat the following sounds:

1. pa pa pa . . .
2. ba ba ba . . .
3. ta ta ta . . .
4. da da da . . .
5. ka ka ka . . .
6. ga ga ga . . .
7. la la la . . .
8. fa fa fa . . .
9. va va va . . .
10. θa θa θa . . .
11. ða ða ða . . .
12. sa sa sa . . .
13. za za za . . .
14. ʃa ʃa ʃa . . .
15. ʒa ʒa ʒa . . .
16. tʃa tʃa tʃa . . .
17. ʤa ʤa ʤa . . .

B. Rote

Now count from 1 to 10.

C. Sentences

Now say these sentences:

1. Naughty Neil saw a robin in a nest.
2. Tiny Tim is putting a hat on.
3. My Daddy mended a door.
4. I saw Sam sitting on a bus.
5. Funny Sean is washing a dirty dish.
6. Cheeky Charlie's watching a football match.
7. Jolly John's got a magic badge.
8. Happy Karen is making a cake.
9. Baby Gary's got a bag of Legos.
10. The puppy is playing with a rope.
11. Bouncy Bob is a baby boy.
12. The phone fell off the shelf.
13. The hamster scrambled up Stewart's sleeve.
14. The nasty boy tossed the basket into the box.

D. Minimal pairs

Please say these words:

1. a sip   a shoe
2. a tore   a chop
3. a Sue   a sheet
4. a top   a chip
5. a sore   a shop
6. a team   a chew
7. a sob   a shore
8. a tip   a cheat
9. a seat   a ship
10. a tomb   a chore

Vowel Intervention

B. May Bernhardt, Joseph P. Stemberger, and Penelope Bacsfalvi

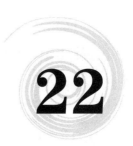

ABSTRACT

This chapter brings together two research streams regarding vowels in phonological intervention: 1) applications of nonlinear phonological theory and 2) the use of articulatory visual feedback, particularly ultrasound. Nonlinear phonological theories posit that 1) vowels are core prosodic elements, and 2) vowels and consonants can either be invisible to each other in phonological patterns because of independent structural representation, or they can affect each other because of prosodic or feature sequence interactions. Two nonlinear phonological intervention studies are presented, showing spontaneous improvement in vowels with some effects of treatment targeting prosodic structure. Vowels may not always improve spontaneously, however. Intervention using visual feedback with technologies such as ultrasound and electropalatography (EPG) may then be assistive, as will be described in the chapter.

INTRODUCTION

Nonlinear phonology encompasses theories that describe the representation of all aspects of phonological form. This chapter presents an overview of nonlinear theories and intervention studies in which vowels were examined (see also Chapter 13). The chapter further describes articulatory visual feedback as an adjunct to phonological intervention for vowels, particularly for individuals with persistent speech impairment deriving from hearing impairment or unknown causes.

The overarching perspective unifying these two streams of research is that phonology and phonetics/articulation are not strictly distinct. Phonology is intermediate between lexical access and motor programming; it deals with categories such as /oʊ/ and [Labial], but not with the fact that the muscular activity involved in producing /o/ is somewhat different following /t/ than following /k/. Nonmodular models of speech production

The authors would like to acknowledge and thank the families and colleagues who have contributed to the clinical application of nonlinear phonology and articulatory feedback intervention. The authors are especially indebted to Bosko Radanov, M.Sc., S-LP(C), for filming the ultrasound DVDs (a supplemental set of DVDs on consonants and ultrasound are available from the first or third authors). We also thank the editors of this book as well as Daniel Santiago and Harry Arnold for DVD editing. We acknowledge the following agencies for funding: BC Medical Services Foundation, BC Health Research Foundation, Canadian Foundation for Innovation, University of British Columbia Humanities and Social Sciences Small Grants and Hampton fund, and British Columbia Ministry of Children and Family Development in conjunction with the Human Early Learning Partnership.

(e.g., Dell, 1986; Nickels, 2001; Stemberger, 1992a) posit, however, that feedback from lower, later levels is necessary for accurate processing at earlier levels, so that phonology affects lexical access, and phonetics affects phonological planning. Thus, strengthening particular phonetic outputs also strengthens the phonology. By including perspectives that are both "phonological" and "articulatory" in the same chapter, we are indicating that both theoreticians and clinicians move back and forth between what is actually articulated and what is "represented," just as the speaker does.

Nonlinear theories provide a comprehensive framework for analysis, goal-setting, and treatment strategies. Articulatory visual feedback facilitates the actual implementation of the treatment plan for individuals who respond slowly to traditional noninstrumental techniques. Each section of this chapter addresses both of these research streams, sometimes in the same subsection, and sometimes in separate subsections.

TARGET POPULATIONS

Primary (and Secondary) Populations

Because nonlinear phonology describes the entire phonological system, principles concerning nonlinear phonological assessment and treatment are pertinent across ages and etiologies (see also Chapter 13). Reports suggest that clients with protracted phonological development (PPD) tend to have relatively greater difficulty learning consonants and word structure than vowels (Stoel-Gammon & Pollock, 2008). However, vowel systems can also be compromised. In particular, languages with large vowel inventories or with specific suprasegmental features realized on vowels (e.g., tone, pitch-accent, vocal quality features) may present developmental challenges for some individuals.

Clients may have difficulty learning specific vowels or vowel features (e.g., lax or round vowels) or specific sequences (e.g., diphthongs or consonant–vowel sequences) (Stoel-Gammon & Pollock, 2008). Beyond the level of the segment (phoneme), clients may show difficulty with resonance (nasal or oral), degree of oral or pharyngeal constriction, vocal quality, intonation, stress or tone—all of which involve vowels. Where suprasegmentals are contrastive (i.e., change meaning), further compromises in intelligibility may be noted. For example, French has both nasal and oral vowels; hypernasality may reduce the oral–nasal distinction in such a language.

A phonological assessment within any framework is incomplete without an evaluation of the vowel system and the associated suprasegmentals. Because nonlinear phonological frameworks address both autonomous and integrated aspects of vowel, consonant, and suprasegmental representations, these frameworks can provide a basis for interpreting patterns of vowel production as both independent entities and in relation to other aspects of speech production.

If assessment determines that vowels are potential treatment targets, intervention may be noninstrumental (using various cues, prompts, and stimuli) or may make use of instrumental feedback, including auditory, visual, or tactile-proprioceptive means. For clients who have difficulty with suprasegmentals, some types of feedback may be more suitable, such as pitch-tracking machines, nasometry, and spectral analysis. Visual articulatory feedback can help clients learn tongue positions and movements (ultrasound) or tongue-palate contact patterns (electropalatography [EPG]). Researchers have used visual articulatory feedback (ultrasound and/or EPG) in vowel intervention for older children and adolescents with severe hearing loss (Bacsfalvi, Bernhardt, & Gick, 2007; Bernhardt, Gick, Bacsfalvi, & Ashdown, 2003) and those with persistent speech impairment (Adler-Bock, Bernhardt, Gick, & Bacsfalvi, 2007; Modha, Bernhardt, Church, & Bacsfalvi, 2008). This chapter briefly describes an articulatory feedback research program, focusing on the ultrasound aspects (see Chapter 21 for an in-depth discussion of EPG). Populations other than those mentioned may also find benefit from vowel intervention using articulatory feedback (both in terms of impairment and age).

ASSESSMENT METHODS FOR DETERMINING INTERVENTION RELEVANCE

Nonlinear Phonological Theories

Bernhardt et al. (see Chapter 13) and Bernhardt and Stemberger (2000) describe assessments based on nonlinear phonological theories. In speech sample elicitations, all vowel targets of the language need to be systematically elicited more than once. The sample needs to provide opportunities to determine 1) whether there are any consonant–vowel interactions, by providing a variety of consonant contexts for each vowel and vice versa; 2) whether stress affects production, by including words with a variety of lengths and stress patterns; 3) for tone or pitch-accent languages, whether there are any differences in these parameters; and 4) the status of suprasegmentals (pitch, loudness, nasality, other vocal features).

Transcription of vowels can be challenging. Clinicians may find it helpful to do specialized training in vowel identification. In Bacsfalvi et al. (2007), for example, a standard audio reference (Ladefoged, 2004) was used to anchor the transcriptions.

Nonlinear vowel analysis involves both inventory and relational descriptions of the vowel segments (phonemes), features, and prosodic units, and may be quantitative or qualitative or both. If vowels are to be included in the intervention plan, specific targets may be selected that dovetail with consonant and word structure targets. (See the section on Nature of Goals in this chapter.)

Articulatory Visual Feedback

This chapter focuses on ultrasound as a method for providing articulatory visual feedback, but EPG is briefly discussed because it was also used in the studies (for more information on EPG, see Chapter 21).

Ultrasound can display static or dynamic images that approximate the tongue's position and movements. The speaker holds a transducer (know as a wand) beneath his or her chin while ultrasound waves are refracted from the air just above the tongue surface. Midsagittal or coronal (tongue surface from left to right) views of all vowels can be displayed. Relative backness of vowels is best seen in the midsagittal view. In tense-lax pairs in most dialects of English (not, however, Australian English), a midsagittal display of /u/ shows an advanced tongue root and greater "height" compared with the lax cognate /ʊ/ in addition to a small difference in relative backness (see Figure 22.1 and the accompanying DVD). Relative height of different vowels can be seen in coronal views by comparing the vowel productions with a reference mark on the computer display.

Assessment of vowels with ultrasound involves both visual and audio recordings. Ultrasound is used to provide visual documentation of tongue shapes and positions in

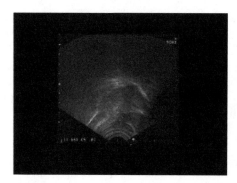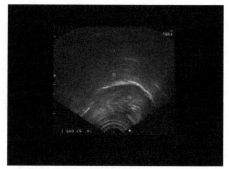

Figure 22.1. Ultrasound displays of a tense-lax high back vowel pair as spoken in Canadian English: /u/ (*left*), and lax vowel /ʊ/ (*right*). The tongue tip is on the right of the midsagittal image.

both the coronal and midsagittal planes for all the vowels of a target language in a variety of contexts (e.g., as isolated phones, in syllables with various consonant contexts, phrases). In addition, simultaneous digital audio recording is used, which may require an external recording system, as described in Bernhardt, Gick, Bacsfalvi, & Adler-Bock, 2005). For clinical purposes, tongue shapes can be described informally by freezing images at the onset, midpoint, and offset of a target and by noting the shape and position of the tongue with respect to an external reference; that is, a predetermined palatal contour obtained through collecting the image of a water swallow (see Bernhardt, Gick, et al., 2005; Stone, 2005). (Various researchers have created quantification methods for ultrasound displays [e.g., Gick, Bernhardt, Bacsfalvi, & Wilson, 2008; Stone, Goldstein & Zhang, 1997; Unser & Stone, 1992; Whalen et al., 2005; Wrench, 2007]; however, at the time of this writing they are not yet easily incorporated into routine speech assessment.)

The client's visually recorded productions can then be compared with the audio recordings of the vowels produced and with stored displays from speakers producing acceptable variants of the targets. The audio recordings also are often analyzed acoustically.

Three features of the assessment require special attention. First, the speech signal must be synchronized exactly with the ultrasound image. Second, the exact location of the transducer beneath the chin plus head movement can affect the display (Whalen et al., 2005; Wrench, 2008a); thus placement is critical. Third, ultrasound machines vary in the degree of resolution possible. The more common, cheaper models record the visual images at a rate of 30 frames per second, whereas the more sophisticated models record at 100 or more frames per second (with no averaging of sampled images). For our clinical studies, the machines could sample at 30 frames per second, which appeared to have been sufficient.

For EPG, the user wears a custom-fit pseudopalate. Electrodes within the pseudopalate record the timing and location of tongue contacts with the hard palate, which appear in real time on a computer screen. EPG shows the degree and location of lateral tongue margin contact in the palatal and velar regions of the oral cavity for the nonlow vowels. Front vowels show greater lateral margin contact (palatal and velar regions) than back vowels (velar contact only). English tense vowels (although not necessarily in Australian English tense vowels) show greater contact further forward than the lax cognates. The WIN-EPG (Wrench, 2008b) allows quantification of the speech patterns, providing a baseline of the degree and location of tongue-palate contact. As with ultrasound, the client's productions can be compared with audio recordings and with displays of speakers with acceptable variants of the target.

THEORETICAL BASIS

Dominant Theoretical Rationale for the Intervention Approach

Nonlinear Phonology

This section highlights vowels in relation to mora theory, onset-rime theory, and feature theories. (See Chapter 13 for a more in-depth discussion of the theories.) It is assumed that impairments in children with protracted phonological development (PPD) are both phonological (representational) and articulatory (implementation of motor programs) and that treatment addresses all levels of production.

A vowel is situated in the phonological hierarchy between the syllable that contains it and the features that compose it. A vowel is not a necessary part of a syllable (because some consonants can be syllabic; e.g., nasals and other sonorants in English) but is generally the *peak* of the syllable. As noted in Chapter 13, there are other levels of representation relevant to vowels: onsets and rimes, and moras. Vowels are the usual nucleus (peak) of the rime, with monophthongs being simple nuclei (having one mora, or weight/timing unit) and long vowels or diphthongs being complex nuclei (having two moras). In languages such as English, which are "weight-sensitive" for stress, complex nuclei attract stress, as may syllables with monophthongs plus codas. The moraic structure of English can be relevant to vowel intervention outcomes, as will be seen later in this chapter.

Description of neighboring (contiguous) vowel sequences varies across accounts and languages; in some languages, contiguous vocalic sequences appear to contain a steady-state vowel and prevocalic (onset) or postvocalic (coda) glide (e.g., /ju/, /waj/ in Kuwaiti Arabic; Bernhardt, Stemberger, Ayyad, Ullrich, & Zhao [in press]; others appear to treat them as consecutive vowels (e.g., /iu/, /waɪ/ in Mandarin; Lee & Zee [2003], although Duanmu [2000] suggested the glides are actually in the onset in at least some dialects). For English, it is generally accepted that the glides /j/ and /w/ are in onset position(except when /j/ occurs with the vowel /u/ after a consonant, as in *cute*, which many researchers assume is a diphthong /ju/); in contrast, diphthongs are treated as consisting of two vowels: /aʊ/, /eɪ/, /oʊ/, /ɔɪ/, /aɪ/, /ju/. Like consonants, vowels can be characterized with three types of features (see Table 22.1): manner (directly under the root node), laryngeal, and place.

The manner features of most vowels are predictable (unmarked defaults) across languages: [−consonantal], [+sonorant], [−nasal], [−lateral], [+continuant]. Some languages (e.g., French) have marked [+nasal] vowels. Laryngeal features are also usually predictable: modal voice is [+voiced], [−spread glottis], [−constricted glottis]. However, some languages have more marked, nondefault laryngeal features: contrastive [+creaky] or [+breathy] voice (e.g., Zapotec; Stemberger, & Lee, 2007) or even allophonically voiceless [−voiced, +spread glottis] vowels (e.g., Japanese). Vowel tones and pitches (although laryngeally controlled) are generally not considered vowel features in current accounts (since Goldsmith, 1979). Instead, they are additional tiers/levels of representation, which can be singly or multiply associated with vowels. Length is also not generally considered a vowel feature but a prosodic aspect of production (moras, as discussed previously).

Table 22.1. Vowels and vowel features for standard adult North American English

Feature	i	ɪ	e*	ɛ	æ	u	ʊ	o*	ɔ	ɨ	ə	ʌ	ɑ/a
+tense	ND		ND		ND	ND		ND				ND	ND
−tense		D		D			D		D	D	D		
Labial						ND	ND	ND	ND				
Coronal	ND	ND	ND	ND	ND								
Dorsal	D	D	D	D	D	D	D	D	D	D	D	D	D
+high	ND	ND				ND	ND			ND			
−high			D	D				D	D		D	D	
−low			D	D				D	D		D	D	
+low					ND								ND

Note: D, default; ND, nondefault (underlying, specified). Where cells are left blank, that feature is considered irrelevant to the particular segment. Note that /ɨ/ is included, although may not be used by some speakers of the standard North American variant. The low back vowel is more fronted in some dialect areas.

*The /e/ and /o/ are the first part of the diphthongs /eɪ/ and /oɪ/ in most North American English dialects.

Regarding place of articulation, older accounts (e.g., Chomsky & Halle, 1968), described vowels in terms of the features [high], [low], [back], and [round]. In current accounts, all vowels continue to be designated as [Dorsal] (with [back], [high] and [low] features), but in addition, the features [Coronal, −anterior], [Labial, +round], and [Guttural] (or [Radical] or [Pharyngeal]) are used. Front vowels are defined as [Coronal], rounded vowels as [Labial], and pharyngealized vowels and /ɑ/ as [Guttural]). The location of the feature [tense] is uncertain; many phonologists consider lax vowels to include pharyngeal constriction and thus place the feature under [Guttural], and refer to it as [−ATR] (nonadvanced tongue root) or [RTR] (retracted tongue root). However, Chomsky and Halle (1968) treated [tense] as more of a manner feature. Accounts also vary on description of features as having one privative (unary) value or two contrasting binary values (+, −). In the Bernhardt and Stemberger framework (1998), the articulator features (Dorsal, Coronal, Labial) are considered unary, and the features that they dominate, binary (e.g., [+high] versus [−high]).

Within the vowel system of a language (or individual), certain vowel features may be defaults (i.e., what is supplied by the system) and other features may need to be learned and represented underlyingly (nondefaults). For adult English, psycholinguistic studies (e.g., Stemberger, 1992b) suggest that /ɛ/ is the default vowel for stressed syllables, with default features thus being [Dorsal, −high, −low], [Coronal, −back], [Labial, −round], [−tense]. The mid-central vowel ə appears to be the default vowel in unstressed syllables: [Dorsal, +back, −high, −low], [Labial, −round], [−tense]. These two vowels tend not to be the earliest learned vowels in English, however (Stoel-Gammon & Pollock, 2008); thus, the default status of features or order of acquisition is not necessarily predictable from the adult phonology. Accounts vary as to which vowels *are* early-appearing; however, taken across studies, children appear to acquire a range of individual vowel features early in development: [Dorsal] for some central or back vowel, [Coronal] for some front vowel, some [+tense] and [−tense] vowels, and some [Labial] vowel(s). Vowel systems in languages with larger vowel inventories (e.g., English) may take longer to acquire than in languages with smaller vowel inventories (Stoel-Gammon & Pollock, 2008); by age 3, however, for English, the defaults appear to be those of adult English (Stemberger, 1993, 2007).

The preceding discussion referenced key phonological features for vowels; that is, features that characterize contrasts between meaningful units. However, vowels have additional characteristics that may provide information to a language learner. Such characteristics include the degree of lip aperture (vertically, as with jaw opening) or the degree of lip spreading (spread /i/ versus neutral /a/). In addition, acoustic distance between vowels may affect learning rate. Languages with smaller vowel inventories and minimal or no overlap in formant plots of different vowels (e.g., Spanish) have very little acoustic ambiguity (Law et al., 2006), whereas languages with larger inventories (e.g., English) have more variability and overlap in formant plots, necessitating the use of additional cues to disambiguate vowels. Vowel systems such as Spanish are thus presumably easier for the learner than the English system, with at least one study confirming that for children with PPD (Goldstein & Pollock, 2000). Because learners may utilize that additional redundant information during acquisition, intervention may also benefit by drawing attention to noncontrastive characteristics.

The use of a common set of vowel and consonant place features, such as that described above, provides a motivation for interaction between the consonant and vowel systems (assimilation or dissimilation, such that a consonant and vowel share a major articulator, [Labial] in [bu] for *do* or [Coronal] in [di] for *bee*). However, consonants and vowels do not always interact with each other. Sometimes, vowels dissimilate or assimilate (vowel harmony) across consonants, or consonants dissimilate or assimilate (consonant harmony) across vowels. Researchers such as Fowler (1980) and Clements and Keyser (1983) have posited that consonant and vowel tiers are separate at some level of representation. Place features, although similar, can be seen as separated into independent C-Place and V-Place units (Bernhardt & Stemberger, 1998). C-Place and V-Place *can* affect each other, but they are not obliged to do so.

Articulatory Visual Feedback

Once a vowel target has been chosen for intervention, the question is what kind of intervention to use. For several decades, articulatory visual feedback has been used as an adjunct in speech habilitation, particularly for clients with compromised auditory perception (e.g., Bernhardt, Loyst, Pichora-Fuller, & Williams, 2000; Dagenais & Critz-Crosby, 1992; Fletcher, McCutcheon, Smith, & Smith, 1989; Keller, 1987; Massaro & Light, 2004; Shawker & Sonies, 1985). Articulatory visual feedback is consistent with the perspective of McGillivray, Proctor-Williams, and McLister (1994) on biofeedback: ". . . a subject can learn to exercise some control over a physiological process if information regarding that process is immediately available" (p. 348). Although the primary processor of the speech signal is the auditory system, not all clients are sufficiently able to use auditory information when trying to match a target. Thus, the inclusion of articulation-focused treatment methods (visual, tactile-kinesthetic) may be necessary to help establish new speech targets. For vowels, visual information about rounding and aperture (vertical or horizontal) can be provided with mirrors while some tactile-kinesthetic information can be provided through palpation of the tissue under the chin. For some clients, these additional cues may be sufficient. However, if they are not, articulatory feedback technologies (particularly ultrasound) can give more detailed information about tongue shape, position, and movements and thus have additional potential to help the learner establish new speech patterns.

Level of Consequences Being Addressed

The assessment and intervention described in this chapter pertains directly to Body Function (impairment) limitations and indirectly to all other levels of the International Classification of Functioning, Disability and Health (ICF; World Health Organization [WHO], 2001). When someone can be understood more readily as a result of effective phonological intervention, social and learning opportunities are enhanced (Bacsfalvi, 2007).

Target Areas of Intervention

The intervention described in this chapter focuses on speech output, but (as noted previously) any phonological intervention that enhances speech production also indirectly has the potential to enhance a client's participation in society.

EMPIRICAL BASIS

Nonlinear Phonological Intervention

Vowel intervention is not the focus of most (English) phonological intervention studies. A small number of studies have addressed vowel intervention specifically, each with only one or a few subjects (e.g., Gibbon, Shockey, & Reid, 1992; Penney, Fee, & Dowdle, 1994; Pollock, 1994; Pollock & Hall, 1991; Robb, Bleile, & Yee, 1999). Some of these studies evaluated vowel changes after consonant intervention, with variable results. For example, Pollock and Hall (1991) followed up three children ages 8–10 years with apparent childhood apraxia of speech and a vowel match of less than 90%. In this study only one child (the most severe) failed to improve notably in vowel production 1 year later. Robb et al. (1999) reported on one child who improved in vowel production after 10 weeks of intervention focusing on voicing of final consonants (and by generalization, on preceding vowel length).

Two nonlinear phonological intervention studies focusing on consonants and word structures (see Chapter 13) supplied vowel data that were examined in post hoc analyses to provide additional information about vowels in phonological intervention. The 16-week studies entailed individual, clinic-based treatment with preschoolers with moderate to severe PPD, with parents actively participating in the 45-minute sessions as well as in home activities. The first study had 19 participants and the second had 15 experimental and 8 control reference participants (all ages 3–5 years).

The objectives of the studies were to enhance speech production and awareness in preschoolers with PPD. Vowels improved significantly pre- to posttreatment in both studies, although treatment targeted only word structure and consonants ($p < .002$ and .001, respectively; t-tests). In the first study (see Chapter 13 and Bernhardt & Stemberger, 2008; Major & Bernhardt, 1998) the group mean vowel match pretreatment (excluding vocalic /ɚ/) was 77.2% (SD, 16.9%, range 24.6%–89.4%) and posttreatment, 90.4% (SD 7.7%, range 72.9%–100%). All vowel types (tense, lax, diphthongs) improved significantly, with the tense vowels /i/, /ɑ/, and /u/ showing a significantly greater gain than lax vowels or diphthongs. The lowest posttreatment match was for diphthongs /aʊ/ and /ɔɪ/ and lax vowel /ɛ/. In the second study, the mean pretreatment vowel match for the experimental group was 75.8% (SD 14.1, range 50.5%–91.9%) and posttreatment was 89.5% (SD 5.4%, range

76.3%–93.8%). All vowels improved, with tense vowels improving most. In comparison, the control reference group for study 2 showed an initial mean vowel match of 85.1% (*SD* 5.6%) and a slight decline to 83.1% (*SD* 7.1%) at the follow-up point. The lack of change for the reference control group suggests that maturation was not the major factor in the experimental participants' vowel improvement. No one factor appeared responsible for the gain in vowel production across the two studies (Bernhardt & Stemberger, 2008). However, as some children acquired codas, their lax vowels also improved. When they had no codas, a bimoraic syllable constraint (common for English) resulted in production of long (tense) vowels instead of lax vowels. After codas were incorporated into the system, lax vowels could be produced to allow a bimoraic syllable. It appears that intervention that does not focus on vowels can have a positive effect on vowel production, particularly if there is some intervention focus on word structure.

Vowels, Ultrasound, and Electropalatography

Articulatory visual feedback technologies, primarily EPG and glossometry, have been used for decades in speech habilitation. Ultrasound has not been used to the same extent, although a preliminary study by Klajman, Huber, Neumann, Wein, and Bockler (1988) evaluated the use of ultrasound in vowel remediation for 18 deaf children ages 8–17 years. They targeted one to four vowels per child in a single session for up to 10 minutes per vowel. Six children produced the target vowels with the ultrasound feedback, 10 showed closer approximations, and two showed no change in this session.

Two vowel intervention studies using both EPG and ultrasound were conducted by the first and third author of this chapter with adolescents with hearing impairment and moderate to severe speech impairment. In the first study, Bernhardt et al. (2003) targeted English high vowels (tense-lax pairs) for four adolescents with moderate to severe hearing impairment (and hearing aids). Before and during the study, the participants were in oral school programs, although they did use pidginized signing with each other and friends. They had both speech-language therapy and assistance from a teacher of the deaf, plus additional practice with teacher aides; speech intervention included primarily traditional speech habilitation methods. Vowels were targeted in three of nine intervention sessions and part of five generalization sessions (which also included liquids and sibilants). Two participants (Pamela, Palmer) received primarily EPG training for vowels, whereas the other two (Peran, Purdy) received primarily ultrasound training for vowels. Two listener studies were performed: In the first study (Bernhardt et al., 2003), two trained listeners completed unblinded phonetic transcription of pre- and posttreatment nonsense-word samples collected in the sentence frame "I'm a _____." In a second study (Bernhardt, Bacsfalvi, Gick, Radanov, & Williams, 2005), 10 untrained listeners rated randomized and blinded pre- and posttreatment vowels (and consonants) of the same nonsense-word samples, as "exactly like," "somewhat like," or "not at all like" the target. According to the transcriptions, all participants except Peran showed significant improvement in production of all vowels (i.e., 15%–47.5% gain in matches, with Peran showing improvement on vocalic /ɚ/). Palmer (who had more EPG training) showed improvement for all treated vowels, whereas Pamela (who also had more EPG training) showed improvement for /i/ and /ʊ/ only. Purdy (who had more ultrasound training) showed improvement for all treatment targets except /i/), whereas Peran (who also had more ultrasound training) showed a gain only for /ʊ/. The untrained listener evaluation agreed that Purdy and Palmer showed the most improved vowels. However, untrained listeners rated

/i/ as most improved across speakers, whereas the trained listeners determined /ʊ/ to be most improved, followed by /i/. Because of this preliminary success and the clients' lack of mastery of the vowels, a second study was undertaken with Peran, Purdy, and Pamela, with both ultrasound and EPG (Bacsfalvi et al., 2007). The tense-lax distinction was again targeted in high vowels, with the lax vowel /ɛ/ being an untreated baseline target. Participants received therapy twice a week for 6 weeks, cycling through the vowel pairs. Ultrasound and EPG were used in most of the sessions and in addition, the SLPs conducted short general lessons on the English vowel system. Real-word monosyllabic stimuli were captured digitally with the EPG and ultrasound equipment, pre- and postintervention in the sentence frame "I'm a _____." The speech samples were transcribed independently by the first and third authors, using the vowel productions on the Ladefoged (2004) CD as an anchoring reference for transcription. In addition, acoustic analyses and EPG contact patterns were evaluated pre- and posttreatment. Across speakers, there were statistically significant gains for /i/ on all three measures (transcription, acoustics, EPG) and for /ʊ/ in terms of EPG contact patterns. Reduction in within-speaker variability was also observed—an important change for speakers with hearing impairment (Ryalls & Larouche, 1992). The untrained /ɛ/ improved less than trained vowels. As in Bernhardt et al. (2003), there were individual differences, with Purdy and Peran showing improvement across all vowels on at least some measures, and Pamela on all vowels but /i/. In order to determine the stability of the observed gains, Bacsfalvi (2007) conducted a follow-up study 3–4 years later, when the participants were 20–23 years old. Speech samples, EPG, and ultrasound data were collected from the participants for selected consonant and vowel targets from the earlier studies. Seven trained listeners unfamiliar with the participants performed blinded ratings of randomized pre- and posttreatment speech samples from the various sampling points. Their ratings indicated that Palmer, Purdy, and Pamela maintained gains for /i/, whereas Peran showed a slight regression. In a qualitative study conducted at the same time, participants and their relatives or associates (Bacsfalvi, 2007) commented that the visual feedback training led not only to improvements in speech production, but also to increased self-confidence and use of oral communication (i.e., enhanced participation in society; the ultimate level of the ICF, 2001).

Summary of Levels of Evidence

In terms of levels of evidence (see Table 22.2), the studies of vowel intervention are best characterized as quasi-experimental, with one study (reported in Bernhardt & Stemberger, 2008) having a nonrandomized control reference group as noted previously.

PRACTICAL REQUIREMENTS

Nature of Sessions

Nonlinear phonological theories do not dictate the number and style of intervention sessions (See Chapter 13 for details on sessions conducted for nonlinear phonological intervention focusing on consonants and word structure.) Considering that vowels may improve spontaneously, they may simply be monitored for spontaneous development. If, however, a child has a very limited segmental inventory at assessment, or shows minimal

Table 22.2. Levels of evidence for studies of treatment efficacy for nonlinear phonology and articulatory visual feedback

Level	Description	References
Ia	Meta-analysis of > 1 randomized controlled trial	—
Ib	Randomized controlled study	—
IIa	Controlled study without randomization	Bernhardt (2007); Bernhardt & Stemberger (2008)
IIb	Quasi-experimental study	Bacsfalvi (2007); Bacsfalvi et al. (2007); Bernhardt, Bacsfalvi, et al. (2005); Bernhardt et al. (2003); Bernhardt & Stemberger (1998, 2000); Major & Bernhardt (1998)
III	Nonexperimental studies, i.e., correlational and case studies	—
IV	Expert committee report, consensus conference, clinical experience of respected authorities	—

Adapted from the Scottish Intercollegiate Guidelines Network (http://www.sign.ac.uk).

progress with vowels after treatment focusing on consonants, vowels may be targeted directly as is discussed further in the Nature of Goals section.

Dosage

Nothing about visual feedback particularly determines the number and style of sessions. The articulatory feedback studies incorporated primarily individual treatment sessions although some group activities were also conducted (e.g., lessons on the English vowel system, generalization practice). Sessions took place over 3–6 weeks, with one to two sessions weekly. Family members or school staff attended occasionally, and helped with between-session activities that did not require visual feedback technology. As in most speech therapy practice, individual client factors, clinician style and knowledge, and service provision restrictions will determine the nature of sessions.

Personnel

Because of the specialist knowledge required for nonlinear phonological intervention and articulatory visual feedback, the speech-language pathologist (SLP) is the primary assessor and program planner. In terms of nonlinear phonological intervention, the SLP may be directly or less directly involved but necessarily oversees any treatment being conducted by others. Because EPG and ultrasound treatment methods are still in early stages of development, the SLP is necessarily the primary interventionist. It can be beneficial to involve caregivers in sessions, to serve as models for the clients, and to receive on-line training to support between-session practice.

KEY COMPONENTS

Nature of Goals

If a client has very few segments or a low vowel match at initial assessment, or shows minimal change in vowels after intervention focusing on consonants and word structure, vowel intervention may be warranted. The following points are a guide to target selection for vowels:

1. *Missing individual vowel features:* Individual vowel features may be absent (e.g., [Labial] or [Coronal] or [+high] or [−tense]) and therefore may be potential targets. For any single feature in English, several vowels might represent that feature target for intervention, e.g., [Labial] implies /oʊ/, /u/, and so forth (see Table 22.1).

   Decisions about which feature(s) to select and which vowels to select for that feature will depend on a number of factors: 1) the client's ability to handle multiple target types simultaneously, 2) needs for consonants and word structures, and 3) the functionality of the particular vowel (frequency, use in common words). Decisions about feature and exemplar vowel selection will also depend on the SLP's perspective concerning goal selection; that is, whether to select complex features and segments (i.e., those for which the client has least phonological knowledge) as suggested in Gierut (1998) or developmentally next targets, as suggested by Rvachew and Nowak (2001), for example. Nonlinear phonological theories do not imply one or the other of these two perspectives exclusively. On the one hand, nonlinear theories suggest that it may be efficacious to target nondefaults (least phonological knowledge) because they *have* to be learned for a language. This requires determining the default status of vowel features for the client. On the other hand, once a set of nondefault features is identified, the most complex (least frequent) or simplest (developmentally next) target may be selected in that set, depending on the client's abilities to handle complexity and on the SLP's perspective.

2. *Restricted vowel feature combinations:* If a particular vowel feature is present in the system, but restricted in terms of its simultaneous combination with other features, then that vowel feature combination is a potential target. For example, if a client matches [−tense] vowels /ɪ/ and /ɛ/ and the [+tense] labial /u/, but does not produce the labials /ʊ/ or /ɔ/, then the feature combination [Labial and −tense] is a potential target. Either one or multiple exemplars of the feature combination target may be chosen for intervention, as described previously for missing individual features. Nonlinear phonology would suggest that a combination of nondefault features might be an optimal target (see Table 22.1). Depending on the status of nondefaults and defaults in the client's system, however, it may not always be possible to use the nondefault–nondefault strategy for targeting feature combinations.

3. *Vowel sequences:* Just as consonant sequences may be intervention targets, so vowel sequences can be intervention targets: 1) diphthongs (contiguous, surface-adjacent sequences and/or 2) across-consonant (heterosyllabic) sequences.

   a. Diphthongs: For many dialects of North American English, there are two simpler same-place vowel sequences (/eɪ/ and /oʊ/) and three more complex sequences that shift in place and height (/aʊ/, /aɪ/, and /ɔɪ/). Similar considerations to those discussed above for individual features pertain to choice of exemplars for intervention. In addition, however, word structures may be relevant. English phonological systems that lack diphthongs may also lack bimoraic syllables composed of lax vowels and codas (Bernhardt, 1990, 1994; Bernhardt & Stemberger, 2008). In this case, it may be efficacious to target diphthongs as one type of word structure target, that is, as a bimoraic syllable (see the case studies).

b. Vowel harmony: Early phonological systems may show evidence of reduplicated syllables, with vowel harmony (e.g., [bib] for /beɪbi/). If so, across-consonant sequences of vowels may be targets: vowels that are present in monosyllables would be potential targets in the new disyllabic sequences.

4. *Prosodic factors:* The accuracy of vowels in stressed versus unstressed syllables is an important factor for English and other stress-timed languages. If analysis shows that stress affects vowel production accuracy, then stress needs to be considered when designing treatment activities (see Description of Activities section later in this chapter). In addition, suprasegmentals associated with vowels (tones, relative pitch, nasality, duration) may need to be targeted, if these are having an impact on intelligibility.

Goal Attack Strategies

Vowels may be integrated as a target into a program with a larger set of goals or be treated as an independent program. A nonlinear phonological framework is compatible with a cyclic approach to goal attack because the overarching objective is to accelerate development of the entire phonological system. (The concept of treatment cycles in the studies described here is based on Hodson & Paden [1991], although both the nonlinear and visual feedback interventions described here differed from that approach both in targets and in cycle length.) The outcomes suggest that the cyclic approach was effective in both the nonlinear and visual feedback studies. Further empirical research is needed to evaluate other goal attack strategies.

Description of Activities

Both awareness/perception and production activities may be assistive in direct vowel intervention. Because vowels are less phonetically precise than consonants, a client may have difficulty producing a match for a target vowel, using traditional noninstrumental auditory, visual, and tactile-kinesthetic cues. Similarly, phonetic placement instructions may not have the desired result. Articulatory visual feedback may enhance the probability of attaining a target if such strategies fail. In the following description of activities, both noninstrumental and instrumental strategies are intertwined (see also the accompanying DVD examples for ultrasound, plus Bacsfalvi et al., 2007; Bernhardt, Gick, et al., 2005; Bernhardt & Stemberger, 2000). The first description concerns phonetic placement, and the second, prosodic manipulation.

One of many possible strategies for phonetic placement of vowels is to hold certain visual cues for vowel characteristics constant while varying others. The example that follows contrasts two vowels. Although certain characteristics are held constant, attention is focused directly on the target feature.

Example. Tense versus lax vowels: e.g., /i/ and /ɪ/ in North American English
Characteristics held constant: Lips spread, minimal jaw opening, tongue body held high, bracing of tongue margins along molars
Cueing for imitation: Tongue retraction (/ɪ/) and advancement (/i/) along with lacing/tensing can be demonstrated by a speaker model.

For noninstrumental facilitation, the client can be encouraged to feel the relative tongue tension and position of the model under the chin right where it joins the neck. Visual supports (diagrams) may also be helpful in showing differences. If ultrasound is used, the clinician or caregiver can model the two vowels so that the difference in relative advancement, height, and root retraction can be seen dynamically and in frozen displays. Specifically, on the midsagittal view, /i/ will be further forward and higher than /ɪ/ and will show an advanced tongue root, whereas on the coronal view, the /i/ will be higher than /ɪ/. If EPG is used, the different amounts of contact (further front, more contact for /i/) can be demonstrated. The client can be asked to identify key parameters on ultrasound or EPG, and/or to draw the different shapes or contact patterns. Silent practice can be helpful as a preliminary to speech imitation. For ultrasound, printouts of the target tongue shapes can be taped to the computer screen so that the model does not need to continuously take the transducer back from the client. For EPG, some displays allow side-by-side client-model comparison. Depending on the client's ability to judge productions aurally, the clinician or other listener can provide more or less verbal feedback about the quality of the production. Once the target has been attained and repeated on successive attempts, the technology can be removed, with the client instructed to try to replicate what was just done, but without technology. Sometimes, closing the eyes and putting the fingers under the chin may facilitate recall of the target patterns. Over time, as in any speech therapy, the targets can be incorporated into words, phrases and conversation, with technology left behind.

Prosodic manipulation can be assistive for diphthongs and stress-timing of vowels. The individual vowels of a diphthong can be highlighted through activities that draw attention to both parts of the sequence in terms of lip and tongue patterns (e.g., spread-round for /aʊ/, low-high for /aɪ/, round-spread for /ɔɪ/) and associated concepts (howling at the moon, *ah-oo*; leaping up for low-high *ah-ee*). Rhythmic attention can be drawn to each of the moras (using drum beats, leaps, claps). For stress-timed languages such as English, some clients need to learn how to vary vowel length across syllables and within phrases to avoid monotonic, monorhythmic production. Rhythmic support (musical) may be helpful. Morse code (alphabets available on the Internet), with its long "DAHS" and short "dits," is illustrative of the changes in speech rhythm and emphasis for short and long vowels and is appealing to older children and adolescents.

Materials and Equipment Required

For assessment, a word list is needed for data collection that includes all vowels of the language within a variety of consonant and word structure contexts. Audio- and (if possible) video-recording equipment is needed as for any phonological evaluation. A set of forms (to track features, as in Table 22.1 or Bernhardt & Stemberger, 2000), and/or a dedicated computer program (e.g., Long, 2006; Masterson & Bernhardt, 2001; Rose & Hedlund, 2008) can assist analysis. There are endless possibilities for therapy materials.

Articulatory technologies discussed in this chapter were two-dimensional dynamic ultrasound and EPG. Ultrasound machines vary in cost from around $10,000 to well over $100,000. One important component is the transducer, which must have sufficient resolution for speech (at least 30 frames per second) yet be able to fit beneath the chin of the client. Stabilization of the transducer (and to a certain extent, the head) is important for doing controlled pre- and postassessments, so that the same part of the vocal tract is being imaged each time. However, in therapy, handheld transducers can be used to reduce fatigue and allow the transducer to pass back and forth from the model to the client (see Gick, Bird, & Wilson, 2005; Stone, 2005). For EPG, the current studies used the Edinburgh WIN-EPG (Wrench, 2008b). However, other EPG machines may be equally effective (in Bernhardt, Bacsfalvi, et al., 2005, for example, a DOS-based Kay Palatometer was used).

ASSESSMENT AND PROGRESS
MONITORING TO SUPPORT DECISION MAKING

Depending on the clinical context, a variety of short probes of trained and untrained words can be administered within the treatment program, either in every session or on some kind of cyclic schedule. Clients themselves, their caregivers, or school or work colleagues and personnel can be encouraged to document progress informally or formally. The SLP can visit the client in nonclinical contexts to monitor conversational use of targets. A major reevaluation may be required after 3 or 4 months of treatment. If a client shows no progress after two treatment cycles, then reevaluation of the program is warranted, with potential development of new targets or intervention strategies. The decision about discharge from intervention depends on the client and restrictions placed on service providers by their employers or those who fund the intervention.

CONSIDERATIONS FOR CHILDREN FROM
CULTURALLY AND LINGUISTICALLY DIVERSE BACKGROUNDS

Before an SLP targets any vowels for treatment, it is very important to find out about vowels of the dialect area and the potential accents of someone who is learning the ambient language. Articulatory displays may be useful for showing differences among dialects and languages in vowel production. For elicitation of a speech sample when no tests exist for a given language, single-word lists can be constructed with a native speaker's assistance, or conversational speech samples can be collected. SLPs are trained in phonetic transcription, and with a native speaker's help in identifying words, they should be able to transcribe the samples and identify overlap and distinctions with the local standard language/dialect. Phonological analysis can be assisted through use of a computer program (e.g., CAPES [Masterson & Bernhardt, 2001], or a freeware program, PHON [Rose & Hedlund, 2008]).

For speakers from diverse linguistic backgrounds, visual feedback may be more facilitative for vowel learning than any words or noninstrumental cues, simply because it is visual, not verbal. The ultrasound machine has been used for speech research in Africa and Mexico, as well as on Native American and First Nations reserves in North America. There is no particular reason not to consider use of visual feedback in speech habilitation for clients outside the European western context.

CASE STUDIES

Nonlinear Phonological Intervention

Bernhardt et al. (see Chapter 13) discuss a 4-year-old child who had a percent vowel match (PVM) of 65% pretreatment. One major target of the word structure intervention module was the syllable as a bimoraic unit, expressed as a diphthong or lax vowel-coda sequence. As the syllable structure improved posttreatment (8% CVC match to 72.7% match), so did the vowels (from 65% to 83.5% PVM).

Another child who had diphthongs as moraic targets was Colin (age 5;0; Bernhardt & Stemberger, 1998, 2000). Pretreatment, his percent consonant match (PCM) was 10.9% and his PVM was 35.3%. Although his initial assessment sample showed matching imitative productions of all English vowels except the rhotic vowel and /ɛ/, he primarily used [a]. One of four treatment targets for the first 6-week treatment block was the syllable as a bimoraic unit, specifically targeted with /aɪ/ and /aʊ/. Attention was drawn to the bimoraic rhythm of the vowel sequence (*ah-ee*, frog leaps, and *ah-oo*, howling at the moon). By the end of the 16-week study, Colin's PVM was 69.2% and his PCM was 34.96%—still low but notably improved.

Articulatory Visual Feedback

For the participants in the articulatory feedback studies, Purdy had the best outcomes overall for vowels and thus more detail is provided about him here. Age 16 at the time of the Bernhardt et al. (2003) study, Purdy had a sloping moderate-to-severe sensorineural hearing loss from birth, with slightly better hearing in one ear. He wore analog-style hearing aids most of the time and used both speech (English, although other family members also spoke Portuguese at home) and signing (learned in high school). His speech was relatively intelligible at the outset of treatment but nonetheless showed a PCM of 37.2% and a PVM of 58.2% (about 10%–20% higher than the PVM of the other three students). Purdy received three 45-minute sessions exclusively with ultrasound for vowels and five sessions that also included consonant targets with both ultrasound and EPG as interventions. The tense-lax high vowel pairs were contrasted during ultrasound training, which included SLP modeling and active imitative practice. At the end of the first study, his vowel scores changed as follows: /u/ from 40% to 70% match, /ʊ/ from 10% to 70% match, /ɪ/ from 40% to 70% match, and /i/ from 60% to 50% match. Treated vowels fared better than untreated vowels (30% overall gain for treated compared with 23% overall gain for untreated vowels). Further intervention was indicated. In a second study (Bacsfalvi et al., 2007), the same vowels were targeted, and with both EPG and ultrasound (independently), during a 6-week period (twice per week). This second intervention period also included general phonetic training about English vowels. All Purdy's vowels again improved, with significant changes in transcriptions, acoustics, and EPG contact patterns across the vowel set. He also showed less variability in tongue-palate contacts posttreatment. In a follow-up study 3 years later, the /i/ was again evaluated, and Purdy's match level had improved to 70% (Bacsfalvi, 2007).

STUDY QUESTIONS

1. What are the key elements in nonlinear descriptions of vowels?

2. What are the possible outcomes of intervention focused on consonants and word structure in terms of vowel development?

3. What types of information does ultrasound provide about vowels?

FUTURE DIRECTIONS

There is much yet to learn about vowels in development and intervention. The authors and others are conducting a cross-linguistic study that will add to our knowledge about vowels in children with typical and protracted phonological development. Currently, one EPG and four ultrasound machines are in clinical settings in British Columbia in addition to the university machines, thus providing more opportunities for clinical intervention and research. Future integration of phonological and phonetic theories and methodologies can only improve the potential outcomes for clients with speech differences.

SUGGESTED READINGS

Bernhardt, B.H., & Stemberger, J.P. (2000). *Nonlinear phonology for clinical application.* Austin, TX: PRO-ED.

Stone, M. (2005, September–November). Ultrasound imaging of the tongue [Special issue]. *Clinical Linguistics and Phonetics, 19*(6–7).

REFERENCES

Adler-Bock, M., Bernhardt, B.M.H., Gick, B., & Bacsfalvi, P. (2007). The use of ultrasound in remediation of /r/ in adolescents. *American Journal of Speech-Language Pathology, 16*(2), 128–139.

Bacsfalvi, P. (2007). *Visual feedback technology with a focus on ultrasound: The effects of speech habilitation for adolescents with sensorineural hearing loss.* Unpublished doctoral dissertation, University of British Columbia.

Bacsfalvi, P., Bernhardt, B.M.H., & Gick, B. (2007). Electropalatography and ultrasound in vowel remediation for adolescents with hearing impairment. *Advances in Speech-Language Pathology, 9*(1), 36–45.

Bernhardt, B.M.H. (1990). *Application of nonlinear phonological theory to intervention with six phonologically disordered children.* Unpublished doctoral dissertation, University of British Columbia.

Bernhardt, B.M.H. (1994). The prosodic tier and phonological disorders. In M. Yavaş, (Ed.), *First and second language acquisition* (pp. 149–172). San Diego: Singular Press.

Bernhardt, B.M.H. (2007, September). *Application of nonlinear phonological theories to intervention: Outcomes studies in British Columbia.* Paper presented at the City University, London.

Bernhardt, B.M.H., Bacsfalvi, P., Gick, B., Radanov, B., & Williams, R. (2005). Exploring electropalatography and ultrasound in speech habilitation. *Journal of the Association of Speech-Language Pathology and Audiology, 29*, 169–182.

Bernhardt, B.M.H., Gick, B., Bacsfalvi, P., & Adler-Bock, M. (2005). Ultrasound in speech therapy with adolescents and adults. *Clinical Linguistics and Phonetics, 19*, 605–617.

Bernhardt, B.M.H., Gick, B., Bacsfalvi, P., & Ashdown, J. (2003). Speech habilitation of hard of hearing adolescents using electropalatography and ultrasound as evaluated by trained listeners. *Clinical Linguistics and Phonetics, 17*(3), 199–216.

Bernhardt, B.M.H., Loyst, D., Pichora-Fuller, K., & Williams, R. (2000). Speech production outcomes before and after palatometry for a child with a cochlear implant. *Journal of the Association of Rehabilitative Audiology, 23*, 11–37.

Bernhardt, B.M.H., & Stemberger, J.P. (1998). *Handbook of phonological development: From a nonlinear constraints-based perspective.* San Diego: Academic Press.

Bernhardt, B.M.H., & Stemberger, J.P. (2000). *Workbook in nonlinear phonology for clinical application.* Austin, TX: PRO-ED.

Bernhardt, B.M.H., & Stemberger, J.P. (2008, June). *Vowel development after nonlinear phonological intervention focusing on consonants.* Paper presented at the International Clinical Phonetics and Linguistics Association Conference, Istanbul.

Bernhardt, B.M.H., Stemberger, J.P., Ayyad, H., Ullrich, A., & Zhao, J. (in press). Nonlinear phonology: Clinical application adaptations for Arabic, German and Mandarin. In J. Guendouzi, P. Loncke, & M.J. Williams (Eds.), *The handbook of psycholinguistic and cognitive processes: Perspectives in communication disorders.* London: Routledge.

Chomsky, N., & Halle, M. (1968). *The sound pattern of English.* Cambridge, MA: The MIT Press.

Clements, G.N., & Hume, E.V. (1995). Internal organization of speech sounds. In J. Goldsmith (Ed.), *The handbook of phonological theory* (pp. 245–306). Cambridge, England: Blackwell.

Clements, G.N., & Keyser, S.J. (1983). *A generative theory of the syllable.* Cambridge, MA: The MIT Press.

Dagenais, P., & Critz-Crosby, P. (1992). Comparing tongue positioning by normal-hearing and hearing impaired children during vowel production. *Journal of Speech and Hearing Research, 37,* 216–226.

Dell, G.S. (1986). A spreading-activation theory of retrieval in sentence production. *Psychological Review, 93,* 283–321.

Duanmu, S. (2000). *The phonology of standard Chinese.* New York: Oxford University Press.

Fletcher, S.G., McCutcheon, M., Smith, S., & Smith, W. (1989). Glossometric measurements in vowel production and modification. *Clinical Linguistics and Phonetics, 3*(4), 359–375.

Fowler, C.A. (1980). Coarticulation and theories of extrinsic timing. *Journal of Phonetics, 8,* 113–133.

Gibbon, F., Shockey, L., & Reid, J. (1992). Description and treatment of abnormal vowels in a phonologically disordered child. *Child Language Teaching and Therapy, 8,* 30–59.

Gick, B., Bernhardt, B.M.H., Bacsfalvi, P., & Wilson, I. (2008). Ultrasound imaging applications in second language acquisition. In J. Hanson Edwards & M. Zampini (Eds.), *Phonology and second language acquisition* (pp. 309–322). Amsterdam: John Benjamins.

Gick, B., Bird, S., & Wilson, I. (2005). Techniques for field application of lingual ultrasound imaging. *Clinical Linguistics and Phonetics, 19,* 503–514.

Gierut, J. (1998). Treatment efficacy: Functional phonological disorders in children. *Journal of Speech, Language, and Hearing Research, 41,* S85–S100.

Goldsmith, J. (1979). *Autosegmental phonology* (Doctoral dissertation, MIT, 1976). New York: Garland Press.

Goldstein, B., & Pollock, K. (2000). Vowel errors in Spanish-speaking children with phonological disorders: A retrospective, comparative study. *Clinical Linguistics and Phonetics, 14,* 217–234.

Hodson, B., & Paden, E. (1991). *Targeting intelligible speech: A phonological approach to remediation* (2nd ed.). Austin, TX: PRO-ED.

Keller, E. (1987). Ultrasound measurement of tongue dorsum movements in articulatory speech impairments. In J.H. Ryalls (Ed.), *Phonetic approaches in aphasia related disorders* (pp. 93–112). San Diego: College-Hill Press.

Klajman, S., Huber, W., Neumann, H., Wein, B., & Bockler, R. (1988). Ultrasonographische Unterstützung der Artikulationsanbahnumg bei gehörlosen Kindern [Ultrasound support for articulation training of hearing-impaired children]. *Sprache-Stimme-Gehör, 12,* 117–120.

Ladefoged, P. (2004). *Vowels and consonants* (2nd ed.). Oxford, England: Blackwell.

Law, F.F., Gilichinskaya, Y.D., Ito, K., Hisagi, M., Berkowitz, S., Sperbeck, M.N., et al. (2006, November). *Temporal and spectral variability of vowels within and across languages with small vowel inventories in different phonetic and prosodic contexts: Russian, Japanese, and Spanish.* Poster presented at the Acoustical Society of America, Honolulu, Hawaii.

Lee, W.-S., & Zee, E. (2003). Standard Chinese (Beijing). *Journal of the International Phonetic Association, 33,* 109–112.

Long, S. (2006). *Computerized profiling.* Retrieved August 1, 2009, from http://www.computerizedprofiling.org

Major, E., & Bernhardt, B. (1998). Metaphonological skills of children with phonological disorders before and after phonological and metaphonological intervention. *International Journal of Language and Communication Disorders, 33,* 413–444.

Massaro, D.W., & Light, J. (2004). Using visible speech to train perception and production of speech for individuals with hearing loss. *Journal of Speech, Language, and Hearing Research, 47*(2), 304–320.

Masterson, J., & Bernhardt, B.M.H. (2001). *Computerized articulation and phonology evaluation system (CAPES).* San Antonio, TX: Pearson PsychCorp.

McGillivray, R., Proctor-Williams, K., & McLister, B. (1994). Simple biofeedback device to reduce excessive vocal intensity. *Medical and Biological Engineering and Computing, 32,* 348–350.

Modha, G., Bernhardt, B.M.H., Church, R., & Bacsfalvi, P. (2008). Case study using ultrasound to treat /r/. *International Journal of Language and Communication Disorders, 43*(3), 323–329.

Nickels, L.A. (2001). Producing spoken words. In B. Rapp (Ed.), *A handbook of cognitive neuropsychology* (pp. 291–320). Philadelphia: Psychology Press.

Penney, G., Fee, E.J., & Dowdle, C. (1994). Vowel assessment and remediation: A case study. *Child Language Teaching and Therapy, 10,* 47–66.

Pollock, K.E. (1994). Assessment and remediation of vowel misarticulations. *Clinics in Communication Disorders, 4,* 23–37.

Pollock, K.E., & Hall, P. (1991). An analysis of the vowel misarticulations of five children with developmental apraxia of speech. *Clinical Linguistics and Phonetics, 5,* 207–224.

Robb, M., Bleile, K., & Yee, S. (1999). A phonetic analysis of vowel errors during the course of treatment. *Clinical Linguistics and Phonetics, 13,* 309–321.

Rose, Y., & Hedlund, G. (2008). *PHON.* Retrieved November 7, 2008, from http://childes.psy.cmu.edu/phon/

Rvachew, S., & Nowak, M. (2001). The effect of target-selection strategy on phonological learning. *Journal of Speech, Language, and Hearing Research, 44,* 610–623.

Ryalls, J., & Larouche, A. (1992). Acoustic integrity of speech production in moderately and severely hearing-impaired children. *Journal of Speech and Hearing Research, 35,* 88–92.

Shawker, T.H., & Sonies, B.C. (1985). Ultrasound biofeedback for speech training: Instrumentation and preliminary results. *Investigative Radiology, 20,* 90–93.

Stemberger, J.P. (1992a). A connectionist view of child phonology: Phonological processing without phonological processes. In C.A. Ferguson, L. Menn, & C. Stoel-Gammon (Eds.), *Phonological development: Models, research, implications* (pp. 165–189). Timonium, MD: York Press.

Stemberger, J.P. (1992b). Vocalic underspecification in English language production. *Language, 68,* 492–524.

Stemberger, J.P. (1993). Vowel dominance in overregularization. *Journal of Child Language, 20,* 503–521.

Stemberger, J.P. (2007). Children's overtensing errors: Phonological and lexical effects on syntax. *Journal of Memory and Language, 57,* 49–64.

Stemberger, J.P., & Lee, F. (2007). San Lucas Quiavini Zapotec speech acquisition. In S. McLeod (Ed.), *The international guide to speech acquisition* (pp. 608–616). Clifton Park, NJ: Thomson Delmar Learning.

Stoel-Gammon, C., & Pollock, K. (2008). Vowel development and disorders. In M. Ball, M. Perkins, N. Mueller, & S. Howard (Eds.), *Handbook of clinical linguistics* (pp. 525–548). Malden, MA: Blackwell Publishing.

Stone, M.L. (2005). A guide to analysing tongue motion from ultrasound images. *Clinical Linguistics and Phonetics, 19,* 455–501.

Stone, M., Goldstein, M.H. Jr., & Zhang, Y. (1997). Principal component analysis of cross sections of tongue shapes in vowel production. *Speech Communication, 22,* 173–184.

Unser, M., & Stone, M. (1992). Automatic detection of the tongue surface in sequences of ultrasound images. *The Journal of The Acoustical Society of America, 91*(5), 3001–3007.

Whalen, D.H., Iskarous, K., Tiede, M.K., Ostry, D.J., Lehnert-leHouillier, H., Vatiokis-Bateson, E., et al. (2005). The Haskins Optically Corrected Ultrasound System (HOCUS). *Journal of Speech, Language, and Hearing Research, 48,* 543–553.

World Health Organization. (2001). *International classification of functioning, disability and health.* Geneva: Author.

Wrench, A.A. (2007, September). *Articulate Assistant Advanced: Ultrasound Module.* Paper presented at Ultrafest IV, Department of Linguistics, New York University, New York.

Wrench, A.A. (2008a). *Ultrasound stabilisation headset users manual: Revision 1.13.* Edinburgh, Scotland: Articulate Instruments.

Wrench, A.A. (2008b). *WIN-EPG.* Edinburgh, Scotland: Articulate Instruments.

Developmental Dysarthria Interventions

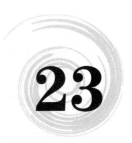

23

Megan M. Hodge

ABSTRACT

This chapter defines developmental dysarthria (DD), describes its potential impact on children with the disorder, and discusses intervention considerations. The neurological impairment underlying DD delays acquisition of speech milestones and reduces control of the muscles used to speak. These factors constrain development of differentiated, precise, dynamic actions of the oral articulators and their coordination with the respiratory-phonatory system to produce clear, efficient speech patterns. Published evidence regarding the effectiveness of interventions designed to increase control of speech muscles and thereby increase intelligibility in children with DD is limited to a few case studies and expert opinion. One case example illustrates use of a bite block to facilitate differentiated tongue movements and establish phonetic placement for lingua-alveolar sounds in a child with athetoid cerebral palsy (CP).

INTRODUCTION

Children with dysarthria have impairments that interfere with signals sent from their brains to the muscle groups (diaphragm, rib cage, abdomen, vocal folds, pharynx, soft palate, tongue, lips, and jaw) that produce the rapid, precise, and coordinated movements of speech. These impairments result in weakness, slowness, and tone abnormalities in the affected muscles and reduce the accuracy and coordination of their actions. Impairments can occur at one or more locations in the nervous system involved in the sensori-motor processes that control speech movements (Hodge & Wellman, 1999). Dysarthria subtypes (spastic, dyskinetic, ataxic, flaccid, mixed) are labeled by the associated site of neural impairment (lesion), observed abnormal neuromuscular signs, and perceived deviant speech characteristics (Duffy, 2005). To date, classification of subtypes of childhood dysarthria follows the conventions used with dysarthria acquired in adulthood (Webb & Adler, 2008). Although some authors question this practice, given the increased complexity and decreased predictability associated with damage to the developing nervous system (Joffe & Reilly, 2004), a standardized system specific to identifying and diagnosing subtypes of DD has not been validated.

DD results from conditions that occur before speech is acquired; that is, the child learns to speak with a mechanism that has impaired neuromuscular function. Examples include CP (when speech muscles are affected), congenital conditions such as Moebius syndrome affecting the cranial nerves (Defeo & Shaefer, 1983), and early onset muscular dystrophy (Nelson & Hodge, 2000). The adverse effect of these conditions on a child's rate of speech acquisition and eventual speech outcome ranges from mild (slight articulatory imprecision and impairments in vocal quality and a somewhat slower speaking rate than expected for age) to profound (can vocalize but does not have functional speech). Children neither "grow out of" nor are "cured" of these neuromuscular impairments. However, the signs of the disorder and the ways in which they are manifested in speech change as the child grows and develops. DD is contrasted with dysarthrias resulting from brain injuries sustained after the child has learned to speak. For example, Morgan and Vogel (2008) included children who acquired dysarthria at 3 years or older in their systematic review of interventions for childhood dysarthria with acquired brain injuries.

Control over the affected muscle groups is also impaired for nonspeech actions in children with DD. Consequently, difficulties drinking, chewing, swallowing, and controlling saliva; abnormal resting postures of the lips, jaw, and tongue; and associated effects on dentition may need to be addressed in the child's therapy program (Hodge & Wellman, 1999; Love, 2000; Workinger, 2005). Problems with these functions may also reduce opportunities for communication if they negatively affect the child's appeal as a conversational partner.

In addition, the neurological impairment that caused DD may affect other nervous system functions. The child also is at risk for impairments in gross and fine motor function, sensory and perceptual processing and language and other cognitive functions. Therefore, although the dysarthric aspect of their speech reflects impaired neuromuscular control, these children may also have constraints on their ability to perceive, process, and remember the sound patterns of their language. Therefore, focus on the impairment affecting the speech muscles must not exclude opportunities and interventions for developing the child's phonological awareness, oral and written language, and social communication skills.

Delayed speech and reduced intelligibility typical of children with speech sound disorders (SSD), including DD, limit their communication opportunities and confidence and success in making their spoken messages understood, with negative consequences for social and language development (Lewis, 2007). This is compounded if a child has motor impairments in other muscle groups that limit communication through gestures or writing, as is observed in some types of CP. In addition, it might be expected that delayed and disordered speech may negatively affect the development of literacy in children with DD. Sandberg (2006) found that children with severe dysarthria have more difficulties acquiring reading and spelling than would be expected from their intellectual level or phonological ability. Based on findings from a longitudinal study of children at ages 6, 9, and 12 years with CP and severe speech production impairments, she concluded that phonological ability does not appear to have the same predictive power for these children as for children with typical speech development. Sandberg identified the need for further studies to elucidate the role of working memory and literacy acquisition strategies for children with severe motor speech disorders and CP. She observed that such studies may also increase our knowledge of the importance of articulatory abilities in early literacy acquisition.

Impact on Speech Acquisition

Like other children in their early years, children with DD are learning to understand and use the sound system (phonology) of their language yet are constrained in their ability to develop control over the movements of muscle groups used in speech. One effect of this is to delay the child's use of prespeech vocalizations and onset of speech behaviors. This limits early sensorimotor experiences with sound making that are needed to establish the perception-action linkages providing a critical foundation for spoken language (Kent & Voperian, 2006). Therefore, an important goal at this stage is to provide multiple, daily opportunities designed to help the child to develop a functional communication system using a combination of eye gaze, facial expressions, gestures, signs, pictures, and vocalizations/early words and to engage in vocal play. According to neuronal group selection theory (Hadders-Algra, 2000), infants are born prewired via multiple groups of neurons for primary functional movements. As development proceeds, some groups of neurons are chosen over others to control a behavior, based on experience and the sensory information produced by the behavior itself. Information acquired from many and variable experiences changes the strength of the synaptic connections within and between neuronal groups, resulting in a variable second repertoire. Frequent experience with trial and error enhances the process of selection. Changes in the connections in the second repertoire allow for situation-specific selection of neuron groups for target skilled behaviors. Many opportunities for active practice enhance processes of selection and therefore better adapted motor behaviors for specific motor functions. Children with DD probably need considerably more repetition of trial-and-error experiences to prime the neural circuitry for prespeech and early speech behaviors than children with typical neuromotor function.

In addition to creating many opportunities for children with DD to gain extensive early sensorimotor experience vocalizing and babbling, it is important to implement a systematic, longer-term plan to develop physiological support for developing spoken language. When speech behaviors emerge, abnormal function of affected muscle groups reduces the spatial and temporal precision of the child's movements to produce and link segments together over time to generate language-specific word shapes and prosodic patterns. That is, the child is learning the phonological system of the language with constraints on his or her speech motor control system. This includes the sensorimotor memory patterns and associations corresponding with the phonetic features of place, manner, and voicing that contrast sounds with one another in the language. Consequently, in addition to being delayed, speech sounds distorted and is often judged to be abnormal in quality and rate. The child's speech is difficult to understand and typically requires extra time and effort to produce, compared with the speech of children without dysarthria.

Depending on the extent of impairment causing the dysarthria, one or more of the speech processes of respiration, phonation, resonance, articulation, and prosody may be affected. Speech characteristics associated with DD can include short breath groups (few words per breath), abnormal voice quality (e.g., harsh, breathy), poor control over pitch and loudness, difficulty using contrastive stress (i.e., all words are perceived as having primary stress), slow speaking rate, hypernasal resonance, nasal air emission, and imprecise articulation affecting vowels and consonants. These children have particular difficulty producing sounds that require more precise control of tongue postures and movements to make vowel and consonant manner and place distinctions (e.g., tense versus lax vowels, monophthongs versus diphthongs, glides versus liquids, stops versus fricatives versus affricates, alveolar versus palatal versus velar place) and the rapid, coordinated movements required for voicing distinctions and consonant clusters (Love, 2000).

Intervention

The focus of intervention for children with DD is twofold. It includes 1) education, support, and specific skills training for family and caregivers to facilitate the child's communication development; and 2) treatment given directly to the child to maximize communication skills (Hodge & Wellman, 1999; Pennington, Goldbart, & Marshall, 2003). In their systematic review of speech-language therapy to improve the communication skills of children with CP, Pennington et al. identified seven child-focused intervention studies that used single case experimental designs. These interventions involved training to increase 1) production of preintentional communication behaviors, 2) requests for objects or actions, 3) responses to others' communication, 4) use of expressive language structures, and 5) relative ease of use of symbol type (iconic communication symbols or Bliss symbols). The authors concluded that despite the studies' methodological flaws, the interventions employed appeared to be associated with increases in the desired behaviors for the individual children studied. Pennington et al. found no experimental studies that focused directly on increasing a child's ability to control and coordinate actions of the respiratory, laryngeal, velopharyngeal, and oral articulatory muscles to speak. Similarly, Morgan and Vogel (2008) concluded that there were too few studies to draw any conclusions about the efficacy of treatment targeting dysarthric speech in children and teenagers with acquired brain injury.

Pennington, Miller, and Robson (2008) observed that textbooks on dysarthria have advocated therapy to reduce motor speech impairments and associated intelligibility limitations in DD. Therapy typically targets all affected speech subsystems: respiration, phonation (loudness and pitch control), nasal resonance, and/or articulation (Love, 2000). Pennington et al. (2008) commented that this approach is based on the assumption that reduction in the child's speech intelligibility, efficiency, and quality reflects all affected speech subsystems, not just oral articulation. For example, Hodge and Wellman (1999) recommended that speech-specific treatment approaches for children with DD follow principles based on the source-filter theory of speech production (Kent & Read, 2002).

Source-filter theory describes speech production as a two-part process. The first part involves creating sound (source). One source is "voice," produced by generating a sustained pressurized air stream from the lungs to push against adducted vocal folds to set them into vibration and keep them vibrating. A second source is "noise," produced by stopping the pressurized air stream at a location in the vocal tract and releasing it suddenly (plosive) or by forcing the air stream through a narrow constriction (fricative), or in combination (affricate). In the second part, the voice and noise sound sources are shaped into the consonant and vowels of the language by the resonant properties of the vocal tract (filter) created by articulation. During speech, actions of the soft palate, pharynx, tongue root, tongue body, tongue tip, jaws (with teeth), and lips change the size, shape, and number of resonating cavities from the vocal folds to the lips and nose.

Treatment that follows principles of source-filter theory focuses on each part. For example, a goal that has a source focus (respiratory and phonatory subsystems) would be to have the child generate a clear, loud voice and sustain this for a few seconds. The objective is to make phonation consistent and loud enough so that the acoustic information it contains is heard easily. Love (2000) suggested that practicing maximum phonation tasks might be effective to accomplish this objective. Other members of pediatric rehabilitation teams may also be involved to optimize the child's seating and positioning for speech breathing. At a later stage, conditioning of the respiratory and phonatory muscle groups may be needed to develop stamina for maintaining loud, clear sound production in connected speech. An example is the application of intensive voice treatment to children with CP (Fox, 2003).

A goal that has a filter focus (velopharyngeal and oral articulatory subsystems) would be to build the child's speech sound repertoire and ability to make sound contrasts

and word shape information as clear and distinct as possible so that listeners can identify these accurately and reliably. This would involve treatment approaches to increase
control of the lips, tongue, and jaw and the coordination of their movements with the actions of the velopharynx, respiratory, and laryngeal muscles. These treatment approaches
fall into the following three categories (adapted from Love, 2000):

- The first includes approaches that are designed to realize a child's potential to produce vowels, consonants, and word shapes that are within the child's physiological
  capability but are delayed in developing. Examples are minimal pairs and nonlinear
  phonological approaches (see Chapters 2 and 13, respectively) to 1) establish sounds
  that are produced correctly in one word position but omitted or misarticulated in others or that are stimulable and 2) eliminate error patterns such as stopping fricatives
  and deleting final consonants.

- The second includes approaches to develop the child's capability to control and coordinate the articulators to make phonemes for which the child is not stimulable. Examples are approaches that use 1) phonetic placement techniques (Secord, Boyce,
  Donohue, Fox, & Shine, 2007) or 2) instrumental feedback such as electropalatography
  (see Chapter 21) to teach the child to control the muscles of the lips and tongue so
  that their movements are better differentiated and more accurate (articulation skill
  training). If a muscle group lacks adequate strength to make a target articulatory
  gesture, exercises to increase strength may be needed prior to therapy to increase
  control of the muscle group for articulation (strength *and* skill training).

- The third includes approaches to develop effective compensatory movements to produce sounds that are recognizable although distorted due to persisting physiological
  limitations. Examples include 1) use of lingua-dental contacts for bilabial sounds by
  children with lip paralysis (Nelson & Hodge, 2000) and 2) production of derhoticized
  /ɹ/ and dentalized lingua-alveolar sibilants. More global compensatory strategies include increasing intelligibility by slowing speaking rate to facilitate coordination
  across speech muscle groups, enhancing other prosodic features such as contrastive
  word stress, and increasing overall speaking effort.

Hodge and Wellman (1999) provided an extensive review of examples of treatment
approaches addressing each of the speech subsystems that might be appropriate for children with DD. As noted by Pennington et al. (2008), although speech-focused intervention for children with DD has been described in textbooks and review articles, no systematic review that evaluates the evidence base for such intervention exists to guide speech
and language clinicians in their treatment decision making.

Hodge and Wellman (1999) observed that a combination of treatment approaches
that address multiple levels of a child's communication disorder are typically used. These
change with the child's and family's needs and as the child's use of effective communication strategies increases. These approaches can be organized according to focus: general
considerations, increasing communicative effectiveness, and developing the child's speech
ability and phonological knowledge (see Table 23.1). The long-term goals of intervention
are to 1) help children with dysarthria accomplish their communication goals as independently as possible across a range of partners and settings, and 2) maximize their potential to use speech as part of their communication system.

Table 23.1.   Guidelines for treatment: Children with developmental dysarthria

General Considerations

- Educate family members, other caregivers, and peers about the nature of the child's speech disorder and ways to communicate effectively with the child.
- Support the child's development of social communication skills and a functional communication system as soon as possible, augmenting speech with developmentally appropriate alternative communication modes.
- Provide receptive and expressive language treatment (both spoken and written) as appropriate and integrate this with speech training activities when possible.
- Address related issues as necessary, including management of any related issues such as attention, lack of motivation, control of drooling, swallowing, oral-dental status, and sensory (auditory-visual) status.

Communicative Effectiveness

- Teach effective use of interaction enhancement strategies.
- Model and promote use of effective conversational repair strategies and speech production self-monitoring skills
- Teach effective cognitive strategies so that the child can use word choice and syntactic structure to maximize listeners' comprehension.
- Promote maintenance of speech production skills that have been established and self-monitoring of communication skills; implement strategies to increase the child's self-confidence and self-esteem in initiating and participating in communication interactions.

Speech Ability and Phonological Knowledge

- Develop the child's phonological and phonetic repertoire with attention to level of development as well as specific profile of muscle group impairment. Phonological and phonetic learning are likely to be delayed by the neurological damage that caused the dysarthria.
- Sound patterns that develop later in typically developing children (e.g., liquids, affricates, consonant clusters) require more demanding control and coordination than earlier developing sounds (e.g., stops, glides) and are also ones that are more difficult for children with speech motor control problems of the oral articulators.
- Voicing contrasts are very difficult for some of these children and may not be a reasonable production expectation. Some children may be able to use effective compensations such as increasing the length of aspiration noise in word initial stops to produce recognizable voiceless stops. Regardless, the child should have opportunities for active listening to voiced-voiceless cognates (e.g., *bat* versus *pat*) to develop phoneme awareness of this contrast.
- Elaborate on word and syllable shape repertoire as soon as the child has some sounds to work with—build on what the child can do.
- Provide opportunities to practice multisyllable productions from the onset of treatment.
- Maintain integrity of phonetic contrasts in multiword utterances and extend utterance lengths. Specific phonological and articulatory training that includes lots of practice opportunities is needed to stabilize sound contrast features, especially in connected utterances where the physiological demands are greater.
- Improve vocal loudness and quality.
- Increase speech intelligibility and naturalness through prosodic training: phrasing, contrastive stress.
- Identify and promote use of effective speech production compensatory behaviors (e.g., slowed rate).
- Build phonological awareness and preliteracy/literacy skills. Later, use regular oral reading practice to maintain speech skills.

TREATMENTS TO INCREASE SPEECH ABILITY BY INCREASING PHYSIOLOGICAL SUPPORT

Because children with dysarthria have impaired physiological support for speech, it has been assumed that they can benefit from treatment approaches designed to increase spatiotemporal control and coordination of speech muscle groups (respiratory, laryngeal, velopharyngeal, lips, tongue, and jaw). The objective of these approaches is to increase movement control for speech production. Clarke (2003) reviewed the theoretical foundations of several neuromuscular treatments and outlined steps to critically evaluate therapies targeting neuromuscular impairments. There is consensus that selection, implementation, and evaluation of these techniques should be made relative to their effect on increasing speech intelligibility and quality. However, little published research supports or refutes the effectiveness of these approaches in changing neuromuscular function or increasing clarity of speech in children with DD. Two approaches that have been evaluated in the past 10 years (intensive voice treatment and phonetic placement followed by surface electromyography) are described in the following sections. A third approach (use of a bite block followed by phonemic practice) has been suggested as a technique to improve articulation in children with motor speech disorders (Crary, 1993) but has not been evaluated specifically with children with dysarthria. The rationale, requirements, and key components of this third approach and a case example are the focus of the final section.

Intensive Voice Treatment

Fox (2003) described the application of intensive voice treatment based on administering Lee Silverman Voice Treatment to children with spastic dysarthria and CP. The treatment was based on principles of motor learning theory (e.g., intensive treatment, high effort exercises, repeated practice trials, and sensory augmentation/sensory awareness training). Treatment consisted of sixteen 1-hour sessions (4 times per week for 4 weeks). In each treatment session the children performed multiple trials of maximum phonation tasks that focused on using a loud voice and then practicing its use in functional phrases. Four children received treatment and one did not. Acoustic measures of voice function, auditory-perceptual analysis of speech samples, and perceptual ratings by parents of participants were obtained during pretreatment and posttreatment and at 6-week follow-up recording sessions. Fox reported that the four treated participants demonstrated a marked change in performance on one or more of the acoustic measures. In addition, there were strong listener preferences for most perceptual characteristics rated in the treated speech samples (posttreatment or follow-up sessions) over pretreatment samples. Parents of these four participants reported improved perceptions on two or more voice, speech, or communication characteristics following treatment, and all had an overall favorable impression of their child's treatment outcome and the treatment approach used. Conversely, no changes were observed in the one participant who did not receive treatment. Fox concluded that her findings suggest that intensive speech treatment changed the output of the speech motor system of the four children who received treatment in a manner that listeners preferred over baseline speech samples. She also observed that her findings highlighted the importance of motor learning principles in treatment focused on changing speech behavior in children with DD and spastic CP.

Phonetic Placement and Surface Electromyography

Marchant, McAuliffe, and Huckabee (2008) described a comparative study of treatment modalities (phonetic placement therapy and surface electromyographic–facilitated biofeedback relaxation therapy) for improving articulation in a 13-year-old girl with severe spastic dysarthria secondary to CP. The authors described phonetic placement therapy (PPT) as an approach to improving articulation that provides direct instruction on where and how to place muscles to produce a speech sound correctly. The authors described surface electromyographic (sEMG) feedback as an approach that attempts to regulate and reduce orofacial spasticity via relaxation, allowing muscles improved range of movement and ultimately, improved articulation. The study design included three baseline sessions, 2 weeks of PPT (45-minutes sessions, five times per week), a posttreatment assessment, 2 weeks with no treatment, 2 weeks of sEMG treatment (45-minutes sessions, five times per week), and a posttreatment assessment.

The consonants /t/, /s/, /f/, /θ/, and /ʃ/ were selected as targets for the PPT intervention. In each session, all sounds were targeted, and one sound was selected as the main focus to receive 30 minutes of treatment. The target sound was identified by an auditory-visual model and corresponding letter(s). A mirror was used to assist with articulatory placement. The child engaged in speech drills with motivating games, and specific feedback was provided after each production attempt. Speech production tasks started with sounds in isolation and progressed to sounds in words when an 80% accuracy rate for a specific sound was attained in isolated production.

A portable sEMG device was used in the biofeedback treatment sessions. The submental and orbicularis oris muscles were targeted for treatment to determine if a reduction in muscle tone resulted in improved articulation. Surface electrodes were placed under the chin (submental muscle) and over the upper lip on the right and left superior orbicularis oris muscles. The first 20 minutes of each treatment session focused on reducing the amplitude of submental EMG activity during rest and nonspeech postures. Software animation provided visual feedback to facilitate motor learning and achievement of the target levels. A target threshold level, chosen by the clinician to ensure success and maintain motivation, was shown on the computer screen during the task. When the child achieved a consistent response below threshold, the target threshold was lowered. The process was repeated multiple times for lingual gestures (tongue protrusion, elevation, depression, and lateralization) and lip pursing and retraction. The second 20 minutes of the session followed the same procedure but focused on bilateral superior orbicularis oris muscles.

Several measures taken in the baseline session and at the end of each of the treatment phases were compared. Results of a single-word intelligibility measure indicated a significant increase in intelligibility post-PPT training (increase of 9%) that was maintained 4 weeks later, following sEMG treatment. Intelligibility at the sentence or paragraph level did not change across the study. No changes to any perceptual articulatory parameters (imprecise consonants, vowel distortions, prolonged phonemes) were observed, and the child's self-perception of her speech impairment did not differ across treatment phases. Acoustic measures of the first (F1) and second (F2) format frequencies for the vowels /ɪ/, /æ/, and /u/ revealed a significant increase in F2 for /æ/ post-PPT training and a significant reduction for /u/ post-sEMG training. No significant differences were found in resting EMG activity across the study, but a reduction in variability of the recording levels during rest was observed post-sEMG treatment. The authors interpreted these results as suggesting that sEMG facilitated greater consistency in lingual and labial functioning that could potentially facilitate improved motor control and articulation with additional training. Significant reductions in EMG activity levels in the nonspeech postures were observed in both submental and orbicularis oris muscles post-sEMG treatment, but this did not result in perceptible changes in the child's speech. The authors concluded that phonetic placement training was effective in improving the child's single-word articulation and suggested that the severity of the child's dysarthria was a factor contributing to the minimal changes observed with treatment.

Discussion

The interventions described by Fox (2003) and Marchant et al. (2008) followed motor learning principles (Strand, 1995). Examples of procedures consistent with these principles are focusing on specific treatment goals, providing frequent treatment sessions per week for a period of at least 2 weeks, maintaining a high rate of responding to provide multiple opportunities for repeated practice within a session on tasks that are closely related to the desired speech behaviors (specificity of training), using sensory-augmented feedback as treatment progresses, and increasing speed to automatize the correct response while maintaining accuracy. The interventions described by Fox and Marchant et al. demonstrated a measurable change in at least one aspect of relevant speech behavior following intervention. Given the chronic nature of the impairment underlying DD, speech-language therapy could be offered on a more or less continuous basis from identification until later adulthood (Love, 2000). However, these two studies suggest that when the goal is to change speech motor skills of children with dysarthria, intensive, short-term treatments focused on achieving specific goals and based on motor learning principles may be more appropriate than less intensive treatment over longer periods. These studies also support the conclusions of Bower, McLellan, Arney, and Campbell (1996) that selecting specific goals for treatment, rather than general aims, and providing intensive, rather than nonintensive, therapy accelerate the acquisition of motor skills in children with CP.

USE OF A BITE BLOCK AND PHONEMIC PRACTICE TO IMPROVE LINGUA-ALVEOLAR CONSONANT PRODUCTION

Target Populations and Assessments for Determining Intervention Relevance

Children with delayed or disordered speech motor control, including those with dysarthria, have difficulty moving the tongue independently of the jaw for lingual sounds, and many children with moderate-to-severe speech disorders have difficulty moving the tip and body of the tongue as separate units for speech (see Gibbon, 1999; Gibbon & Wood, 2003). Love stated "it has been commonly observed that tongue movements, particularly tongue-tip elevation, are difficult for the neurologically impaired child and often require extensive training for improvement" (2000, p. 181). A bite block can be used to give the tongue the experience of moving independently of the jaw and to improve a child's ability to control the tongue to achieve differentiated, precise placements for articulation of lingual-alveolar (e.g., /t, d, n, l/) and velar (/k, g, ŋ/) consonants.

Bite blocks are small blocks that may be fashioned from hard plastic or dental impression material. These blocks are made to fit between the upper and lower teeth, either between the central incisors (Dworkin, 1978) or the molars on one side of the mouth (Netsell, 1985). The child bites (without clenching) with sufficient force to keep the block in place. This holds the jaw stable so that the lips and tongue can experience moving without accompanying movements of the jaw. Workinger (2005) described bite block use with a 7-year-old child with DD and CP to increase lip movement for bilabials. The bite block was used to stabilize the jaw while practicing bilabial consonants in isolation, consonant-vowel syllables, and syllable strings. When the child could achieve accurate bilabials with the block, the same activities were accomplished without it. After therapy progressed to production of bilabials in all positions in words and blends, contexts of increasing difficulty were introduced.

Dworkin (1978) described the use of a bite block to improve lingua-alveolar articulation in four 6- to 8-year-old children with age-level school achievement. These children 1) had normal oral structures, 2) used exaggerated mandibular excursions that appeared to interfere with differential placement of the tongue during lingua-alveolar consonant production, and 3) were assumed to have weakness and incoordination of the tongue musculature. The children were not identified as being dysarthric but were described as having lingua-alveolar valving difficulties that resulted in distortion of lingua-alveolar consonants at all levels of speech. Dworkin's procedure provides the basis for the following description of bite block use in treatment.

No standardized assessments are available to determine the appropriateness of using a bite block. Several factors to consider include the following:

1.   The child's safety, comfort, and willingness to cooperate in holding the bite block in place in the mouth—A bite block is not appropriate for children who are resistant to having it in their mouth or who are at risk of choking or swallowing it.

2.   The child's stimulability for lingua-alveolar consonants (e.g., /t, d, n, l/) that are contrastive with velar /k, g, ŋ/ consonants—If the child is readily stimulable for these sounds without the block, it is likely unnecessary. However, a bite block may be useful if the child 1) has difficulty controlling the tongue to make clear, contrastive productions of alveolar and velar consonants, especially if these movements are accompanied by excessive movements of the mandible; and 2) shows signs of lingual weakness and reduced coordination of tongue movements on an oral mechanism exam. If tongue weakness or excessive movement of the mandible is observed during the oral mechanism exam, and the child is cooperative, the examiner can determine if the child can elevate the tongue tip against the alveolar ridge and maintain this position, depress the tongue tip, and move the tongue from side to side with a block in place. If tongue movement is linked to the jaw, the child will have difficulty making these movements when the jaw is constrained by the block.

Crary (1993) described how bite blocks might be used diagnostically on speech diadochokinetic tasks. He suggested that if performance on these tasks deteriorates with the bite block in place, the child may be using excessive jaw movement to accomplish the task. Conversely, if performance improves with the bite block in place, the block may increase jaw stability and decrease interfering jaw movements.

3.   The child's rate of progress in achieving accurate, well-differentiated alveolar and velar sounds, especially when both alveolar and velar sounds are in the same syllable (e.g., *duck* and *coat*) when the clinician uses other approaches such as PPT or sound approximation techniques (Secord et al., 2007)—If progress is slow and production is inconsistent, especially at higher levels of phonetic complexity, a bite block may be effective to develop better differentiated tongue movements and placements for these sounds, resulting in more precise, consistent consonant production.

Theoretical Basis

Dworkin's (1978) rationale for using a bite block was that it would 1) inhibit excessive mandibular activity and 2) develop independent lingual movements that would improve lingua-alveolar consonant production. The few publications addressing therapeutic use of bite blocks have not specified a theoretical basis for their use. Crary (1993) described a bite block as an example of a disruptor that alters the habitual manner of speech production and challenges the talker to use a different pattern of articulatory movement to accomplish a given speaking task. From this perspective, a bite block might be considered a type of constraint-induced movement therapy (CIMT). Therefore, the theoretical basis of CIMT, as used in physical and occupational therapy, and conceptualizations of neuroplasticity (how the brain changes structurally as a result of new learning and experience; Kleim & Jones, 2008) appear relevant.

CIMT (Taub, Uswatte, & Pidikiti, 1999) helps individuals with central nervous system damage regain use of affected limbs. The focus of CIMT lies with forcing the individual to use the affected limb by restraining the unaffected one. The affected limb is then used intensively for several hours a day for at least 2 weeks. As a result of repetitive exercises with the affected limb, the individual's brain grows new neural pathways. The developers of CIMT argue that after a neurological insult such as a stroke, individuals stop using the affected limb because they are discouraged by the difficulty. As a result, a process called "learned nonuse" sets in, furthering the deterioration. It is this process that CIMT seeks to reverse. Similarly, a child who may have difficulty developing and refining control over the lips or tongue continues using jaw movements to compensate for these difficulties. This prevents the child from gaining experience using more varied and sophisticated lip and tongue movements. By constraining the jaw, a bite block forces the child's brain to reorganize to learn to use the lips and tongue in a new way. As a result of the child engaging in appropriate, repetitive exercises using the lips and tongue, the brain grows new neural pathways corresponding to new movement capabilities of the lips and tongue that are independent of jaw movement. These movement capabilities reflect the movement experiences gained in the exercises.

Using the terminology of the International Classification of Functioning, Disability and Health (World Health Organization, 2001), use of a bite block to increase the variety and control of tongue movements for speech targets the level of impairment. The functional limitation on a child's activity of speaking is reduced when tasks are practiced to establish these new movement capabilities in a child's articulatory patterns for production of well-differentiated, precise lingual consonants at various levels of phonetic complexity.

Bite block use focuses on changing a child's speech output by increasing movement capabilities of the tongue to improve articulatory precision and efficiency. A secondary effect of improved articulatory precision may be improved speech discrimination abilities for lingual consonants.

Empirical Basis

Only one published study (Dworkin, 1978) was identified that described the use of a bite block in children with SSD. As noted previously, the purpose of this exploratory study was to determine the feasibility of a bite block to inhibit hypermandibular activity and thereby improve lingua-alveolar valving and lingua-alveolar phoneme production in four school-age children for whom other approaches were unsuccessful. The study describes a technique that the author developed for articulation intervention in children with persisting distortion of lingua-alveolar sounds, which corresponds to level 5 on the continuum of intervention evidence described by Ingram (1998). The children were selected for the study based on their persistent speech errors on lingua-alveolar sounds, despite 3 months of intensive articulation therapy that focused on auditory discrimination and phonetic training. Treatment was similar for each of the four cases and had three parts:

1.   One 90-minute orientation session to help the child understand the concepts of 1) lingua-alveolar valving and hypermandibular movement that interfered with lingua-alveolar valving, in relation to the child's speech and 2) normal production of lingua-alveolar phonemes /t, d, n, l, s, z/. Audio and visual (mirror) feedback was provided to help the child identify articulatory errors, lingua-alveolar valving difficulties, and excessive mandibular movements.

2.   Four 45-minute sessions of bite block training. The bite block was constructed of a piece of round inflexible plastic (length and diameter of 0.5 inch) with a small hole drilled in the middle to accommodate a handle. The 5-inch-long plastic handle was designed to allow the clinician to control the bite block and prevent accidental swallowing. In each training session, the bite block was positioned in the child's mouth upright between the upper and lower central incisors. The child was instructed to move the tongue tip from the floor of the oral cavity to the alveolar ridge and then down again. Trials were repeated over four 3-minute sets with each set consisting of 40 repetitions (total of 160 repetitions). Children were positioned in front of a mirror to view their tongue movements. Measures of lingua-alveolar valving abilities were based on 160 trials using a six-category system (unable to raise tongue-tip to alveolar ridge, raised mandible, lateral shifts of mandible, lowered mandible, exaggerated mandibular movements, and correct valving). Pretraining, the number of trials classified as "correct valving" ranged from 0 to 21 for the four children. After the fourth session of bite block training, the number of trials classified as correct valving ranged from 122 to 154 across the children.

3.   A phonemic practice program in which the children received individual treatment for three 1-hour sessions a week for 40–48 sessions. The six phonemes (/t, d, n, l, s, z/) were trained individually. Training began with single CV syllables (e.g., /tʌ/). Once this level was mastered, training progressed to single CVC syllables (e.g., /taːp/). Then bi- and tri-syllable words and blends with the target phoneme in the initial position were introduced, followed by similar procedures for medial and final positions. Once phoneme production was acceptable in words, conversational speech was elicited, audio recorded, and narrowly transcribed. If no errors occurred for the target phoneme, training began on the next phoneme. For phonemes in which errors occurred in conversation, training stages were reviewed. The decision to terminate treatment was based on narrow phonetic transcription of each participant's performance during conversational speech and on the subtests of the Goldman-Fristoe Test of Articulation Sounds in Words and Sounds in Sentences (Goldman & Fristoe, 1969). The criterion for dismissal was no detectable errors during lingua-alveolar phoneme production. Evidence for the treatment efficacy of using a bite block to increase lingua-alveolar phoneme accuracy in children with reduced control of tongue movements includes nonexperimental studies and clinical experience of respected authorities (see Table 23.2).

Practical Requirements

Dworkin (1978) described placement of the block between the upper and lower central incisors, whereas Netsell (1985) described procedures for creating a bite block to position between the upper and lower molars on one side of the mouth. The placement to one side between the molars blocks jaw action on both sides and has the advantage that the tongue can be viewed without obstruction when the block is in place.

Prior to training, the clinician needs to provide the child and caregiver with a short, clear explanation of the bite block and a demonstration of how it works. Consent for use

Table 23.2. Levels of evidence for studies of treatment efficacy using a bite block to increase lingua-alveolar phoneme accuracy in children with reduced control of tongue movements

Level	Description	References
Ia	Meta-analysis of > 1 randomized controlled trial	—
Ib	Randomized controlled study	—
IIa	Controlled study without randomization	—
IIb	Quasi-experimental study	—
III	Nonexperimental studies, i.e., correlational and case studies	Dworkin (1978)
IV	Expert committee report, consensus conference, clinical experience of respected authorities	Crary (1993); Netsell (1985); Workinger (2005)

Adapted from the Scottish Intercollegiate Guidelines Network (http://www.sign.ac.uk).

should be obtained from the caregiver and child. The child needs to understand the bite block's placement and cooperate in holding it in place while attempting tongue movement. A ready-made block can be used or a custom one can be constructed. Procedures for using a bite block are described in the video demonstration included in the accompanying DVD. In some cases, it may be more effective to work collaboratively with the child's dentist to construct a block. Once the block has been constructed, standard procedures for handling, cleaning, and storing it need to be followed, as for any object that is put into a child's mouth.

Nature of Sessions

The bite block training described by Dworkin (1978) was delivered on an individual basis at school in 45-minute sessions. Although frequency of sessions per week was not specified, it is assumed that the four sessions occurred within 1–2 weeks. According to motor learning principles, if new motor skills are to be acquired, treatment must occur on an intensive schedule (Strand, 1995). Following bite block training, three 1-hour phoneme practice programs were delivered on an individual basis weekly.

Personnel

A clinician must gain experience constructing and using bite blocks before recommending or using them in treatment. It is recommended that training be delivered by the clinician because intervention using the bite block is expected to be intensive and short term and requires a relationship of cooperation and trust with the child. The author of this chapter has trained highly motivated parents to conduct home practice sessions for bite block training between therapy sessions. This included educating the parent about the careful use of the bite block and modeling how to instruct the child to make the desired tongue movements. Then the parent observed the clinician conducting six sets of the exercises with at least 10 repetitions each (with short breaks between sets). Following this, the parent practiced positioning the block and instructing the child for three sets of 10 repetitions of the exercise, under the clinician's supervision. Parent and child questions were discussed and they were provided with a score card to record two practice sessions each day, each with three sets of 10 repetitions. At the beginning of the next therapy session, the clinician reviewed the score card with the parent and child, addressed any questions or concerns, and then observed while the parent and child demonstrated what they did at home for 10 repetitions. The clinician provided any needed corrective feedback. This format continued for the remaining bite block treatment, with the clinician providing and modeling treatment for six sets of 10 repetitions each, while the parent observed, then having the parent and child engage in supervised practice for another three sets of 10 repetitions each. The parent and child were then asked to follow the practice schedule described previously. The same strategy could be used to train a therapy assistant to provide practice sessions between clinician-directed sessions. Once bite block training is completed, phonemic training could follow the same format, with the clinician providing treatment and either a trained caregiver or therapy assistant providing practice between treatment sessions.

Key Components

Goals and Activities

The goal of bite block intervention is to have the child attempt to move the tongue tip to touch up behind the upper front teeth, with the bite block in place. The child is encouraged to develop skill in moving the tongue to this placement and holding it there for a few seconds.

When the child can perform the movement task easily and consistently, the clinician moves to phoneme training for lingua-alveolar consonants (e.g., /d, n, l, t/). Using a sequential approach initially, the clinician starts with a phoneme for which the child is stimulable. With the bite block in place, the child imitates the clinician's model of the target phoneme in a CV syllable (e.g., /nʌ/; containing central vowel initially) for multiple repetitions over several sets. When the child can make the sound easily and consistently, multiple productions of the CV (3–5) in a series (e.g., /nʌnʌnʌ/) are required. Then without the bite block in place, the child practices the same task until achieving consistency.

If the child had a pattern of backing lingua-alveolar phonemes, activities should include activities to facilitate differentiation of lingua-alveolar versus velar cognates. First, with the bite block in place, have the child alternate place of production in CV syllables within CV syllable chains (e.g., /dʌkʌdʌkʌdʌkʌ/). Repeat this until the child can maintain accuracy across syllables within a trial over several sets of 10 trials each. This may be difficult at first, but with practice, especially in repeated syllable chains, hearing the feedback of the correct target sounds, and with encouragement from the clinician, the child can learn to use the tongue to make these sounds distinct. Once the child can do this easily and consistently, repeat the same training task without the bite block in place. When the child can maintain accurate production over several sets of 10 repetitions without the bite block, introduce minimal pair therapy targeting the place contrast. Minimal pair activities (e.g., *dough:go; tea:key; thin:thing*) provide opportunities for the child to engage in active problem solving to practice the newly established articulatory placement.

At this point, typical articulation therapy techniques can be used to stabilize production of the target sound in various positions in words, consonant blends, and word combinations. Once the first alveolar phoneme is mastered, another would be targeted following the same steps but with the expectation that successive phonemes will take less time to train.

Materials and Equipment Required

The following materials are needed for bite block training:

- Bite block with strong handle attached (e.g., plastic fishing line tied securely around the block) that the clinician can hang on to for safety reasons

- Tissues (the bite block may stimulate increased saliva production)

- A mirror

- Score cards to record completion of each set of 10 repetitions

- Stickers or other motivators to recognize/reward completion of the exercises

- Disposable gloves, liquid dish soap, hot water, paper towels, and a clean storage container for handling, cleaning, and storing bite block between uses

- Picture/text stimuli for lingua-alveolar target phonemes in sounds, syllables, words, and minimal pairs with velar sounds (/d-g; t-k; n-ŋ/)

Several procedures for constructing a bite block are described in the video demonstration included in the DVD. A guideline for size is a block that keeps the jaws apart at a distance that is about one-third of the child's maximal jaw excursion. Measure the maximal jaw excursion and determine one-third of this. Then notch a tongue depressor to this width. Insert this between the upper and lower central incisors and use this position of the jaw to determine the approximate height of the bite block. When using dental impression materials, a fixative is combined with dental putty. The mixture is shaped into an oblong block. A knife is used to make a groove around the block to attach fishing line. A long end of the fishing line is left to hang out of the mouth to hang on to for safety. The soft block of material is placed in the mouth, posterior to the lower canine incisor. With the tongue depressor in place at midline between the upper and lower incisors, the child bites down until maximum closure is obtained against the tongue depressor. The molars will press into the soft bite block. The block is then removed from the mouth, allowed to harden, and then excess material is trimmed away with a knife. This technique provides a bite block that has the impression of the individual's teeth, which helps it to stay in place. When ready to use, the bite block is put in the mouth in the same place it was made (the dental imprint fits the child's teeth).

Mouth protectors from a sporting goods store can provide an alternative to dental impression material. These are firm, plastic dental inserts that soften when placed in hot water. A piece of the guard is cut away, softened in boiling water for about 45 seconds, removed with rubber gloves, fashioned into a bite block, and secured with fishing line in much the same way as described for the dental compound.

Assessment and Progress Monitoring to Support Decision Making

The child's performance raising the tongue to the alveolar ridge and holding the position for at least 2–3 seconds with the bite block in place can be recorded for each repetition within a set. After 2 weeks (four treatment sessions with intervening daily practice sessions), determine if the child can perform the task without the bite block in place and without raising or other extraneous movements of the mandible. If the child can do this at least 80% (24 of 30) of trials (over three sets with 10 repetitions each), move to phoneme training. If not, continue with one or two more sessions of bite block training. In phoneme training, continue to record the child's performance on the target phoneme for each repetition of a task within a set at the relevant level of production (syllable, word, phrase). For each phoneme, start training with the bite block in place. When the child can accomplish the target activity (lingua-alveolar CV in isolation, in strings of 3–5 CV syllables, or alternating lingua-alveolar CV syllables) with the bite block in place and maintain 80% accuracy over three sets of 10 trials, remove the bite block and repeat the activity. When the child can perform the production task without extraneous movement of the tongue at or greater than 80% correct over three sets of 10 trials without the bite block, move to the word level of production (initial position, then final position, then in multisyllable words, all positions). Use the same criterion to determine when to move to the next level. When the criterion is met for multiple syllable words, move to the next phoneme to train. It is expected that with each new phoneme, the number of trials to meet the criterion will decrease. If the child shows a pattern of velar fronting, implement a minimal pair approach to contrast lingua-alveolar and velar place of articulation, starting at the syllable level with bite block training. Terminate treatment when the child demonstrates at least 80% accurate articulation of lingua-alveolar sounds in connected speech (12-minute sample).

Considerations for Children from Culturally and Linguistically Diverse Backgrounds

The use of a bite block described in this chapter focuses on increasing movement capabilities of the tongue for lingua-alveolar consonants, which are found in most languages. The intervention is appropriate for children who have poor control over tongue movements in speech. Children with these characteristics are found in all cultures. However, clinicians who are considering use of a bite block need to be sensitive to child and parent concerns about putting a foreign object in the child's mouth and how it will be handled and cleaned.

CASE STUDY

C had a diagnosis of severe athetoid CP. He was essentially nonverbal until age 6 years, at which time he demonstrated a strong desire to speak. Augmentative communication systems had been introduced in his preschool years, but he showed little interest in using these for functional communication at home or school. He was a very social child and used eye gaze, facial expressions, body language, and differentiated vocalizations to communicate, supported by the use of yes-no questions from his communication partners. He attended his community school in a classroom at grade level for his age but followed an adapted program with an aide. At age 7 years, he started receiving outpatient speech services at the local children's rehabilitation hospital. Testing by a reading consultant indicated that C's reading comprehension and recognition were significantly below age level (preprimer). His independent mobility was very limited, and he was learning how to use a power wheelchair. He was able to sit functionally with support from shoulder straps on his wheelchair.

Assessment Results

All of C's speech subsystems were affected. He could generate and sustain phonation for only 2–4 syllables per breath and had difficulty regulating vocal pitch and loudness. At rest, C's mouth posture was typically open and he drooled excessively. He had an anterior open bite and used a tongue-thrust swallowing pattern. He demonstrated sufficient strength to close his jaws on command but appeared to lack the control or sensory feedback to keep them occluded at rest. He demonstrated the ability to round, retract, purse, and close his lips, but lip movements during speech were limited in range. C was unable to elevate the anterior part of his tongue to make contact with the alveolar ridge. His tongue movements during speech were accompanied by excessive mandibular movements.

Analysis of a 50-word spontaneous speech sample in conversation with his clinician (78 single-word imitation task that sampled vowel, consonant, and syllable contrasts of English words) and the Test of Children's Speech Intelligibility Measures (Hodge & Wellman, 1999; a 20-sentence [80 words] imitation task) indicated that C had the following consonants in his repertoire: /p, b, f, v, m, w, θ, j, k, g, ŋ/. Inconsistent omission of these sounds was evident, especially in medial and final word positions and as phonetic complexity and utterance length increased. Consonant sounds not in C's repertoire included /t, d, n, tʃ, dʒ/ produced as velar stops or pharyngeal fricatives; liquids /ɹ/ and /l/ produced as glides (/w/ for /ɹ/; /j/ for /l/), and fricatives /s, z, ʃ/ produced as the interdental fricative /θ/. He was stimulable for all vowels and diphthongs but reduced his vowel space in connected speech. Inconsistent voicing errors were noted on obstruent consonants, and intermittent mild hypernasality was apparent during connected speech. Intelligibility was further reduced by inconsistent syllable omission in multisyllabic words and utterances, more frequently at the end of words and breath groups. He did not produce any consonant blends and used a restricted number of syllables shapes (V, CV, CVC, VC).

C's parents indicated that they could understand about 60% of his communicative attempts and estimated that his teacher understood between 25% and 50% of these, depending on context. They stated C would get upset, give up, repeat, or use a gesture when not understood and judged him to be successful about 20% of the time at fixing a message so that it could be understood (depending on the listener's age and experience). They estimated that people unfamiliar with C understood between 10% and 20% of his speech in context.

Intervention

Treatment was scheduled twice weekly for 45-minute sessions over 12 weeks. Overall goals of treatment were to increase intelligibility and communicative effectiveness. Strategies included increasing the consistency of use of the consonants in his phonetic repertoire (all word positions in 1–3 syllable utterances), establishing movement capability for lingua-alveolar place of articulation and production of identifiable lingua-alveolar phonemes /l, n, t, d/ in the initial position in key words in nonimitative speech production tasks, developing effective use of a letter board to repair communication breakdowns that occurred during treatment sessions via modeling and cuing (linked with reading and spelling levels at school), and decreasing drooling by increasing use of a closed-lips resting posture using established procedures of oromyofunctional therapy.

Activities were incorporated in each session to accomplish the various objectives. The amount of time spent on each activity varied across sessions, depending on C's attention and progress. Only procedures specific to lingua-alveolar training are described here due to space limitations. Bite block training modified from Dworkin (1978) was used to develop C's ability to control his tongue tip to lift and hold it up behind the alveolar ridge for increasingly longer durations. A bite block was made from a sports mouth guard because C could not tolerate having dental impression material in his mouth while it hardened. In the first session, the clinician demonstrated and explained how she planned to use the bite block to help C learn to move the front of his tongue. Then she attempted to position the block on the left side between his upper and lower molars, which C tolerated after several trials. In the second session, the time he maintained the block in position increased from 3 to 10 seconds. Once he could maintain the block in place comfortably for at least 10 seconds, he was coached to attempt to raise his tongue tip to touch behind the alveolar ridge. This was initially very difficult, but with practice and much encouragement, C developed control to hold it in position for at least 2 seconds. Once he could do this over three sets of 10 trials, the time to maintain tongue elevation per trial was increased. When C could hold the position for at least 10 seconds, he repeated this task with the bite block removed. At the end of six treatment sessions, he was able to sustain an elevated tongue tip position for at least 5 seconds per trial over a set of 10 trials without the bite block.

At this point, training lingua-alveolar phonemes was introduced, starting with /l/. Auditory and visual models of single /lV/ syllables using low vowels were provided. Once he could imitate these single syllables accurately (80% over three sets of 10 trials), these production tasks were introduced: initial /lV/ syllables in chains of 3–5 syllables and then CVC words containing /l/ in initial position with central or low vowels and labial or velar consonants (sounds he could produce correctly) in final position (*log, lamb, laugh*). Printed cards were used to elicit the syllable chains, and cards with pictures and text were used to elicit the CVC words. Game-like activities were used to sustain C's motivation and cooperation. Pictures of appropriate tongue positions for alveolar versus velar place of articulation were discussed and displayed as reminders during treatment. C was encouraged to find the letter *L* on his alphabet board at the beginning of each session to remind him of the goal and what the tongue needed to do. A mirror provided C with visual feedback. Initially C produced each target following the clinician's spoken model. When he reached 80% accuracy over three sets of 10 utterances, a model was provided only as needed to maintain a high success rate. After C was successful in producing /l/ without models in the three key words, three more initial /l/ CVC words were introduced. The same procedures were repeated for /d/, /n/, and then /t/. With each new phoneme, training time decreased.

During training, C overgeneralized and started to front velar consonants. To help him establish differentiated alveolar versus velar placements, production of a series of minimal pair CV syllables (e.g., *duh* versus *guh; tuh* versus *kuh*) in alternating order was practiced, first with the bite block, then with it removed. This was followed by practicing minimal pair CVC words (with contrastive lingua-alveolar and velar sounds in word initial position) presented in random order, without the bite block, to consolidate accurate, differentiated production of these sounds in the appropriate locations for the target words. When C was 80% accurate in nonimitated productions of words containing initial lingua-alveolar and alveolar sounds, phrase-level production was introduced in functional phrases (e.g., "I like to ____"). Words with initial /l/ clusters and high-use words containing alveolar sounds (e.g., *gorilla*, *Titanic*, *eleven*) were introduced in the final three sessions. A card game was created to play at home using cards with a picture of a favorite topic (Titanic) on the back of each card. Two cards were made for eight rhyming words, targeting initial alveolar phonemes, one initial /l/ cluster, and a velar foil (*bow, blow, dough, toe, no, go, so, low*). The game was played following a script. The active player asked, "Do you have ____?" If the answer was "yes," the other player gave the requested card. If the answer was "no," the other player stated this, then said, "Go fish."

The intervention was designed to build on C's existing capabilities and to focus on functional goals (speech-specific skills). Negative practice was avoided by choosing training words that contained sounds in C's repertoire, with the exception of the target phoneme.

Outcome

At the end of the 12 weeks, C was stimulable for accurate production of /l, n, t/, and /d/ in all positions in words. On re-administration of the 78-word imitation task, C's production of these four lingua-alveolar phonemes was judged to be 80% accurate when scored by a clinician not familiar with his speech and blind to the treatment goals. Correct instances of these sounds occurred in his spontaneous speech on the key words trained during the sessions and in his card game. C spontaneously changed his error pattern of substituting velar stops for affricates to a more typical pattern of substituting lingua-alveolar stops for affricates (e.g., *tin* rather than *kin* for *chin*). He increased his frequency of letter board use and acquired sight reading vocabulary for the training targets. With reminders, he was able to maintain a lips-together resting posture and reduced his drooling substantially during the sessions.

STUDY QUESTIONS

1. What distinguishes children with DD from children with other SSD?

2. Will increasing the strength of a muscle result in skilled articulatory movements of the same muscle for specific speech sounds without speech skill–specific training? Justify your response. (See Clarke, 2003 for an additional study resource.)

3. Describe the characteristics of children for whom bite block training may be appropriate and contrast these with characteristics of children for whom it is not appropriate.

4. Summarize the nature of the evidence base for the efficacy of treatment to increase the speech intelligibility of children with dysarthria, and identify one implication of this for clinical practice.

FUTURE DIRECTIONS

No controlled studies were identified that determined if a short period of intensive bite block training can increase a child's ability to develop correct articulation of lingua-alveolar sounds and maintain these in connected speech. Given the heterogeneity of children in the target population, modest, well-controlled single-subject, small-group, or combined single-subject–group studies appear to be feasible first steps to determine its efficacy (see Morgan & Vogel, 2008; Wambaugh, 2006). If positive effects are found, these need to be replicated. An additional consideration is that bite blocks are relatively inexpensive compared with electropalatography and ultrasound, which are also designed to increase a child's ability to produce differentiated tongue movements and increase articulatory accuracy. If bite block training is found to be efficacious, studies comparing bite block training with these other approaches are a potential area for future research to determine, if for at least some children, bite block training followed by phoneme-specific articulation training results in comparable outcomes.

From a broader perspective, no systematic review of the effectiveness of treatments to increase speech ability in children with DD has been published to date (Pennington et al., 2008). According to these authors,

> Speech and language therapists therefore have little evidence on which to base treatment decisions. Some may provide intervention as there is no evidence to show that the treatment does not work or causes harm. Others may withhold treatment because there is no evidence showing its effectiveness. (p. 2)

Pennington et al. (2008) proposed a protocol for a systematic review of studies of speech therapy for children with onset of dysarthria prior to 3 years of age. The objectives are to determine if direct treatment to improve these children's speech is more effective than no intervention and if specific types of intervention are more effective than others at improving their speech intelligibility. The authors list measures of primary and secondary treatment outcomes for their review that are relevant for future research. The former include those that address aspects of speech production (respiration, phonation, nasality, articulation, sound pressure level, and intelligibility), further classified according to the International Classification of Functioning, Disability and Health (World Health Organization, 2001), and the latter address satisfaction of the child and family with treatment; noncompliance with treatment; direct costs of treatment; and adverse events, including time missed from education. The results of this proposed review will provide a foundation and direction for future research in speech therapy for children with DD.

One of the barriers to treatment research in childhood dysarthria is the heterogeneity of the population. It is expected that the systematic review of speech treatment studies for children with dysarthria onset up to 3 years of age, proposed by Pennington et al. (2008), will reflect findings similar to those reported by Morgan and Vogel (2008), who reviewed treatment studies targeting speech in children who acquired dysarthria after 3 years of age. This review demonstrated a critical lack of studies addressing treatment efficacy and suggested that contributing factors included the lack of understanding of characteristics or natural history of dysarthria in children, lack of a diagnostic classification system, and heterogeneity in the etiology and resulting dysarthria types in the target population. The possible co-occurring perceptual, cognitive, and linguistic processing impairments in children with dysarthria present an additional barrier for group studies. Immediate challenges for future treatment research in DD are to 1) provide adequate descriptions of participants that can be replicated across investigators and 2) design and conduct studies that have adequate experimental controls for internal and external validity to ensure that the treatment was responsible for observed changes.

SUGGESTED READINGS

Clarke, H.M. (2003). Neuromuscular treatments for speech and swallowing: A tutorial. *American Journal of Speech-Language Pathology, 12*, 400–415.

Hodge, M.M., & Wellman, L. (1999). Management of children with dysarthria. In A. Caruso & E. Strand (Eds.), *Clinical management of motor speech disorders in children* (pp. 209–280). New York: Thieme.

Kleim, J.A., & Jones, T.A. (2008). Principles of experience-dependent neural plasticity: Implications for rehabilita-

tion after brain damage. *Journal of Speech, Language, and Hearing Research, 51*, S225–S239.

Netsell, R. (1985). Construction and use of a bite block for the evaluation and treatment of speech disorders. *Journal of Speech and Hearing Disorders, 50*, 103–106.

Strand, E. (1995). Treatment of motor speech disorders in children. *Seminars in Speech and Language, 16*(2), 126–139.

REFERENCES

Bower, E., McLellan, D.L., Arney, J., & Campbell, M.J. (1996). A randomised control of different intensities of physiotherapy and different goal-setting procedures in 44 children with cerebral palsy. *Developmental Medicine and Child Neurology, 38*, 226–237.

Clarke, H.M. (2003). Neuromuscular treatments for speech and swallowing: A tutorial. *American Journal of Speech-Language Pathology, 12*, 400–415.

Crary, M.A. (1993). *Developmental motor speech disorders.* San Diego: Singular Publishing Group.

Defeo, A.B., & Shaefer, C. (1983). Bilateral facial paralysis in a pre-school child: Oral-facial and articulatory characteristics. In W.R. Berry (Ed.), *Clinical dysarthria* (pp. 165–186). San Diego: College-Hill Press.

Duffy, J.R. (2005). *Motor speech disorders: Substrates, differential diagnosis and management* (2nd ed.). St. Louis: Mosby-Year Book.

Dworkin, J.P. (1978). A therapeutic approach for the improvement of lingua-alveolar valving abilities. *Language, Speech, and Hearing Services in Schools, 9*, 169–175.

Fox, C.M. (2003). Intensive voice treatment for children with spastic cerebral palsy (Doctoral dissertation, University of Arizona, 2003). *Dissertation Abstracts International, 63*(12), 5796-B–5797-B.

Gibbon, F.E. (1999). Undifferentiated lingual gestures in children with articulation/phonological disorders. *Journal of Speech, Language, and Hearing Research, 42*, 382–397.

Gibbon, F.E., & Wood, S.E. (2003). Using electropalatography (EPG) to diagnose and treat articulation disorders associated with mild cerebral palsy: A case study. *Clinical Linguistics and Phonetics, 17*, 365–374.

Goldman, R., & Fristoe, M. (1969). *Goldman-Fristoe Test of Articulation.* Circle Pines, MN: American Guidance Service.

Hadders-Algra, M. (2000). The neuronal group selection theory: Promising principles for understanding and treating developmental motor disorders. *Developmental Medicine and Child Neurology, 42*, 707–715.

Hodge, M., & Wellman, L. (1999). Management of children with dysarthria. In A. Caruso & E. Strand (Eds.), *Clinical management of motor speech disorders in children* (pp. 209–280). New York: Thieme.

Ingram, D. (1998). Research-practice relationships in speech-language pathology. *Topics in Language Disorders, 18*(2), 1–9.

Joffe, B., & Reilly, S. (2004). The evidence base of the evaluation and management of motor speech disorders in children. In S. Reilly, J. Douglas, & J. Oates (Eds.), *Evidence-based practice in speech pathology* (pp. 219–257). London: Whurr.

Kent, R.D., & Read, C. (2002). *The acoustic analysis of speech* (2nd ed.). Clifton Park, NY: Thomson Delmar Learning.

Kent, R.D., & Voperian, H.K. (2006). In the mouths of babes: Anatomic, motor and sensory foundations of speech development in children. In R. Paul (Ed.), *Language disorders from a developmental perspective: Essays in honor of Robin S. Chapman* (pp. 55–81). Mahwah, NJ: Lawrence Erlbaum Associates.

Kleim, J.A., & Jones, T.A. (2008). Principles of experience-dependent neural plasticity: Implications for rehabilitation after brain damage. *Journal of Speech, Language, and Hearing Research, 51*, S225–S239.

Lewis, B. (2007). *Short- and long-term outcomes for children with speech sound disorders*. Retrieved March 15, 2009, from http://www.literacyencyclopedia.ca/pdfs/topic.php?topId=23

Love, R.J. (2000). *Childhood motor speech disability* (2nd ed.). Toronto: Maxwell Macmillan Canada.

Marchant, J., McAuliffe, M.J., & Huckabee, M.-L. (2008). Treatment of articulatory impairment in a child with spastic dysarthria associated with cerebral palsy. *Developmental Neurorehabilitation, 11*, 81–90.

Morgan, A.T., & Vogel, A.P. (2008). Intervention for dysarthria associated with acquired brain injury in children and adolescents. *The Cochrane Database of Systematic Reviews*, (3). doi:10.1002/14651858.CD006279.pub2

Nelson, M., & Hodge, M. (2000). Effects of facial paralysis and audiovisual information on stop place identification. *Journal of Speech, Language, and Hearing Research, 43*, 158–171.

Netsell, R. (1985). Construction and use of a bite block for the evaluation and treatment of speech disorders. *Journal of Speech and Hearing Disorders, 50*, 103–106.

Pennington, L., Goldbart, J., & Marshall, J. (2003). Speech and language therapy to improve the communication skills of children with cerebral palsy. *The Cochrane Database of Systematic Reviews*, (3). doi:10.1002/14651858.CD003466.pub2

Pennington, L., Miller, N., & Robson, S. (2008). Speech therapy for children with dysarthria acquired before three years of age. *The Cochrane Database of Systematic Reviews*, (1). doi:10.1002/14651858.CD006937

Sandberg, A. (2006). Reading and spelling abilities in children with severe speech impairments and cerebral palsy at 6, 9, and 12 years of age in relation to cognitive development: A longitudinal study. *Developmental Medicine & Child Neurology, 48*, 629–634.

Secord, W.A., Boyce, S.E., Donohue, J.S., Fox, R.A., & Shine, R.E. (2007). *Eliciting sounds: Techniques and strategies for clinicians* (2nd ed.). Clifton Park, NY: Thomson Delmar Learning.

Strand, E. (1995). Treatment of motor speech disorders in children. *Seminars in Speech and Language, 16*(2), 126–139.

Taub, E., Uswatte, G., & Pidikiti, R. (1999). Constraint-induced movement therapy: A new family of techniques with broad application to physical rehabilitation: A clinical review. *Journal of Rehabilitation Research and Development, 36*(3), 237–251.

Wambaugh, J.L. (2006). Treatment guidelines for apraxia of speech: Lessons for future research. *Journal of Medical Speech-Language Pathology, 14*(4), 317–321.

Webb, W., & Adler, R. (2008). *Neurology for the speech-language pathologist* (5th ed.). St. Louis: Mosby.

Workinger, M.S. (2005). *Cerebral palsy: Resource guide for speech-language pathologists*. Clifton Park, NY: Thomson Delmar Learning.

World Health Organization. (2001). *International classification of functioning, disability and health*. Geneva, Switzerland: Author.

Nonspeech Oral Motor Intervention

Heather M. Clark

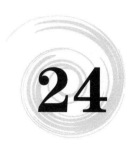

ABSTRACT

Oral motor exercises (OMEs) target underlying sensorimotor functions thought to underlie speech sound production. This chapter explores a select number of OMEs targeting strength, somatosensory function, and motor control. The physiological responses to these interventions are described along with a discussion of how the techniques apply to the unique neurophysiology of the speech mechanism. A review of the evidence supporting the use of OMEs will reveal that the interventions that have been most carefully researched are not necessarily those typically employed by speech-language pathologists (SLPs) and that much more extensive and higher quality treatment literature is needed to determine the conditions under which OMEs are most beneficial, as well as the therapeutic mechanisms underlying their effectiveness.

INTRODUCTION

Oral motor exercises (OMEs), purported to address underlying physiological functions supporting speech production, are a common component of intervention for childhood speech sound disorders (SSDs; Lof & Watson, 2008). OMEs may target muscle strength, range of motion (ROM), control, and sensory functions such as somatosensory detection and perception. This chapter describes OMEs that target musculature relevant to speech sound production (i.e., lips, tongue, jaw, and velar muscles), although many compilations of OME techniques include interventions that further target phonatory and respiratory functions.

TARGET POPULATIONS

Although OMEs have been included in intervention recommendations for children displaying a variety of difficulties including speech sound production disorders, hypernasality, and drooling, the individuals most likely to benefit from OMEs are those whose speech difficulties arise from sensorimotor impairments.

PRIMARY POPULATIONS

Impairments in orofacial strength, ROM, and somatosensory function have been described for a number of populations. Surprisingly, the populations for which neuromuscular impairments are most obvious (e.g., children with cerebral palsy, children with Down syndrome) have been studied to delineate the nature of neuromuscular impairments affecting the speech mechanism.

Children with Down syndrome typically exhibit weakness and hypotonia of the extremities (Morris, Vaughan, & Vaccaro, 1982). Similar impairments in the orofacial musculature are presumed, although empirical evidence of these impairments is lacking in the literature. In particular, low muscle tone in the tongue musculature is cited as contributing to speech and swallowing impairments (Carolina Pediatric Dysphagia, 2008) as well as to sleep apnea (Kavanagh, Kahane, & Kordan, 1986; Limbrock, Castillo-Morales, Hoyer, Stover, & Onufer, 1993; Veldi, Vasar, Hion, Vain, & Kull, 2002). Some authors (e.g., Lashno, 2003) further argue that somatosensory impairments contribute to impaired function in Down syndrome. Although the supposition that such sensorimotor impairments are characteristic of Down syndrome is apparently widely accepted, clinical research is needed to characterize these impairments and their relationship to speech sound production.

Cerebral palsy is another condition for which significant sensorimotor limitations are presumed to underlie speech impairments (Love, 2000; Mecham, 2002). Children with spastic cerebral palsy are typically described as exhibiting hypertonia of the orofacial musculature, resulting in speech movements that are slow and poorly controlled (Darley, Aronson, & Brown, 1975). In contrast, ataxic cerebral palsy is generally believed to be associated with orofacial hypotonia that limits the speed and accuracy of speech sound production (Ingram & Barn, 1961). Although no studies have demonstrated orofacial tone variations in *children* with cerebral palsy, a study of lingual tone in *adults* with spastic cerebral palsy failed to identify the presence of spasticity in the tongue muscles (Neilson, Andrews, Guitar, & Quinn, 1979). Finally, somatosensory impairments are not thought to be a primary contributor to speech impairments in cerebral palsy, and systematic research exploring the presence and nature of such impairments is limited (Ingram & Barn, 1961). The lack of research data detailing sensorimotor impairments of the speech musculature in these and other childhood conditions affecting the motor system highlights the need for careful assessment of sensorimotor function before considering OMEs.

A third population for which OMEs are recommended are children who exhibit oral myofunctional disorders (OMD), including tongue thrust. OMD includes maladaptive resting postures or movement patterns of the mouth that negatively affect oral growth patterns and dental occlusion (Nelson, 2001). There is no a priori assumption of sensorimotor dysfunction in OMD; that is, children with intact somatosensory function, strength, and muscle tone may exhibit OMD. Nonetheless, OMD may reflect an imbalance in orofacial strength (Nelson, 2001) or impaired perception of tongue position (Wood, 1971). Children with tongue thrust, a phenomenon in which the tongue protrudes anteriorly during the swallow or has a resting posture protruding beyond the anterior teeth, are generally thought to be at risk for developing speech sound production disorders, particularly frontal lisps and interdental articulation of alveolar stops (Mason & Proffit, 1974).

Because many OMEs do not require volitional responses from the child, these techniques have been described for children as young as neonates. Indeed, for passively applied interventions, the primary limitation is not age but the child's tolerance of orofacial stimulation. The OMEs that require volitional responses from the child are appropriate for children who can follow verbal instructions or imitate a visual model.

Secondary Populations

Although it is not immediately clear why it would be so, OMEs are also employed with children who do not exhibit neuromuscular impairments (e.g., developmental phonological disorders) or who demonstrate impairments not amenable to the techniques employed (e.g., childhood apraxia of speech; Lof & Watson, 2008). Rationales for recommending OMEs for these children may include an intention to "warm up" the speech musculature, to enhance awareness of the articulators, or as a means of simplifying complex movement patterns (Forrest, 2002; Lof & Watson, 2008). A discussion of these rationales is included in the Theoretical Basis section later in this chapter.

ASSESSMENT METHODS FOR DETERMINING INTERVENTION RELEVANCE

In spite of rather widespread belief that children with SSD exhibit sensorimotor impairments (Lof & Watson, 2008), clinical methods for identifying these impairments are scarce. Because each OME addresses one or more specific underlying impairments, it is critical that appropriate assessments are conducted to ensure that intervention does not target impairments that are not present.

Strength

Orofacial strength, defined as the ability of a muscle group to produce force, is most commonly assessed subjectively by having the child attempt to move an articulator against resistance provided by the examiner. For example, the clinician may have the child protrude his or her tongue while pressing back against the tongue with a tongue blade or have the child hold his or her lips closed, not allowing the clinician to insert the blade between the lips. Objective measures of orofacial strength are also available. Perhaps the most widely used in clinical settings is the Iowa Oral Performance Instrument (IOPI; Blaise Medical, Inc., Hendersonville, TN). This device measures pressure generated against a soft, air-filled bulb. Lingual elevation strength may be assessed by positioning the bulb along the hard palate. The child is instructed to elevate the tongue against the bulb with maximum effort. Motivated trials in which the clinician cheers "Push! Push! Push!" are thought to yield the highest pressure readings (Ballard, Solomon, Robin, Moon, & Folkins, 2009). The IOPI bulb can be coupled with attachments that allow measurement of lingual protrusion and lateralization, cheek compression, and lip compression strength (Clark, Solomon, O'Brien, Calleja, & Newcomb, 2008). Adequate normative data are lacking for both objective and subjective measures of orofacial strength in children; thus, clinicians rely primarily on their own experiences. In the case of the IOPI, clinicians may refer to the small number of studies reporting strength measures of typically developing children ages 5–12 years (Murdoch, Attard, Ozanne, & Stokes, 1995; Robin, Somodi, & Luschei, 1991).

Range of Motion

ROM, often cited as a function improved by OMEs, may be influenced by muscle strength as well as other neuromuscular factors such as hypertonia and joint hypomobility. As is true for strength, ROM is typically assessed subjectively. The clinician instructs the child to move the target articulator as far as possible in specific directions. For example, the child may be asked to "try to touch your nose with the tip of your tongue" or "smile as wide as you can." For such tasks, no resistance is applied, and ROM is gauged relative to subjective standards based on the clinician's experience or, for selected movements, with respect to symmetry (e.g., do the right and left sides of the mouth retract to the same extent?).

Objectifying measures of ROM is possible for many orofacial movements. For example, a labial goniometer (Stefanakos, 1997) quantifies the degree of deviation from horizon exhibited by the lips at rest or while actively sustaining a posture. ROM of the lips and tongue might also be assessed with a flexible measuring tape positioned to quantify distance from resting to fullest extended position.

A limitation of both subjective and objective ROM measures is that no norms exist to assist the clinician in identifying performance outside of the normal range. Moreover, ROM is strongly influenced by the size and shape of the orofacial structures, such that it may not be clear if quantifiably smaller ROM suggests neuromuscular impairment or appropriate function within the child's unique structural configuration. Symmetry of ROM may thus be the most meaningful measure available because the child serves as his or her own reference, although the degree to which departure from symmetry is associated with impaired function has also not been quantified.

Muscle Tone

The assessment of muscle tone has been largely overlooked by traditional oral motor assessment protocols (e.g., Shipley & McAfee, 2008). Tone of the limb musculature is typically assessed subjectively by the examiner passively moving the articulator (e.g., arm, wrist, lower leg) and judging the resistance provided by the resting muscle. Similar procedures have been described for the tongue and lips (Dworkin & Culatta, 1996); however, normative data are not available that characterize the range of normal resistance provided by these articulators in the various directions they might be passively moved. Moreover, given the overlapping and interconnected architecture of the orofacial muscles, these techniques will identify the resistance provided by muscle groups but not by individual muscles.

Beckman (1988) described a method for assessing the response of orofacial tissue to passive displacement. Although the techniques are purported to assess strength at intensity levels described as "minimal competence" (Beckman, 1988), the methods are most consistent with the operational definition of muscle tone as opposed to muscle strength. Beckman's assessment procedures suffer from the same limitation as other subjective measures, in that normative data defining the normal range of function are lacking, and no validation of the method through comparison of objective and subjective measures has been conducted.

A final subjective measure of muscle tone utilized by some clinicians is visual inspection of resting orofacial postures. Facial droop and enlarged structures are often considered signals of reduced muscle tone. Retraction of the lips and/or tongue is thought to indicate increased muscle tone. Unfortunately, no studies have examined orofacial muscle tone in children with altered resting postures, so these presumptions remain unsubstantiated.

Objective measures of orofacial muscle tone have been described within research contexts (Clark & Solomon, 2004; Leonard et al., 2003; Seibel & Barlow, 2007; Veldi, Vasar, Vain, & Kull, 2004) but have not been adopted for standard clinical practice. These tools typically measure some aspect of tissue displacement in response to an external load applied to the cutaneous tissue directly above a muscle (Leonard et al., 2003; Veldi et al., 2004) or to orofacial structures controlled by target muscles (Seibel & Barlow, 2007). The development of clinically feasible versions of these objective measures is limited by cost and portability; thus, the options for valid clinical assessment of muscle tone are quite limited.

Somatosensory Function

Assessment of somatosensory integrity is complicated by the vast range of unique functions (e.g., single-point touch threshold, oral stereognosis, position judgments) that may be targeted for assessment. This discussion will be limited to the perception of jaw position, a somatosensory skill particularly relevant to accurate speech sound production. Readers are referred to other sources for a thorough review of the myriad techniques described for both subjective and objective measures (Boliek et al., 2007; Snyder, Prescott, & Bartoshuk, 2006; Williams & Lapointe, 1971).

The richness of proprioceptive receptors (e.g., muscle spindles) in the jaw musculature suggests that such afferents are relevant to muscle control during speech, chewing, and/or swallowing. The ability of individuals to judge the position of the jaw has been studied extensively by speech and dental scientists, providing a literature describing methods for assessing proprioceptive acuity. These measures frequently involve sophisticated instrumentation (e.g., Broekhuijsen & van Willigen, 1983; De Nil & Lafaille, 2002) not available to clinicians; however, the general principles may be adapted for the clinical setting. For example, one method for assessing jaw proprioception is to have the child repeatedly open the jaw to a predetermined position. Whereas researchers judge accuracy through the use of strain gauges, clinicians might use a ruler to measure the distance between the lips or the edges of the upper and lower incisors. Alternatively, bite blocks of varying thickness can be placed between the molars to stabilize the mandible at a specific height, and the child can be asked to judge the degree of jaw opening through comparisons (e.g., "Is this one bigger or smaller than the last one?"). Direct magnitude estimation may also be used, in which a specific degree of opening is designated as the referent (e.g., "This is a five") and all judgments of jaw opening are made relative to that referent, with wider openings assigned ratings higher than five and narrower openings rated lower than five. These methods are not appropriate for young children who cannot understand the instructions or for children unable to stabilize a bite block. Moreover, like many other subjective assessments, no norms are available to help clinicians identify subnormal performance.

THEORETICAL BASIS

Dominant Theoretical Rationale for the Intervention Approach

The primary purpose of OMEs is to influence underlying sensorimotor capabilities supporting effective speech production. In addition, some clinicians use OMEs to "warm up" the speech musculature or to heighten awareness of oral structures (Lof & Watson,

2008). In all cases, the underlying assumption guiding the use of OMEs is that facilitating sensorimotor function of the speech musculature during nonspeech activities will enhance sensorimotor control for speech sound production.

The theoretical foundations underlying OME are complex given the array of physiological impairments targeted and the number of techniques described to address those impairments. The discussion in this chapter will be limited to three broad areas of OME: strength training, muscle tone-altering interventions, and motor control techniques.

Strength Training

Strength training is arguably the most common application of OMEs, perhaps because weakness is common to a number of childhood conditions and because weakness is relatively easy for clinicians to identify. Before discussing the theoretical models informing the development of strength-training programs, it is first necessary to consider how weakness impacts speech sound production.

There is no question that speech sound production requires the production of some level of force by the various articulators. What is less clear is what degree of weakness is necessary to negatively affect articulatory accuracy. The forces produced during normal speech are much smaller (e.g., 20%) than the forces that can be produced by the articulators during nonspeech maximum contractions (see Kuehn & Moon, 2000 for review). Luschei (1991) argued that the unique physiology of the lingual musculature may cloud the relationship between forces produced and strength required for clear articulation. Specifically, because the lingual muscles exert force by displacing tissue fluids rather than leveraging around a joint, Luschei argued that high levels of strength may be required to move the tongue quickly. Nonetheless, empirical investigations have failed to demonstrate a clear relationship between strength and speech clarity. For example, in adult speakers, individuals with lingual strength at approximately 50% of normal demonstrated 100% intelligible speech (Solomon, Clark, Makashay, & Newman, 2008). Moreover, it wasn't until strength levels were less than 30% of normal that all participants demonstrated reduced intelligibility. In addition, at least one investigation found that children with speech sound errors demonstrated greater lingual strength than children without sound errors (Sudberry, Wilson, Broaddus, & Potter, 2006). Thus, the use of strength training in the intervention of speech sound production disorders remains controversial.

The relationship between strength and speech notwithstanding, OMEs targeting underlying weakness must adhere to standard principles of strength training arising from the exercise science and rehabilitation literature (Clark, 2003). This chapter highlights three key principles: specificity, overload, and recovery.

Training specificity refers to the observation that the effects of strength training are limited to movements that very closely match the exercises completed (Jones, McCartney, & McComas, 1986; Schmidt & Lee, 1998; Schmidt & Wrisberg, 2000). A number of exercise characteristics are subject to specificity, but this discussion highlights only those characteristics of greatest relevance to OMEs. Contraction velocity is an exercise characteristic subject to specificity. In other words, the movements that comprise the exercise must closely match the speed of the movements used in the target behavior. As indicated previously, although speech does not require the production of high forces, it does require fast movements (Barlow & Burton, 1990), suggesting that OMEs targeting strength should utilize exercises requiring relatively rapid movement of the articulators.

Integration of movement is also relevant for speech production. Because motor program schemas incorporate all of the relevant muscle actions contributing to functional movement outcomes (e.g., throwing a ball requires stabilization by the trunk muscles in addition to the actions of the arm and shoulder), exercises should incorporate all muscle groups pertinent to the target outcome (Schmidt & Lee, 1998; Schmidt & Wrisberg, 2000). Because speech production involves activation of respiratory, phonatory, resonatory, and articulatory musculature, OMEs targeting speech sound production should involve exercises that engage all of the relevant musculature, even if all muscle groups are not targeted for strength training.

The second principle of strength training relevant to OMEs is the concept of overload. Muscle strength increases only when exercise taxes the targeted muscle beyond its typical level of use (Cerny, Sapienza, Lof, & Robbins, 2007). When muscle requirements exceed their typical use, the motor control system responds by increasing motor unit recruitment. Over time, prolonged overload will result in muscle hypertrophy, further increasing strength. Increased strength and muscle hypertrophy has been demonstrated for the lingual musculature when exercise is conducted at 80% of maximum (Robbins et al., 2005, 2007).

Finally, the issue of recovery is pertinent to OMEs targeting increased strength. When a muscle is exercised to the point of overload, waste products accumulate within the muscles, and muscle tissue may even be degraded. Ample time after exercise is required for the body to remove metabolic waste and rebuild muscle tissue (Kisner & Colby, 1996). If exercise is repeated before recovery is complete, strength will be gained at a slower rate. For the muscles of the extremities, research supports the recommendation that an interval of approximately 48 hours be allowed between exercising the same muscle group. Unfortunately, similar research investigating optimal exercise intervals has not been conducted on the speech musculature. Nonetheless, studies incorporating tongue exercise conducted daily (Clark, O'Brien, Calleja, & Newcomb, in press), three days per week (Clark, Barber, & Irwin, 2004; Robbins et al., 2005, 2007), and five days per week (Lazarus, Logemann, Huang, & Rademaker, 2003) have demonstrated increased lingual strength. Moreover, exercising as little as once per day (Clark et al., 2004; Clark et al., in press) or as often as five times per day (Lazarus et al., 2003) has also shown benefit. More systematic study of exercise intensity is needed to provide clear guidance regarding the most appropriate exercise schedule.

Muscle Tone-Altering Interventions

A number of OMEs purportedly target alterations in muscle tone. The theoretical foundation for these interventions focuses on the response of muscle spindles to sensory stimulation. Muscle spindles are sensory receptors that respond to changes in muscle fiber length. In most limb muscles, stimulation of the muscle spindle elicits a stretch reflex, in which the muscle that is lengthening reflexively contracts (Levin & Feldman, 1994; Stejskal, 1979). The resistance provided by this reflexive contraction is a primary contributor to observed muscle tone, which is defined as the amount of resistance a muscle provides to passive stretching.

Techniques that stimulate the muscle spindle and thus evoke a stretch reflex are commonly used to increase muscle tone, particularly in the case of flaccidity (Trombly, 1983). Similarly, techniques that inhibit activation of the stretch reflex are employed to reduce muscle tone in the case of spasticity (Gracies, 2001). Limiting the utility of these interventions is the presence and function of muscle spindles in the orofacial musculature. Specifically, only the jaw closing muscles demonstrate stretch reflexes typical of limb muscles (Cooper, 1960). Thus, techniques that stimulate or inhibit stretch reflexes of this muscle group would be expected to influence tone. However, muscle spindles are largely lacking from the lips and facial muscles; therefore, such interventions would not be expected to influence tone of these muscle groups (Neilson et al., 1979). Finally, although muscle spindles are present in the lingual musculature, stretch reflexes are not observed, thus interventions targeting the stretch reflex would not be expected to be beneficial (Cooper, 1953; Neilson et al., 1979).

Motor Control

The theoretical foundations for OMEs targeting motor control arise from the motor learning literature. When OMEs are employed to enhance motor control, the general assumption is that breaking down complex speech movements to their component parts (e.g., lip closure) allows the motor system to plan simpler movement patterns and gradually develop skilled control of more complex movement patterns. Unfortunately, limited evidence exists to support the notion of part-to-whole transfer of motor skills (Schmidt & Lee, 1998). Instead, motor learning appears to be task specific and goal oriented. When movements (e.g., lingual elevation) are decontextualized by removing them from the larger movement pattern (e.g., production of /t/) and target outcome (e.g., intelligible speech), very little transfer of motor learning should be expected (Schmidt & Lee, 1998; Schmidt & Wrisberg, 2000).

Levels of Consequences Being Addressed

OMEs, by definition, address underlying sensorimotor physiology rather than directly targeting speech production. Specifically, OMEs target the International Classification of Functioning, Disability and Health constructs of Muscle functions (b730–b749), Movement functions (b750–b789), Sensations related to muscles and movement functions (b780), and Additional sensory functions (b250–b279) (World Health Organization, 2001).

Target Areas of Intervention

Within the construct of Muscle and Motor Functions, OMEs target muscle power (strength), tone, and endurance, as well as motor reflex functions, control of voluntary movements, and sensations related to muscles and movement function. Within the construct of Sensory Functions, OMEs target proprioception and touch functions.

EMPIRICAL BASIS

Research Outcomes

The broad range of OME techniques and the array of populations to whom they have been applied make it difficult to provide a succinct review of literature addressing their benefit. This section highlights evidence from the peer-reviewed literature, with an acknowledgment that lower levels of evidence have been disseminated in other forms (e.g., conference presentations or books).

American Speech-Language-Hearing Association Systematic Review

In recognition of the need for clinicians to have ready access to treatment literature relevant to clinical management decisions, the American Speech-Language-Hearing Association (ASHA) National Center for Evidence-Based Practice has undertaken to conduct systematic reviews of the evidence related to select interventions. One such systematic review targeting OMEs examined the peer-reviewed literature addressing the use of nonspeech OMEs across populations (Arvedson et al., 2007). Only those studies identified by the ASHA systematic review that relate to childhood speech sound production disorders (McCauley, Strand, Lof, Schooling, & Frymark, 2009) are reviewed here.

Oral Myofunctional Disorders

Three controlled trials (Baskervill, 1976; Christensen & Hanson, 1981; Korbmacher, Schwan, Berndsen, Bull, & Kahl-Nieke, 2004) and one exploratory study (Ray, 2003) failed to identify significant differences in speech production accuracy or lingual movements following nonspeech OMEs. A single exploratory study reported that the proportion of children and young adults exhibiting a lisp decreased following OMEs (Daglio, Schwitzer, Wuthrich, & Kallivroussis, 1993). In each of these studies, the exercise provided was a variation of "tongue thrust therapy," an approach that typically emphasizes lip closure and lingual positioning during speech and swallowing movements.

Down Syndrome

The efficacy studies addressing the benefit of OMEs for children with Down syndrome examined the use of palatal plates to stimulate sensorimotor function (Backman, Grever-Sjolander, Bengtsson, Persson, & Johansson, 2007; Carlstedt, Henningsson, & Dahllöf, 2003; Carlstedt, Henningsson, McAllister, & Dahllöf, 2001). Although no benefit for perceptual accuracy of speech sounds or parental rating of intelligibility was revealed, one study reported that children treated with the palatal plate demonstrated significantly more consistent lip rounding during speech than did children in the control group (Carlstedt et al., 2001).

Cerebral Palsy

The OMEs just described—tongue thrust intervention and palatal plates—have also been administered to children with cerebral palsy. In an exploratory study, Ray (2001) found that although tongue thrust intervention failed to increase diadochokinetic rate, intelligibility was significantly improved. The exploratory study examining the benefit of palatal plates for children with cerebral palsy failed to provide adequate information about speech outcomes (Fischer-Brandies, Avalle, & Limbrock, 1987), so it is unknown if this approach should be considered for children with cerebral palsy. However, given that palatal plates did not improve the speech sound accuracy of children with Down syndrome, there appears to be very limited reason to expect this OME to improve the speech of children with cerebral palsy.

Cleft Palate

Sucking and blowing exercises are a common recommendation to improve velopharyngeal valving. However, the single exploratory study that examined the benefit of these techniques for reducing hypernasality in children with repaired clefts failed to demonstrate significant differences in perceptual ratings of nasality during speech sound production (Powers & Starr, 1974).

Functional Speech Sound Production Disorder

In an exploratory study, Dworkin (1978) described four children (age range 6–8 years) with jaw instability that was judged to be preventing accurate productions of lingua-alveolar consonants. Following several months of traditional articulation-focused intervention yielding limited progress, intervention was supplemented with bite blocks (this technique is described in detail later in this chapter). Following 40–48 sessions of bite block intervention conducted three times per week for up to 4 months, speech sound accuracy improved to within normal limits. The author concluded that although bite blocks would be unlikely to benefit all children with SSD, the presence of jaw hypermobility may signal the need for OMEs.

Finally, a single exploratory study (Fischer-Brandies et al., 1987) reported that children with developmental SSD failed to reduce the number of errors on a standardized articulation test after intervention with an oral motor approach (Strode & Chamberlain, 1997).

Nonspeech Oral Motor Exercises Versus Oral Motor Exercises Plus Speech

The systematic review conducted by ASHA included only those studies that did not utilize speech movements as a component of the intervention. The rationale for excluding "mixed treatment" studies is that such reports cannot differentiate intervention effects of OMEs from that of speech practice. However, as suggested earlier and as emphasized by OME proponents (Marshalla, 2008), OMEs are in fact most likely to have benefit within the context of speech movements. Thus, it might be argued that the ASHA review is not comprehensive and may have overlooked literature relevant to the discussion of OMEs. For example, an exercise program (described in Practical Requirements section) that exercises the velum during speech production has been demonstrated to be beneficial for reducing hypernasality in a series of exploratory studies (Kuehn, 1991; Kuehn et al., 2002). Nonetheless, until research is conducted with appropriate controls that allow readers to determine the effects of OMEs beyond those provided by speech practice alone, we must rely on studies that do not incorporate speech at all.

Summary of Levels of Evidence

See Table 24.1.

PRACTICAL REQUIREMENTS

It is beyond the scope of this chapter to discuss the implementation of every possible OME. Instead, the discussion will focus on general principles that arise from the theoretical and empirical bases reviewed previously.

Nature of Sessions

OMEs should never be the primary focus of a complete session. Instead, OMEs may be incorporated, as appropriate, into sessions of which the majority of time is used to elicit speech behaviors directly.

Table 24.1. Levels of evidence for studies of treatment efficacy for oral motor exercises

Level	Description	References
Ia	Meta-analysis of > 1 randomized controlled trial	—
Ib	Randomized controlled study	Carlstedt et al. (2001, 2003); Christensen & Hanson (1981); Korbmacher et al. (2004)
IIa	Controlled study without randomization	Backman et al. (2007); Baskervill (1976)
IIb	Quasi-experimental study	Fischer-Brandies et al. (1987); Guisti Braislin & Cascella (2005)
III	Nonexperimental studies, i.e., correlational and case studies	Daglio et al. (1993); Dworkin (1978)*; Powers & Starr (1974); Ray (2001*, 2003)
IV	Expert committee report, consensus conference, clinical experience of respected authorities	Boshart (1998)*; Chapman Bahr (2001)*; Marshalla (2000)*; Rosenfeld-Johnson (2001)*

Adapted from the Scottish Intercollegiate Guidelines Network (http://www.sign.ac.uk).
*Publications that support the use of OMEs for improving speech sound production

Personnel

Depending on the goals for which OMEs are employed, the SLP or other individuals may be responsible for administering the intervention. For example, the SLP or speech-language pathology assistant is most likely to administer OMEs when the purpose is to direct the child's attention to the orofacial mechanism as a component of the regular session. Alternatively, if the goal of OMEs is to strengthen the speech mechanism, parents may also be trained to administer the procedures outside of the formal intervention session.

Clinicians wishing to learn specific techniques for OMEs may choose to take advantage of workshops offered in the area of OMEs. Unfortunately, the methods touted by such workshops are not equally valid. Therefore, clinicians should critically appraise all information provided at workshops, determining how the recommended procedures adhere to principles guiding sensorimotor interventions and the level of evidence available to support their use.

When appropriate, clinicians may recommend that parents administer OMEs. In this case, the clinician must ensure the parent understands the purpose of the intervention, the appropriate procedures for applying the intervention (or eliciting the target behavior), and the type of feedback to be provided or observations to be made following the application of the intervention. It will be useful to have the parents describe the response to intervention so that the clinician may recommend modifications to the protocol as appropriate.

KEY COMPONENTS

The specific strategies encompassing OMEs are numerous and variable depending on the muscle group or sensory system targeted and the intended impact on sensorimotor function. This chapter addresses only select examples of interventions targeting strength, muscle tone, and motor control.

Nature of Goals

The general goal of OMEs is to normalize sensorimotor function of the speech mechanism. Ideally, goals will specify a target level of performance (e.g., "Julie will produce peak interlabial pressures of 20 kPa on three of five trials"). Unfortunately, because some sensorimotor functions are not easily quantified in the clinical setting, goals may be qualitative and/or subjective (e.g., "Julie will exhibit a resting tongue position where no part of the tongue is visible between the incisors").

Goal Attack Strategies

Although no empirical data exist to direct the sequencing of targets for OMEs, general principles may be drawn from the literature addressing neuromotor rehabilitation of the limb musculature, typical sensorimotor development, and approaches developed to treat sensorimotor impairments in adults.

Many individuals may experience two or more co-occurring impairments. For example, children with spastic cerebral palsy may exhibit weakness, hypertonicity, and hyper-responsivity to sensory stimulation. Although the relationships among strength, tone, and somatosensory function are yet to be illuminated for the speech musculature, it might be speculated that hypertonia contributes to muscle weakness by preventing optimal length-tension relationships (Folkins & Linville, 1983). Indeed, reducing hypertonia through icing or stretching prior to beginning exercise is a long-standing principle in rehabilitation of limb spasticity (Levine, Kabat, Knott, & Boss, 1954). Moreover, to the extent that a child's hypersensitivity to tactile stimulation exacerbates his or her spasticity, it may be appropriate to address sensory targets as one component of normalizing muscle tone.

In addition to prioritizing sensorimotor impairments, clinicians should also consider the order in which muscle groups should be targeted. Again, in the absence of empirical evidence, clinicians must rely on theoretical models to guide intervention selection. One such model (Dworkin, 1991) posited that the articulatory and phonatory systems are highly dependent on respiratory and resonatory functions. Thus, within this framework, the oral musculature, supporting articulation, would not be targeted until adequate airway support, velopharyngeal valving, and phonatory efficiency are established (Marshalla, 2000). Likewise, given that jaw control is the earliest developing oral motor skill, followed by lip differentiation and finally lingual control (Green, Moore, & Reilly, 2002; Morris & Klein, 2000), it might be recommended that the sensorimotor function of these articulators be targeted in the observed developmental sequence (Marshalla, 2000; Rosenfeld-Johnson, 2001). Systematic research is needed to determine the validity of these recommendations.

Description of Activities

The following sections are not intended to be an exhaustive description of all possible OMEs. Instead, they provide examples of OMEs that are most consistent with physiological models and empirical evidence.

Strength Training

As suggested earlier, the rationale for strengthening the orofacial musculature to improve speech sound production is limited. Nonetheless, if the clinician has sufficient reason to believe that speech movements are limited by weakness, OMEs to increase strength may be warranted. Consistent with the principles detailed previously in this chapter, exercises most likely to lead to functional changes in speech production must systematically overload the muscle group exhibiting weakness while integrating all related movements of the target outcome. A strength-training program that successfully addresses these issues is the constant positive airway pressure (CPAP) protocol designed to strengthen the velopharyngeal musculature (Kuehn, 1991; Kuehn et al., 2002). CPAP is a device that delivers air at a predetermined pressure through a nasal mask into the nasopharynx. The CPAP adds to the standard resistance provided by gravity and tissue stiffness to achieve overload. The pressure can be adjusted over the course of intervention accommodating progression as the velopharyngeal mechanism is strengthened. The exercise performed when the CPAP is in place is speech production of syllables, words, and sentences, effectively incorporating all the related movements of the target outcome: speech. The protocol specifies that exercises should be performed once daily, allowing ample recovery time between training sessions.

Exercise protocols that similarly overload other individual muscle groups while incorporating all movements inherent to the target behavior are largely lacking. Clark, Barber, and Irwin (2004) described a protocol in which adult participants produced the /t/ phoneme at targeted lingual pressures monitored by a biofeedback device. Similar exercises could be designed in which the pressure sensor was placed interlabially as a means of targeting lip strength. A limitation is that in both of these cases the presence of the pressure transducer changes the somatosensory context of the speech movements and obstructs natural speech movements somewhat.

A popular OME program targeting increased strength of the speech musculature is the straw/horn hierarchy described by Rosenfeld-Johnson (2001). As is true for speech, straw drinking and horn blowing require coordinated, integrated movements of the lips, tongue, velum, and respiratory musculature. This program systematically overloads the muscle groups by applying a hierarchy of straws/horns that offer progressively higher resistance. Unlike many other OMEs that isolate movements of single articulators with limited added resistance, the straw/horn hierarchy incorporates a number of features (e.g., overload, co-activation of related muscle groups) consistent with principles of strength training. The greatest limitation of this program is that the exercise does not incorporate speech. Thus, although many muscle groups active during speech are strengthened for sucking/blowing movements, carryover to speech movements would be expected to be less than if speech movements were exercised.

Regardless of the exercise selected, the training protocol should be based on proven schedules, such as three sets of 10 repetitions daily or three times per week (Clark et al., 2004). Although training protocols described for the limb musculature often suggest training to the point of fatigue (Kisner & Colby, 1996), evidence suggests that the speech musculature is remarkably resistant to fatigue (Kuehn & Moon, 2000; Solomon, 2004, 2006). Thus, it is more likely that individuals performing orofacial exercise will report a sense of exertion rather than exhaustion.

Muscle Tone-Altering Interventions

As suggested previously, because tone-altering interventions target stretch reflex actions of the muscle spindle, only the jaw closing musculature (i.e., masseter) is an appropriate target for these OMEs. The jaw musculature may demonstrate either hypo- or hypertonicity, thus OMEs that address each of these impairments are described.

Children with Down syndrome may exhibit hypotonicity, contributing to a low resting position of the mandible and an open-mouth posture. If hypotonicity is judged to limit jaw stability for articulation (Rosenfeld-Johnson, 2001), applying OMEs that stimulate the masseter muscle spindles may be appropriate. Two interventions that evoke muscle spindle reflexes are vibration and tapping. Because these modalities are largely absent from the treatment efficacy literature, it is not possible to recommend a particular schedule of intervention or intensity of application. Nonetheless, some cautions apply to the use of these techniques. Most notably, vibration can cause breakdown of fragile facial skin (Farber, 1982; McCormack, 1996) and should thus be applied only in short durations (Taylor, Anderson, & Patil, 2004). Also, vibration can exacerbate extrapyramidal and cerebellar symptoms such as those common in athetoid and ataxic cerebral palsy, respectively (McCormack, 1996).

Hypertonicity of the mandibular muscles may limit jaw excursion and thus negatively influence speech sound production. Icing and massage are techniques used to reduce muscle tone. The masseter is a relatively superficial and thus accessible muscle for these interventions. Icing helps to normalize tone by reducing nerve conduction velocities (Hedenberg, 1970; Miglietta, 1973). It should be noted that nerve conduction for volitional movements is also slowed, which may cause unintended weakness. Massage, in contrast, adds no risk of weakness, but may reduce muscle tone by facilitating central and peripheral relaxation (Cyriax, 1980). Massage to reduce muscle tone should be firm but not so intense as to cause discomfort, as pain may induce muscle spasms exacerbating hypertonicity (Earley, 2000; Michlovitz, 1986; Weber & Brown, 1996).

Motor Control

It is clear that both somatosensory and motor functions contribute to overall motor control. There is evidence to suggest that both vibrotactile (touch) and muscle spindle receptors contribute proprioceptive inputs to the motor control systems (Barlow, 1999). OMEs that stimulate these proprioceptive inputs have been suggested as a means of establishing stability for speech movements (Rosenfeld-Johnson, 2001). One technique for heightening the proprioceptive input associated with jaw position is the use of bite blocks (Crary, 1993; Rosenfeld-Johnson, 2001). A bite block is a small, solid structure that is held between the molars and secured with string or other tether to prevent accidental choking or swallowing. When a bite block is in place, added proprioceptive information about jaw position is provided by the sensory input to the teeth stabilizing the bite block. Typically, the child completes speech activities with the bite block in place (Crary, 1993). This technique addresses the important training principle of specificity by using speech as the movement(s) practiced. Moreover, if a large bite block is used, it provides an opportunity to simultaneously target lingual ROM as the tongue compensates for the immobilized mandible. The greatest limitation of bite block OME is that the somatosensory information utilized during practice (i.e., dental pressure) is not available during normal speaking tasks and in fact serves to disrupt or "perturb" natural somatosensory processing (Folkins & Zimmerman, 1981). If the child becomes dependent on atypical somatosensory feedback for accurate speech sound production, generalization to speaking situations outside of intervention may be minimal.

Materials and Equipment Required

The plethora of materials and programs available for OMEs is seemingly disproportionate to the empirical and theoretical support for their use. This is perhaps a reflection of the entertainment value of many of these materials (e.g., horns, bubbles) rather than an implicit need for a broad range of materials to adequately address potential sensorimotor impairments. Nonetheless, some devices may prove more useful than others. For example, equipment that serves to overload one or more articulators while providing for speech production (e.g., continuous positive airway pressure or CPAP) would be expected to be more effectual than materials that elicit nonspeech movements.

ASSESSMENT AND PROGRESS MONITORING TO SUPPORT DECISION MAKING

The ultimate goal of OMEs is improved speech sound production, thus performance at this level is most relevant to judgments of progress. Nonetheless, given the presumption that speech improves as a result of normalized sensorimotor function, documenting changes in strength, muscle tone, and/or somatosensory integrity is also warranted. Unfortunately, small changes in sensorimotor function may be imperceptible by subjective methods (Solomon & Clark, 2008). Thus, objective tools (e.g., IOPI) are necessary to detect therapeutic changes.

The literature provides very limited guidance regarding what degree of change in sensorimotor function is clinically relevant. Experiments examining strength training of the lingual musculature suggest that increases of 5%–25% may be expected after 4–9 weeks of training (Clark et al., 2004; Clark et al., in press; Robbins et al., 2005, 2007). However, the rate or degree of increase that is necessary to effect change in speech production is still unknown. Even less information is available to guide judgments of therapeutic changes in somatosensory function or muscle tone. These limitations further highlight the need for clinicians to use improvements in speech sound production accuracy as the primary measure of progress. However, because OMEs are always used in combination with other interventions, clinicians must be mindful that improvements in speech production cannot be attributed solely to improved sensorimotor function unless a carefully designed research protocol is incorporated as part of the intervention methodology.

CONSIDERATIONS FOR CHILDREN FROM CULTURALLY AND LINGUISTICALLY DIVERSE BACKGROUNDS

No data are available to suggest that OMEs have differential effects on speakers from culturally or linguistically diverse backgrounds. Nonetheless, clinicians choosing to include OMEs should be cognizant that some cultures may be more or less accepting of interventions that invade the oral space or involve the clinician touching the child's face.

CASE STUDY

The following case study is fictitious, but based on a reported case study of a young adult whose speech improved following OME (Stierwalt & Robin, 1996). Starla is a 9-year-old child who sustained a severe traumatic brain injury during a motor vehicle accident when she was 6. Upon emerging from a coma, she demonstrated severe spastic-ataxic dysarthria characterized by pronounced orofacial weakness and reduced range and speed of lingual movements.

Her speech was largely unintelligible and limited to weakly differentiated vowels. Language was relatively spared, and Starla communicated primarily through writing and typing on a personal digital assistant (PDA). She received 26 months of traditional speech therapy targeting articulatory accuracy and overall comprehensibility, after which intelligibility had improved to approximately 25% with familiar listeners and her speech sound repertoire had expanded to include labials as well as more clearly differentiated vowels. At that point, her progress plateaued and she was dismissed from intervention.

Starla's parents sought additional services through a nonprofit clinic. At the time of assessment, Starla's lingual strength was assessed objectively utilizing the IOPI, with which she was able to generate 15 kPa of pressure by elevating the tongue against the palate. This performance is significantly below the expected range of 40–60 kPa. Performance on the Speech Intelligibility Test (SIT; Yorkston, Beukelman, Hakel, & Dorsey, 2007) was 28%. At this point, Starla began a tongue-strengthening program that included lingual elevation exercises using the light display on the IOPI as feedback regarding generated pressures. She performed the exercises daily in her home while continuing to attend twice weekly intervention sessions targeting articulatory placement, speech rate, and phrasing.

Following 3 months of intervention, Starla's lingual strength had increased to 38 kPa. Articulatory accuracy for /t/, /d/, and /n/ during word-level treatment probes was 85%; however, intelligibility outside of intervention was judged by her parents to be largely unchanged. After 3 additional months of intervention, lingual strength had improved to within normal limits (45 kPa), and articulatory accuracy for /t/, /d/, and /n/ was 95% during structured conversation. Additional articulatory targets—/s/, /ʃ/, /l/, /k/, and /g/—had been introduced and were produced with 70% accuracy in word probes and 45% accuracy in structured conversation. SIT performance increased to 65%. Because lingual strength was now within normal limits, tongue strengthening was discontinued. Starla resumed speech therapy within the public school setting, three sessions weekly, and attended one additional session per week through the clinic. The focus of intervention at this point was accuracy of speech sound production, as speech rate and phrasing were judged to be optimal for intelligibility. Following a final 3 months of intervention through the clinic, Starla's lingual strength remained within normal limits (48 kPa), articulatory accuracy of lingual phonemes was greater than 70% for each phoneme in structured conversation, and SIT performance was 82%. At this point, intervention through the clinic was discontinued; however, Starla continued to receive speech intervention from the school SLP.

STUDY QUESTIONS

1. What evidence is available from this case study to suggest that Starla's speech sound production was limited by the presence of lingual weakness? Was this the only limitation?

2. Was it appropriate to discontinue strength training when lingual strength had improved to within normal limits? Why or why not?

3. Does this case study support the use of OMEs in isolation?

FUTURE DIRECTIONS

This chapter has highlighted a number of questions surrounding the use of OMEs for improving speech sound production. Nonetheless, many clinicians with success in treating speech sound production disorders consider OMEs to be a necessary component of a comprehensive intervention program, particularly for children with suspected sensorimotor impairments and/or persistent speech sound production difficulties (Lof & Watson, 2008).

Given the disparity between evidence and theory and practice, rigorous study is needed to 1) provide strong evidence documenting the benefit or lack of benefit from these techniques and 2) elucidate the physiological mechanisms contributing to identified therapeutic benefits. Clinicians employing OMEs can contribute to these efforts by implementing carefully controlled single-subject designs. Indeed, such studies incorporating appropriate physiological outcomes in addition to speech outcomes may address both the question of benefit as well as the therapeutic mechanisms affecting the speech outcomes.

Randomized controlled trials involving larger groups of children are also needed; however, such research is costly and time consuming. Although funding for treatment research is limited and often prioritized according to theoretical rationale for study, qualified researchers must continue to seek opportunities to study these techniques, thus providing information that can be used by clinicians as they make clinical management decisions.

One development that will likely serve to advance the study of OMEs is the establishment of the Oral Motor Institute. This nonprofit organization was founded by clinicians for the express purpose of promoting research that "demonstrate[s] the scientific basis of oral sensory and motor techniques" (Oral Motor Institute, 2007). Such clinician-led movements underscore the ecological validity of OME research and may ultimately lead to a response by funding agencies to prioritize funds for this line of study.

SUGGESTED READINGS

Clark, H.M. (2003). Neuromuscular treatments for speech and swallowing: A tutorial. *American Journal of Speech-Language Pathology, 12*, 400–415.

Forrest, K. (2002). Are oral-motor exercises useful in treatment of phonological/articulatory disorders? *Seminars in Speech and Language, 23*(1), 15–25.

Hodge, M. (2002). Nonspeech oral motor treatment approaches for dysarthria: Perspectives on a controversial clinical practice. *Perspectives on Neurophysiology and Neurogenic Speech and Language Disorders, 12*(4), 22–28.

Lof, G.L. (2003). Oral motor exercises and treatment outcomes. *Language Learning and Education, 10*, 7–11.

Shuster, L. (2001). Oral motor training and treatment for apraxia of speech. *Perspectives in Neurophysiology and Neurogenic Speech and Language Disorders, 11*, 18–20.

REFERENCES

Arvedson, J.C., Clark, H.M., Lazarus, C., Lof, G.L., McCauley, R.J., Strand, E., et al. (2007, November 16). *The effectiveness of oral-motor exercises: An evidence-based systematic review.* Paper presented at the Annual Convention of the American Speech-Language-Hearing Association, Boston.

Backman, B.A.C., Grever-Sjolander, A., Bengtsson, K., Persson, J., & Johansson, I. (2007). Children with Down syndrome: Oral development and morphology after use of palatal plates between 6 and 48 months of age. *International Journal of Paediatric Dentistry, 17*, 19–28.

Ballard, K.J., Solomon, N.P., Robin, D.A., Moon, J., &

Folkins, J. (2009). Nonspeech assessment of the speech production mechanism. In M. McNeil (Ed.), *Clinical management of sensorimotor speech disorders* (2nd ed., pp. 30–45). New York: Thieme.

Barlow, S.M. (1999). *Handbook of clinical speech physiology.* San Diego: Singular Thomson Learning.

Barlow, S.M., & Burton, M.K. (1990). Ramp-and-hold force control in the upper and lower lips: Developing new neuromotor assessment applications in traumatically brain injured adults. *Journal of Speech and Hearing Research, 33,* 660–675.

Baskervill, R.D. (1976). The effects of special speech therapeutic procedures involving individuals with sibilant distortions: A pilot study. *International Journal of Orofacial Myology, 2*(4), 86–92.

Beckman, D. (1988). *Beckman oral motor interventions.* Course pack accompanying oral motor assessment and intervention workshop (2001). Charlotte, NC: Author.

Boliek, C.A., Rieger, J.M., Li, S.Y., Mohamed, Z., Kickham, J., & Amundsen, K. (2007). Establishing a reliable protocol to measure tongue sensation. *Journal of Oral Rehabilitation, 34*(6), 433–441.

Boshart, C.A. (1998). *Oral motor analysis and remediation techniques.* Temecula, CA: Speech Dynamics.

Broekhuijsen, M.L., & van Willigen, J.D. (1983). Factors influencing jaw position sense in man. *Archives of Oral Biology, 28*(5), 387–391.

Carlstedt, K.G., Henningsson, G., & Dahllöf, G. (2003). A four-year longitudinal study of palatal plate therapy in children with Down syndrome: Effects on oral motor function, articulation and communication preferences. *Acta Odontologica Scandinavica, 61*(1), 39–46.

Carlstedt, K.G., Henningsson, G., McAllister, A., & Dahllöf, G. (2001). Long-term effects of palatal plate therapy on oral motor function in children with Down syndrome evaluated by video registration. *Acta Odontologica Scandinavica, 59*(2), 63–68.

Carolina Pediatric Dysphagia. (2008). *Feeding and swallowing difficulties in children with Down syndrome: Frequently asked questions.* Retrieved May 17, 2008, from http://www.feeding.com/images/Down%20Syndrome%20Feeding.doc

Cerny, F., Sapienza, C., Lof, G.L., & Robbins, J. (2007, November 15). *Muscle training principles and resulting changes to speech and swallowing.* Paper presented at the annual convention of the American Speech-Language-Hearing Association, Boston.

Chapman Bahr, D. (2001). *Oral motor assessment and treatment: Ages and stages.* Boston: Allyn & Bacon.

Christensen, M.S., & Hanson, M.L. (1981). An investigation of the efficacy of oral myofunctional therapy as a precursor to articulation therapy for pre-first grade children. *Journal of Speech and Hearing Disorders, 46*(2), 160–167.

Clark, H.M. (2003). Neuromuscular treatments for speech and swallowing: A tutorial. *American Journal of Speech-Language Pathology, 12,* 400–415.

Clark, H.M., Barber, W.D., & Irwin, W. (2004, March 18–20). *Specificity of training in the lingual musculature.* Paper presented at the Conference on Motor Speech, Albuquerque, NM.

Clark, H.M., O'Brien, K., Calleja, A., & Newcomb, S. (in press). Effects of directional exercise on lingual strength. *Journal of Speech, Language, and Hearing Research.*

Clark, H.M., & Solomon, N.P. (2004). *Effect of vibration and icing on muscle tissue compliance.* Manuscript in preparation.

Clark, H.M., Solomon, N.P., O'Brien, K., Calleja, A., & Newcomb, S. (2008, March 6–9). *Lingual and buccal strength: Innovations in clinical assessment.* Poster presented at the Biennial Conference on Motor Speech, Monterey, CA.

Cooper, S. (1953). Muscle spindles in the intrinsic muscles of the human tongue. *Journal of Physiology, 122,* 193–202.

Cooper, S. (1960). Muscle spindles and other receptors. In G.H. Bourne (Ed.), *The structure and function of muscle* (pp. 381–420). New York: Academic Press.

Crary, M.A. (1993). *Developmental motor speech disorders.* San Diego: Singular.

Cyriax, J.H. (1980). Clinical applications of massage. In J.B. Rogoff (Ed.) *Manipulation, traction and massage* (pp. 152–169). Baltimore: Williams & Wilkins.

Daglio, S.D., Schwitzer, R., Wuthrich, J., & Kallivroussis, G. (1993). Treating orofacial dyskinesia with functional physiotherapy in the case of frontal open bite. *International Journal of Orofacial Myology, 19,* 11–14.

Darley, F., Aronson, A., & Brown, J.R. (1975). *Motor speech disorders.* Philadelphia: W.B. Saunders.

De Nil, L.F., & Lafaille, S.J. (2002). Jaw and finger movement accuracy under visual and nonvisual feedback conditions. *Perceptual and Motor Skills, 95*(3), 1129–1140.

Dworkin, J.P. (1978). A therapeutic technique for the improvement of lingua-alveolar valving abilities. *Language, Speech, and Hearing Services in Schools, 9,* 169–175.

Dworkin, J.P. (1991). *Motor speech disorders: A treatment guide.* St. Louis: Mosby.

Dworkin, J.P., & Culatta, R. (1996). *Dworkin-Culatta Oral Mechanism Examination and Treatment System.* Nicholasville, KY: Edgewood Press.

Earley, D. (2000). Superficial heat agents. In A.G. Bracciano (Ed.), *Physical agent modalities* (1st ed., pp. 49–62). Thorofare, NJ: Slack.

Farber, S.D. (1982). *Neurorehabilitation: A multisensory approach.* Philadelphia: W.B. Saunders.

Fischer-Brandies, H., Avalle, C., & Limbrock, G.J. (1987). Therapy of orofacial dysfunctions in cerebral palsy according to Castillo-Morales: First results of a new treatment concept. *European Journal of Orthodontics, 9*(2), 139–143.

Folkins, J.W., & Linville, R.N. (1983). The effects of varying lower-lip displacement on upper-lip movements:

Implications for the coordination of speech movements. *Journal of Speech and Hearing Research*, *26*(2), 209–217.

Folkins, J.W., & Zimmerman, G. (1981). Jaw muscle activity during speech with the jaw fixed. *Journal of the Acoustical Society of America*, *69*, 1441–1445.

Forrest, K. (2002). Are oral-motor exercises useful in treatment of phonological/articulatory disorders? *Seminars in Speech and Language*, *23*(1), 15–25.

Gracies, J.M. (2001). Physical modalities other than stretch in spastic hypertonia. *Physical Medicine and Rehabilitation Clinics of North America*, *12*(vi), 769–792.

Green, J.R., Moore, C.A., & Reilly, K.J. (2002). The sequential development of jaw and lip control for speech. *Journal of Speech, Language, and Hearing Research*, *45*(1), 66–79.

Guisti Braislin, M.A., & Cascella, P.W. (2005). A preliminary investigation of oral motor exercises among children with mild articulation disorders. *International Journal of Rehabilitation Research*, *28*(3), 263–266.

Hedenberg, L. (1970). Functional improvement of the spastic hemiplegic arm after cooling. *Scandinavian Journal of Rehabilitative Medicine*, *2*, 154–158.

Ingram, T.T., & Barn, J. (1961). A description and classification of common speech disorders associated with cerebral palsy. *Cerebral Palsy Bulletin*, *3*, 57–69.

Jones, N.L., McCartney, M., & McComas, A.J. (1986). *Human muscle power*. Champagne, IL: Human Kinetics.

Kavanagh, K.T., Kahane, J.C., & Kordan, B. (1986). Risks and benefits of adenotonsillectomy for children with Down syndrome. *American Journal of Mental Deficiency*, *91*(1), 22–29.

Kisner, C., & Colby, L.A. (1996). *Therapeutic exercise foundations and techniques* (3rd ed.). Philadelphia: F.A. Davis.

Korbmacher, H.M., Schwan, M., Berndsen, S., Bull, J., & Kahl-Nieke, B. (2004). Evaluation of a new concept of myofunctional therapy in children. *International Journal of Orofacial Myology*, *30*, 39–52.

Kuehn, D.P. (1991). New therapy for treating hypernasal speech using continuous positive airway pressure (CPAP). *Plastic and Reconstructive Surgery*, *88*, 959–966.

Kuehn, D.P., Imrey, P.B., Tomes, L., Jones, D.L., O'Gara, M.M., Seaver, E.J., et al. (2002). Efficacy of continuous positive airway pressure for treatment of hypernasality. *Cleft-Palate-Craniofacial Journal*, *39*, 267–276.

Kuehn, D.P., & Moon, J.B. (2000). Induced fatigue effects on velopharyngeal closure force. *Journal of Speech, Language, and Hearing Research*, *43*, 486–500.

Lashno, M. (2003). Sensory integration: Observations of children with Down syndrome and autism spectrum disorders. *Disability Solutions*, *3*(5-6), 31–35.

Lazarus, C., Logemann, J.A., Huang, C.F., & Rademaker, A.W. (2003). Effects of two types of tongue strengthening exercises in young normals. *Folia Phoniatrica et Logopaedica*, *55*(4), 199–205.

Leonard, C.T., Deshner, W.P., Romo, J.W., Suoja, E.S., Fehrer, S.C., & Mikhailenok, E.L. (2003). Myotonometer intra- and interrater reliabilities. *Archives of Physical Medicine and Rehabilitation*, *84*(6), 928–932.

Levin, M.F., & Feldman, A.G. (1994). The role of stretch reflex threshold regulation in normal and impaired motor control. *Brain Research*, *657*(1–2), 23–30.

Levine, M.G., Kabat, H., Knott, M., & Boss, D.E. (1954). Relaxation of spasticity by physiologic techniques. *Archives of Physical Medicine and Rehabilitation*, *35*, 214–223.

Limbrock, G.J., Castillo-Morales, R., Hoyer, H., Stover, B., & Onufer, C.N. (1993). The Castillo-Morales approach to orofacial pathology in Down syndrome. *International Journal of Orofacial Myology*, *19*, 30–37.

Lof, G.L., & Watson, M. (2008). A nation-wide survey of non-speech oral motor exercise use: Implications for evidence-based practice. *Language, Speech, and Hearing Services in Schools*, 392–407.

Love, R.J. (2000). *Childhood motor speech disability* (2nd ed.). Boston: Allyn & Bacon.

Luschei, E.S. (1991). Development of objective standards of nonspeech oral strength and performance. In C.A. Moore, K.M. Yorkston, & D.R. Beukelman (Eds.), *Dysarthria and apraxia of speech: Perspectives on management* (pp. 3–13). Baltimore: Paul H. Brookes Publishing Co.

Marshalla, P. (2000). *Oral motor techniques in articulation and phonological therapy*. Kirkland, WA: Marshalla Speech and Language.

Marshalla, P. (2008). "Oral motor treatment" vs. "nonspeech oral motor exercises." *Oral Motor Institute*, *2*(2). Retrieved August 12, 2009, from www.oralmotorinstitute.org

Mason, R.M., & Proffit, W.R. (1974). The tongue thrust controversy: Background and recommendations. *Journal of Speech and Hearing Disorders*, *39*, 115–132.

McCauley, R.J., Strand, E., Lof, G.L., Schooling, T., & Frymark, T. (2009). Evidence-based systematic review: Effects of non-speech oral motor exercises on speech. *American Journal of Speech-Language Pathology*. doi:10.1044/1058-0360(2009/09-0006)

McCormack, G.L. (1996). The Rood approach to treatment of neuromuscular dysfunction. In L.W. Pedretti (Ed.), *Occupational therapy: Practice skills for physical dysfunction* (pp. 377–399). St. Louis: Mosby.

Mecham, M. (2002). *Cerebral palsy* (3rd ed.). Austin, TX: PRO-ED.

Michlovitz, S.L. (1986). Biophysical principles of heating and superficial heat agents. In S.L. Michlovitz & S.L. Wolf (Eds.), *Thermal agents in rehabilitation* (pp. 99–118). Philadelphia: F.A. Davis.

Miglietta, O. (1973). Action of cold on spasticity. *American Journal of Physical Medicine*, *52*, 198–205.

Morris, S., & Klein, M.D. (2000). *Pre-feeding skills: A comprehensive resource for mealtime development* (2nd ed.). San Antonio, TX: Therapy Skill Builders.

Morris, A.F., Vaughan, S.E., & Vaccaro, P. (1982). Measurements of neuromuscular tone and strength in Down's syndrome children. *Journal of Mental Deficiency Research, 26*(1), 41–46.

Murdoch, B.E., Attard, M.D., Ozanne, A.E., & Stokes, P.D. (1995). Impaired tongue strength and endurance in developmental verbal dyspraxia: a physiological analysis. *European Journal of Disorders of Communication, 30*, 51–64.

Neilson, P.D., Andrews, G., Guitar, B.E., & Quinn, P.T. (1979). Tonic stretch reflexes in lip, tongue and jaw muscles. *Brain Research, 178*(2–3), 311–327.

Nelson, R.M. (2001). *OMD explained.* Retrieved May 19, 2008, from http://www.southwestoralmyo.com/omd-info.htm

Oral Motor Institute. (2007). *About the OMI.* Retrieved May 17, 2008, from http://www.oralmotorinstitute.org/about.html

Powers, G.L., & Starr, C.D. (1974). The effects of muscle exercises on velopharyngeal gap and nasality. *Cleft Palate Journal, 11*(1), 28–35.

Ray, J. (2001). Functional outcomes of orofacial myofunctional therapy in children with cerebral palsy. *International Journal of Orofacial Myology, 27*, 5–17.

Ray, J. (2003). Effects of orofacial myofunctional therapy on speech intelligibility in individuals with persistent articulatory impairments. *International Journal of Orofacial Myology, 29*, 5–14.

Robbins, J., Gangnon, R.E., Theis, S.M., Kays, S.A., Hewitt, A.L., & Hind, J.A. (2005). The effects of lingual exercise on swallowing in older adults. *Journal of the American Geriatric Society, 53*(9), 1483–1489.

Robbins, J., Kays, S.A., Gangnon, R.E., Hind, J.A., Hewitt, A.L., Gentry, L.R., et al. (2007). The effects of lingual exercise in stroke patients with dysphagia. *Archives of Physical Medicine and Rehabilitation, 88*(2), 150–158.

Robin, D.A., Somodi, L.B., & Luschei, E.S. (1991). Measurement of tongue strength and endurance in normal and articulation disordered subjects. In C.A. Moore, K.M. Yorkston, & D.R. Beukelman (Eds.), *Dysarthria and apraxia of speech: Perspectives on management* (pp. 173–184). Baltimore: Paul H. Brookes Publishing Co.

Rosenfeld-Johnson, S. (2001). *Oral motor exercises for speech clarity.* Tuscon, AZ: Ravenhawk.

Schmidt, R.A., & Lee, T.D. (1998). *Motor control and learning: A behavioral emphasis* (3rd ed.). Champaign, IL: Human Kinetics.

Schmidt, R.A., & Wrisberg, C.A. (2000). *Motor learning and performance: A problem based learning approach* (2nd ed.). Champaign, IL: Human Kinetics.

Seibel, L.M., & Barlow, S.M. (2007). Automatic measurement of nonparticipatory stiffness in the perioral complex. *Journal of Speech, Language, and Hearing Research, 50*(5), 1272–1279.

Shipley, K.G., & McAfee, J.G. (2008). *Assessment in speech-language pathology: A resource manual.* Florence, KY: Cengage Learning.

Snyder, D.J., Prescott, J., & Bartoshuk, L.M. (2006). Modern psychophysics and the assessment of human oral sensation. *Advances in Otorhinolaryngology, 63*, 221–241.

Solomon, N.P. (2004). Assessment of tongue weakness and fatigue. *International Journal of Orofacial Myology, 30*, 8–19.

Solomon, N.P. (2006). What is orofacial fatigue and how does it affect function for swallowing and speech? *Seminars in Speech and Language, 27*(4), 268–282.

Solomon, N.P., & Clark, H.M. (2008). Assessment of orofacial strength in adults with dysarthria. *Journal of Medical Speech-Language Pathology, 16*, 251–258.

Solomon, N.P., Clark, H.M., Makashay, M.J., & Newman, L.A. (2008, March 6–9). *Orofacial strength and speech in normal and disordered adults.* Paper presented at the Conference on Motor Speech, Monterey, CA.

Stefanakos, K.H. (1997). *U.S. Patent No. 5678317.* Washington, DC: U.S. Patent and Trademark Office.

Stejskal, L. (1979). Postural reflexes in man. *American Journal of Physical Medicine, 58*(1), 1–25.

Stierwalt, J.A.G., & Robin, D.A. (1996, February). *Tongue strengthening in the treatment of severe dysarthria: A single-subject study.* Paper presented at the Eighth Biennial Conference on Motor Speech, Amelia Island, FL.

Strode, R., & Chamberlain, C. (1997). *Easy does it for articulation: An oral motor approach.* East Moline, IL: LinguiSystems.

Sudberry, A., Wilson, E., Broaddus, T., & Potter, N. (2006, November 17). *Tongue strength in preschool children: Measures, implications, and revelations.* Paper presented at the Annual Convention of the American Speech-Language-Hearing Association, Boston.

Taylor, M., Anderson, E., & Patil, P. (2004, March 18–20). *Clinical applications of vibrotactile stimulation: Theoretical bases, techniques, and case findings.* Paper presented at the Conference on Motor Speech, Albuquerque, NM.

Trombly, C.A. (1983). *Occupational therapy for physical dysfunction.* Baltimore: Williams & Wilkins.

Veldi, M., Vasar, V., Hion, T., Vain, A., & Kull, M. (2002). Myotonometry demonstrates changes of lingual musculature in obstructive sleep apnoea. *European Archives of Otorhinolaryngology, 259*(2), 108–112.

Veldi, M., Vasar, V., Vain, A., & Kull, M. (2004). Obstructive sleep apnea and ageing myotonometry demonstrates changes in the soft palate and tongue while awake. *Pathophysiology, 11*(3), 159–165.

Weber, D.C., & Brown, A.W. (1996). Physical agent modalities. In R.L. Braddom (Ed.), *Physical medicine and rehabilitation* (pp. 449–463). Philadelphia: W.B. Saunders.

Williams, W.N., & Lapointe, L.L. (1971). Correlations between oral form recognition and lingual touch sensitivity. *Perceptual and Motor Skills, 32*(3), 840–842.

Wood, J. (1971). Tongue thrusting: Some clinical observations. *Journal of Speech and Hearing Disorders, 36,* 82–89.

World Health Organization. (2001). *International classification of functioning, disability, and health.* Geneva: Author.

Yorkston, K.M., Beukelman, D.R., Hakel, M., & Dorsey, M. (2007). Speech Intelligibility Test for Windows [Computer software]. Lincoln, NE: Institute for Rehabilitation Science and Engineering at Madonna Rehabilitation Hospital.

Interventions for Children with Speech Sound Disorders

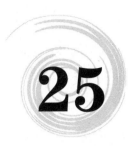

25

Future Directions

Rebecca J. McCauley, A. Lynn Williams, and Sharynne McLeod

ABSTRACT

This chapter shares conclusions we have reached about interventions for children with speech sound disorders (SSD). Many of these conclusions may prove valuable for four specific audiences with interests in children with SSD: students of speech-language pathology, clinicians, professors, and parents— the audiences addressed at the beginning of the book. In general, however, these conclusions are addressed specifically to clinicians and to a fifth group— researchers interested in SSD. Although sharing much in common with the other audiences, researchers have an overriding interest not only in the current state of interventions for children with SSD but also in the development of more effective and efficient intervention strategies for the future. Through a brief discussion of the implications of this book for clinical practice and future research, we revisit many topics introduced in Chapter 1, including the structure and classification of interventions, evidence-based practice (EBP), and the International Classification of Functioning, Disability and Health: Children and Youth Version (ICF-CY; World Health Organization, 2007).

OVERVIEW

Anything we may recommend in this final chapter runs the risk of undermining the perspective of EBP we have tried to foster with this book. Consequently, before we continue, we offer a word of caution. Although based on our immersion in the content of this book and an accumulation of about 60 combined years of clinical and research experience, our observations here fall at the lowest level of the Scottish Intercollegiate Guideline Network (SIGN) system of evidence appraisal. Specifically, we are offering our expert *opinion* on the subjects we discuss. Given this perspective, you might think we would choose to keep our thoughts to ourselves as having no utility because of their falling at such a low level of evidence. Instead, we remind readers that it is equally—and sometimes more important—to face squarely the realities of evidence quality, use available evidence with its limitations in mind, and continue forward to seek better evidence. Not only do we take that view as we conclude our writing but we also urge you to adopt the same view as you finish reading this book and continue your work and interactions with children affected by SSD.

CLINICAL PRACTICE FOR CHILDREN WITH SPEECH SOUND DISORDERS

We base our concluding reflections on the content of this book as well as on our work with children with SSD, beginning clinicians, and seasoned veteran clinicians who talk to us about their clients. These reflections lead us to offer advice in the form of a three-step process that we would recommend to clinicians who want to refine their practice:

1. Find one well-developed intervention approach that has been devised for the clients you serve and the need(s) they have.

2. Learn to use that approach masterfully.

3. Repeat steps one and two.

Although brief, these three steps sum up a strategy that clinicians can use to hone their craft and advance their science within the constraints of busy work lives.

Step 1: Find One Well-Developed Intervention Approach

At first reading, this step may seem most appropriate for a beginning clinician. Few seasoned clinicians would be pleased with the view that they have a single strategy; in fact, they will have many—some, that they find valuable; others, that they wish they could improve or replace outright. For both the experienced and inexperienced clinician, then, a focused strategy for improving clinical practice may prove best. Such a strategy seems realistic and encouraging of conscientious execution. In particular, the iterative nature of the process (i.e., Step 3) is intended to ensure an agenda for advancement that is not begun whole-heartedly, then abandoned. For experienced clinicians, the "one well-developed intervention" might be identified to address a common client need they would like to meet better or a group of clients (e.g., children with motor speech disorders or cleft palate) whom they serve infrequently but want to serve better. In contrast, for more beginning clinicians (including students), that *one* intervention might be a multicomponent approach that could be used for a broadly defined group and that addresses several related needs (e.g., intelligibility and speech sound acquisition, speech sound generalization and phonological awareness).

The value of this first step hinges on two elements contained within it—the extent to which an intervention is seen as well-developed and the extent to which it fits specific types of clients and their need(s). Readers undoubtedly may anticipate that *well-developed* means an intervention for which high-quality evidence has been obtained, but it does not mean *only* that. Rather, it means the highest quality evidence *relative* to that available for alternative interventions currently being used or being considered. Within the intervention chapters, a summary of relevant evidence is not limited to the Empirical Basis section. It is also presented in the Theoretical Basis section, in which readers can examine the assumptions and indirect sources of research evidence that they can then test against their clinical judgment and experience. Similarly, less direct evidence is presented in other sections that allows you to estimate "on-the-ground" validity; that is, the extent to which you believe you can faithfully implement core elements of the approach in your own work setting, with the resources and skills you possess. Our hope is that this book facilitates direct comparisons of evidence quality for those interventions we were able to include. In addition, we hope that the methods and metrics to which you have been introduced or reintroduced here (e.g., evidence tables, levels of evidence) can guide you through further comparisons—either by dent of your individual efforts or through group efforts (e.g., within a school district or clinic department).

Estimating an intervention's *fit* with your clients and their needs might seem to be a completely straightforward element within Step 1. However, developing clear ideas about the nature of your clients is almost always complicated by a myriad of particulars that make each person unique, such as age, the severity of their SSD, related problems, as well as their culture and language, to name a few. When seeking to identify a client's need(s), the ICF-CY (WHO, 2007) provides strong support for considering the most complete view of who that client is. Even a brief consideration of that classification system makes it clear that, although we may expect "trickle down" effects from working on particular sounds or sound patterns to the benefit of larger concerns such as communicative effectiveness, there are times when directly basing our intervention choices on needs as they are experienced and valued by the child and his or her family results in the most significant impact. Thus, for example, when a preteen with cerebral palsy, moderate developmental dysarthria, and associated drooling comes to our attention, initial attention to social acceptability and intelligibility may trump needs involving a specific phoneme distortion. Conceptualized client needs based on the ICF-CY (or a simplified version of it) may increase not only the child's self-image and the family's satisfaction with our work but also our efficiency and therefore the quality of our working life.

Consideration of client preferences is one of three components of EBP (Dollaghan, 2007; Sackett, Rosenberg, Gray, Hayes, & Richardson, 1996); however, client preference has been the least studied component within speech-language pathology practice. In the case of children with SSD, the client often includes the child, his or her family, teachers, and significant others. In a national study, 67% of speech-language pathologists (SLPs) reported that they involve parents in planning intervention; however, only 38% reported that they allowed parents to make final decisions about intervention goals (Watts Pappas, McLeod, McAllister, & McKinnon, 2008). When parents were asked about their preferences for intervention, they reported more satisfaction with services that were respectful, supportive, accessible, coordinated, and provided in a family-centered manner; conversely they were more dissatisfied if these factors were not a part of intervention (Watts Pappas & McLeod, 2009).

To date, in pediatric speech-language pathology practice for children with SSD, the child's parent(s) is more likely to be invited to share his or her preference, rather than the child. The rights of children to have a voice in matters that affect them have been upheld by the United Nations since 1989 (UNICEF, 2008). However, within the profession of speech-language pathology, we are only beginning to listen to children's views. Children's views have been sought on their attitudes toward intervention (Owen, Hayett, & Roulstone, 2004) and insights into living with speech and language impairment (McCormack, McLeod, McAllister, & Harrison, 2010). Innovative methods have been used to respectfully listen to children in child-friendly ways. These have included asking children to draw (Holliday, Harrison, & McLeod, 2009; McLeod, Daniel, & Barr, 2006), asking questions (McLeod, 2004; Vanryckeghem & Brutten, 2006), and interviewing children (McCormack et al., 2010; Owen et al., 2004). One insight from a group of 4- to 5-year-old children with SSD is that they have not perceived that they have a problem with their speech, but that the problem lies in the ears of the listener.

> The findings of this research suggest the strategies and advice SLPs provide to children with speech impairment and their families need to go beyond changing children's speech production to incorporate ways to enhance listeners' understanding and ways to address the frustration experienced by both communication partners. (McCormack et.al., in press, p. 33)

Readers can probably identify several sections in each chapter intended to help them judge the fit between the client/client needs and the intervention because many sections answer somewhat different but relevant questions on this issue. Of course, a first-approximation answer to the overall question of fit comes from the Target Populations section. Other valuable sections, however, include Empirical Basis (Does the research evidence include clients such as mine?), Assessment Methods for Determining Intervention Relevance (What pattern of test results should I consider as indicators that the intervention is appropriate?), and Considerations for Children from Culturally and Linguistically Diverse Backgrounds (Can I modify this approach so it better fits my client's background?). Even the Theoretical Basis section may prove pertinent (Did the developers consider skills or related problems I see as important for my clients when they developed this approach?). Many clinicians will also find viewing the DVD samples informative to questions of appropriateness for a client or clients. Once an empirically supported intervention's fit with an intended client or clients has been judged acceptable, implementation is the obvious—but not necessarily simple—next step.

Step 2: Learn to Use That Approach Masterfully

The process of improving clinical practice for children with SSD described in Step 1 falls squarely under the banner of EBP. In fact, much of what was described is no more than a compression of recent characterizations of EBP in speech-language pathology. For example, EBP[3] has been defined as "the conscientious, explicit, and judicious integration of (a) best available external evidence from systematic research, b) best available evidence internal to clinical practice, and c) best available evidence concerning the preferences of a fully informed patient" (Dollaghan, 2007, p. 2). This definition, and most like it, may leave the impression that "all is well" once decisions about the direction of intervention have been made using these integrated sources of high-quality information. Step 2 in the process we recommend is intended to call attention to clinicians' core and enduring contribution to EBP in SSD interventions.

Beginning clinicians are keenly aware of how challenging it can be to integrate descriptions and observations of new methods with previous knowledge and individual styles of interaction. New terms, concepts, and even values must be remembered, understood, and translated into new behaviors and habits. Otherwise, they cannot meaningfully serve as the basis for planning, implementing, and evaluating the effectiveness of an intervention moment by moment and session by session over the course of therapy. In addition, although seasoned clinicians are also seasoned learners, they too recognize the special challenges involved in modifying or shifting away from engrained practice patterns to adopt new ones.

In her formulation of EBP[3], Dollaghan (2007) discussed E[2] and E[3] as evidence deriving from clinical practice and client preferences, respectively—both of which she acknowledged as being relatively poorly understood when compared with E[1], external evidence from systematic research. In her discussion, she stressed the importance of clinical data as part of E^2 in determining the actual value of any intervention to the particular client (what we termed *on-the-ground validity* previously). This importance stems from the fact that research evidence can only suggest what outcomes will *probably* take place for future treated groups of clients rather than predicting what outcomes *will* take place for a given person—or child with SSD, in our case. Actual outcomes must be carefully observed and acted upon individually as guides to ongoing intervention decisions.

E^2 represents the logical extension of EBP to *practice-based evidence* (PBE). In line with this idea, Justice and Fey (2004) called for "scaling up," which is a concept that refers to efforts to close the research-to-practice gap through a two-step process. First, *scaling up of research* involves research at the third stage of the research continuum described in this book and elsewhere as *effectiveness studies*. Research at this stage examines real-world clinical problems implemented within clinical settings. The complementary second process involves the *scaling up of practices*, which facilitates the translation of research to clinical practice. Although this process includes the clinicians' scrutiny of available evidence, it also speaks to the importance of accountability of our practices, as well as the need for clinicians and researchers to work in tandem in investigating interventions and their outcomes to design more efficient and more effective approaches that are robust regardless of the intervention context (laboratory or clinic) or intervention agent (researcher or clinician).

Dollaghan (2007) introduced the topic of treatment fidelity (i.e., the faithfulness with which an intervention is executed by individual clinicians) within her discussion of evidence from clinical practice (E^2). However, she elaborated on that topic very little. From the clinician's vantage point, this concept encompasses the range of challenges faced when using personal interactions for clinical purposes—challenges that warrant self-reflection regardless of whether one is a novice or veteran. Such challenges exist because adoption of a new intervention draws not only upon cognitive resources (e.g., based on the amount of online complex decision making or multitasking required by an intervention) but upon effective resources as well (e.g., the immediacy of the effects that can be expected, the degree of vigilance needed for adapting input based on the child's response). Although external feedback about clinical practice is routinely provided in some form for students or new employees, this is less so for experienced clinicians. Consequently, there may be self-evaluation strategies clinicians can use to promote achievement of treatment fidelity while preserving the potential additional benefits of one's unique clinical style.

At present, there is little research on the nuts and bolts of how clinicians practice, much less on variables affecting treatment fidelity in SSD (Justice, 2010). However, treatment fidelity and its effects on intervention effectiveness have begun to be studied for practicing teachers (e.g., Justice, Mashburn, Pence, & Wiggins, 2008; Pence, Justice, & Wiggins, 2008) and are likely beginning for SLPs as well, especially as demands for accountability increase (Justice & Fey, 2004). In their 2008 study, Pence et al. reported on 14 teachers who were randomly assigned to learn a structured language enrichment program and were followed at three points over an academic year. Their training in that program consisted of an intensive 15-hour (3-day) format followed by a half-day refresher workshop, which included having them watch and self-evaluate recordings made in their own classrooms. Fidelity was examined by observers using checklists at three points in time to document—among other aspects of the teachers' implementation—the frequency and quality with which they applied the specific language stimulation techniques used in the program (e.g., recasts, open-ended questions). One finding of interest here was that although trained teachers tended to use a greater number of techniques than comparison teachers, trained teachers still did not use these techniques very frequently. Trained teachers did, however, use the techniques more over time—a finding that was at least partially attributed to the follow-up training they received. This study is mentioned because it points out the difficulty involved in adopting new methods and because it suggests several potential avenues by which professionals may enhance their application of new interventions.

Whereas in the longer term, research can help the profession learn how to support clinicians as they adopt new interventions, in the meantime, acknowledging the role we as clinicians play in the quality of intervention outcomes can serve as a solid first step. Ideas that arise from the research described previously include 1) reflecting seriously on whether aspects of an intervention will pose such serious barriers to our implementation that we should seek alternatives, 2) listing procedures we think may be difficult to implement before we decide to use an intervention so that we can brainstorm methods for tackling them or verifying their implementation, and 3) periodically developing and using checklists on key procedures to aid self-evaluation from videotapes.

Although demanding, scrutinizing our actual use of interventions makes it possible to add another set of operational variables (ones that are related to our implementation of specific procedures) to the list of variables that can be altered substantially or minimally when improvements in children's targeted behaviors do not exist or are not as large as desired. In addition, whereas reactions to intervention complexity or the novelty of an intervention's methods and terminology have probably always tacitly influenced clinicians' decisions in choosing SSD interventions, explicit recognition that intervention complexity should be considered when making a choice about whether to adopt an approach may improve our practice—and may provide important feedback to the developers of interventions as well.

Step 3: Repeat Steps 1 and 2

This step was included in recognition of the pressing need for clinicians to increase the scope, quality, and efficiency of interventions they provide to children with SSD—all while they also increase the scope, quality, and efficiency of interventions and other services they provide to all the other children they serve. In fact, continuous improvement of clinical practice occurs against a backdrop that might sometimes best be described as "one great blooming, buzzing confusion" (James, 1890/1983, p. 462). Not surprisingly, much of the skepticism about EBP that is often expressed by colleagues seems to stem from an impression that EBP obligates clinicians to make *every* clinical decision solely on the basis of external evidence—at a point in time when such evidence is scanty and resources to underwrite the process are minimal. Fortunately, when EBP is explored more fully, selectivity and rationality in choosing *when* to seek external evidence is recognized as a vital necessity.

A typical first step in outlines of the EBP process consists of framing an important and answerable question. When we consider interventions for SSD in this context, something such as a cost-benefit analysis comes to mind. The *benefit* portion of the analysis is reflected in the importance of the question—in this case, a question about what intervention is best to use for a certain child or group with SSD. Importance, for most clinicians, is probably related to impact—that is, the number of children in their practice who might be helped by the intervention, the degree of improvement they might expect for individual children, and the number and identity of areas in which improvements might be seen (e.g., more accurate speech sound use, increased intelligibility, improved phonological awareness). The *cost* portion of the cost-benefit analysis includes the time it will take to employ an EBP search for a new intervention, subsequent training time, the time and number of paid interventionists involved in ongoing use of the intervention (including any additional time that may be required to make sure that they are implementing it correctly), and actual purchases of materials or technology, as required. Consequently, in Step 3 of our recommended process, we encourage clinicians to consider both costs and benefits as they begin to develop ideas about the next new intervention they will seek.

With the time demands that every SLP works within, we realize that it will be difficult to undertake this step without support. Though it is not our goal to discuss or present the vast number of publications and tutorials that are available to assist clinicians in learning the steps of EBP, we would like to mention a couple of resources that will be particularly beneficial. A recommendation made by Baker and McLeod (2008) was for SLPs to create or join an EBP network. As a working example of an EBP collaborative, they cited the New South Wales Speech Pathology EBP Network (http://www.ciap.health.nsw .gov.au/specialties/ebp_sp_path/). SLPs meet on a quarterly basis to identify clinical questions to be addressed and researched. Topics that have been reviewed are posted at this site for use by other SLPs. Another resource that has been available since 2006 is the peer-reviewed journal *Evidence-Based Practice (EBP) Briefs* (http://www.speechand language.com/ebp/), which is a free quarterly electronic publication that addresses a variety of clinical questions that have been systematically examined using the steps of EBP. Finally, Baker and McLeod also referenced a very useful speech pathology database for best interventions and treatment efficacy, known as speechBITE (http://www.speech BITE.com). These resources are offered as ways for clinicians to "jump start" the EBP process, as well as models for conducting EBP individually or in collaboration with colleagues.

In the spirit of this step in our recommended three-step process, we undertook this book with the hope that it would be an ongoing resource for readers, not only in the information provided on specific interventions within individual chapters, but especially in the form of the tabular summaries we included in Chapter 1 and in the section overviews. Granted, the information contained here will need to be supplemented as researchers continue to study and advance their interventions yielding timely additional evidence. Still, given the relatively slow pace of research in smaller behavioral fields and the tightly organized nature of the descriptions offered by chapter authors, we are confident that this book will serve a valuable beginning point for some time to come.

FUTURE RESEARCH NEEDS

Some readers of this book may have shaken their heads in chagrin when they failed to find a chapter on an approach that they consider immensely valuable—for example, the traditional articulation approach (Secord, 1989; Van Riper, 1963) or dynamic temporal and tactile cuing for children with severe childhood apraxia of speech (Strand, 2009; Strand & Debertine, 2000). We, too, wish we could have been exhaustive in our coverage of interventions that can reasonably claim compelling research, or even well-framed theory as a starting point, for support. Nonetheless, the 23 interventions included here represent a great many of the exciting alternatives now available for the remediation of SSD.

As a window on intervention research in SSD, the 23 intervention chapters reflect the prevailing methods being used and varied levels of support being provided. In addition, their authors offer persuasive insights on directions for future research, both concerning their target intervention and SSD interventions as a whole. A recurring theme in their comments is the need for additional research that is of higher quality for a greater range of children with SSD. In our concluding comments on research needs, we choose not to spend much time in reiterating those basic and incontrovertible calls for more extensive and rigorous research. Instead, we will briefly outline two additional directions for research: 1) research on clinicians' contributions to treatment outcomes, and 2) research on critical ingredients for SSD interventions.

Research on Clinicians' Contributions to Treatment Outcomes

In a 2004 paper, Justice and Fey commented, "EBP requires clinicians to seek answers to . . . questions, and it requires researchers to do more to help them to find the answers." Here we would add that when those answers and questions have led to the adoption of a well-supported intervention, EBP also requires researchers to do more to help clinicians learn to implement those interventions in a manner likely to yield the biggest benefits to clients—that is, they need to do more to help clinicians ensure treatment fidelity. Without such research, the push toward EBP-oriented selection of interventions, even if fully embraced, may only be followed by what could be called piecemeal implementation.

Clinicians are incredibly busy people who may intentionally or unintentionally adopt a pick-and-choose attitude toward new methods, causing them to use some aspects of a studied intervention but not others (Lancaster, Keusch, Levin, Pring, & Martin, 2009). This seems especially likely when clinicians are unsupported in the steps that follow judicious adoption of cutting-edge interventions, such as those described in this book. Not surprisingly, in larger professions, there is a growing body of work aimed at identifying ways in which professionals (e.g., pediatricians, hand surgeons, nurses, teachers) can be assisted with such workplace complexities (e.g., Courtlandt, Noonan, & Feld, 2009; MacDermid & Graham, 2009; Resnick et al., 2005; Stein, 2008). For example, in 2007, Atul Gawande, a prominent surgeon and writer, wrote about the significant contribution to reducing death rates and complications in surgical settings made by using a safety checklist (see also, Haynes et al., 2009). Although lapses in clinical performance and treatment fidelity may not be associated with the level of risks in speech-language pathology as they are in surgical interventions, the documented value of a 19-item surgical checklist demonstrates that support for clinicians' treatment fidelity does not necessarily require complex programs or even extensive continuing education.

In a smaller profession such as ours, research on how best to support treatment fidelity may be seen as lower in priority than the development of new and improved interventions. However, diminished treatment fidelity seems likely to threaten both quality of care *and* quality of the workplace (Harris, Prater, Dyches, & Heath, 2009). Threats to quality of care follow directly from failures to achieve the conditions that resulted in the positive outcomes associated with an empirically supported intervention. Workplace quality may be threatened if diminishments in positive outcomes and clinicians' guilt over their own clinical methods—which may aspire to EBP, but *feel*, and in fact *be*, more like agglomerative mishmash—undermine a clinician's professional self-concept and job satis-faction. Granted, lapses in treatment fidelity may not be shown to have *widespread* neg-ative effects on clinicians themselves—that is an empirical question, awaiting further data. However, if they do, they may also indirectly contribute to the field's considerable difficulties in recruitment and retention (American Speech-Language-Hearing Associa-tion [ASHA], 2004; Edgar & Rosa-Lugo, 2007). Finally, even if neither of these postulated effects on individual clinicians or the field as a whole are confirmed, the threat of reduced fidelity to client outcomes makes its investigation for SSD interventions an important pri-ority for this research community.

So far in this section, our discussion of research needs related to SSD interventions has focused on ways in which clinicians can limit outcomes. Clearly, however, there is equal reason to study the ways that clinicians contribute positively to outcomes, inde-pendent of which intervention they use. Naively, anyone who has participated in or ob-served SSD interventions develops an awareness of the role that the clinician can play in motivation—an area that can be central to positive outcomes for children with SSD (Kwiatkowski & Shriberg, 1993). Particularly for older children with SSD, who may have participated in interventions for much of their lives, identifying clinician attributes and behaviors that enhance motivation could represent a boon to outcomes. The importance of research on clinicians as a variable affecting treatment outcome has emerging value in the area of stuttering (Zebrowski, 2007). Given the frequency with which SSD appears in the caseloads of SLPs who work with children, such work also holds promise for this area of speech-language pathology.

Research on Critical Ingredients for Speech Sound Disorder Interventions

Careful reading of the 23 intervention chapters, or even a cursory look at their summary tables, reveals numerous similarities across interventions. The structural model of inter-vention (based on Fey, 1986, 2008) that is illustrated in Figure 1.1 suggests numerous major elements that may be shared across interventions. Whereas some of these common elements may be accidental or reflect only the shared constraints of providers or settings, others—especially those from interventions with the greatest research support across multiple types of clients—may reflect what can be described as "active ingredients," ele-ments of interventions that contribute most directly to positive outcomes, such as dosage or intervention setting, to name a few.

Examination of effectiveness has almost always occurred at the level of the individ-ual intervention. However, research in related areas (e.g., Garland, Hawley, Brookman-Frazee, & Hurlburt, 2008; Kasari, 2002), as well as our own observations of recurring themes in interventions described in this book, suggests the possible benefits of identify-ing common elements of well-developed interventions. By looking across empirically supported interventions for such elements, researchers may more quickly develop in-novative plans for 1) beneficial modifications to established interventions or 2) new in-terventions designed to incorporate promising elements for use with as yet unserved subgroups of clients. Once tentatively identified, a number of methodologies within single-subject experimental designs (e.g., Barlow, Nock, & Hersen, 2009; McReynolds & Kearns, 1983) are available to confirm the value of such ingredients to the efficacy of par-ticular interventions. In addition, comparison studies in which two well-supported interventions are pitted against each other can be studied within rigorous group designs that are considered by many to represent particularly powerful evidence supporting intervention selections (e.g., Kasari, 2002).

Efforts to identify active ingredients are seen as vital to future advances in behavioral interventions in a variety of disorder areas, even those marked by client heterogeneity, such as autism spectrum disorder. In 2002, Kasari evaluated the quality of research conducted on 10 comprehensive interventions for young children with autism. She observed that the absence of detailed descriptions of the intervention approaches (e.g., updated treatment manuals and specific guidelines for instruction) made comparisons across studies impossible in many important areas. She further observed that this could be a problem even for studies that indicated use of a single treatment manual (Lovaas, 1981, as cited in Kasari, 2002), especially when ongoing revision of the intervention itself was evident (Lovaas, 1993, as cited in Kasari, 2002). At a minimum, the absence of detailed descriptions of specific interventions in associated research thwarts a major process associated with the scientific process, namely replication of that research by independent researchers. In addition, it may compound the problems clinicians face in achieving treatment fidelity for adopted interventions. Finally, as Kasari noted in her review, insufficient description of interventions in research seems likely to frustrate attempts to identify key ingredients. Despite this difficulty, Kasari considered evaluation of the active ingredients of existing approaches to be a major issue for future studies of autism interventions.

Evaluation of the active ingredients may also represent a very productive direction for research on SSD interventions. A number of the interventions in this book, especially those designed for children with motor speech disorders (e.g., Chapters 7, 19, 24), cited "principles of motor learning" as a theoretical foundation and source of many elements within their intervention. Inspection of the numerous principles comprising this influential body of evidence regarding the frequency, timing, and nature of feedback, frequency of scheduling, and so forth, may provide one source of clues to likely key ingredients. There are undoubtedly many others.

In this book, we have begun a process in which 23 SSD interventions have been carefully, if not exhaustively, described and have incorporated the use of a chapter template, summary tables, and a structural model of intervention, all of which ease the task of making comparisons across interventions. Although we did not consciously consider the value of these methods for the identification of key ingredients in SSD intervention, clearly they can contribute to hypothesis formation and thus to the design of appropriate research.

A complete list of research directions suggested by this book is beyond our capacity to summarize in this final chapter. Many of the directions we have recommended explicitly or implied in this chapter involve extensions of work on individual interventions, especially those with existing empirical support, including the following:

- Studies using research designs or improved methods (e.g., larger samples) associated with higher levels of evidence than currently reported for that intervention

- Replications of high-quality studies

- Studies designed to determine efficacy for groups of children with SSD for which the intervention has not yet been studied, such as those of different cultural or linguistic backgrounds, or with different diagnoses

- Studies designed to identify barriers to treatment fidelity during their implementation by practicing clinicians as well as methods to surmount them

  Some of our recommendations, however, have been based on issues that cross several interventions, such as

- Studies examining clinician characteristics associated with improved client motivation and outcomes

- Studies designed to identify key ingredients examining the role of hypothesized key ingredients on interventions containing them

- Group studies comparing interventions intended for similar populations of children with SSD

Readers may recognize omissions from these lists and can probably identify a myriad of other recommendations made within their favorite intervention chapters. Most certainly, however, over the course of their studies, readers will have arrived at many exciting ideas for future studies that have not been anticipated by either intervention chapter authors or ourselves. We hope these readers will 1) test the logic of their ideas and hypotheses with others who care about SSD and 2) consider preparations for pursuing them through research.

FINAL REFLECTIONS

Preparation of this book and work with its numerous authors have provided rich opportunities for learning about SSD, including some in which we have considered the needs of clinicians and researchers frankly and, we hope, compassionately. We have done so with particular vigor in this chapter. Of course, however, the principal needs that have inspired this book and prompted the sustained efforts of authors and editors alike over the many months of this project are those of children with SSD and their families. These children's needs and their families' desires for them include the need to produce speech more accurately, to communicate more effectively through spoken language, to participate more fully in their worlds, and to apply and extend that knowledge as they acquire written language. Our final hope, therefore, is that as readers approach the end of this book, they will find themselves better able to participate in the community of professionals and others who work to help children with SSD achieve their goals.

REFERENCES

American Speech-Language-Hearing Association. (2004). *Evidence-based practice in communication disorders: An introduction.* Retrieved September 4, 2009, from http://www.asha.org/docs/html/TR2004-00001.html

Baker, E., & McLeod, S. (2008, November). *EBP and speech sound disorders: What do we know?* Seminar presentation at the American Speech-Language-Hearing Association Annual Convention, Chicago.

Barlow, D.H., Nock, M.K., & Hersen, M. (2009). *Single case experimental designs: Strategies for studying behavior change* (3rd ed.) Boston: Allyn & Bacon.

Courtlandt, C.D., Noonan, L., & Feld, L.G. (2009). Model for improvement: Part 1. A framework for health care quality. *Pediatric Clinics of North America, 56*(4), 757–778.

Dollaghan, C.A. (2007). *The handbook for evidence-based practice in communication disorders*. Baltimore: Paul H. Brookes Publishing Co.

Edgar, D.L., & Rosa-Lugo, L.I. (2007). The critical shortage of speech-language pathologists in the public school setting: Features of the work environment that affect recruitment and retention. *Language, Speech, and Hearing Services in the Schools, 38*, 31–46.

Fey, M.E. (1986). *Language intervention with children*. Boston: Allyn & Bacon.

Fey, M.E. (2008, November). *Practice in child phonological disorders: Tackling some common clinical problems*. Seminar presentation at the American Speech-Language-Hearing Association Convention, Chicago.

Garland, A.F., Hawley, K.M., Brookman-Frazee, L., & Hurlburt, M.S. (2008). Identifying common elements of evidence-based psychosocial treatments for children's disruptive behavior problems. *Journal of the American Academy of Child and Adolescent Psychiatry, 47*(5), 505–514.

Gawande, A. (2007, December 10). Annals of medicine: The checklist. *The New Yorker*. Retrieved September 13, 2009, from http://www.newyorker.com/reporting/2007/12/10/071210fa_fact_gawande

Harris, S.F., Prater, M.A., Dyches, T.T., & Heath, M.A. (2009). Job stress of school-based speech-language pathologists. *Communication Disorders Quarterly, 30*(2), 103–111.

Haynes, A.B., Weiser, T.G., Berry, W.R., Lipsitz, S.R., Breizat, A.S., Dellinger, E.P., et al. (2009). A surgical safety checklist to reduce morbidity and mortality in a global population. *New England Journal of Medicine, 360*(5), 491–499.

Holliday, E.L., Harrison, L.J., & McLeod, S. (2009). Listening to children with communication impairment talking through their drawings. *Journal of Early Childhood Research, 7*(3), 244–263.

James, W. (1890/1983). *The principles of psychology*. Cambridge, MA: Harvard University Press.

Justice, L.M. (2010). When craft and science collide: Improving therapeutic practices through evidence-based innovations. *International Journal of Speech-Language Pathology, 12*(2), 79–86.

Justice, L.M., & Fey, M.E. (2004, September 21). Evidence-based practice in schools: Integrating craft and theory with science and data. *ASHA Leader, 4–5*, 30–32. Retrieved October 12, 2009, from http://www.asha.org/publications/leader/archives/2004/040921/f040921a.htm

Justice, L.M., Mashburn, A., Pence, K.L., & Wiggins, A. (2008). Evaluation of a preschool language curriculum: Influence on children's expressive language skills. *Journal of Speech, Language, and Hearing Research, 51*(4), 983–1001.

Kasari, C. (2002). Assessing change in early intervention programs for children with autism. *Journal of Autism and Developmental Disorders, 32*(5), 447–461.

Kwiatkowski, J., & Shriberg, L. (1993). Speech normalization in developmental phonological disorders: A retrospective study of capability-focus theory. *Language, Speech, and Hearing Services in Schools, 24*(1), 10–18.

Lancaster, G., Keusch, S., Levin, A., Pring, T., & Martin, S. (2009). Treating children with phonological problems: Does an eclectic approach to therapy work? *International Journal of Language and Communication Disorders, 29*, 1–12.

MacDermid, J.C., & Graham, I.D. (2009). Knowledge translation: Putting the "practice" in evidence-based practice. *Hand Clinics, 25*, 125–143.

McCormack, J., McLeod, S., McAllister, L., & Harrison, L.J. (2010). My speech problem, your listening problem, and my frustration: The experience of living with childhood speech impairment. *Language, Speech, and Hearing Services in Schools, 41*, 379–392.

McLeod, S. (2004). Speech pathologists' application of the ICF to children with speech impairment. *Advances in Speech-Language Pathology, 6*(1), 75–81.

McLeod, S., Daniel, G., & Barr, J. (2006). Using children's drawings to listen to how children feel about their speech. In C. Heine & L. Brown (Eds.), *Proceedings of the 2006 Speech Pathology Australia National Conference* (pp. 38–45). Melbourne: Speech Pathology Australia.

McReynolds, L.V., & Kearns, K.P. (1983). *Single subject experimental designs in communicative disorders*. Baltimore: University Park Press.

Owen, R., Hayett, L., & Roulstone, S. (2004). Children's views of speech and language therapy in school: Consulting children with communication difficulties. *Child Language Teaching and Therapy, 20*(1), 55–73.

Pence, K.L., Justice, L.M., & Wiggins, A.K. (2008). Preschool teachers' fidelity in implementing a comprehensive language-rich curriculum. *Language, Speech, and Hearing Services in Schools, 39*, 329–341.

Resnick, B., Inguito, P., Orwig, D., Yahiro, J.Y., Hawkes, W., Werner, M., et al. (2005). Treatment fidelity in behavior change research. *Nursing Research, 54*(2), 139–144.

Sackett, D.L., Rosenberg, W.M.C., Gray, J.A.M., Hayes, R.B., & Richardson, W.S. (1996). Evidence-based medicine: What it is and what it isn't. *British Medical Journal, 312*, 71–72.

Secord, W.A. (1989). The traditional approach to treatment. In N.A. Creaghead, P.W., Newman, & W.A. Secord (Eds.), *Assessment and remediation of articulatory and phonological disorders* (pp. 129–158). Columbus, OH: Charles E. Merrill.

Stein, M.L. (2008). Scaling up an early reading program: Relationships among teacher support, fidelity of implementation and student performance across sites and years. *Educational Evaluation and Policy Analysis, 30*(4), 368–388.

Strand, E.A. (2009). Child-centred dynamic assessment. In C. Bowen (Ed.), *Children's speech sound disorders* (pp. 263–264). Oxford, England: Wiley-Blackwell.

Strand, E.A., & Debertine, P. (2000). The efficacy of integral stimulation with developmental apraxia of speech. *Journal of Medical Speech-Language Pathology, 8*(4), 295–300.

UNICEF. (2008). *The Convention on the Rights of the Child.* Retrieved August 10, 2009, from http://www.unicef.org/crc

Van Riper, C. (1963). *Speech correction: Principles and methods* (4th ed.). Upper Saddle River, NJ: Prentice Hall.

Vanryckeghem, M., & Brutten, G.J. (2006). *KiddyCat: Communication attitude test for preschool and kindergarten children who stutter.* San Diego: Plural Publishing.

Watts Pappas, N., & McLeod, S. (2009). Parents' perceptions of their involvement in allied health intervention. In N. Watts Pappas & S. McLeod (Eds.), *Working with families in speech-language pathology* (pp. 73–110). San Diego: Plural Publishing.

Watts Pappas, N., McLeod, S., McAllister, L., & McKinnon, D.H. (2008). Parental involvement in speech intervention: A national survey. *Clinical Linguistics and Phonetics, 22*(4), 335–344.

World Health Organization. (2007). *International classification of functioning, disability and health: Children and youth version.* Geneva: Author.

Zebrowski, P.M. (2007). *Beyond technique: What makes therapy work.* Presentation at the Annual Meeting of the Council of Academic Programs in Communication Sciences and Disorders, Palm Springs, CA.

Glossary

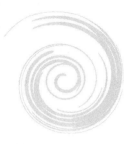

2 Minimal Pair Intervention

conventional minimal pairs   Pairs of meaningful words produced as homonyms by a child, whereby those words typically contain few or minimal opposition features (e.g., *tip* and *sip*) or are near minimal pairs (e.g., *tip* and *trip*).

homonym   Words with different meanings that share the same pronunciation.

semantic confusion   A conversational phenomenon that occurs when a speaker's intended word is heard by the conversational partner as a different word, resulting in communication breakdown.

3 Multiple Oppositions Intervention

homonymy   Production of two or more words that sound alike but have different meanings (e.g., [tu] for *two*, *coo*, *chew*, and *stew*).

idiosyncratic rule   An unusual or atypical rule that the child exhibits (e.g., a child's production of *Lee* for *see* and *she*).

phoneme collapse   A phonological error pattern that reflects broader systemic rules of substitution or deletion that might cover several different sound classes (i.e., stops, fricatives, and affricates), places of production (i.e., alveolar, velar, palatal), and/or linguistic units (i.e., singletons and clusters).

phonological processes   Labels used to describe sound change, generally within a single aspect of production (i.e., place, voice, or manner) or to describe deletion patterns (i.e., final or initial deletions or reduction of clusters to a singleton); classified as substitution, deletion, or assimilation processes. These descriptive labels reflect more narrow sound correspondence error patterns between the child and adult sound systems.

4 Complexity Approaches to Intervention

absolute linguistic universal   A phonological characteristic or trait occurring across all languages (e.g., all languages have stops).

complexity   An abstract concept useful for studying systems, the constituent parts of systems, and how system parts interact in a hierarchically organized way.

complex phonological intervention targets   Intervention targets that are typically nonstimulable, later-developing phonetically more complex marked segments or clusters associated with least productive phonological knowledge for an individual child.

implicational universal/relationship   The existence of one characteristic or trait implying the existence of another characteristic or trait (e.g., fricatives imply stops).

markedness A linguistic concept referring to the relative existence of phonological characteristics or traits across languages, whereby common or universal characteristics are unmarked and universally rarer or uncommon characteristics are marked. Typically, marked traits imply the existence of unmarked counterparts.

phonological generalization Change in a phonological system (e.g., addition of singleton phonemes or consonant clusters, addition of distinctive features) implicationally related to a treated phonological skill.

5 Core Vocabulary Intervention

case study research A method of investigation that emphasizes detailed contextual analysis of a limited number of events or conditions and their relationships. Although often considered exploratory investigations, a series of intervention case studies often provide the best evidence that do not incur many of the problems that can emerge in large scale randomized controlled trials (RCT).

core vocabulary intervention Core vocabulary intervention involves children with inconsistent speech sound disorder (SSD) learning to consistently say a set of high-frequency, functionally powerful words that target the underlying phonological planning deficit. The long-term goal of intervention for children who make inconsistent errors is to establish consistent (as opposed to correct) production of words in spontaneous speech.

efficacy research A method of investigation in which specific models and specific therapeutic protocols are examined with the criteria/goals of achieving empirically supported therapy status; often referred to as the original "purist" laboratory efficacy research.

effectiveness research A method of investigation involving naturalistic implementation of interventions which attempts to understand not only the ways therapy is practiced in the real world, but also to identify those factors and dynamics that influence therapy; it also strives to increase the effectiveness of therapy, regardless of models, protocols, or specific techniques used.

inconsistent SSD A speech disorder characterized by inconsistent pronunciation of the same words and phonological features not only from context to context but also within the same context. Inconsistent SSD due to a deficit in phonological assembly involves an impaired ability to plan the sequence of phonemes that make up a word, in the absence of any oromotor signs of childhood apraxia of speech (CAS).

6 The Cycles Phonological Remediation Approach

critical age hypothesis The premise that children are at a major risk for literacy problems if severe speech difficulties have not resolved by age 5 ½ years.

cycles phonological remediation approach Approach that involves targeting phonological patterns in a cyclical fashion.

intelligibility The degree to which others can understand a person's speech.

Matthew effects Stanovich (1986) compared achievement levels of children who are poor beginning readers with their peers and noted that the gap widens over the years (i.e., the rich get richer and the poor get poorer).

metaphonological awareness Explicit awareness of the sound/pattern structure of spoken words (independent of meaning)

phonological deviations Speech sound/ pattern changes (e.g., omissions) that result in productions that differ from the standard.

phonological patterns Accepted groupings of sounds within an oral language (e.g., consonant clusters) that a child needs to produce to be understood.

7 The Nuffield Centre Dyspraxia Programme

developmental verbal dyspraxia Term used in the United Kingdom for the condition now known as *childhood apraxia of speech* (CAS). ASHA (2007) defines CAS as "a neurological childhood (pediatric) speech sound disorder in which the precision and consistency of movements underlying speech are impaired in the absence of neuromuscular deficits (e.g., abnormal reflexes, abnormal tone) . . . The core impairment in planning and/or programming spatio-temporal parameters of movement sequences results in errors in speech sound production and prosody." (p. 1)

lexical representations Include information on semantics, grammar, and orthography, as well as the phonological representation and motor program. The phonological representation includes the information necessary to identify a given word, as produced by a range of speakers.

motor planning The stage at which a plan for the whole utterance is formed within the Stackhouse and Wells (1997) model (e.g., "I want a cup of tea"). It involves retrieving motor programs for individual words and assembling the different gestural targets in the correct sequence, incorporating grammatical structures and prosodic features.

motor programming An online output process, through which new motor programs can be created. It is thought to include a store of phonological units, which can be combined to create new motor programs for unfamiliar words. For example, motor programming is utilized when asking a child to gently blend /s/ with /i/, to create the new motor program *sea* (for a child who can articulate /s/ as a single sound, but usually replaces /s/ with /t/ in words).

motor programs Include part of the stored lexical representations and consist of a series of gestural targets for the articulators, designed to achieve an acceptable pronunciation of the word. For example, accurate production of the word *tea* would require the following instructions: Initiate airstream, close velopharyngeal sphincter, make closure with margins of tongue to alveolar ridge, release closure, assume raised front tongue body posture, spread lips, and initiate voice.

picture cues NDP3 has a set of picture cues to represent all of the consonant and vowel phonemes in standard British English. For example, a picture of a *tap* is used to represent the sound /t/, and a picture of an *eye* is used to represent the sound /aɪ/. This helps the child retain and retrieve the motor program for the sound, thus making an abstract concept of *a sound* more concrete. The picture cues are also used to prompt the child to produce the sound at word level.

phonotactic structures The permitted combinations of phonemes and syllable structures in a given language. These are typically expressed as combinations of C and V, in which C = consonant and V = vowel. Examples of phonotactic structures include CV, for a word such as *two*, and CVCV, for a word such as *baby*. The term *syllable structure* may be used as a synonym for phonotactic structure.

psycholinguistic approach A child's speech difficulties are viewed as being derived from a breakdown at one or more levels of a speech processing model, consisting of input and output channels and stored linguistic information (lexical representations). This enables the SLP to create a psycholinguistic profile for an individual child, detailing his or her strengths and weaknesses in processing (Stackhouse & Wells, 1997).

8 Stimulability Intervention

joint attention When clinician (or other adult) and child are both focused on a similar object or item of interest at the same time.

multimodal Use of cues across a variety of domains, including auditory, visual, and tactile.

palindrome generalization probe List of untrained words that are read the same way in either direction (e.g., *pop*).

stimulability Ability of a client to correctly imitate a sound that was previously produced in error when provided with auditory and visual cues by the clinician.

9 Psycholinguistic Intervention

lexical representations Knowledge stored about a word including its meaning, what it sounds like, how it is produced, how it is written, and how it can be used in sentences.

literacy Ability to read (decode and comprehend what has been read) and write/spell.

persisting speech difficulties Difficulties with any aspect of speech processing or production that have not resolved by the time a child starts formal schooling.

psycholinguistics Study of the psychological factors involved in processing and producing language; the study of the relationship between language in its different forms (e.g., spoken, written, or signed) and the mind.

speech processing The complex psycholinguistic skills encompassing input speech processing, storage of representations in the lexicon, and output speech production that enable us to make sense and produce speech and to develop phonological awareness skills for literacy.

speech processing profile A practical tool that can be used to organize assessment data from a child into appropriate processing levels in order to evaluate his or her speech processing strengths and weaknesses.

10 Metaphonological Intervention: Phonological Awareness Therapy

metaphonological intervention An approach to therapy that encourages a child to reflect on word structure and the characteristics of his or her own speech in order to understand the need for change and the means of achieving it.

phoneme awareness Awareness of the individual phonemes in words.

phonological awareness The ability to pay conscious attention to the sound structure of language.

phonological representation Information, held in long-term memory, about the phonological form of words. Detailed and accessible phonological representations are thought to underlie accurate speech production, reading, and spelling.

11 Computer-Based Interventions

computer-based interventions The use of computer software programs to deliver a specific intervention approach at the computer or to print out stimulus materials to be used in intervention away from the computer.

motor program Stored set of instructions for the pronunciation of a particular word.

phoneme blending Identification of a word from given phonemes presented in sequence.

phoneme detection Identification of individual phonemes within a given word or nonword.

psycholinguistic intervention An approach to intervention based on a model of speech processing involving input, stored lexical representations, and output.

speech processing All the skills involved in understanding and using speech.

stored lexical knowledge Information held about a word, including phonological representation, semantic representation, motor program, grammatical representation, and orthographic representation.

12 Speech Perception Intervention

phonological processing involves the recognition and/or manipulation of phonological units in speech input. Measures of phonological processing ability include spoken word identification, phonological awareness, and nonword repetition tasks.

speech perception the process of transforming a continuously changing acoustic signal into discrete linguistic units. Although models of speech perception vary widely in their details, most models assume a multistage process in which extraction of the acoustic details is accomplished by means of basic auditory processing mechanisms, and then the acoustic representation is transformed into phonetic units, and finally a hierarchically organized phonological representation is constructed that is subsequently used in the process of lexical access.

13 Nonlinear Phonological Intervention

coda A syllable-final consonant.

default What the phonological system gives for free; what is not learned but is provided if no nondefault learned feature or element is used.

feature The smallest component of speech sounds that combine and recombine to form segments. Features describe place, manner, and laryngeal characteristics of speech sounds.

foot A grouping of one stressed and one or several unstressed syllables. Position of the stressed syllable defines the prominence pattern of the syllable as left-(trochaic) or right-prominent (iambic).

mora A rhythmic, weight unit of the rime of the syllable that designates one phonological beat ("When a V or C get a beat in the tree, that's a mora . . . ").

nonlinear phonology Phonological theories that describe the hierarchy of phonological form from the feature to the prosodic phrase.

onset Consonants before the peak (usually the vowel) of a syllable.

quantity-sensitive language A language in which stress is assigned by weight of a syllable (i.e., syllables with more than one mora tend to get stressed).

rime The peak of the syllable (usually a vowel) and any consonants following it.

14 Dynamic Systems and Whole Language Intervention

dynamic systems accounts of oral and written language development The theoretical framework proposing that phonological development interacts with development of larger language patterns including discourse structures, sentences, words, and grammatical morphemes; closely related to connectionist theories of mental processing.

MorphoPhonic faces A graphic device used in dynamic systems and whole language intervention in which a phonic face represents the first letter sound of the most frequently occurring words in children's storybooks.

Phonic Faces Drawings used in dynamic systems (whole language) intervention that incorporate letters within the faces of characters who are producing speech sounds.

whole language accounts of oral and written language development The theoretical framework proposing that children develop oral and written phonological abilities as a natural consequence of their communicative interactions with adults, including interactive storybook reading.

15 Morphosyntax Intervention

cloze task A fill-in-the blank type of elicited production task in which the clinician creates a context for a particular morpheme to be used, begins an utterance, and pauses strategically for the child to complete the sentence by using the target form.

finite morphemes A class of grammatical morphemes that are particularly challenging for children with specific language impairment. Finite morphemes, which are marked for both tense and agreement, include copula and auxiliary *be*, auxiliary *do*, regular past tense, and third person singular regular.

focused stimulation A facilitation technique in which a clinician provides numerous contextually appropriate examples of a target form (e.g., grammatical form or vocabulary target). The clinician responds naturally or recasts when the child attempts to use the target, but the child is not explicitly required to produce the target.

forced choice An elicited production technique for which a clinician presents a child with two possible choices, both of which include the target form. An example of forced choice for a past tense morpheme may be, "Tell me what the frog did: he *jumped* or he *leaped*."

generalization Indirect changes that occur in different forms or contexts than those that are the focus of communication intervention.

morphosyntax The relationship between the language domains of syntax and morphology. Many individuals who have deficits in one of these domains also will have deficits in the other. For example, individuals who omit morphemes are likely to have related deficits in sentence structure.

preparatory set An elicited production technique for which a clinician models a target form, typically at the sentence level, and then creates an opportunity for the child to use the same target but in a slightly different context (i.e., the child may use the same grammatical target, but with different vocabulary words than what the clinician used).

speech sound disorder Individuals with SSD, for a variety of possible etiologies, have difficulty producing speech sounds to a greater extent than would be expected for their peer group. In the preschool years, many children with SSD also may have co-occurring deficits in language.

16 Naturalistic Intervention for Speech Intelligibility and Speech Accuracy

naturalistic speech intervention A responsive intervention that includes play activities within everyday conversational contexts; it is an alternative child-led approach to imitation and drill methods for teaching individual phonemes that can be applied to a wide variety of individual goals.

speech accuracy   The accuracy with which individual speech sounds (phonemes) are produced.

speech intelligibility   The degree to which the listener understands what the speaker says when the target is uncertain.

17   Parents and Children Together (PACT) Intervention

SFWF   Syllable-final word-final position (e.g., the position of /g/ in *bag*).

SFWW   Syllable-final within-word position (e.g., the position of /t/ in *Batman*).

SIWI   Syllable-initial word-initial position (e.g., the position of /l/ in *laugh*).

SIWW   Syllable-initial within-word position (e.g., the position of /m/ in *Batman*).

therapy block   A period of therapy attendance; in PACT this usually means one intervention session per week, 1 week apart, for 10 weeks.

therapy break   A period of therapy nonattendance, usually of about 10 weeks duration, during which families involved in PACT continue to apply skills and strategies learned during therapy blocks.

18   Enhanced Milieu Teaching with Phonological Emphasis for Children with Cleft Lip and Palate

elicited imitation   Sound productions that occur as a result of prompting strategies used by clinicians to encourage vocalizations; over time, the treatment goal is to transition to strategies that facilitate spontaneous production.

EMT/PE   Naturalistic intervention strategy designed to simultaneously facilitate vocabulary and speech sound production in young children. Enhanced milieu teaching with phonological emphasis adds speech recasting to the EMT prompting options to provide correction strategies for target sounds.

phonetic awareness   An awareness of place of articulation features for target sounds. This differs from phonological awareness that emphasizes the awareness and manipulation of syllable and phonemic segments of words.

recasting   A clinical strategy designed to promote concurrent learning of language and speech forms. The clinician or trained parent repeats the child's utterance using correct grammatical and/or phonological forms.

spontaneous production   Child-initiated vocalizations facilitated by clinical strategies that support naturalistic intervention.

target vocabulary   Established for each child based on performance on consonant inventories and language samples. The target vocabulary guides the clinical intervention by including words and sounds that are both inside and outside the child's current ability. Use of the target vocabulary provides a sense of success for the child to scaffold production of new sounds and words.

19   PROMPT: A Tactually Grounded Model

attractor state   Regarded as behaviors within a range of contexts and biological conditions that will retain dynamic stability or overall task orientation and offer resistance to minor perturbations (Thelen & Fogel, 1987).

mapping   In a word or phrase form provides feed-forward information about motor plans, their variations, and associations of motor movements to cognitive-linguistic information. In mapping, the clinician maps in the motor-phoneme movements using surface prompts, but expects either nothing back from the client or a production that is clearly within that individual's current motor capacity.

motor equivalence   Ability of the speech production system to reach "end-target" positions, and/or accompanying acoustical correlates by varying the degree of muscular contraction and aerodynamic contributions.

motor-phoneme   Motoric requirements and interactions which produce acoustic characteristics that represent cognitive-linguistic constructs, retain meaning. and symbolize language and language change.

motor speech schema   A well-developed, unconscious or conscious speech-motor action (e.g., mouth opening or closing when speaking the word *mama*).

parameter estimation   Ability of the motor speech system to determine the amount and degree of movement and the coordinated effort needed by all speech support systems to produce acceptable end-target productions.

planes of movement   Within the intraoral space, the articulators move in several global directions. The articulators include the mandible, facial muscles, and tongue. These movements are within the vertical (superior/inferior), horizontal and anterior (anterior/posterior), or lateral (lateral/medial) planes.

speech-motor template   A speech-motor template may be thought of as a static representation defining the properties or features of a phoneme that are required to differentiate it from another in a language. These features define the tactual input given in PROMPT and how it is applied differentially across sounds.

synergies   May be described as classes of movement patterns involving collections of muscle or joint variables that act as basic units in the regulation and control of movement, thereby reducing the degrees of freedom to achieve motor equivalence.

tactual-kinesthesia   The perception of muscular movement and tension, derived from the functioning of afferent nerves connected with muscle tissue, skin, joints and tendons; also called "muscle sense."

20   Family-Friendly Intervention

family   The notions of what constitutes a family and a parent differ between cultures and change over time. Family types include nuclear, extended, foster, adoptive, reconstituted, blended, homosexual, and sole parent forms. Within a family, the parent(s) of a child may be the biological mother or father or another adult who has assumed responsibility for the child's care.

family-centered practice   Family-centered practice focuses on supporting and strengthening the child's whole family, and a key concept is the acceptance of the family as the client rather than just the child. Family-centered practice acknowledges the parent's and family's right to make the final decisions about their child's intervention. Synonymous terms are *family empowerment; family-focused intervention;* and *family-centered service, practice,* or *care.*

family-friendly practice   A form of practice in which families are supported to be involved in intervention provision and planning; however, the professional leads the intervention, thereby fulfilling his or her responsibility to provide evidence-based and effective intervention to the child.

parent   A primary caregiver of a child who may or may not be the child's biological parent. In some cases more than one parent or other family members may be primarily involved in the child's intervention.

21 Visual Feedback Therapy with Electropalatography

CLEFTNET A national collaborative initiative in the United Kingdom that allows children with cleft palate to receive assessment and intervention with electropalatography from trained clinicians in geographically distributed centers that have access to technical experts at a central site for data analysis and interpretation and technical support.

electropalatography (EPG) A visual feedback technology that displays images of tongue-palate contacts on a computer screen. The user wears a custom-fit plate (sometimes called a pseudopalate) with electrodes that indicate contact points.

facilitative contexts Specific phonetic contexts in which components of a preceding or following sound facilitate correct production of the target sound; these correct productions can then be practiced to promote correct production in other contexts.

palatograms Two-dimensional representations of tongue-palate contact (also called EPG frames), which are used to model correct tongue postures and provide clients with feedback about their actual tongue–palate contacts during speech.

undifferentiated gesture A type of articulation error that occurs during productions of lingual consonants in which tongue-palate contact lacks clear differentiation among the tongue tip/blade, the tongue body, and the lateral margins of the tongue rather than being limited to contact areas appropriate to the target sound (e.g., tongue tip and tongue blade contact for alveolar consonants).

22 Vowel Intervention

ultrasound A visual feedback technology that displays images of tongue shape and movement in one of two views (midsagittal: the tongue tip to the root; coronal: a view of the tongue's surface at one point) when a transducer probe is held beneath the chin.

23 Developmental Dysarthria Intervention

bite block A small block made of hard plastic, acrylic, or a dental impression material that is positioned between the upper and lower teeth to stabilize (block) movement of the jaw and can be used to elicit lip or tongue movement, independent of the jaw, during speech.

constraint induced movement therapy A form of therapy that helps people with central nervous system damage regain the use of an affected limb by forcing the client to use it by restraining the unaffected limb.

dysarthria A speech disorder resulting in brain damage that disrupts control over the movements used to produce the sound patterns of speech.

hypermandibular activity Excessive or exaggerated movements of the lower jaw that interfere with accurate placement of the tongue for lingual phonemes.

neuroplasticity The brain's ability to reorganize itself by forming new neural connections throughout life. Neuroplasticity allows the neurons (nerve cells) in the brain to compensate for injury and disease and to adjust their activities in response to new situations and experiences or to changes in their environment.

source-filter theory A theory that describes speech production as a two-stage process involving the generation of a sound source with its own spectral shape and structure, which is then shaped or filtered by the resonant properties of the vocal tract.

24 Nonspeech Oral Motor Intervention

flaccidity Reduced muscle tone characterized by lack of resistance to passive stretch.

muscle spindle Sensory receptors that respond to changes in muscle fiber length.

muscle tone Resistance of muscle to passive stretch.

overload Characteristic of exercise in which muscles are forced to perform at levels higher than typical of every day movements.

recovery Interval between exercise sessions in which nutrients are restored to and wastes are removed from the muscles.

spasticity Increased muscle tone characterized by exaggerated resistance to rapid passive stretch.

specificity Characteristic of training in which benefits are limited to those movements that most closely match the trained exercise.

strength training Exercises causing muscles to produce overloaded forces for the purpose of increasing strength.

stretch reflex Reflex resulting in stimulation of the muscle spindle, causing a contraction in the stimulated muscle.

THE INTERNATIONAL PHONETIC ALPHABET (revised to 2005)

CONSONANTS (PULMONIC)

	Bilabial	Labiodental	Dental	Alveolar	Postalveolar	Retroflex	Palatal	Velar	Uvular	Pharyngeal	Glottal
Plosive	p b			t d		ʈ ɖ	c ɟ	k ɡ	q ɢ		ʔ
Nasal	m	ɱ		n		ɳ	ɲ	ŋ	N		
Trill	ʙ			r					ʀ		
Tap or Flap		ⱱ		ɾ		ɽ					
Fricative	ɸ β	f v	θ ð	s z	ʃ ʒ	ʂ ʐ	ç ʝ	x ɣ	χ ʁ	ħ ʕ	h ɦ
Lateral fricative				ɬ ɮ							
Approximant		ʋ		ɹ		ɻ	j	ɰ			
Lateral approximant				l		ɭ	ʎ	ʟ			

Where symbols appear in pairs, the one to the right represents a voiced consonant. Shaded areas denote articulations judged impossible.

CONSONANTS (NON-PULMONIC)

Clicks		Voiced implosives		Ejectives	
ʘ	Bilabial	ɓ	Bilabial	ʼ	Examples:
ǀ	Dental	ɗ	Dental/alveolar		
ǃ	(Post)alveolar	ʄ	Palatal	pʼ	Bilabial
ǂ	Palatoalveolar	ɠ	Velar	tʼ	Dental/alveolar
ǁ	Alveolar lateral	ʛ	Uvular	kʼ	Velar
				sʼ	Alveolar fricative

VOWELS

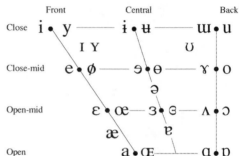

Where symbols appear in pairs, the one to the right represents a rounded vowel.

OTHER SYMBOLS

ʍ Voiceless labial-velar fricative
w Voiced labial-velar approximant
ɥ Voiced labial-palatal approximant
ʜ Voiceless epiglottal fricative
ʢ Voiced epiglottal fricative
ʡ Epiglottal plosive

ɕ ʑ Alveolo-palatal fricatives
ɺ Voiced alveolar lateral flap
ɧ Simultaneous ʃ and x

Affricates and double articulations can be represented by two symbols joined by a tie bar if necessary.

k͡p t͡s

SUPRASEGMENTALS

ˈ Primary stress
ˌ Secondary stress   ˌfoʊnəˈtɪʃən
ː Long   eː
ˑ Half-long   eˑ
˘ Extra-short   ĕ
ǀ Minor (foot) group
ǁ Major (intonation) group
. Syllable break   ɹi.ækt
‿ Linking (absence of a break)

DIACRITICS

Diacritics may be placed above a symbol with a descender, e.g. ŋ̊

̥	Voiceless	n̥ d̥	̤	Breathy voiced	b̤ a̤	̪	Dental	t̪ d̪
̬	Voiced	s̬ t̬	̰	Creaky voiced	b̰ a̰	̺	Apical	t̺ d̺
ʰ	Aspirated	tʰ dʰ	̼	Linguolabial	t̼ d̼	̻	Laminal	t̻ d̻
̹	More rounded	ɔ̹	ʷ	Labialized	tʷ dʷ	̃	Nasalized	ẽ
̜	Less rounded	ɔ̜	ʲ	Palatalized	tʲ dʲ	ⁿ	Nasal release	dⁿ
̟	Advanced	u̟	ˠ	Velarized	tˠ dˠ	ˡ	Lateral release	dˡ
̠	Retracted	e̠	ˤ	Pharyngealized	tˤ dˤ	̚	No audible release	d̚
̈	Centralized	ë	̴	Velarized or pharyngealized	ɫ			
̽	Mid-centralized	e̽	̝	Raised	e̝ (ɹ̝ = voiced alveolar fricative)			
̩	Syllabic	n̩	̞	Lowered	e̞ (β̞ = voiced bilabial approximant)			
̯	Non-syllabic	e̯	̘	Advanced Tongue Root	e̘			
˞	Rhoticity	ɚ a˞	̙	Retracted Tongue Root	e̙			

TONES AND WORD ACCENTS

LEVEL			CONTOUR		
e̋ or	˥	Extra high	ě or	ˇ	Rising
é	˦	High	ê	ˆ	Falling
ē	˧	Mid	e᷄	˧˥	High rising
è	˨	Low	e᷅	˩˧	Low rising
ȅ	˩	Extra low	e᷈	˧˩˧	Rising-falling
↓		Downstep	↗		Global rise
↑		Upstep	↘		Global fall

Index

Throughout this index, *t* indicates a table and *f* indicates a figure.

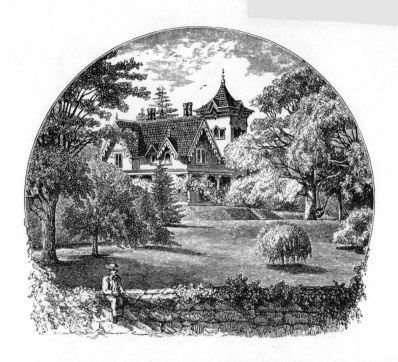

VICTORIAN GARDENS

The Art of Beautifying Suburban Home Grounds

A Victorian Guidebook of 1870 by Frank J. Scott

LIBRARY OF VICTORIAN CULTURE
AMERICAN LIFE FOUNDATION
Watkins Glen, New York
1982

First Edition

ISBN: 0-89257-023-7

THE AMERICAN LIFE FOUNDATION is a non-profit, educational in-
stitution specializing in the acquisition and dissemination of
knowledge through publications. Open to the study of all aspects
of American life, it is especially interested in the relationships of
things and ideas and how the social functions of artifacts from
the past relate to those of today. Recently, it has been repub-
lishing many nineteenth-century stylebooks about architecture
and the decorative arts to assist old house owners and other
preservationists. For a free listing write:

American Life Books, Box 349, Watkins Glen, NY 14891.

Design and production by
Walnut Grove Graphics
Watkins Glen, NY 14891.

Printing and binding by
Valley Offset, Inc.
Deposit, NY 13754.